Sir Harold Ridley
AND HIS FIGHT FOR SIGHT
He changed the world so that we may better see it

David J. Apple, MD

Professor of Ophthalmology and Pathology
Director of the David J. Apple, MD Laboratories for Ophthalmic Devices Research
Moran Eye Center, Department of Ophthalmology and Visual Sciences
Salt Lake City, Utah, USA
Distinguished Senior US Scientist Awardee, Alexander von Humbolt Foundation
Doctor of Science (honoris causa) China Medical University
Shenyang, People's Republic of China
Member, Deutsche Akademie der Naturforscher
(German Academy of Research in the Natural Sciences)

Formerly: Professor and Chairman Emeritus of Ophthalmology and Pathology
Pawek-Valloton Chair of Biomedical Engineering
Director, Ocular Pathology Laboratory and Center for Research on
Ocular Therapeutics and Biodevices
Director, World Health Organization (WHO) Collaborating Center for Prevention of Blindness
Albert Florens Storm Eye Institute
Medical University of South Carolina
Charleston, South Carolina

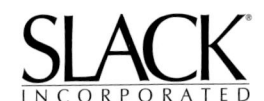

SLACK
INCORPORATED
Delivering the best in health care information and education worldwide
6900 Grove Road • Thorofare, NJ 08086

A website has been created specifically for *Sir Harold Ridley and His Fight For Sight: He Changed the World So That We May Better See It*. Please visit **www.haroldridley.com.**

Front cover images: Top, Sir Harold Ridley at Stonehenge, about 10 miles from his Wiltshire retirement cottage. Photograph by David J. Apple. Bottom, Royal Air Force Squadron 601, in 1937.

For the complete list of photo credits, see page 309.

www.slackbooks.com

ISBN 1-55642-786-7
ISBN-13 978-1-55642-786-2

Copyright © 2006 by SLACK Incorporated

All rights reserved. No part of this book may be reproduced, stored in a retrieval system or transmitted in any form or by any means, electronic, mechanical, photocopying, recording or otherwise, without written permission from the publisher, except for brief quotations embodied in critical articles and reviews.

The procedures and practices described in this book should be implemented in a manner consistent with the professional standards set for the circumstances that apply in each specific situation. Every effort has been made to confirm the accuracy of the information presented and to correctly relate generally accepted practices. The authors, editor, and publisher cannot accept responsibility for errors or exclusions or for the outcome of the material presented herein. There is no expressed or implied warranty of this book or information imparted by it. Care has been taken to ensure that drug selection and dosages are in accordance with currently accepted/recommended practice. Due to continuing research, changes in government policy and regulations, and various effects of drug reactions and interactions, it is recommended that the reader carefully review all materials and literature provided for each drug, especially those that are new or not frequently used. Any review or mention of specific companies or products is not intended as an endorsement by the author or publisher.

SLACK Incorporated uses a review process to evaluate submitted material. Prior to publication, educators or clinicians provide important feedback on the content that we publish. We welcome feedback on this work.

Published by: SLACK Incorporated
                6900 Grove Road
                Thorofare, NJ 08086 USA
                Telephone: 856-848-1000
                Fax: 856-853-5991
                www.slackbooks.com

Contact SLACK Incorporated for more information about other books in this field or about the availability of our books from distributors outside the US.

Apple, David J., 1941-
  Sir Harold Ridley and his fight for sight: he changed the world so that we may better see it / David J. Apple.
    p. ; cm.
  Includes bibliographical references and index.
  ISBN-13: 978-1-55642-786-2 (alk. paper)
  ISBN-10: 1-55642-786-7 (alk. paper)
  1. Ridley, Harold, Sir, 1906-2001. 2. Ophthalmologists--Great Britain--Biography. 3. Intraocular lenses--History. 4. Cataract --Surgery--History. I. Title.
  [DNLM: 1. Ridley, Harold, Sir, 1906-2001. 2. Ophthalmology--Great Britain--Biography. 3. History, 20th Century--Great Britain. 4. Lenses, Intraocular--history--Great Britain. 5. Ophthalmologic Surgical Procedures--history--Great Britain. WZ 100 R545a 2006]
  RE36.R53A67 2006
  362.197'75240092--dc22
                                                        2006019613

For permission to reprint material in another publication, contact SLACK Incorporated. Authorization to photocopy items for internal, personal, or academic use is granted by SLACK Incorporated provided that the appropriate fee is paid directly to Copyright Clearance Center. Prior to photocopying items, please contact the Copyright Clearance Center at 222 Rosewood Drive, Danvers, MA 01923 USA; phone: 978-750-8400; website: www.copyright.com; email: info@copyright.com

Printed in the United States of America.

Last digit is print number: 10 9 8 7 6 5 4 3 2 1

"Throughout the centuries there were men who took first steps down new roads armed with nothing but their own vision. Their goals differed, but they all had this in common: that the step was first, the road new, the vision unborrowed, and the response they received—hatred. The great creators—the thinkers, the artists, the scientists, the inventors—stood alone against the men of their time.

Every great new thought was opposed. Every great new invention was denounced. The first motor was considered foolish. The airplane was considered impossible. The power loom was considered vicious. Anesthesia was considered sinful. But the men of unborrowed vision went ahead. They fought, they suffered, and they paid. But they won."

Ayn Rand
The Fountainhead
1944

"As a former flight surgeon in the Air Force, I can compare our mission as eye surgeons with the one to conquer outer space. The evolution of contemporary cataract surgery involved overcoming many professional and governmental obstacles through the creative genius and tenacity of many true pioneers. Consider how cataract patients are treated today in your OR, and you will appreciate what we have accomplished in the past 45 years. We are now space-walking in the operating room."

Herve M. Byron, MD
Flashback
Cataract Surgery Modern History

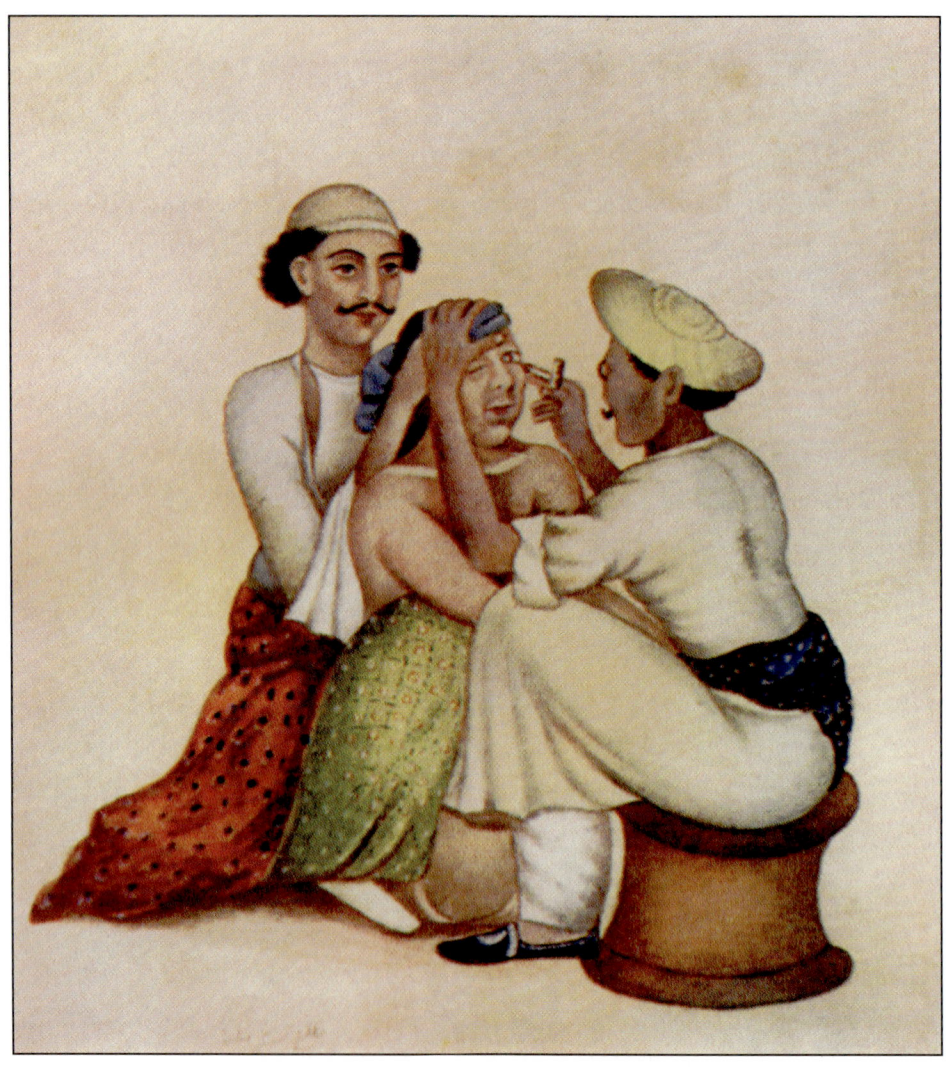

This gruesome procedure called "couching"—intended to dislodge the opaque cataractous lens by insertion of a long needle into the eye—was the only surgical means for treating cataracts for over 6000 years. It has a very high complication rate, especially with hemorrhage and infection. It is still practiced in some regions today.

An early written description of couching came from Sushrata (also spelled Susrata or Sushrutha), an Indian surgeon circa 600 BC.

DEDICATION

To those closest to Sir Harold and myself who for years provided unyielding support as we pursued our busy careers.

To Sir Harold's wife Elisabeth and their children, Nicholas, Margaret, and David. Elisabeth supported him through a world war, and all were there during his struggle as he advanced his "cure of aphakia."

To my wife Ann. We married in 1995, and soon thereafter she was forced not only to manage the usual stress of being a doctor's wife, but also had to assume the duties of a caregiver and nurse (very lovingly and successfully, I might add) as I struggled with a series of severe illnesses.

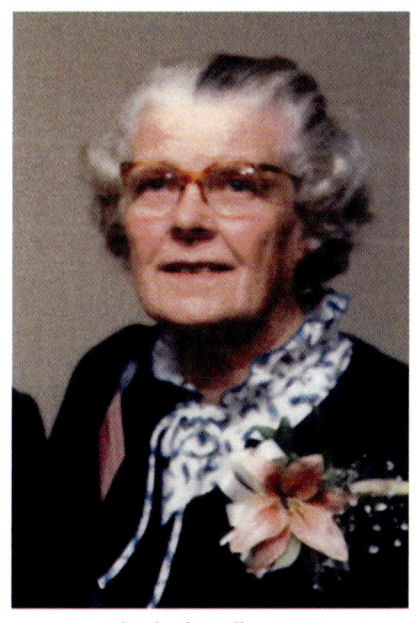

Elisabeth Ridley, UK

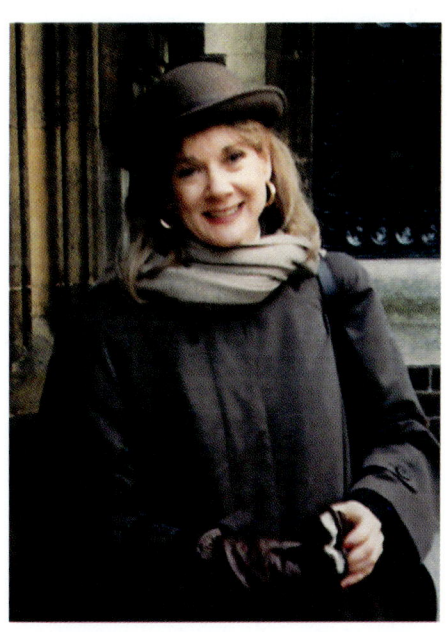

Ann Apple, Salt Lake City, UT/Charleston, SC. (Photograph taken by the author in Cambridge, UK.)

Contents

Dedication .... *vii*
Acknowledgments .... *xiii*
About the Author .... *xv*
Foreword by Jim Mazzo .... *xvi*
Foreword by I. Howard Fine, MD .... *xvii*
Foreword by Emanuel Rosen, Bsc, MD, FRCSE, FRCOphth, FRPS .... *xviii*
Foreword by Christopher Morgan .... *xx*
Preface .... *xxi*

Chronology of Sir Harold Ridley .... **xxix**

Chapter 1 **The Secret Code: The "Extra-Capsular Ext."** **2**
　　　　　　London. November 29, 1949 2
　　　　　　A Gift to the World 6
　　　　　　Why Did It Take So Long? 10

Chapter 2 **From Darkness to Light** **14**
　　　　　　Eye Surgery in the Dark Ages; Perforation of the Eye With a Needle 16
　　　　　　The "Black Hole" 17
　　　　　　From Darkness to Light 19
　　　　　　Cataract—The Most Common Cause of Visual Loss 21
　　　　　　Cataracts May Cause Morbidity in Addition to Simple Vision Loss 24
　　　　　　Colors and the Cataracts of Claude Monet 25

Chapter 3 **Roots of a Modest Giant of Science** **30**
　　　　　　The Ridleys: 1555 32
　　　　　　The Parkers: "Do It and It's Done." 34
　　　　　　The World Harold Was Born Into 35
　　　　　　The Early Years 39
　　　　　　School Days and Medical Training 43

Chapter 4 **"David, Mr. Ridley Wants to Meet You"** **52**
　　　　　　July 1980 to May 1989: Arrival to a New Job 52
　　　　　　Summer, 1985: A Summons to Visit Mr. Ridley 58
　　　　　　From the Old Country to America's Heartland, My Ancestors,
　　　　　　　　Origins, Childhood, and Medical Training (1941-1985) 61
　　　　　　History and Heroes 63
　　　　　　Entering the Field of Medicine—The Eyes Have It 65
　　　　　　Charleston and the Apple Korps 67
　　　　　　Triumphs and Tragedies: 1989-Present 72
　　　　　　Summary 73

Chapter 5 **River Walks** **78**
　　　　　　The Quest for a Complete Cataract Operation 79
　　　　　　Clinical Diagnosis of Cataract 80
　　　　　　Three Surgical Methods to Remove a Cataract 91

CONTENTS

Chapter 6 **Adlertag: The Quest for a Complete Cataract Operation, Step 2: Visual Rehabilitation with the IOL** **98**
    Casanova, Quacks, Progressives, and Prophets 102
    The "Airplane Story" Unfolds: "A Story Too Good to Be True" 104
    The Setting: Royal Air Force Tangmere and Surrounding Hospitals 106
    The Players 109
    "Mouse" Cleaver and the Pilots of the 601 Squadron 111
    Fury Across Europe 116
    Adlertag: "You Will Wipe the British Air Force From the Sky" 118
    Coming Full Circle: One Piece of Plastic Is Replaced with Another 120
    What Was Flight Lieutenant Cleaver's Precise Role in the Development of the IOL? 122
    The Invention of the IOL: The Actual Sequence of Events, ca 1935 to 1951 123
    Epilogue: It's Plastic! 125

Chapter 7 **A Simple Question, Mobilization** **128**
    The Pilot 130
    The Student 130
    The Optician and the Chemist: The Cure of Cataract 133
    The Surgeon 138

Chapter 8 **The Operation: November 29, 1949** **140**
    The "Brave Londoners" 142
    A Lingering Question 147

Chapter 9 **Rapid Descent Into a Period of Doldrums** **150**
    A Mistake Leads to an Early Unveiling 151
    A Prophet in His Own Country 152
    Harold's First Rebuff 154
    Sir Stewart Duke-Elder 155
    D.E. 160
    A Fast Downhill Slope 161
    "Put Out to Pasture" 162
    Chicago 163
    A Rejection From a Colleague in Ocular Pathology 164
    A Different Outcome? 165

Chapter 10 **A Gradual Ascent to a New Revolution in Surgical Eye Care** **166**
    "Who Would Support Me Before Peter Choyce?" 168
    Other Supporters and Pioneers 171
    The Philadelphia Story 172
    Munich, 1966 173
    Paris, 1974 174
    "America's Doctor" Prescribes the IOL to the FDA 175
    Unstoppable Forward Movement 177

Chapter 11 **The Good, the Bad, and the Ugly: Evolution of IOLs, Ups and Downs** **180**
    IOL Design: Haptics and Loops: Solving the Problem of Decentration 184
    Material Problems 187
    Secondary Cataracts (Posterior Capsular Opacification) 188

Infections (Endophthalmitis) 190
Evolutionary Excellence 191

Chapter 12 *Let's Get Rid of Our Glasses* 192
Corneal Refractive Surgery..196
Intraocular Lens Refractive Surgery...198
Svyatoslav Fyodorov...200
Phakic Intraocular Lenses..200
Bifocal and Multifocal Intraocular Lenses 201
The Start of Something Big 202

Chapter 13 *Innovations in Addition to the Intraocular Lens* 204
Tropical Ophthalmology: Onchocerciasis (River Blindness) and Cataract-IOL Surgery
in the Developing World 205
Shipped Out 209
Attacking River Blindness 209
Applying Laboratory Technology to Cataract-IOL Surgery in the Developing World................212
Bringing Light to the Underprivileged World:
Introducing the Modern Cataract-IOL Operation 215
Ridley Establishes a Foundation..217

Chapter 14 *Released Prisoners of War in Thailand and Burma*................................... 220
Nutritional Amblyopia: Involvement of the Optic Nerve and Macula...................221

Chapter 15 *Technical Applications from World War II* 228
Televising Eye Operations 230
Noninvasive Diagnosis of the Retina and Optic Nerve..231

Chapter 16 *Biomedical Engineering and Artificial Organ Transplantation* 239

Chapter 17 *Honors, Many Received "Long After I Should Have Been Gone"* 244
A Book Signed by Grateful Surgeons 246
Election to the Royal Society 246
An Honorary Doctor's Degree 248
Celebrating the Intraocular Lens' 50th Anniversary at the Royal Albert Science Museum 249
Election to Ophthalmology Hall of Fame 251
A Long and Illustrious List..251

Chapter 18 *Knighthood and the End*.. 252
"What Was a Miracle Yesterday Remains a Miracle Today and Forever" 253
Success at Last...255
Confronting Old Age...256
The End of a Long and Fruitful Journey 258
The Farewell 258
Words of Respect 259
A Fitting Place for a Memorial Service..260

CONTENTS

Chapter 19 A Service of Thanksgiving and Redemption on
Battle of Britain Sunday, September 18, 2005 262

Appendices

Glossary 271
Map of England 281
Map of London 283
Landmark Articles 285
The Ridley Foundation 289
Publications: Sir Harold Ridley, MD, Cantab, FRCS, Eng. FRS 291
Sir Harold Ridley: Memberships, Presentations, and Honors 297
David J. Apple, IOL-Related Articles, Early Phase (1984-1986). 299
Articles, Editorials, and Obituaries written by David J. Apple about Sir Harold Ridley 303
List 1: Visual Acuity Measurements 305
List 2: World Health Organization Classification of Visual Impairment (Simplified) 307

Photo Credit List 309

Index 311

Acknowledgments

Dr. Kensaku Miyake of Nagoya, Japan (pictured at right) was a strong supporter of Sir Harold, and a good friend and research collaborator. The value of the Miyake-Apple Posterior Photographic/Video technique is that the research findings on eyes obtained post-mortem have translated into valuable clinical applications.

Ms. Ann Curran, my administrative assistant, labored many dozens of hours in layout, preparation, and typing of the manuscript.

Jim Gilman, CRS and Beth Snodgrass, both of Ophthalmic Imaging at the University of Utah, accomplished a humongous task. I had collected over 1200 photographs and other visual material. They took charge of arranging these according to chapter number and provided "print ready" scans to the publisher.

I thank the Ridley Family (Harold's wife Elisabeth and their children Nicholas, Margaret, and David) for the wonderful support of this book and their kind sharing of written material and photographic images.

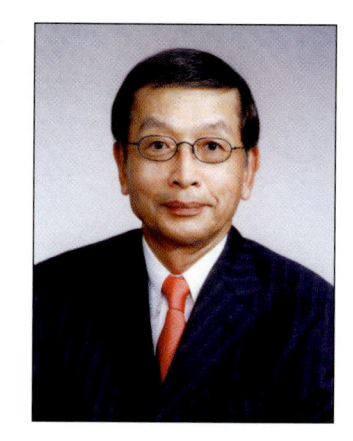

Others who provided some of the direct, hands-on efforts that were indispensible during various phases of book production included:

- Mr. Chuck Dew
- Ms. Joyce Edmonds
- Dr. Macella Escobar-Gomez
- Ms. Christine Ford
- Reva Hurtes
- Dr. Guy Kleinmann
- Mrs. Sandi Mohlmann
- Dr. Irmi Neuhann
- Dr. Qun Peng
- Lauren Plummer, Editor, SLACK Incorporated
- Mr. Norman Rasmussen
- Mrs. Tracy Strauss
- Dr. Nihti Visehook
- Mr. Brian Zaugg

A special thanks to my colleague who has worked with me for over two decades in the field of intraocular lenses, Dr. Randall Olson.

Especially thanks to all 200+ members of the Apple Korps, of whom Harold was very fond.

Finally, thanks to the many colleagues, publishers, surgeons, and contemporaries of Sir Harold who provided valuable information and material through interviews and by providing visual images:

- Mrs. Jane Adams
- Daniel Albert
- Mr. Joe Anderson
- Dr. Steven Archinoff
- Professor Eric Arnott
- Mr. Steven Arnott
- Dr. and Mrs. David Austin
- Drs. Ehud and Ayala Assia
- Dr. Gerd Auffarth
- Dr. Cornelius Binkhorst
- Dr. Michael Blumenthal
- Kevin Buehler
- Dr. Herve Byron
- Dr. Jerry Cagle
- The Late Dr. Peter Choyce and Dianna
- Ian Collins
- Dr. Neil Dallas
- Dr. Jim Davidson
- Dr. Edward Epstein
- Dr. Jerry Freeman
- Dr. Howard Fine
- Dr. Svyatoslav Fyodorov
- Dr. Howard Gimbel
- Dr. T. Hara
- Dr. Ken Hoffer
- Dr. Norman Jaffe
- The Late Dr. Charles Kelman
- Warwick Kitt
- Dr. Richard Kratz
- Jacki Lindstrom
- Dr. Richard Lindstrom
- Dr. Charles Letocha
- Dr. Martin Mainster
- Dr. Barry Masters
- Jim Mazzo
- Christopher Morgan
- Donnie Munro Giulia Newton
- Dr. O. Nishi
- Mrs. Doreen Ogg
- Dr. Stephen Obstbaum
- Dr. Richard Packard
- The late Dr. Maurice Rabb
- Dr. Buddy Ratner
- Dr. Michael Roper-Hall
- Dr. Emanuel Rosen
- Dr. Steven Schallhorn
- Dr. Steven Shearing
- Dr. William Simcoe
- Dr. Robert Sinskey
- Dr. Richard Troutman
- Mr. J. P. Wayenborough
- Dr. Hugh Williams
- Dr. Jan Worst

RAF Tangmere Museum

ABOUT THE AUTHOR

David J. Apple, MD is the Director of the David J. Apple, MD Laboratories for Ophthalmic Devices Research, Moran Eye Center, Department of Ophthalmology and Visual Sciences at the University of Utah in Salt Lake City. A noted international lecturer, Dr. Apple is recognized for his contributions to research on intraocular lenses. In addition to writing 23 books, 71 book chapters, and 529 original articles, he has made over 1400 scientific presentations worldwide. He and his wife Ann currently reside in both Salt Lake City, UT and Sullivan's Island, SC.

Dr. Apple can be reached through SLACK Incorporated, Health Care Books and Journals, 6900 Grove Road, Thorofare, NJ 08086.

FOREWORD BY JIM MAZZO*
CHAIRMAN, PRESIDENT, AND CEO OF ADVANCED MEDICAL OPTICS, INC.

In our busy lives, most of us take much for granted. We don't think about how inventions and products that make our lives easier and more enjoyable came to be. But if we took the time to explore the circumstances that led to their invention, we would certainly uncover some fascinating details.

Such is the case with Dr. David Apple's brilliantly written *Sir Harold Ridley and His Fight For Sight: He Changed the World So That We May Better See It*. David tells the compelling story of a British ophthalmologist, Harold Ridley, who revolutionized cataract surgery after seeing a Royal Air Force (RAF) pilot who sustained injuries during the Battle of Britain. Fragments of the plane's cockpit canopy were embedded in both of his eyes. He proved that the same material used to create the canopy could be used to manufacture intraocular implants, and went on to invent and implant the world's first intraocular lens (IOL).

Ridley would pioneer several other medical breakthroughs in vision care that have improved the quality of people's lives for generations since his first cataract-IOL procedure was first performed in 1949. His innovative thinking, painstaking research, unwavering determination, and steadfastness against opposition continue to be an inspiration today.

David's long friendship with Ridley began in 1985, when he pioneered the combined field of ophthalmology and pathology with studies on the biocompatibility of implant materials. David's ophthalmic device research helped optimize the safety of Ridley's invention and drive the adoption of IOLs. He considered Ridley a mentor, and the two were personal friends until Ridley's death in 2001. David, recognized around the world as a leading expert in ocular pathology, was a co-founder of the Center for Intraocular Lens Research, now designated the David J. Apple, MD Laboratories for Ophthalmic Devices Research at the University of Utah. This center has received international acclaim for its studies. He has contributed extensively to ophthalmic literature, having authored including 23 textbooks, 71 chapters in textbooks, and more than 529 journal articles in the refereed scientific literature.

Please enjoy *Sir Harold Ridley and His Fight For Sight: He Changed the World So That We May Better See It*, as you take a journey through an amazing career that revolutionized the ophthalmic industry and forever changed the lives of millions.

---

* Author's note: The preparation of a book covering the life and works of a prolific clinician and innovator and my relationship with him as we worked to gain acceptance of him and his innovations required a huge outlay of resources, time, energy, and finances. It could not have been accomplished without backing, logically from one who clearly understands the relevance of Sir Harold Ridley's work. I salute Jim Mazzo, Chairman, President, and CEO of Advanced Medical Optics, Inc. (AMO) for his time and commitment—with no conditions or restrictions attached. Without his support there is no way that the complete story of this man—until now almost a footnote to history—could have been told.

Foreword by I. Howard Fine, MD
Clinical Associate Professor, Oregon Health Sciences University
Past President, American Society of Cataract and Refractive Surgery
Eugene, Oregon

"He (Ridley) changed the world."

I. Howard Fine, MD, New York Times, 2000

(From the perspective of an American surgeon.)

This book is about an almost-forgotten man—indeed an almost forgotten GREAT MAN. Professor David Apple, MD developed a personal and professional relationship with Sir Harold Ridley that lasted from 1985 until Ridley's death in 2001. In my opinion, it was not only based on pure medical considerations, but also one of father and son—perhaps not unlike that beautifully and professionally revealed in *Tuesday with Maurie*. There is no doubt that Ridley, the inventor of the intraocular lens, probably would have remained a minor footnote in history were it not for the work of David Apple. In his research directed toward developing better IOL materials and designs, as well as optimizing surgical techniques, Dr. Apple uncovered and publicized the role of Sir Harold Ridley in the development of intraocular lenses and other important innovations.

While working with Dr. Apple on lab studies, which helped confirm the clinical usefulness of my surgical technique, cortical cleaving hydrodissection, I recall and can personally attest to the enthusiasm he often expressed when discussing their friendship.

Cataract surgery is the miracle of 20th century medicine. There are over 2.5 million cataract surgeries performed each year in the United States and at least 9 million annually world-wide, probably even more. Prior to the availability of the intraocular lens implants, surgeons were reluctant to operate and patients were reluctant to undergo cataract surgery because of the dangers inherent in some of the early techniques and the multiple disadvantages of coke-bottle cataract spectacles.

There are a variety of sources that have recognized and publicized the problems cataracts create for patients. The Framingham study in Massachusetts has shown us that there is a statistically significant increase in falls associated with hip fractures in senior citizens who have cataracts in just one eye. A report in the *Journal of the American Medical Association* showed that there was a marked increase in automobile accidents among senior citizens with cataracts who opted to delay surgery compared to those who underwent cataract surgery. Studies by healthcare economists in Sweden have documented that patients who delay cataract surgery to the point that they have to give up cherished activities, whether it is driving, sewing, or painting, very frequently after visual rehabilitation following cataract surgery never go back to those activities. Jonathan Javitt, in a study for the World Bank, has documented that cataract surgery was the most cost efficient surgical procedure in medicine and had the highest quality-of-life-years value for society. A large number of senior citizens living in nursing homes were disabled primarily because of limited vision due to a cataract. More recently, with special "high-tech" visual examinations such as contrast sensitivity testing and wavefront aberrometry, we have come to recognize that even with early cataracts, changes in spherical aberration within the human lens can dramatically compromise functional vision.

The lifestyle limitations and disadvantages caused by cataracts can be eliminated by early surgery with IOLs. Today patients come for cataract surgery earlier than ever before and enjoy enhanced visual acuity as a result of continuously improving IOL technology. Cataract surgery is the only surgery that not only restores but enhances vision over what existed prior to the detrimental effects of disease or aging. In a rapidly emerging new area within cataract surgery, refractive lens exchange, patients may elect to undergo removal of their crystalline lens and replacement by an IOL prior to the development of cataracts. By doing this their functional vision is enhanced, they enjoy a decreased dependence on spectacles, and they are freed from ever developing cataracts.

The above reasons, and many more, are the reasons that this book, an account of one of the most important developments in the history of eye surgery, must be published. It is important that Harold Ridley not be forgotten. Dr. Apple has very carefully assembled his material with a focus on accuracy, using the combined techniques of a medical researcher, a detective, and an investigational reporter. This was necessary to accurately document facts, including events that occurred 50 to 60 years ago, the time frame of Ridley's most productive output of great innovations. It is also a panoramic view of all of the personal, professional, political, economic, and social forces that control events—forces that interact to either retard or suppress or to facilitate and enhance any truly new and innovative development. Reading this book is a rewarding adventure for all audiences, not only eye surgeons and medical personnel, but all people who are awed by the miracles of modern medicine.

Foreword by Emanuel Rosen, BSc, MD, FRCSE, FRCOphth, FRPS
Visiting Professor, University of Manchester Department of Visual Sciences
Past President, International Intraocular Implant Club, 2000-2002
Past President, European Society of Cataract & Refractive Surgeons, 1987-1992
Co-Editor, Journal of Cataract & Refractive Surgery

(From the perspective of a British surgeon.)

Following completion of my training as an eye surgeon in the early 1970s, I established a practice working in the treatment of retinal diseases. For me, a young surgeon moving forward in a fascinating speciality, it was a thrill to be able to help patients with the treatment using tools we had available at that time. Although my focus was on the retina, my colleagues and I did all types of eye operations.

In the summer of 1973, I performed a cataract operation and, for the first time, implanted an intraocular lens (IOL). This was almost 25 years after Ridley's invention. The lens that I used was a modification that had been designed by two colleagues from Holland, Dr. Cornelius Binkhorst and Dr. Jan Worst, affectionately called the Dutch Duo. The positive result that was achieved that day in the operating room and the effect on the patient was so dramatic that I became an instant convert to IOLs. The work of Binkhorst and Worst, as well as several of their contemporaries helped bring credibility to Mr. Ridley's invention, which was still much disparaged at that time—almost three decades after its invention.

There was still severe resistance to Ridley's technological breakthrough in the profession, especially from the academic establishment. Many of us who were converted to implants were sometimes isolated from participation in various meetings, and indeed Ridley and Choyce had already formed the Intraocular Implant Club (IIIC) in 1966. We also formed a European organization designed to help in the understanding and advancement of implants, the European Intraocular-Ocular Implant Council (EIIC), which eventually set a pattern of meeting in different European countries each year. The EIIC graduated to a Society format, becoming the European Society of Cataract and Refractive Surgeons.

I had realized from that first day in 1973 that I was about to participate in the transformation of intraocular implant surgery, which had attracted such a hostile birth as Ridley did his early work. Implants then passed through a stage of infancy and childhood, maturing into an adolescence and maturity that was soon to deliver joy to patients and surgeons alike.

Understanding the pathophysiology of lens implantation (for example, how does the procedure work? how does one prevent complications?) was a fundamental need and requirement. Surgeons always need to understand what they are doing, and what are the correct indications and contraindications for intervention. How does one comprehend adverse events and counter them and, most importantly, how do they prevent their occurrence?

Beginning in about 1981-82, David Apple and his team, the Apple Korps, started to provide the answers needed. They continue to do so today, having celebrated the 25th year of existence of the Apple Laboratory. They deserve incalculable thanks from a full generation of patients and surgeons. I had the pleasure of working with David and his team on several occasions. I recall a notable one where we were studying means of assuring safety during surgery by the introduction in 1980 of a product called Healon (Advanced Medical Optics, Santa Ana, California), an agent which helps "lubricate" and thus protect tissues within the eye during the implant procedure. This material, termed a viscoelastic agent, has become a universally accepted tool used to help assure the safety of all types of eye operations.

The decade from 1975 to 1985 stimulated the entrepreneurial energies of cataract surgeons whose implant fantasies were realized. Their hopes always were to improve on Mr. Ridley's lens and many devised various forms and designs of implants, some unfortunately based on incomplete theory and causing significant morbidity, as the profession sought the "final solution" of a safe and durable implant. Sorting this out required conceptual originality as well as knowledge of biomaterials and biomechanics—this was the forte of the Apple Laboratory. Eventually the mix of clinical hard earned experience and basic science performed in the laboratory led to lasting and safe solutions.

An ultimate goal was finally reached by the late 1980s. Surgeons were able to securely and permanently implant and sequester the IOL into its correct location—the actual site where the normal lens was normally situated, a site clinically termed the "lens capsular bag." These improvements immediately helped decrease the incidence of cataract-IOL surgery complications.

We should all be grateful to a few contemporaries of Ridley who had the vision to immediately recognize the value of his work. I salute Peter Choyce, Edward Epstein, and Salvo Fyodorov, among others, whose vision for their patients and their profession was outstanding. Harold Ridley himself of course encountered intense hostility. Colleges from the generation after Ridley often were criticized as they tried to improve and modernized the cataract-IOL operation. I, myself, was criticized as I tried to bring various modern techniques for cataract and refractive surgery to my region—most of which have been successful and are used routinely today. I know that David Apple often met with resistance as he commonly had to confront both surgeons and companies. Their individual persistence helped counter the animosity of many academic ophthalmologists, both in Britain, on the European Continent, and across the Atlantic.

These pioneering ophthalmic surgeons and researchers can be well satisfied that the hostilities surrounding this development, which lasted for almost four decades, have been overcome. The efforts begun by Ridley, these few early pioneers, and presently by a whole new generation of surgeons have initiated a major subspecialty of ophthalmology, namely the subspecialty of cataract-IOL-refractive surgery.

I am sure that my contemporaries, as well as myself, are now very proud that we have participated in and contributed to what David Apple has termed the "golden age of ophthalmology and the visual sciences."

Sir Harold Ridley in his final years may have written:
> "It was a barren time at best
> Its fruits were few
> Life has not since been wholly in vain
> For now I hear a wisdom plucked from joy and pain
> Before I go to take some slender share."

FOREWORD BY CHRISTOPHER MORGAN
CHAIRMAN, RAYNER & KEELER, LTD.*

This is the story of one remarkable man's perseverance against many odds in his mission to complete the cure of cataracts, an achievement that must surely rank as one of the greatest medical and scientific breakthroughs of the 20th century. Yet, though he had received honours from many quarters and was elected a member of the Royal Society in 1986, it was not until the new millennium that he received belated civil honours in Britain, when he received a knighthood at age 93, a year before his death.

My first and only meeting with Harold Ridley (as he then was) was on the occasion of the 50th anniversary of the very first intraocular lens (IOL) operation, performed by him on 29th November 1949 at St. Thomas' Hospital, London. The lens was "manufactured" (used here in the literal sense of hand-crafted) by Rayner in Brighton, close to its present IOL plant, from an ultra pure form of Perspex developed by ICI for the construction of fighter plane cockpit windows in the late 1930s. The design was the result of close collaboration between these companies and Ridley. Appropriately, the event was held on the roof of the London Science Museum, amongst the Spitfires and other wartime aircraft. Sadly, David Apple himself was prevented through ill health from being there on that occasion.

This fascinating book, enlivened with carefully assembled photographs, shows how Ridley's patient genius brought together his observations on wounded World War II pilots with his expertise and knowledge as an ophthalmic surgeon, to draw some remarkable conclusions. No one could be better qualified to write this definitive account of Sir Harold Ridley's life and achievements than Professor David Apple, MD. His admiration for his subject shines throughout his work. It is based on thorough research and first-hand experience through frequent contacts with Ridley himself, as well as visits to the sources from which the latter drew his inspiration.

Many millions of cataract sufferers in the world have had their vision restored through IOL implantation. Back in 1942 Ridley had also discovered the cause of river blindness, afflicting countless people in Africa, a disease now curable and preventable. Characteristically, Ridley wanted as many people as possible to benefit from IOL implantation and declined any royalties from his invention. This wish was respected by Rayner, who have also donated thousands of lenses to teams of eye surgeons visiting some of the poorest areas of the world.

The year 2006 marks the centenary of Ridley's birth and in four years' time, Rayner will itself be celebrating its centenary. Nothing gives us more pride than our association with Ridley over those pioneering post-war years. My great uncle F W Ewart Morgan was chairman of our group at that historic time in November 1949, as was my father Geoffrey Morgan in 1965 when a technology transfer agreement allowed the lenses to be made in the USA, and also in 1981 when FDA approval was first granted. My present-day colleagues will want to join me in wishing the author the success he deserves with this book. Particularly I should mention Ian Collins and his successor as managing director of our IOL company, Donald J. Munroe, who in 2005 was elected to join the author as a member of the elite Intraocular Implant Club, formed by Ridley as its first president.

---

* Author's note: Rayner & Keeler, Ltd. was the company that manufactured the first IOL, 1948-1949.

Preface

Sir Harold Ridley (1906-2001) invented the intraocular lens (IOL) during the period between the 1930 and 1950s, based in part on his World War II experience with airplane pilots' eye injuries.

For the first time in history it was possible to achieve a successful restoration of sight for the millions of patients who were partially or totally blind with the condition we term a cataract—a clouding of the affected patient's lens. This is the most common cause of blindness in the world; 50 million individuals suffer from this condition. In some regions waiting-lists for cataract surgery are growing at a rate of 14,000 per day. For over 6,000 years there was no treatment of this condition except for an unsatisfactory procedure termed couching (see Frontispiece preceding the Dedication).

The IOL has made possible a real solution to this problem so that this condition, which was so long considered untreatable, is now eminently treatable and, as stated by Dr. Howard Fine, citing the work of Jonathan Javitt: "Cataract surgery is the most cost-effective and efficient surgical procedure in medicine and has the most quality-of-life-years value for society." Today there are over 10 million patients annually who are now receiving an IOL—and still the number is growing.

Harold succeeded by working with a superb team, including optical specialists at Rayner & Keeler, Ltd. (UK), experts in the field of plastics at Imperial Chemical Industries (UK), and others. He himself did not become a household name. For example, although I entered the field of vision care in 1968, I had not even heard of him until over 10 years later. I did a few dozen implants during my residency; the only teaching I received was from a senior resident at the local Veterans Administration Hospital. This resident was actually termed "too aggressive" by our faculty, but he kindly provided me instructions in a rote fashion (mostly from the company's brochure) so that I could proceed. Later, during my early years as an attending surgeon, I did perhaps 100 cases just as a return to posterior chamber IOLs was beginning—the type of fixation that Sir Harold had preferred all along. The patients did fine.

By the early 1980s when I moved to Utah I finally began working with IOLs in our research laboratory (see Chapter 4). I was pleasantly surprised! The skepticism, which had been drilled into us by our professors and the international doyens of ophthalmology for many years, vanished from my mind. Almost overnight I changed first to a positive frame of mind—soon thereafter, to outright enthusiasm. So many people had always been so negative about so many aspects of the IOL—but our research efforts changed our opinions on what we had heard constantly from the ophthalmic establishment. From the laboratory viewpoint, which in some ways may be as or more reliable than some clinical studies, our findings did show that the IOL worked!

Our published research findings, beginning with IOL #1 (see page 52) and three others that appeared in rapid succession in 1984-1985, were well-received and helped to contribute to further improvements in the quality of IOLs and helped them survive at a time when they were facing much criticism, much of it unwarranted. By 1985 Harold had apparently had become familiar with our first four published research articles.* I was dumbfounded but honored when he invited (summoned) me to visit him in England. That summer, while in Europe, I flew to London and then took a train to his beautiful retirement cottage near Salisbury. You can't believe my excitement and pride as I stepped out of the train and walked down to meet him outside the station.

However, I was immediately stunned! His visage showed sadness and frustration—the appearance of a very unhappy and depressed man. He soon appeared very happy to see me and this increased by the hour.

---

* These four studies from 1984-1985 are cited here. See the appendix for several more publications that rapidly came off the press from 1984-1986, as well as books and book chapters.
1. Apple DJ, Craythorn JM, Olson RJ, Little LE, Lyman JB, Reidy JJ, Loftfield K. Anterior segment complications and neovascular glaucoma following implantation of posterior chamber intraocular lens. *Ophthalmology*. 1984;91:403-419.
2. Apple DJ, Mamalis N, Loftfield K, Brady SE, Olson RJ, et al. Complications of intraocular lenses. A historical and histopathological review. *Surv Ophthalmol*. 1984;29:1-54.
3. Apple DJ, Mamalis N, Brady SE, et al. Biocompatability of implant materials: A review and scanning electron microscopic study. *J Am Intraocul Implant Soc*. 1984;10:53-66.
4. Apple DJ, Reidy JJ, Googe JM, Mamalis N, et al. A comparison of ciliary sulcus and capsular bag fixation of posterior chamber intraocular lenses. *J Am Intraocul Implant Soc*. 1985;11:44-63.

PREFACE

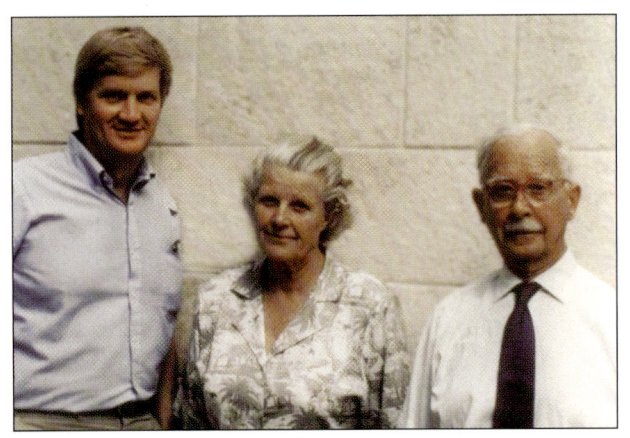

My first meeting with the Ridleys was in summer of 1985—the beginning of a wonderful personal and professional relationship. Elisabeth is in the middle, flanked by me on her right, with Harold on her left.

We began a good personal and professional friendship that lasted until his death. His invention was a true gift to humanity and I thought it was an incredible injustice that he was not only not being honored, he was being ignored. The events set in motion on that summer day in 1985 are the essence of what we will chronicle in this book, ie, the long voyage (over 60 years) of a man and his innovation through periods of very rough waters to a safe harbor.

I started thinking about Sir Harold's biography on the day I met him. I quickly realized that this would not just be an honor, but was a duty. Although it was not particularly easy to reach his idyllic cottage in Stapleford in Wiltshire near Salisbury, I made a point to visit his home two to three times each year, alone in the early years and later almost always with my wife, Ann, after our marriage in 1995.

We would often do river walks (see Chapter 5) and then would retire to his living room and then his upstairs. We would transcribe the information exchanged during our river walks and also fetched different memorabilia and papers, which we copied and expanded over a period of 15 years. We continually jotted down notes (which he refered to as "jottings"), which he would then type himself on his tiny word processor. A few years before he died he asked me to formalize all of this in his biography and I signed a contract to become his official biographer. After his death, his sons kindly sent me additional photographs and text material.

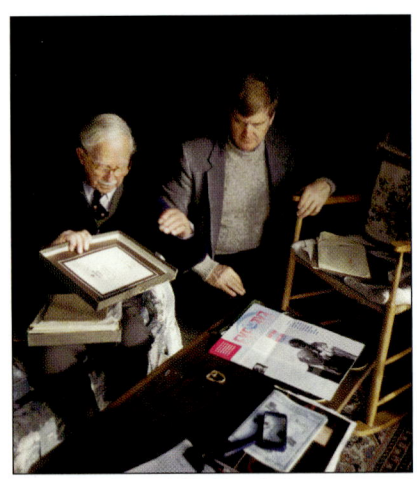

Organization of Sir Harold's papers and memorabilia at his home near Salisbury, UK. On each visit, which averaged about three per year, we prepared drafts for the future preparation of the Memoirs of the Royal Society, which I was able to write for editorials and for this biography. In 2001, he and his wife Elisabeth signed a document designating me his official biographer.

The origins of the IOL seem sometimes to have remained shrouded in mists as thick as a London fog. In this book I have explored the topic, using interviews with many of his contemporaries to catalogue as many events as possible. I have explored the actual origins of his first discussions of the IOL in the 1930s, the role of the "pilot," the role of the "student," the events leading to the first implantations, the early presentations and subsequent attacks which led to depressions, and the later positive events which led to a rekindling of interest in the lens and respect for Sir Harold, who was eventually knighted.

In addition to focusing on the IOL, I also have taken care to describe events and discoveries in his career that have generally remained almost unknown to most of us, ranging from his work on onchocerciasis to the use of electronic techniques derived from World War II.

Throughout the years, by far the three most common questions I have been asked regarding Sir Harold have been 1) is the "airplane story" really true?, 2) what caused the delay in widespread implementation of the IOL and why was he sometimes depressed and in conflict with one person?, and 3) was he a smart man, even a genius, or a "modest giant of science" as noted on page 31 of the text—and should we regard him as a hero, or was he an average surgeon who lucked out and appeared at the right time and place?

I will cover each of these in detail in the text and will provide a few introductory comments now.

Is the "Airplane Story" Really True?

By far the most common question I receive regarding Sir Harold relates to the "Spitfire" story. The first response I always must give is that if it is a true story connected with Sir Harold, it was not a "Spitfire," it was a Hurricane. He was adamant about that differentiation. For years I was very confused about the "airplane story" and didn't know how to fit it into the entire pattern. The story was too good to be true. In addition, Mr. Ian Collins, former Managing Director of Rayner & Keeler, Ltd., has noted that some reasons for a lack of clear-cut documentation are that most of the records regarding the early design and manufacture of the IOL (between 1949-1960) has sadly been lost. The manufacturer, Rayner & Keeler, Ltd., had two moves of their Head Office, where the records were kept and also were victims of two floods. Therefore, ample surviving records from the company only exist from 1957 and later.

The invention of the intraocular lens by Sir Harold is not nearly as simple as often believed; in fact, it was a complex evolutionary process. The standard belief is that he observed a downed World War II pilot with eye injuries due to fragments of Plexiglas from the cockpit canopy becoming embedded in the eyes, after which he had a sudden flash of genius and came up with the idea.

It was far more complex than that—a process that lasted for over at least two decades from the time he first seriously considered the idea of a IOL until his first implantation in the mid-20th century.

In fact, the episode(s) regarding the pilot(s) was but one of many factors, albeit a very significant one. In determining the sequence of events of the invention of the IOL (see Chapter 6), I found that the "airplane story" was one of six factors. The examinations of the injured pilot(s) in effect provided a hugely important phase, the "pre-clinical" study—seemingly not planned ahead of time, but initiated after the surgeon's realization that the injury could be used to provide evaluations necessary for future implantations. We are fortunate that at least some military and medical records of at least one pilot, Flight Lieutenant Gordon "Mouse" Cleaver, have been preserved. Many other pilots had such injuries, but reliable records are no longer available in virtually all of those cases. I have chosen to tell the story of Flight Lieutenant Cleaver and his squadron in detail to illustrate how the pilot's injury provided a means to study the biocompatibility (tolerance) of the material Harold had chosen for his IOL.

What Caused the Delay in Implanting the IOL and Why Was He Sometimes Depressed and in Conflict With Some Colleagues, Especially One?

"I had 25 years in the wilderness and a whole generation of cataract patients who might have enjoyed full visual rehabilitation instead suffered the abnormalities of aphakia."

Harold Ridley

As he started his voyage to perfect and disseminate his idea—which he knew was a good one, he thought, and hoped that he would have smooth sailing.

Something went very wrong!!

Within a few years the few kind and complimentary words that he heard from several close and supportive colleagues had largely been drowned out by a deluge of criticisms and vilifications from any naysayers, mostly emanating from the "academic establishment" of the time.

A few of many examples of these are as follows:

"This operation should never be done."
"The first report was a layman's magazine."
"This operation offends the first principle of eye surgery."
"A foreign body can cause sympathetic ophthalmia and malignant disease."
"Rayner should be prosecuted for supplying implants."
"Would you have one of these things put in your son's eye?"
"Dr. Ridley, why don't you GO HOME."
"If any of you ever use an IOL in a hospital that I control, I will most certainly testify against you in legal process."
"The IOL and the phacoemulsification procedure that goes with it represent a time bomb."

PREFACE

If I, David Apple, had presented a new invention to the world and if such criticism had been leveled at me personally, I know that I would have shriveled up and disappeared. It is no wonder that Sir Harold on more than one occasion required antidepressant therapy, but he did hang in there.

After I met him I noticed how unknown a figure he was. Even in his little tiny village of Stapleford, the taxi driver, the butcher, the nearby farmers—all who were good friends—had no idea what he was or had done. What was really serious was the fact that the various naysayers of his era were in part responsible for blocking the implementation of his invention, not just for a few months or years, but for well over two decades! Harold was right with his comment "a whole generation of cataract patients… suffered…" There was some patriotic component to his depression.

> *"As a result of the failure of British Ophthalmology to join and support the pioneers Britain lost its rightful place in a new and developing field. Through this failure a whole generation of British men and women who underwent cataract surgery between 1951 and 1975 were denied the full treatment which was then becoming available."*
>
> *Harold Ridley*

Finally, this did turn around… "all's well that ends well."

Was He a Smart Man, Or Even a Genius and Should We Regard Him as a Hero, or Was He an Average Person Who Just Lucked Out and Appeared at the Right Time and Place?

There were many contemporaries of Harold back in the 1940s to 1960s who considered him anything but a hero. They certainly did not like the fact that they were being forced to change the way they did their surgery. We will speak about the huge paradigm shift that he brought about, in essence forcing doctors to place a foreign body into the eye in contrast to the well established dictum of taking things out of the eye.

Many at that time considered his approach to be cavalier, if not unethical. This feeling persists in some circles even today and some feel that he should have been thrown into jail at that time and still should be today if he exhibited the same behavior by moving forward without "oversight" of his operation.

The naysayers' main complaint was that he did not do proper and careful basic and pre-clinical (laboratory) studies in anticipation of this operation. This is a good try, but I respectively submit that it isn't true. First, one has to remember that his work was going on in postwar heavily-bombed London where the niceties of such experimentation were difficult. But most importantly, he was actually—perhaps without not even realizing it—doing the best of all possible preclinical studies—on humans!

Therefore, was he smart? How many of us could figure out how to do a preclinical study on an invention that had not yet been invented? And how about the following? We will see in Chapter 15 that Harold was the inventor of the concept of the scanning laser ophthalmoscope (SLO)—long before the invention of the laser! I have the impression that it would require a very smart man to accomplish this. Look also at the list in the figure on the next page—a number of therapeutic options that his invention unlocked for us in later generations of clinicians and scientists to develop, again reflecting the work of a very competent man. There is no doubt that immense energy and intelligence were packed in that tiny frame that stood barely five feet high.

Back to the question "was he a hero?", I would disagree with his contemporaries who would say "no." In Chapter 4 I emphasized how I was raised in a mid-western community where I was strongly influenced by "heroes" who had lived in and around my community and environment, ranging from Abraham Lincoln to Mark Twain. Therefore, having spent two decades analyzing what Harold did, it was a very short and easy step for me to consider him a hero.

Finally, I have no doubt that each of the 10 million people who receive an IOL worldwide each year, who have absolutely no idea who Sir Harold was, would consider their unknown benefactor to be a hero.

PREFACE

1949

For the first time the lens capsular bag became accessible for visual and therapeutic implantations.

1. Classic IOLs
2. Refractive/vision enhancing devices (Super Vision); phakic IOLs
   a. Toric lenses
   b. Multifocal IOLs
   c. Accomodative IOLs
   d. IOLs to correct wavefront aberrations (high order Zernike polynomials)
3. Low vision IOLs (eg, Galilean telescopic devices)
4. "Sun block" IOLs
5. "Piggyback" IOLs
6. Pediatric IOLs
7. Drug delivery systems
   a. Anti-PCO-IOLs
   b. General intraocular therapy
8. Intraocular plastic surgery (artificial colored implants)
9. Implant site for various retinal stimulators ("artificial eyes")

Sir Harold's mid-20th century invention of the IOL initiated a major paradigm shift regarding eye surgery as follows:

Not only did he invent the basic IOL with the primary purpose of restoring vision to the partially or totally blind, he achieved more.

First, he "opened up the capsular bag" which made possible the use of many other patient procedures, lenses, and devices that considerably broadened the capabilities of the operation. Second, he in essence became a pioneer in the nascent field of biomedical engineering. He contributed to the new clinical subspecialty of organ, tissue, and artificial prosthesis implantation. He started with the lens, but many continued on with the heart, kidney, and many others.

Some Goals

"Having spent some time with Cornelius Kees Binkhorst, the great surgeon and teacher, in the Netherlands, I asked him if I could copy some of his slides before going back to my country, hoping to receive a few slides from his vast collection. The very next day, my true teacher brought a suitcase full of slides! 'Those are my slides,' he said, 'copy what you need!'

"Moral of the story: Medical facts should be open. Patients deserve to know the facts and be able to understand any disease they, their relatives and friends may have so that they may be able to choose the best possible medical care."

Modified from C. Huber, Switzerland

I want the facts about Sir Harold to be "open," as was so well stated by Dr. Huber. As I tell his story, including my long-term professional and personal association with him, I will cover to the best of my ability the true history and facts regarding his invention of the IOL and other innovations. My goal is to do what a good teacher should do, namely, to provide not only the basic story, but also to provide ample didactic material about the various eye diseases and therapies that we will cover.

Many friends and colleagues suggested that I present this almost as a novel, but I have decided to keep this book totally nonfiction with no intent to move into the realm of historical fiction in order to embellish the contents.* Sometimes

---

* The reader who is not an ophthalmologist or trained eye health care provider will soon realize that most discussions and associated photographs regarding the eye and eye diseases will involve an always-difficult and often-bewildering vocabulary with a special jargon. This will also include many difficult-to-comprehend images. Please do not be discouraged!

A major goal of this book is to inform and teach by providing easy-to-understand descriptions of the eye, its diseases, and the treatments initiated by Sir Harold that will lead to better understanding of these. I have structured the text and photographs so that it should be easy for the eye care professional to skip over the various non-challenging sections if he or she so desires. Similarly, there are some sections that are probably only comprehensible in entirety to a trained professional. In chapters where the content is highly technical and difficult for the non-ophthalmologist to comprehend, I would suggest that the reader peruse the photographs of that section but pass over some or most of the text—and not get bogged down.

I have prepared the book so that it should be useful, interesting, and informative to anyone who has one or more of the eye diseases under discussion. I am sure that an individual who is about to have cataract-IOL surgery will find much of interest.

PREFACE

truth is stranger than fiction. I have arranged things the way Harold would have liked it. I have made liberal use of quotes and comments from the master himself, done in italics throughout the text. Harold was a firm believer in crediting those who preceded him (or who also worked concurrently with him) in his various projects. That is the basic reason for the inclusion of Chapter 5, River Walks. Also, it was during the river walks that I came up to speed with Harold's thoughts and activities prior to 1985, before I met him. Events after that were usually first hand. There are certain segments that might appear out of place as a straight forward biography, eg, discussions of the Apple Korps or discussions of Charleston, SC. However, they are included because these and others are topics the Ridleys enjoyed.

After very difficult years of rejection, he was often depressed and his visage was very commonly similar to that seen on the left, below. As we continued to work together and as his life's work finally was more and more accepted, the happy man that we see in the illustration on the right, below, emerged and remained. Many people ask me what my most pleasing accomplishments were in my career. The answer is two-fold—helping improve the cataract-IOL procedure that he began and helping him become the satisfied man we see in the final photograph.

These two photographs speak volumes about Harold's mood over the years as we worked together.
LEFT: Early on, his sadness was apparent and dominant in his personality.
RIGHT: As things were sorted out in his final years and his innovations and contributions were finally recognized, we thankfully saw this positive change in his demeanor. Observing this turnabout as we grew closer and closer together has been one of the most satisfying events of my career.

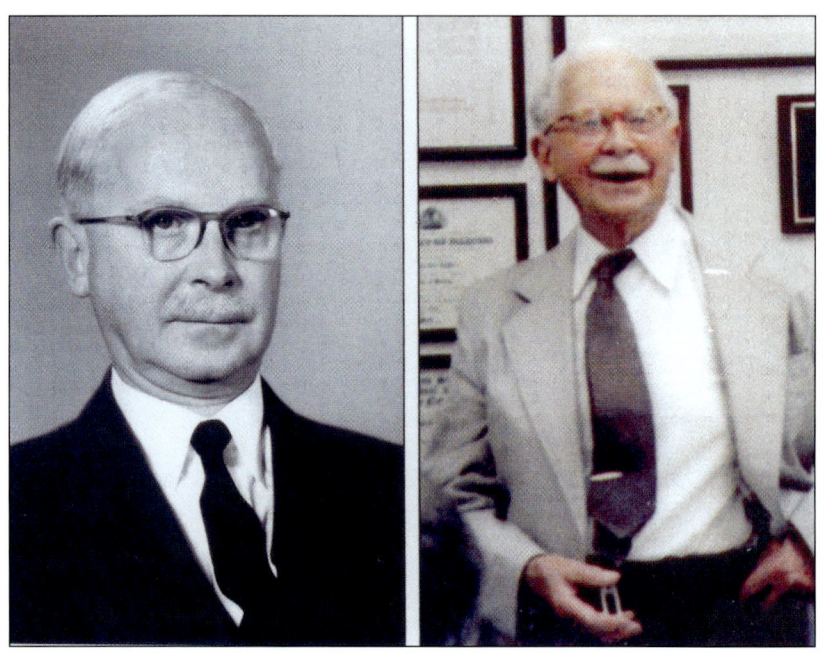

Chronology of Sir Harold Ridley

Early 15th century — Nicholas Ridley, a collateral ancestor of Harold and future Bishop of London was born in Northumberland. He entered Pembroke College, Cambridge, 1518; Fellow, 1825. Chaplain to Archbishop Cranmer, 1537; Chaplain to King Henry VIII, 1540; Bishop of London, 1550. Denied amnesty by Queen Mary ("Bloody Queen Mary"), 1553. Martyred at Oxford on October 16, 1555.

1748 — Jacques Daviel of France, invented the procedure of extracapsular cataract surgery (ECCE), which for the first time would give surgeons an alternative to couching. Finally there was a means of extracting the opaque lens rather than pushing it deeply into the eye. This set the stage for Harold's later invention that brought visual rehabilitation.

1863 — Birth of Nicholas Charles Ridley (Harold's Father), at Bratott, Lincolnshire on April 6th.

1889 — On August 27th, Nicholas Ridley was commissioned into the Royal Navy by Admiral Arthur Hood. However, he had to leave the service in 1891 because of complications of hemophilia.

1906 — Birth of Harold Ridley (Future Sir Harold Ridley, KT, MD, FRS) on July 10th in Kibworth, Beauchamp in Leicestershire. He was the oldest son of Margaret Parker and Nicholas Ridley.

1909 — The family moved to Oadby, a nearby village where his father had his practice. He also practiced at the Leichester Royal Infirmery. Harold attended elementary school in Hove.

1910 — At age 4, Harold sat on Florence Nightingale's knee. This occurred during a visit of his mother to her friend, the world-renowned nurse.

1911 — The 1911 Nobel Prize in medicine was awarded to Alvar Gullstrand for mapping the anatomy and mechanisms of the optical system. This set the stage, but it was not until about 40 years later that his scientific findings were applied to Harold's IOL.

1912 — On July 25th, at age 6, Harold was present with his father at a post-flight gathering honoring the successful flight by the French pilot, Louis Bleriot, from Calais, France to Dover, England. This was the first crossing of the English Channel by a powered air craft. No longer was Britain completely separate from the continent. It was "no longer an island"—an important influence on Harold's life and career.

CHRONOLOGY OF SIR HAROLD RIDLEY

1914-18	World War I. Harold was too young to serve. He belonged to the "lost generation," so named because of the carnage of the war during which so many young men just older than him had been killed.
1920-23	Attends Charterhouse School in Godalming, Surrey, with superior achievement in the sciences and mathematics.
1924-27	Pembroke College, Cambridge (MA, MD with Tripos [honors]).
1932	Ship's tours of the Far East and Eastern Europe.
1930s	Accompanied his father to Vienna, Budapest, and other central European countries to observe their (for the period) advanced surgical techniques. Most cataract surgery on the continent at that time was intracapsular cataract extraction (ICCE). Harold noted, even during these early years, that Germany was making preparations for war.
1930	Completed basic medical training at Saint Thomas' Hospital.
1930	Ophthalmic registrar (resident) at Saint Thomas' Hospital. Two highly respected mentors were 1) Mr. Geoffrey Doyne and 2) A. C. Hudson (Huddy). Geoffrey Doyne was the son of Robert Doyne (1957-1916). The latter was the discoverer of Doyne's Honeycomb Retinal Dystrophy and Founder of the Oxford Ophthalmological Congress.
1933	Sir Stewart Duke-Elder knighted.
1934-36	Registrar at the Royal London Ophthalmic Hospital (RLOH), later named Moorfields Eye Hospital. By 1936 Harold was the only registrar.
1935	First mention of implants by Harold, in connection with discussions he had with his father and professors. They politely rejected this idea and he shelved it until the 1940s, when he began observing and performing surgery on various injured pilots. We are able to trace in detail the records of Flight Lieutenant Gordon "Mouse" Cleaver. These observations (between 1940 and 1948) became a pre-clinical study to evaluate the biocompatibility of the cockpit material that Ridley and his colleagues later used to manufacture the first implant.
1935	Received a laudatory letter of recommendation from Sir Stewart Duke-Elder in support of his application for a staff appointment at the Royal Eye Hospital.
1935	First negative encounter with Sir Stewart Duke-Elder. In his capacity in overseeing the eye clinics at Moorfields Hospital, Harold insisted that all consultants, including Duke-Elder, follow the regulations and staff their clinics in person. This apparently offended Duke-Elder. Harold forever lamented that he had not been more lenient and politically correct.
1937	Death of Harold's father.
1938	Appointed full surgeon and consultant at Moorfields Hospital.
1939	Consultant at both Moorfields and Saint Thomas' Hospitals. The Germans invaded Poland on September 3, 1939 and also conquered Czechoslovakia and the low countries. They then prepared to attack France. The waiting period was called the "Phony War." They did attack France on May 10, 1940. (The Battle of France lasted from May 10, 1940 to June 22, 1940). France was divided up into zones, including a zone directly occupied by Germany and a zone ruled by their puppets, the Vichy Government.
1940	Dunkirk, the end of the "Battle of France," soon to be followed by the German attack over the English Channel, "The Battle of Britain."
1940	July to September-October, the Battle of Britain was fought by "The Few." Harold, not yet inducted into the Royal Army, worked as a civilian at several hospitals in the South very near the heavily attacked channel. The main St. Thomas' Hospital in London was partially evacuated in anticipation of the invasion. Many were transferred to satellite hospitals that were established in the South where Harold worked ("I saw many casual-

ties," he said). These facilities included the military facility at Aderholt, Saint Luke's Hospital in Guildford, and a St. Thomas' facility in Godalming. Harold treated patients evacuated from RAF Tangmere, the base airport of the 601 Squadron.

1940   August 14th, Adlertag (Eagle Day), the turning point of the Battle of Britain where the RAF eventually began its ultimate repulse of the German air invasion. On August 14th, Flight Lieutenant "Mouse" Cleaver flew two sorties, the morning one being uneventful and in his own Hurricane. A second "scramble" was ordered; he had to seek a second plane as his own aircraft was being serviced. He forgot his goggles in the rush. He was hit by German fire, and parachuted safely even though he was acutely blinded in both eyes by fragments of plastic shrapnel.

August 15th was the beginning of years of follow up treatment of Flight Lieutenant Cleaver's injured eyes, in essence a pre-clinical study. Some have suggested that this was the symbolic birthday of the intraocular lens. In reality, Harold's decade long follow-up of him and no doubt other pilots represented a pre-clinical study of an invention that Harold was considering but had not yet been invented.

1941   Formally inducted into the Royal military service as a temporary Major.

1941   On May 10th Harold married Elisabeth Jane Weatherhill (born August 16, 1916 in Surrey). Bombs were falling during the wedding. They subsequently had 3 children—Margaret in 1942, Nicholas in 1943, and David in 1951.

1943   Assigned to service in Ghana by Sir Stewart Duke-Elder, who was in charge of ophthalmology assignments for the British Military. He did important clinical work on two very important diseases that affected the eye: onchocerciasis (river blindness) and vitamin A deficiency.

1944-45   Transferred to the Thailand-Burma theater of war, where he began treatment of released prisoners of war suffering from nutritional eye deficiencies (amblyopia). He made a very important observation that has not been credited to him. He recognized that such lesions are not just optic nerve lesions, but put forth the hypothesis that the choriocapillaris (small vessels) coursing to the central macular region may play a role in the etiology or pathogenesis of some maculopathies—possibly a model for "age-related macular degeneration" (ARMD). He utilized multivitamin therapy.

1945   Publication of his classic monograph on onchocerciasis in the *British Journal of Ophthalmology*. This was based on work he had completed during his service in Ghana. He described the "Ridley Fundus."

1946   Appointed consultant surgeon at Moorfields Hospital.

1947   Discharged from military service.

1947-71   Civilian consultant in ophthalmology to the Ministry of Defense (army).

1940-50   Throughout the decade of the 1940s he did research on a number of topics besides the intraocular lens. During and after World War II, he recognized the numerous possibilities of supplying new technological innovations and discoveries from the war to peaceful uses. These included experiments with the relatively new video technology in conjunction with the Marconi Wireless Company. Some of the work was applied to developing non-invasive means of diagnosis of retinal and optic nerve diseases. He developed the groundwork for modern scanning laser ophthalmology (SLO), even before the laser was invented! He was ably assisted at St. Thomas' by Mr. Peter Styles, an electronic technologist.

1948   Harold obtained the first video images of the interior of the eye and televised eye operations.

1948   A young medical student named Mr. Stephen Perry, who knew little about ophthalmology, asked Harold a simple, but important question after seeing Harold do the standard cataract surgery of the period. He asked "why not replace the extracted lens with another one?" That single question gave Harold the courage to proceed with an idea to design and implant an IOL.

CHRONOLOGY OF SIR HAROLD RIDLEY

1948	He mobilized an excellent team and for the next two years, he and his team—Pike of Rayners, Holt of ICI, and others, began the process and efforts that led to Operation #1 on November 29, 1949. The details are not clear, but the two operations were done by Harold himself: 1) November 29, 1949 and 2) February 8, 1950.
1949	November 29th, the date formally regarded as the first cataract-IOL operation. It was performed by Harold Ridley at Saint Thomas' Hospital in London, officially known as Operation #1.
1950	Purchased a house, Keeper's Cottage, Stapleford in Wiltshire in 1950, initially for weekend fishing (angling) and later for retirement.
1950	Showed monochrome and color fundus (retinal) pictures for the first time at the Oxford Ophthalmological Congress. He developed what he termed "intraocular television." He was an early advocate of telediagnosis.
1950	The first cataract-IOL operations were done in the highest secrecy. One patient erroneously reported for a postsurgical examination to the office (rooms) of Mr. Fredrick Ridley, who of course noted the well-implanted IOL. "The secret was out, the cat was out of the bag," Harold said. This necessitated an early announcement of the project.
1951	The first scientific publication of the IOL and Harold's operation appeared in the *Bulletin of St. Thomas' Hospital Reports* in 1951;Vol. 7:pp. 12-14.
1951	On July 9th, Harold made his first formal presentation of findings on his cataract-IOL operation at the annual meeting of the Oxford Ophthalmological Congress. He brought two very successfully operated patients to the meeting. However, he was severely rebuked by Sir Stewart Duke-Elder and others.
1952	Presentation of his findings in Chicago. He implanted the first IOL in America at that time.
1952	The first implant done by an American was performed by Dr. Warren Reese of Philadelphia. After he had seen Harold do the very first implant on American soil in Chicago in 1952, Reese immediately flew back to Philadelphia where he did the operation. He and his friend and partner, Dr. Turgut Hamdi, both of Wills Eye Hospital in Philadelphia, became ardent supporters of Harold and his technique. Hamdi and Reese (1962) were among the first, if not the first, ophthalmologists to suggest the possibility of bi-multifocal IOLs, a very visionary suggestion since they have now apparently come into their own.
1952	American Academy of Ophthalmology and Otolaryngology in Chicago, first comments of Dr. Derrick Vail (later published in the *American Journal of Ophthalmology*, 1952;Vol. 35:pp. 1701-1703). He severely criticized Harold. A close friend of Sir Harold Ridley, he later died in Duke-Elder's 63 Harley Street home in London.
1951	Negative comments regarding a histopathological report on an intraocular lens was published by Dr. Georgiana Dvorak Theobald, Chicago in 1951. She asserted that IOLs could be very damaging to the eye. She also criticized (unfairly) that he had had inappropriately published articles in the lay press, eg, *Time Magazine*, which at that time was deemed "unscientific and unprofessional by the ophthalmic establishment."
1950-51	Some of the earlier supporters of Harold and indeed true pioneers of the implant included Dr. Peter Choyce, UK; Dr. Edward Epstein, South Africa; Dr. Svyataslav Fyodorov, former USSR; and Dr. Cornelius Binkhorst, The Netherlands.
1950s	First pediatric implants performed by Drs. Edward Epstein and Peter Choyce.
1962	Purchased a house and office (rooms) at 53 Harley Street from Henry Stallard.
1966	After rejection from full participation in the International Congress of Ophthalmology (ICO) scheduled for Munich in 1966, Peter Choyce, the organizer of a tiny group of pioneer implant surgeons of the day, did an "end run." With Harold as the first president, they formed the Intraocular Implant Club (IIC) in London. Their first meeting was on Bastille Day, July 14, 1966, at the Royal Society of Medicine in London.
1972	Scientific meeting of the IIC in Budapest.

CHRONOLOGY OF SIR HAROLD RIDLEY

1971	On July 10th Harold retired from hospital service.
1974	The International Congress of Ophthalmology's 1974 meeting was held in Paris in 1974. Choyce was again provided only a half-hearted acceptance of his group by the meeting organizers. He then found an adjacent room near the Convention Center and hosted a huge group of ophthalmologists, including many Americans who were interested in hearing about IOLs. Harold was a "surprise visitor" at the IIC. Because of its growth, it was renamed the International Intraocular Implant Club (IIIC).
1978	At AAO in San Francisco, Harold was given a book with the signatures of 4000 grateful surgeons.
1986	On March 22nd, Harold was elected to the Royal Society, Britain's highest scholarly accolade.
1986	Harold received the Golden Medal, awarded by the Worshipful Society of Apothecaries London (1614).
1987	Flight Lieutenant "Mouse" Cleaver has an eye operation in London. Professor Eric Arnott replaced the fragments of plastic in one of his injured eyes with an IOL! Things had come full circle.
1992	Harold received the Gullstrand Medal from the Swedish Ophthalmological Society.
1989	Harold received an honorary degree from the Medical University of South Carolina, Storm Eye Institute, Charleston, SC, in May 1989. The degree was presented by the author. This was Harold's first award from an academic institution. He also later received an honorary degree from the University of London.
1989	In Washington, DC harold was honored by American Society of Cataract and Refractive Surgery.
1992	Harold received the Gullstrand Medal from the Swedish Ophthalmological Society, Stockholm.
1994	The Gonin Medal was conferred to Harold by the Club Jules Gonin, Lausanne, Switzerland.
1997	Harold was honored by the delegates at the Oxford Ophthalmological Congress in tandem with a lecture given by the author at the time. This meeting symbolically brought Harold's experiences at Oxford around full circle, from 1) an in initial prewar pleasant visit accompanying his father in the 1930s, to the 2) very difficult first presentation of his IOL on July 1951, to this latter one, 3) a final outpouring of gratitude and applause of long duration.
1999	Fiftieth Anniversary Celebration of the IOL, sponsored by Rayner Intraocular Lenses, Ltd., held at the Royal Victoria and Albert Science Museum in London.
1999	A Special Honor Award was presented to Harold by the American Society of Cataract and Refractive Surgery, and he was inducted into the Ophthalmology Hall of Fame at their annual 1999 meeting. He also received a special honor from Rayner Intraocular Lens, Ltd.
2000	In February, Knighthood was conferred by Queen Elizabeth II to Harold in London. The author and others had sent letters to Prime Minister Tony Blair and his wife Cherie.
2001	Harold died peacefully at 5:30 PM on May 25, 2001 at Salisbury District Hospital, UK of complications of a severe cerebral vascular disease (stroke).
2002	The Queen Mother Elizabeth Bowes (April 4, 1900 to March 30, 2002) passed away. She had had a very successful IOL implantation by Dr. John Pearce a few years earlier with excellent result.
2004	The "Ridley Walk," in honor of Bishop Nicholas Ridley (died 1555) and Sir Harold Ridley (1906-2002), was established at Pembroke College, Cambridge.

St. Thomas' Hospital, London.
TOP: Artist's painting of the hospital shortly after its construction in the Italianate style in the 1860s.
BOTTOM: The hospital and Westminster Bridge after the Blitz. The white arrow shows a heavily damaged portion of the building; the ophthalmology ward and surgical suites (theatres) were in this block. The long street that courses along the river bank is the Albert Embankment. The artist Monet lived and worked there sporadically between 1901 and 1903.

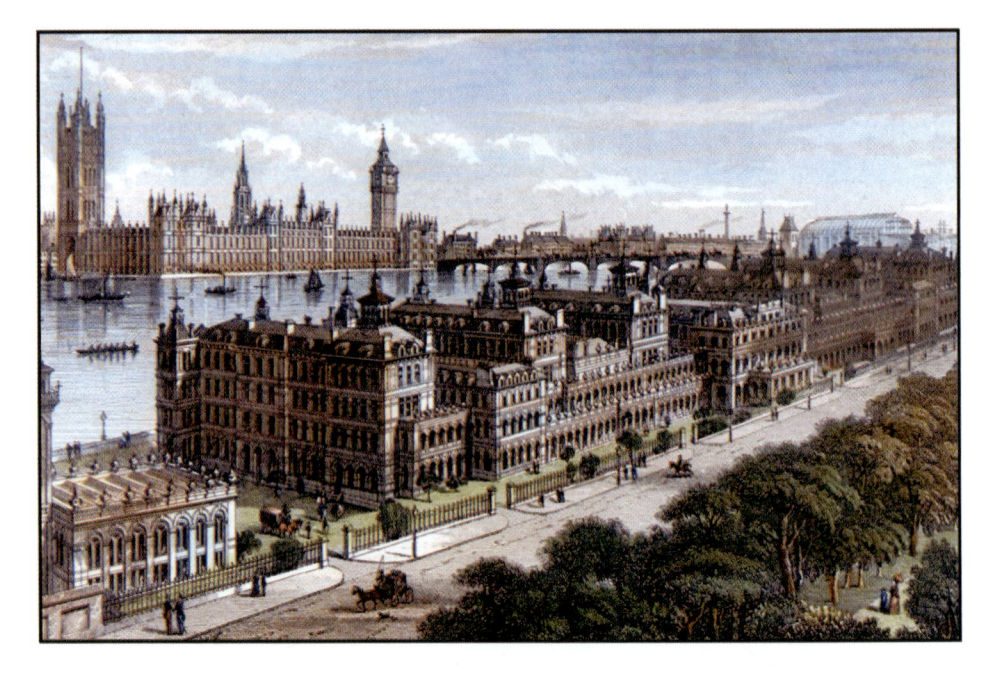

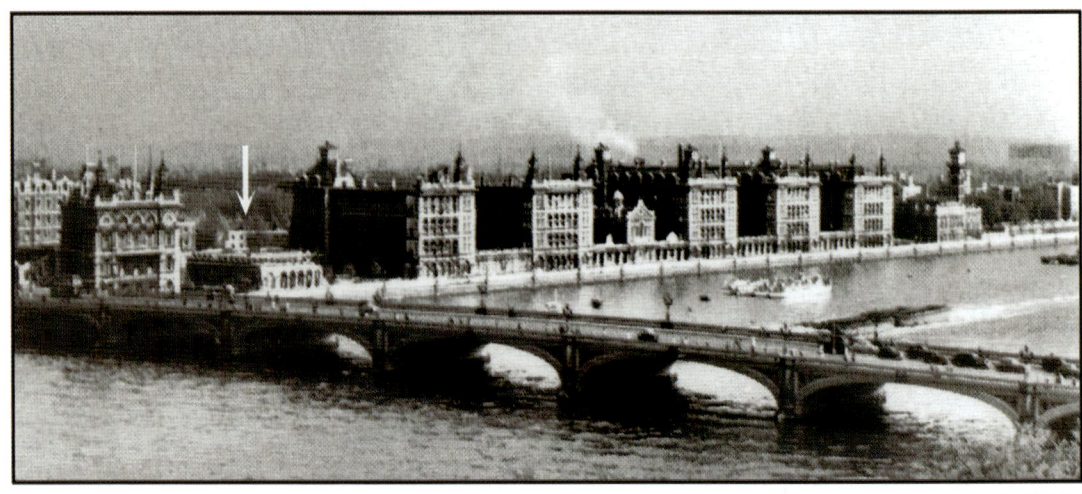

1

The Secret Code: The "Extra-Capsular Ext."

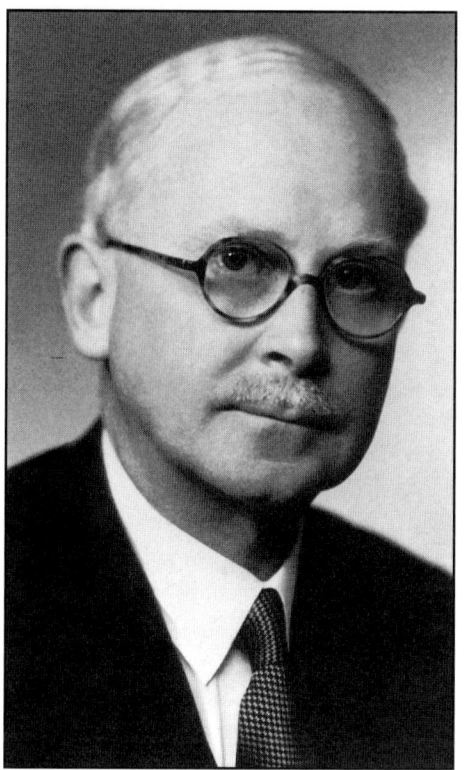

Harold Ridley, ca. 1948, age 42. This is the time period when he was doing research on intraocular lenses as well as many other projects simultaneously, including the application of television to ophthalmology. He was busy assembling a team of colleagues to prepare for his November 29, 1949 cataract-IOL operation.

"God has been indeed been kind to me, for He gave me a job to do, which was really worth doing and He made me a member of the team from the Eye Department of our venerable Hospital, which has indisputably accomplished a World First by completing the cure of cataract."

Harold Ridley

LONDON. NOVEMBER 29, 1949

Early risers were treated to a crisp, fair morning—a welcome change from the drizzly, overcast weather that occurs in Britain during the season's passage from fall to winter. It had been almost four and a half years since Victory in Europe (VE) Day, marking the end of World War II. Repairs and renovations were a constant reality as the city labored to deliver itself from the wreckage of war.

Since the end of the awful days of the Blitz bombardments in the early 1940s, articles in London's newspapers, such as *The Times of London*, documented the efforts of a brave and tenacious citizenry to rebuild their city.

One of the most notable events documented in the *Times* on that quiet November day was a notice that the plans for the final design of the Chapel of St. Paul's Church in Central London had been completed. The new construction was dedicated to the bond that Britain and the United States had forged during the conflict. Previously known as the Jesus Chapel, it was to be renamed the American Memorial.

CHAPTER 1

Further perusal of the newspaper headlines on that November day revealed no evidence that an earthshaking event had occurred or was impending. All seemed quiet and routine. *Actually, nothing could have been further from the truth!*

Early in the afternoon of this otherwise "ordinary" day, the prominent London eye surgeon, Mr. Harold Ridley (in England, surgeons are referred to as "Mr.") and a small cluster of colleagues assembled in an operating room (theatre) at St. Thomas' Hospital. Some of them did not realize it, but they were preparing for a momentous eye operation that was destined to change not only ophthalmology but also medicine in general and, indeed, the world.

It was not by chance that Ridley chose St. Thomas' Hospital, impressively situated on the Thames at Westminster Bridge, for what he believed would be a revolutionary operation. He had trained there for many years with fine leaders, including Mr. Jeffrey Doyne and Mr. A. Cyril Hudson.

This hospital was and is renowned for many reasons, both medical and nonmedical. It was founded in the Middle Ages. The top image on the first page of this chapter was painted in the 1860s, shortly after a new construction and modernization in an elegant Italianate architectural style. It had been the workplace of Florence Nightingale. Ridley's mother, Margaret Parker, had been a nurse (Sister).

It is not well known that Claude Monet, the great French artist and one of the founders of Impressionism, enjoyed working from a base he had established in the hospital. He outfitted a room in the hospital facing the Thames and the Houses of Parliament. During three sojourns in London between 1901 and 1903, he immortalized the river site of the adjacent buildings and bridges near the hospital in numerous paintings. The century-old operating rooms destroyed in the Blitz were rebuilt just a few hundred paces away from the previous site of Monet's rooms.

Monet himself developed an eye problem during the early 1920s. The lenses of both of his eyes had a condition that caused them to cloud—the very common visually disabling or blinding disease termed a cataract. During Monet's time surgeons were only able to partially treat

TOP: This is a photograph of the ophthalmology ward prior to the war.
LOWER LEFT: The ophthalmology ward was badly damaged during the bombings.
LOWER RIGHT: The operating rooms were made sufficiently functional for Harold Ridley's landmark operation on November 29, 1949.

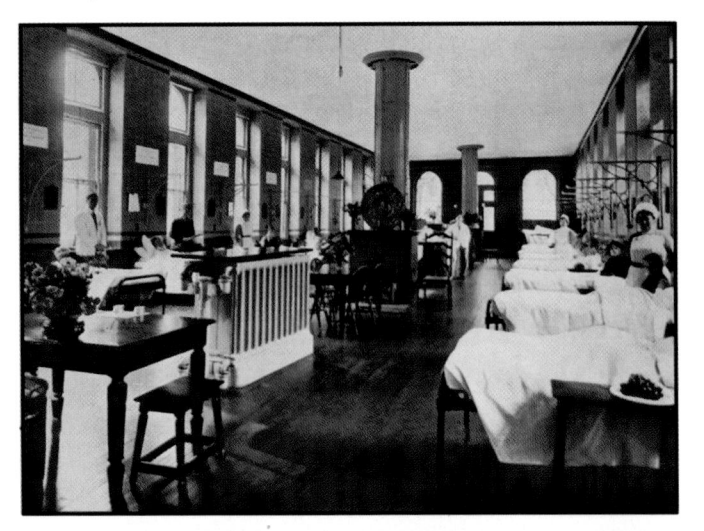

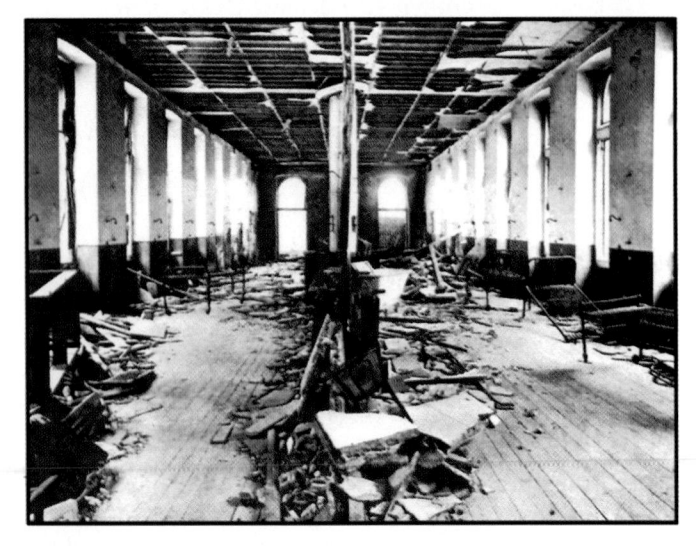

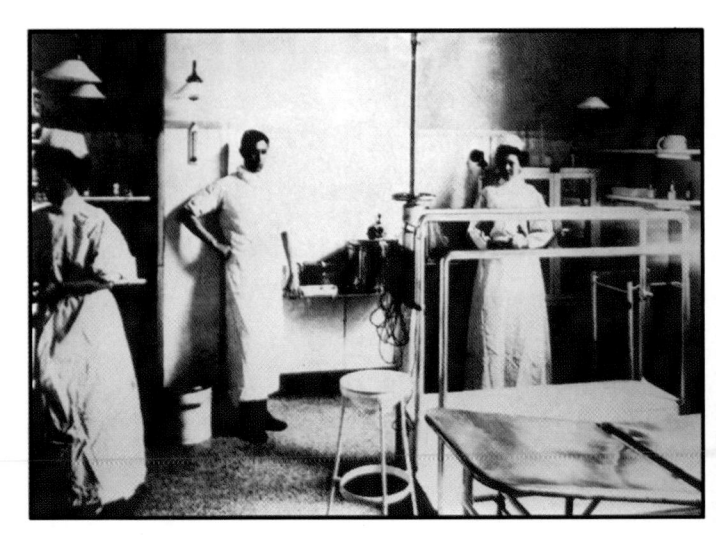

THE SECRET CODE: "THE EXTRA-CAPSULAR EXT."

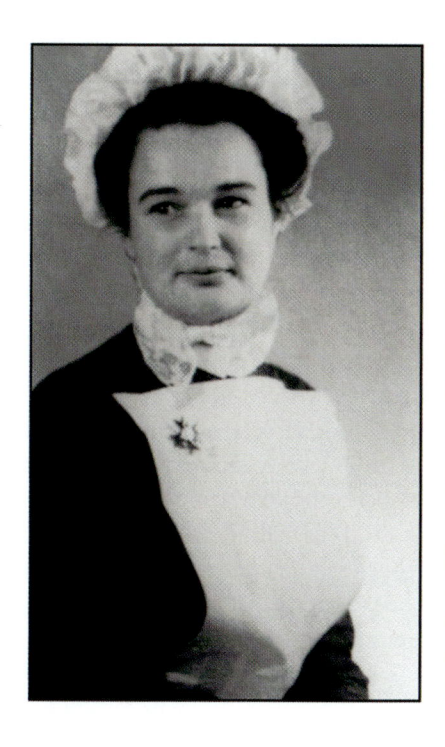

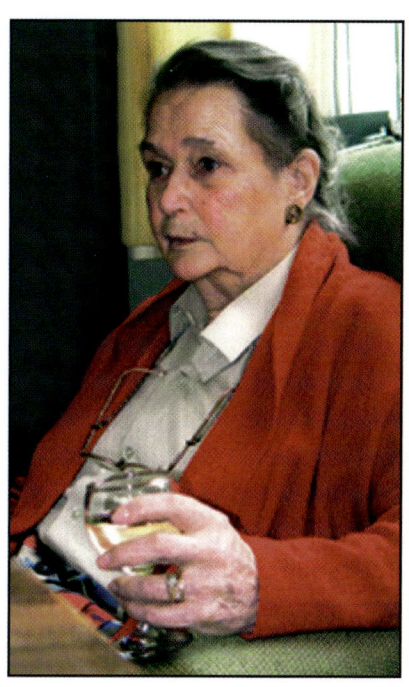

LEFT: Doreen Clarke (married name Ogg), at the time of Ridley's operation, November 29, 1949. She had trained as a Florence Nightingale Nurse. Harold had given her the highly responsible task of holding and guiding the flashlight (torch) that illuminated the operating field.
RIGHT: Mrs. Ogg is comfortably retired in Hampshire and has clear memories of that first operation. (Photograph taken by Ann Apple.)

a cataract; they could only remove the cloudy, cataractous (opaque) lens. Prior to Ridley, there were no satisfactory means to replace the extracted, diseased lens with a healthy or functional one. Monet would have been ecstatic if he had been the benefactor of the gift that Harold Ridley was about to deliver a half century later: the intraocular lens (IOL). As an artist who depended on quality of vision and color perception, he would have benefited greatly from Ridley's efforts.

During the Blitz of World War II some of the hospital buildings had been damaged or destroyed, including the ophthalmology (Greek: ophthalmo = eye; ology = study) ward and the eye operating room. Rapid postwar reconstruction had succeeded in restoring some of these facilities to functional operation by 1949, just in time to become the site of Harold Ridley's now famous "top secret" operation.

Harold's* team began performing their assigned duties around the operating table on that November day. Miss Doreen Clarke proudly assumed her very important role as the nurse who, in addition to the many assignments that were inherent in doing any eye operation, was responsible for the illumination of the operative field. At that time they did not have operating microscopes with high-power magnification and built-in illumination. She used a simple flashlight (torch).

The operation Harold had been preparing for 4 months was performed in secrecy. The brave person who volunteered to be operated on was a 49-year-old hospital nurse named Elisabeth A., who had a total cataract in one eye. This operation and the series of operations performed soon thereafter by Harold's team were the very first of their kind. They were hugely important in that they were needed to prove the feasibility, potential safety, and efficacy of the IOL—the invention that finally brought us a complete cure for cataract.

---

* From our meeting in 1985 until his death in 2001 Harold and I remained close personal and professional friends; I will refer to him from now on as Harold.

CHAPTER I

The only documentation of this first procedure was Miss Clarke's entry in the surgical log book: "Extra-capsular ext." "Extra-capsular ext." is the abbreviation for the formal designation of extracapsular cataract extraction (ECCE), the operation necessary before Harold's IOL could be properly implanted. She did not mention the implant. It was Harold's plan to keep any mention of the IOL in this and the other early operations under wraps for as long as two years as he collected clinical and scientific data on the results of the surgery.

The procedure he started that day is now recognized as one of the greatest innovations in the history of eye care. The operation for cataracts had been muddled in stagnation for over 6,000 years. Some improvements in the cataract removal technique had been made by a few insightful surgeons, most notably beginning in the 18th century in France. Harold created the modern miracle of lens replacement, thus truly rendering a **complete** cure for this disease. This operation, broadly termed the cataract-IOL operation, has since brought sight to many millions of people throughout the world.

The magnitude of visual loss and/or blindness caused by unoperated cataract is staggering. The number of people who will benefit from this operation will continue to increase because nearly all individuals on this planet will develop cataracts if they live long enough. Of course, people are living much longer now than in previous decades.

Harold not only launched this powerful and irreversible forward movement in the field of ophthalmology and the visual sciences, but also in the exciting new field of artificial implant surgery applied to many other organs and tissues of the body. He, therefore, helped create the new specialty of biomedical engineering. In addition, without intending or knowing it, he changed the practice styles and economics of his field and, in fact, all fields of medicine.

A portion of the surgical log book from the St. Thomas' Eye Operating Room. Miss Clarke had, per Harold's instructions, designated the operation as an "extra-capsular ext." She was instructed not to mention an implant at this time. He desired that the operation remain confidential, while he gathered the results of his first several cases for open presentations and publications.

A Gift to the World

The Ridley Lens

Harold's initial lens was a circular disc design, impeccably manufactured by Rayner & Keeler, Ltd, UK, a prominent optical company in the United Kingdom. It was made of plastic, the same basic material used to manufacture cockpit canopies in airplanes of that era. It was intended to mimic a patient's natural (crystalline) lens.

A major paradigm shift was set in motion on that November day. There was a new concept that was difficult for some surgeons at that time to grasp.

Prior to November 29, 1949, surgeons were always trained to take things *out* of the eye (ie, cataracts, blood, puss, foreign bodies that had penetrated into the eye, etc).

Now, after November 1949, surgeons were about to be asked to put a foreign material *into* the eye—light years ahead of what had been reality to most in the past.

This change would cause extensive controversy for many years as people attempted to either criticize or rationalize the operation. Prior to this, no one had seriously even considered the concept of putting different kinds of artificial solid or semisolid substances into the eye, as was being advocated. Today, it all seems so simple, but 50-plus years ago, accepting this idea required a huge leap of faith.

THE SECRET CODE: "THE EXTRA-CAPSULAR EXT."

The ancients had called the region in the interior of the eye, behind the iris and where they could not see into, "a black hole" or "terra incognito" (forbidden territory). Of course, by 1949, surgeons had long since learned to see into this region but had gained little or no experience in introducing any kind of foreign object into the interior of the eye.

Harold's innovation was an operation that needed widespread publicity (ie, a campaign to convince the many unbelievers in the world that his ideas made sense). There was intense competition to find people to listen. One must remember that this invention was made in an era before, during, and shortly after World War II, when innovations in many fields were being made, eg, (1) the discovery of penicillin; (2) atomic energy-related discoveries such as the initiation of the first chain reaction in Chicago, and shortly thereafter, the creation of the atom bomb in the Manhattan Project; and (3) Watson and Crick's, and others' elucidation of the structure of the DNA molecule in 1953. These and other high-profile events made the headlines; the IOL did not.

Before we begin this narrative of Harold Ridley's long voyage through often tumultuous seas, later accompanied by myself, I would like to introduce a few more examples of IOLs. These range from his very first design to some ultra modern implants now being implanted with excellent results. This will provide the reader an introduction as to what, in fact, an IOL is and looks like. At first glance, an IOL reveals what appears to be a deceptively simple design or configuration, without, for example, electronics or gadgetry within its substance. However, the implant itself, and especially its planned interaction with the surrounding tissues in the eye, was and remains far from simple.

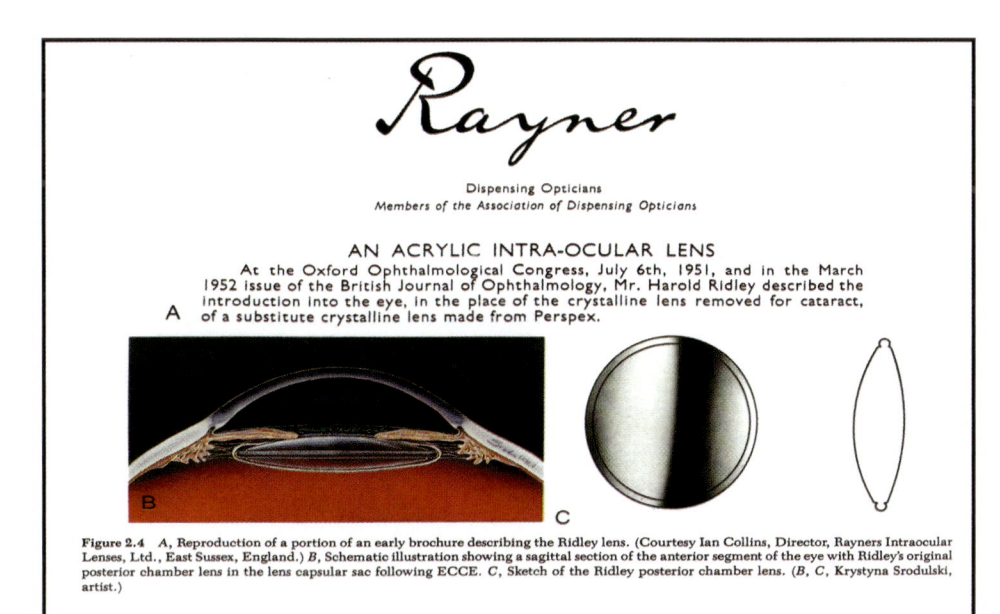

Figure 2.4 A, Reproduction of a portion of an early brochure describing the Ridley lens. (Courtesy Ian Collins, Director, Rayners Intraocular Lenses, Ltd., East Sussex, England.) B, Schematic illustration showing a sagittal section of the anterior segment of the eye with Ridley's original posterior chamber lens in the lens capsular sac following ECCE. C, Sketch of the Ridley posterior chamber lens. (B, C, Krystyna Srodulski, artist.)

The very first IOL design implanted by Harold Ridley in his series of operations beginning on November 29, 1949 was a simple, but very well manufactured biconvex disc fabricated from a plastic material (acrylic, PMMA)—a material still used today. These are sketches of the lens derived from the brochure and from my 1989 textbook showing the desired ideal appearance of the IOL after placement into the eye. It was manufactured by a company in England, Rayner & Keeler, Ltd., a company that heretofore specialized in spectacle manufacture.

Modern IOLs

No doubt in early years some authorities may not have taken the lens seriously because, at first glance, it may have appeared to be "too simple," not loaded with "bells and whistles," not loaded with electronic gadgetry, etc that might have drawn more attention to the press and public. Such assumptions were incorrect. It took many years (ca. 25 years) for lens manufacturers to design the IOLs that we use today. Lens designers and

CHAPTER I

manufacturers learned that the addition of extensions from the optic component of the lens help provide secure and long term fixation of the IOL in the eye. They help stabilize the lens.

Harold's basic lens was therefore modified and modernized to the point that we now have the very fine vision-restoring lenses commensurate with what we expect as we move forward in the 21st century. It has not been an easy process. Over the years, IOLs have been modified; sometimes improved, sometimes not.

Most IOLs today have a special shape and configuration (as seen on this page). Like their predecessors from Ridley's era, the lens' central optical component (simply termed the *optic*) was and still is made of plastic material. However, by the 1980s, researchers began to use soft foldable materials so that the optic could be folded like a taco and inserted through a very small incision. When surgically situated in place in the desired location, the lens is designed to open naturally and remain permanently in the eye. Such small incision surgery is analogous to the well-known arthroscopic surgery commonly done on injured limbs, for example, on people who have had ski injuries.

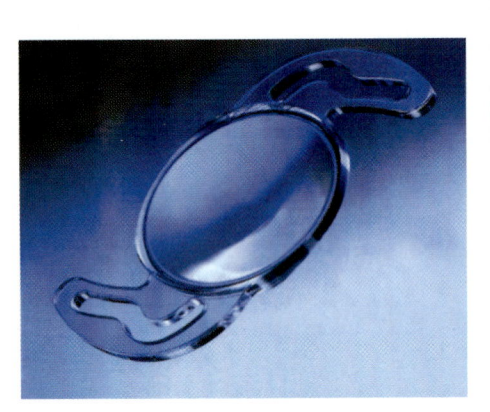

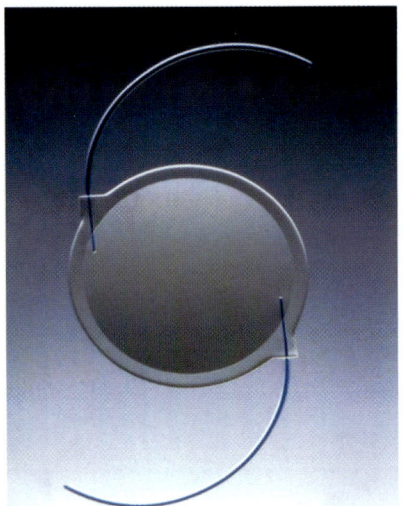

Even at this early stage in the text, I will comment on IOL morphology from Harold's original disc design to the modern lenses used today. These illustrations here show the two lens types that evolved based on type of manufacture: these include 1) the so called one-piece designs (left) and 2) the three-piece designs (three pieces because the central optic is one and the two adjacent C-shaped loops, or haptics, are another two, totaling three).

All of these additions have lens stabilization as a primary function. The haptics help provide and secure long term fixation of the IOL in the eye, preferably within the lens capsular bag. Harold originally envisioned this, but was unable to achieve it all of the time because many surgical instruments on hand were still vintage 19th century.

The photographs on this page show the important supporting elements that help permanently secure the entire implant in its intended location—namely, the site of the patient's original lens. Today, these supporting structures are commonly designated as "loops" or "haptics." They help fixate the lens and, in doing so, help it to "hold still"—a very important consideration. The technical details of these things are beyond the scope of this chapter but will be considered later.

Bi-Multifocal IOLs

"Ridley's IOL* may be viewed as a sincere attempt to evaluate the daring and dramatic replacement which is so simple in concept that, like many other great discoveries, one wonders why it was not thought of earlier.

"If it, or any of its modifications, prove feasible—and we believe they will—its benefits can hardly be calculated.

"Eyes now considered lost from an industrial standpoint will be saved, and patients engaged in work demanding binocular vision will have their livelihood restored.

---

* This must be one of the earliest, if not the earliest, mentions of the concept of a bi-multifocal IOL. The value of this visionary comment has been confirmed by that fact that multifocal IOLs are now in high demand and are highly successful. Reese and Hamdi had been adamant and vocal supporters of Ridley since the early 1950s.

THE SECRET CODE: "THE EXTRA-CAPSULAR EXT."

"Who knows but what in days to come some ingenious surgeon may not only replace the cataractous lens but may devise some means of changing its focus or making it bifocal, so that from an ocular standpoint it will really result in rejuvenation."

Warren S. Reese and Turgut N. Hamdi
Philadelphia, Pa, 1962

One of the great advances that has occurred since "day one" (November 29, 1949) and has assumed great importance today is the added possibility of achieving both near and far vision capability within a single implant—mimicking the process of accommodation that normally occurs with our natural lenses. Examples of correcting for near and far vision are seen in the bifocal spectacles that many of us wear. These provide correction for both near (reading) vision and for distance vision.

In 1962, the American surgeons Dr. Warren Reese, the first American to implant an IOL after having been instructed in 1951 by Ridley himself, and his very reliable and prolific colleague Dr. Turgut Hamdi (both of Philadelphia) may have been the first to suggest the possibility of manufacturing an IOL with a bifocal (or multifocal) correction into an implantable IOL (see the Footnote on the previous page).

In the 1980s, a protégé of Harold's in England, the late Mr. John Pearce, made an early prototype of a bifocal IOL, as illustrated on this page. He instructed a manufacturer to fabricate a more powerful (thicker) lens in the center of a basic Ridley IOL. With this model, patients could achieve vision at both near and far. Unfortunately, the quality of vision with this early design was not satisfactory for widespread use.

Fortunately, Reese and Hamdi's and Pearce's comments have blossomed today into *multifocal* IOLs—defined as a single IOL that can focus through multiple layers in space from near to far. Special concentric rings are fabricated onto the optic's surface and thus provide the basis of this amazing technology. These are now manufactured by several companies and may hold at least one of the keys to the long-awaited dream of "getting rid of glasses." It is fascinating to note that some types of such special lenses have been designed based on principles gained from using the specialized lenses (Fresnel prisms) used in the past to increase the intensity of the beams emitted from costal lighthouses.

This advancement from Harold's very first lens to modern multifocal designs represents a clear demonstration of the perseverance of both Harold and those who believed in his ideas, as opposed to some naysayers who only criticized IOLs and did not work to improve them.

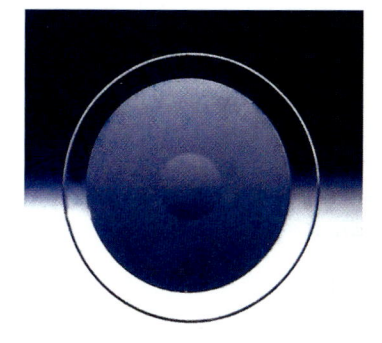

Some brilliant ideas to make the Ridley design even more useful appeared very early. For example, Drs. Reese and Hamdi in Philadelphia, were perhaps the first to mention the possibility of using bifocal IOLs.

In the 1980s Mr. John Pearce, an English surgeon who I believe played a significant role in my life by introducing me to Harold Ridley, designed a Ridley-style lens that had one special modification. In the center the lens was given increased magnification, intended to function as a bifocal to allow better reading at close distances, in addition to normal distance vision. To my knowledge, this is the first attempt to utilize the optic of Ridley's IOL in order to create a platform that can undergo various modifications that can change and indeed improve the characteristics and uses of a given IOL.

John Pearce should also be credited with being one of the first (1975) to strongly recommend a return to posterior chamber lenses, which is now the lens type selected by most surgeons today.

CHAPTER 1

Multifocal IOLs.

These represent a significant modernization of Ridley's first design, to modern "space age" creations. His lens had no fixation elements. Sixty years later, it has been transformed by simply adding a few features. The lenses here are made by three different companies and are now manufactured from materials that allow them to be folded so they can be put in the eye through very small incicisions (which makes for a safer operation).

The concentric rings that have been manufactured into the optics seen in all three of these lenses (although they are hard to visualize in the third image) have rendered multifocality to each of them so that the patient receives a benefit that almost appears to be a miracle, namely the ability to see well at both near and far with one lens.

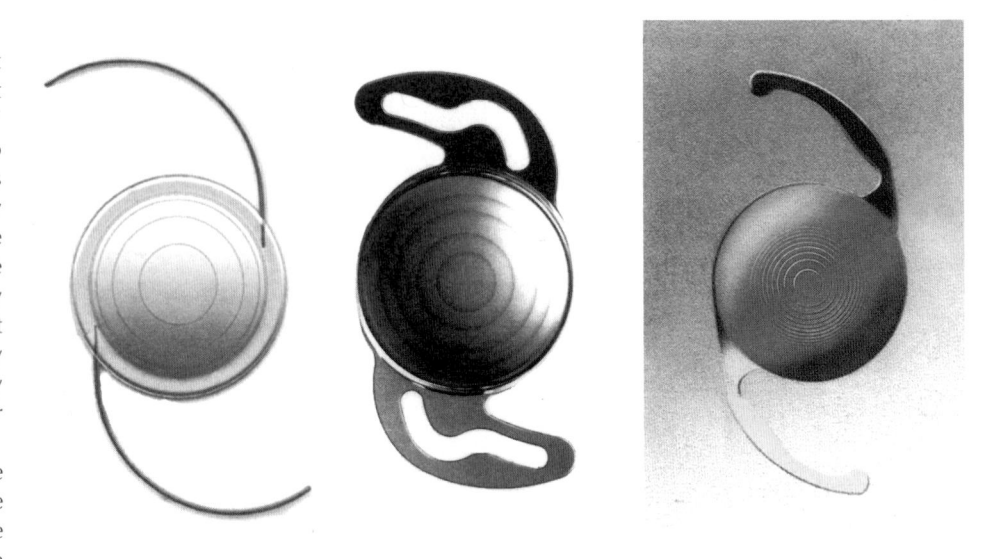

WHY DID IT TAKE SO LONG?

"I had twenty-five years in the wilderness and would have been spared much suffering if David Apple, the one who at last took the trouble to read and analyze all the early implant papers, had appeared in the 1950s, for a whole generation of cataract patients might then have enjoyed full visual rehabilitation instead of suffering the abnormalities of aphakia."

Harold Ridley, 1989

IOLs have come a long way and, in spite of many glitches during the evolutionary processes, we all agree that "alls well that ends well." However, something went wrong in the meantime. The IOL did not bring Harold an immediate and universal acclaim. On the contrary, many of his colleagues, especially in what we term "the academic establishment,"* strongly rejected him and his work. Many people looked for anything negative they could find. I have long been bothered by a comment Harold penned in 1951 when describing the reaction to his first presentation of his new invention at Oxford:

"Until the Oxford lecture of 1951, most surgeons were guided by a contented, self-important 'club' comprised mostly of unswerving department chairmen who were satisfied with the cataract operation of the early 1900s and still depended on unsatisfactory thick spectacles or contact lenses to serve as a replacement of the removed opaque lens.

"When the presentation of the paper and its film ended, there was surprisingly little comment, attributable no doubt to the impact of a new and revolutionary idea. At later meetings, some wounding comments were made.

---

* We will refer often to the "establishment," defined in the *Oxford English Dictionary* as follows: "a social group exercising power generally, or within a given field or institution, by virtue of its traditional superiority, and by the use esp. of tacit understandings and often a common mode of speech, and having as a general interest the maintenance of the status quo."

THE SECRET CODE: "THE EXTRA-CAPSULAR EXT."

"This delayed the cure of aphakia (aphakic = no lens) for 25 years, so that an entire generation of cataract patients needlessly suffered aphakia."

Were the remarks made by Harold in Oxford and elsewhere reflections of a bitter man or was there, in fact, a real delay in implementation that Harold laments in these comments?

To help address this question of why there was such a delay in implementing the mainstream use of IOLs, I asked a colleague from Alcon Laboratories, Fort Worth, Texas, Mr. Kevin Buehler, Vice President of Marketing, to prepare the graph illustrated below. It shows a tabulation of the number of IOLs implanted annually on a worldwide basis, beginning with Harold's first few patients in 1949/1950. The graph reveals what I now consider an amazing and disturbing finding. There was virtually no increase in the annual numbers of IOL implantations for over 25 years after "day one." Harold's words were not, therefore, those of a bitter man; he was correct!

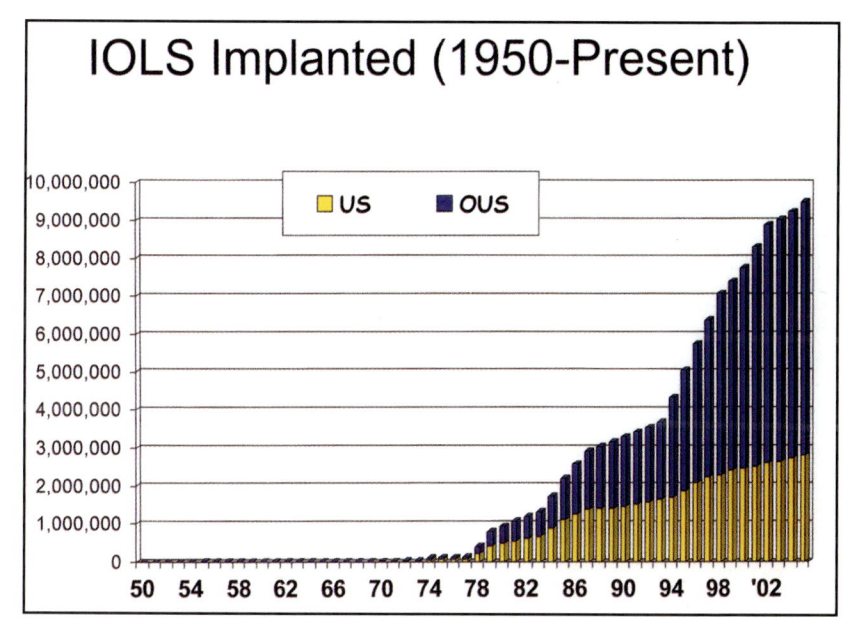

This graph shows the number of IOL implants done annually on a world-wide basis, beginning at the very start in 1949-50 when Harold did his first few cases. Although there were some problems with both the lens and the surgical technique of the time, my research and analysis of the literature shows that good results could indeed be obtained with this lens. However, note that virtually nothing happened between 1950 and until almost 1980. Thereafter, a gradual ascent in usage of IOLs occurred, in part assisted by innovative clinicians and also by research from our laboratory (see Chapter 4).

A key point here is that an entire generation of patients who had cataract surgery with no implant between approximately 1950 and 1980 were not given the opportunity to enjoy the advantages of this invention.
US = United States; OUS = outside the US.
(Graph prepared by Kevin Buehler, Alcon Laboratories.)

This graph answers the question that greatly concerned me for many years: why did IOL implant surgery stagnate during the long time period between 1948 and 1950 until almost 1980, precisely the time period when, as he lamented, an entire generation was deprived of a complete cure of cataracts—an operation that would have changed their lives.

Was this delay because the original and early IOLs were hopelessly bad? That answer is easy, at least in regard to Harold's original model. A firm "no"! Other researchers and I have shown that the quality and, hence, the basic safety of the very first IOL itself was good, if not perfect. Harold's first Ridley lens and all those thereafter more than met the stringent Food and Drug Administration (FDA) standards of today!

We have already seen that the original Ridley lens did not yet have the important supporting haptics that were added later by others. However, when patients underwent surgery by good surgeons such as Harold himself, good results were usually achieved. Even the decentrations that sometimes occurred with the Ridley lens were not severe enough to have caused the long delay of 25 years that occurred.

CHAPTER 1

Further evidence that the IOL quality was not a cause of the long delay was provided by Dr. Charles Letocha and colleagues of Pennsylvania who did a clinical research project on patients implanted with Ridley lenses during the very early years. Dr. Letocha acquired photographs showing several patients who had lived many years with Ridley lenses in their eyes. In some cases, the IOLs had been in place for over 50 years.

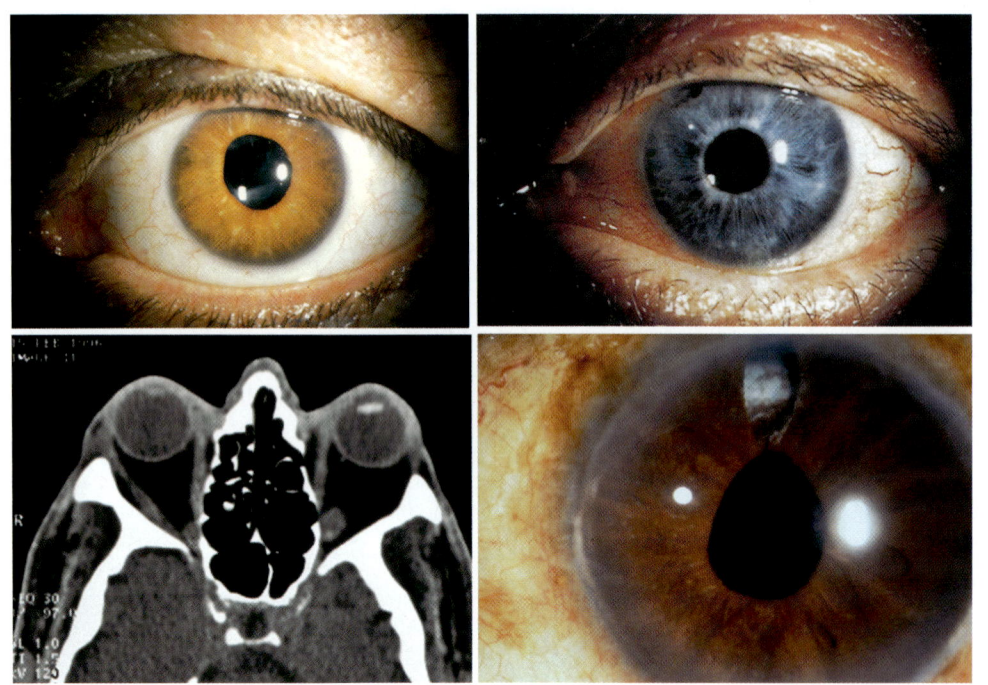

Three of the four patients noted in the photograph on this page are still alive after over 50 years with the implant in their eyes. The fourth patient had a Ridley lens in his eye 40 years until his death. The point is that these lenses were very compatible and generally well tolerated.

It is clear that the 25- to 30-year delay was in part caused by many *nonmedical* reasons (eg, interpersonal conflicts, ophthalmic politics, jealousy, fear of the unknown, and many other issues). One goal of this book is to show the struggle of an often-depressed Harold Ridley, working in the early years after 1950 with colleagues including Peter Choyce and Svyatoslav Fyodorov, and working later, after 1985, with many others including myself to assure the acceptance of his invention and to help him receive the recognition that he deserved. We will explore some of these reasons in order to set the record straight, to find out why this happened, and to provide information that might help prevent future innovations from suffering the same fate.

This montage set of photographs shows the eyes of four patients who had Ridley lenses in the early years (1950 to 1960). They are clustered here to exemplify that perfectly good results did occur with each lens and good longevity could be expected. Three of the four eyes seen in this montage are in patients who have had Ridley lenses in their eyes for over 50 years and remain fine today. The patient illustrated in the upper right photograph died after 30 successful years with the Ridley lens. (Courtesy of Dr. Charles Letocha.)

Harold, his coworkers, and the companies with whom he worked (most importantly Rayner & Keeler, Ltd) were not enriched by these original IOLs. He did not patent them. It was his goal to provide a gift to humanity, and he succeeded at great cost. In addition to dealing with the huge academic establishment of the time, he always had a fear of possible legal actions if there were problems or complications, in spite of the fact that malpractice litigations were rare in the 1950s.

Harold endured numerous attacks and rejections, often leading to periods of depression that required medication. Eventually, the ordeal came to an end; he was vindicated. I am grateful that I was able to join Harold during some of the lean years and to have been with him as he finally, albeit too briefly, could enjoy the fruits of his labors.

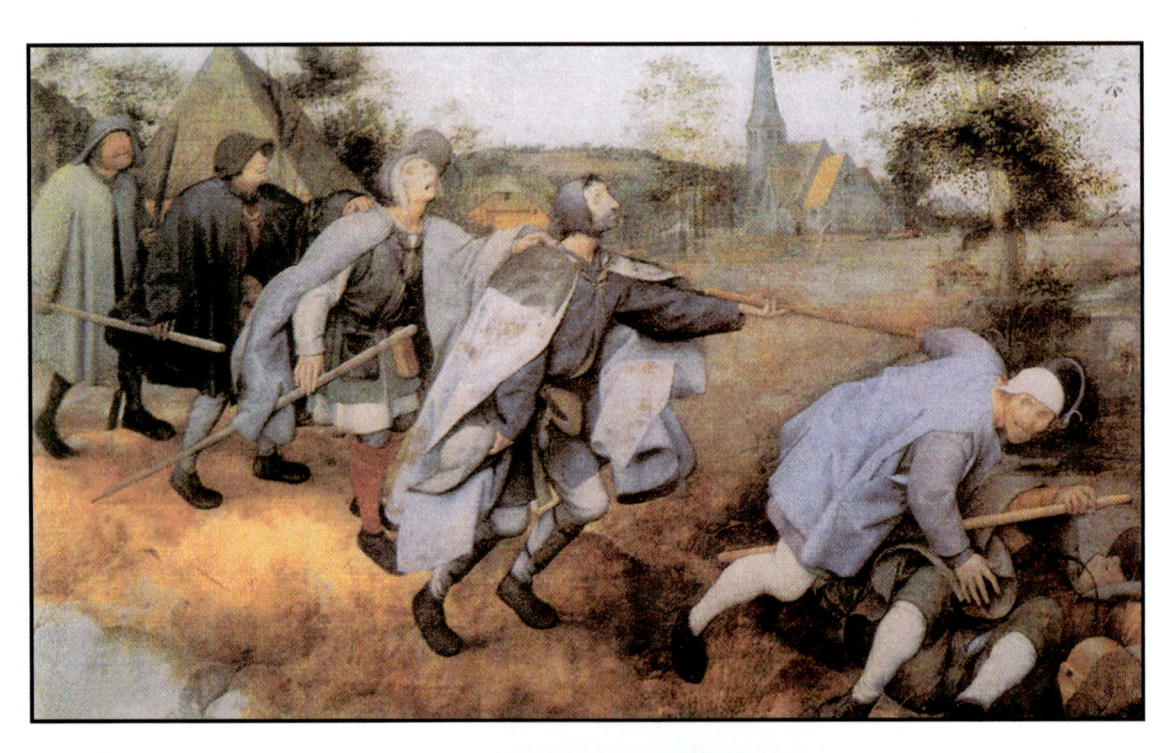

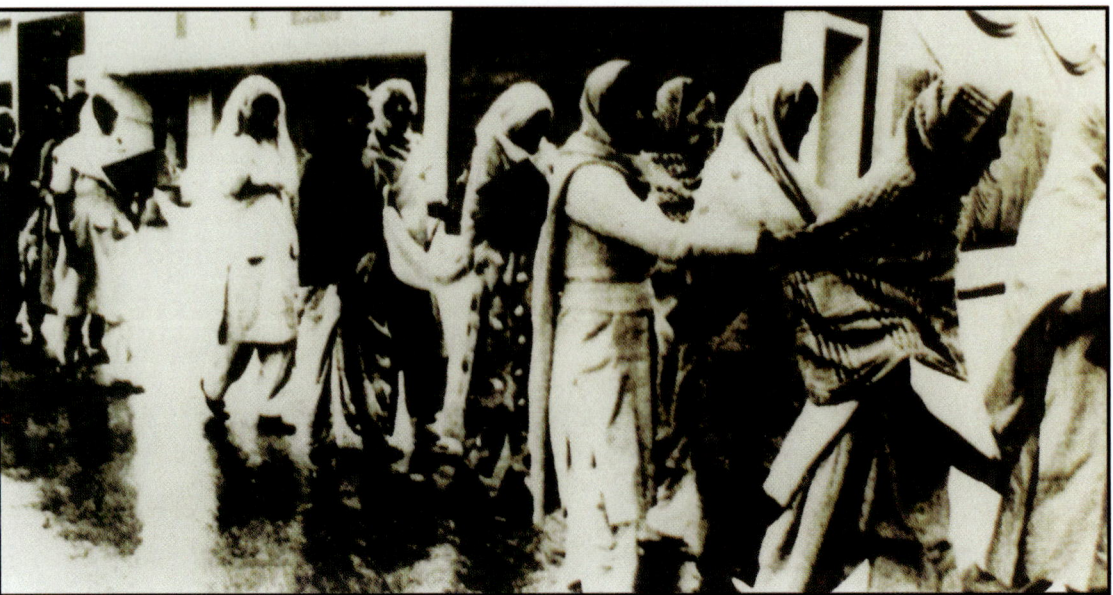

The scourge of blindness: the blind leading the blind.
TOP: A painting by Pieter Brueghel, the elder, 1568.
BOTTOM: Dismal weather makes things even worse for patients with visiual loss from cataracts. These patients must be led around by friends, relatives, and colleagues if they wish to survive, not unlike the situation seen in the top figure. This photograph was taken in the 1990s. A huge cataract backlog unfortunately still exists and is growing each day at an exponential pace.

2

From Darkness to Light

"I am entirely deprived of sight. I do not see anymore. I am plunged into the darkness of night."

Rosalba Carriera, artist, Venice ca. 1757

In Chapter 1 I introduced the concept of cataract-IOL surgery and showed images of some examples of intraocular lenses (IOLs), the artificial lenses designed by Harold Ridley to replace the discarded opaque lens that has to be surgically removed. We will now briefly look at the status of eye research and surgery in the past, the nature of the actual human lens (the crystalline lens), the process of cataract formation, and the various sequelae (after effects) of this disease.

For at least 6,000 years very little progress had been made in the theory or practice of eye surgery. The images on the previous page are two renditions of the concept of "the blind leading the blind" separated in time by 400 years. They are poignant reminders of the misery associated with blindness. Finally, by the 18th century, some new procedures were introduced, such as the ECCE operation introduced in France by Jacques Daviel. However, it was Harold's invention of the IOL that finally provided the first real opportunity for *complete* restoration of vision in operated patients.

This was and remains hugely important because of the magnitude of this condition. Over half of all world blindness (blindness is defined as vision worse than 20/2400 [3/60]) is from cataract—over 25 million individuals. Furthermore, 110 million individuals suffer from cataract-induced visual impairment worse than 20/2200 (6/60). In some regions of the world, the waiting list for cataract surgery continues to grow at a rate of 14,000 new cases a day, or 600 per hour. It has been impossible for surgeons to keep up with the backlog.

CHAPTER 2

Eye Surgery in the Dark Ages;
Perforation of the Eye With a Needle

Historically, cataracts were removed—if they were removed at all—by a very unsatisfactory procedure called "couching." It is believed that this operation was popularized by a man who was considered the father of Hindu surgery, the Indian physician Susruta. Couching was the only means of treating cataract blindness for many millennia and has been performed on millions if not billions of people. In this procedure, a practitioner takes aim with a needle and literally punctures the eye with it. He or she then attempts to push the cloudy lens out of its normal location with the tip of the needle. The ultimate goal is to dislodge the lens and move it away from the patient's visual axis or line of sight.

With lots of luck, a surgeon could remove the visual obstruction. However, by definition, this operation would leave the patient's eye without a *functioning* lens. The lens, of course, is what focuses light onto the retina at the back of the eye. The haziness and poor vision caused by the cloudy lens is, of course alleviated, but the ultimate vision was usually not really better because everything was out of focus and was often worse. By the 17th century, eyeglasses were devised to help the minority of patients who had successful cataract operations to focus the light coming into the eye

The technique of couching with a needle from Georg Bartisch, 16th century.
LEFT: Needles are pierced into the eye in the hope of pushing the cataractous, opaque lens out of the visual axis so that it falls to the bottom of the eye and sits harmlessly within the interior. This was a lofty goal but not often achieved. More common were the complications of hemorrhage and infection.
RIGHT: A series of ornamental couching needles designed for this operation.

The technique of couching with a needle.
LEFT: The surgery was gruesome. Patients often had to be literally tied down since the pain was usually uncontrollable (from Georg Bartisch, 16th century).
RIGHT: Even today, couching remains in vogue in some regions of the world.

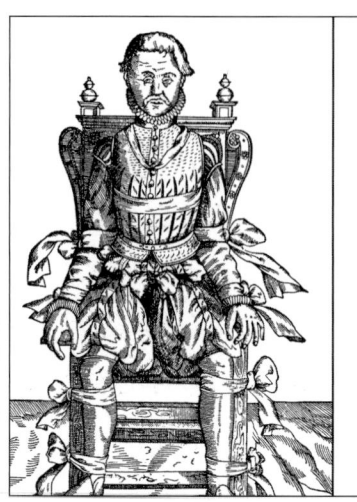

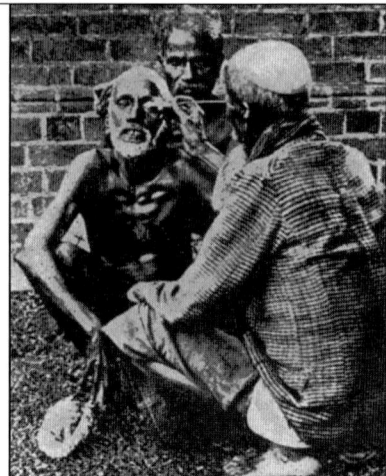

in lieu of his or her surgically displaced lens. These glasses, termed aphakic spectacles, had to be terribly heavy and thick, like the bottoms of glass pop bottles. They caused many types of distortions—like looking into a carnival "funny mirror"—producing imperfect vision at best.

Beyond the fact that a poke in the eye with a needle can be excruciatingly painful, couching was often a disaster because of two common complications. First, blood vessels in and around the eye were often punctured after the insertion of a needle, often causing uncontrollable bleeding. Second, infections were often caused by the insertion of a dirty, unsterile needle. I doubt very much that the surgeons themselves were confident in this procedure. A common practice was for the surgeon, who for many years typically traveled from city to city to locate patients (termed itinerate surgeons), was to do the operation, dress and patch the eye, and then leave town!

It should not be surprising that the cynical two-liner quoted below came into existence in the years when couching was the predominant surgical technique and, to make matters worse, during the years prior to Harold and his sight-restoring IOL:

"The most common cause of blindness in the world is untreated cataract. The second most common cause of blindness in the world is 'treated cataract.'"

Source Unknown

THE "BLACK HOLE"

Why did the field of eye care and surgery remain in the dark ages for so long? For centuries, scientific and clinical understanding of the interior of the eye was hindered. Without special instrumentation and special pharmacologic agents that could be administered in eye drops, physicians and research scientists could not see well if at all behind the plane of the pupil and iris. The inside, or back, of the eye behind the pupil nearly always appeared black when observed without special aids, just as it always does as we view people in our daily existence.

The region behind the pupil, which we now know contains important structures such as the retina, macula, optic nerve, blood vessels, and much more, was literally a

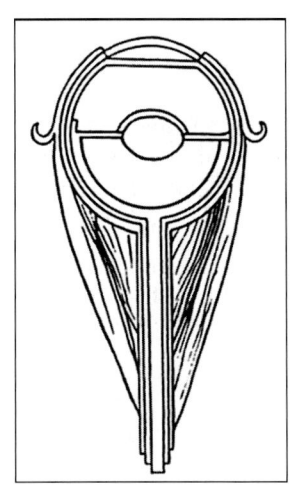

It is important for scientists to understand the anatomy (structure) of the eye in order to have any hope of treating any disease affecting it. Such understanding has been very slow to come. For example, many early researchers were not even sure where the lens was situated within the globe.

Note, for example, this ancient drawing in which the investigator mistakenly determined that the lens was in the middle of the eye (in the vitreous space) rather than toward the front. Mistakes like this were made because artifacticious dislocations of the lens commonly occurred in early times when modern tools of examination were not available.

CHAPTER 2

"black hole," a forbidden territory or "terra incognota." For centuries, many eye diseases were difficult to understand and diagnose and, therefore, considered incurable. Ophthalmologists could not expect to cure diseases of an organ they could not see or understand. For various reasons, including the fact that the eye is very small with a complex structure, it was difficult to study it in a coherent scientific fashion. Observers began to view it not as a functioning visual organ, but more as a mystical or religious symbol, as a supernatural entity, or as a beautiful object to be painted by artists.

Indeed, scientific investigations often gave way to preoccupations with mystical concepts. Deep symbolism was ascribed to the eye, depending on the religious interests, superstitions, and many other inclinations of the examiner. Sometimes, "studies" of the eye were used for evil purposes even as late as the 20th century.

Scientific study of the eye was sometimes replaced by artistic, religious, and mystical considerations of this "exotic organ."
LEFT: Eye of Hora (Egypt). Because much of the structure and function of the eye remained a mystery over centuries, the eye more often attracted the attention of artists and mystics rather than scientists.
RIGHT: A beautiful Renaissance engraving on a panel of a door in Florence, Italy.

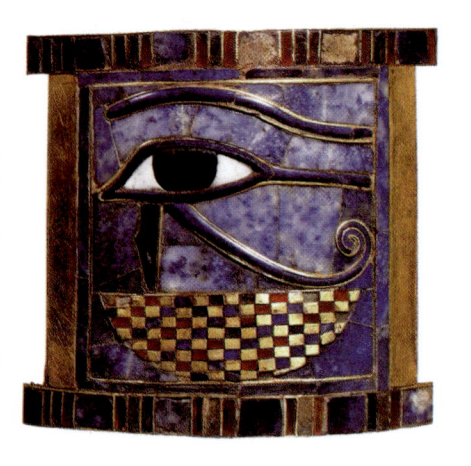

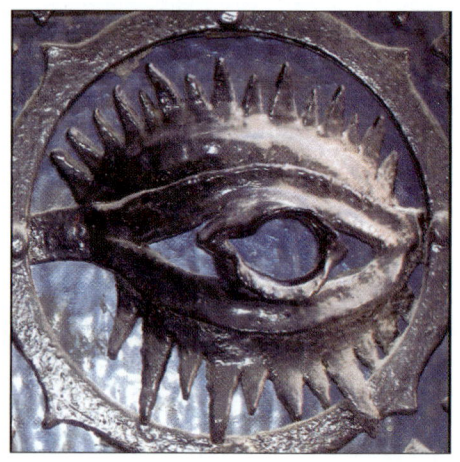

Most unfortunately a pernicious and non-sensical use of an eye's characteristics was devised in order to "classify individuals according to race."
LEFT: In the Nazi era the results of eye examinations were sometimes instrumental in deciding life or death. The shape and measurements or even the color of the iris were used to separate individuals, sometimes condemning them to death.
RIGHT: A chart was used by a German "ophthalmologist" to classify individuals utilizing various eye forms, shapes, and colors. This was used to separate "undesirables" from "Aryans."

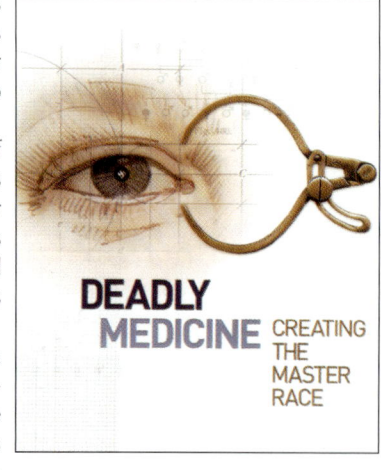

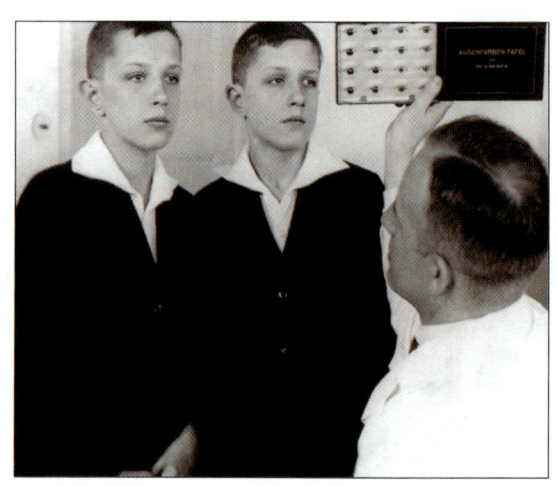

From Darkness to Light

Over time, the human will to uncover mysteries began to cut through the secrets of the eye, revealing its true nature, especially its structure and function. By the 17th century, from about the time of Sir Isaac Newton, scientists turned their attention back to scientific studies on the eye. Newton's work on optics, the study of how light moves and is focused, showed, among other things, the movements of light rays in and out of the eye. His contributions are still used in hospitals and offices on a daily basis by eye specialists working with optical aids such as spectacles, contact lenses, IOLs, and even lasers.

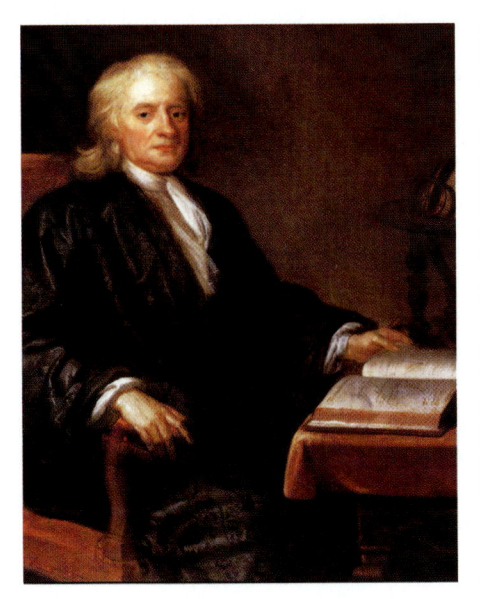

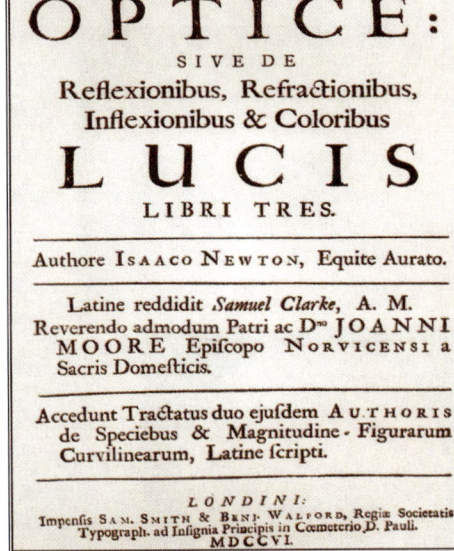

By the 17th Century, scientists were beginning to make progress in scientific evaluations of the eye.
LEFT: Sir Isaac Newton did much to enhance our understanding of how the eye functions and how rays of light are transformed into vision, the first step in the march toward attacking and curing various disease processes.
RIGHT: This is Newton's classic treatise on *Optics*, Latin ed. This work was translated into multiple languages.

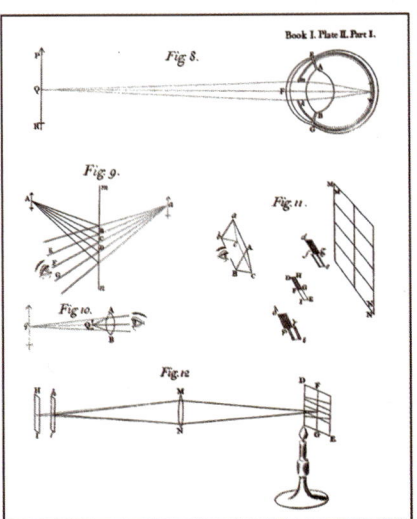

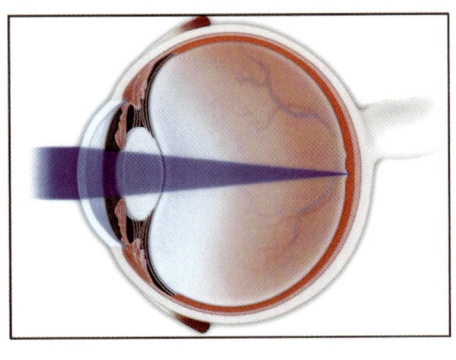

Simple diagram showing the fruits of the work of Newton and many of his colleagues, including René Decartes, the great geometrist.
LEFT: In his work, *Optics*, Newton provided diagrams showing how the rays of light traversed in and out of the eye.
RIGHT: All of us who work in the field of ophthalmology and vision care apply the work of Newton daily on the job. This drawing shows how a light ray from the outside (left) passes through the various components of the eye and focuses to a point on the retina (right). Compare the configuration of this drawing of the rays (in blue) with Newton's original drawings that he termed figure 8 at the top of the illustration on the left.

An invention in 1851 by the German physicist Hermann von Helmholtz constituted a huge breakthrough in clinical diagnosis of eye diseases. Actually, he and a not-so-well-known Charles Babbage of England independently invented the ophthalmoscope. For the first time it visually exposed to the examiner the once-hidden territory behind the living pupil. This invention made it possible for researchers to understand the physical eye and

CHAPTER 2

Finally, a view into the interior of the eye.
LEFT: The interior of this eye remains "hidden" behind the dark pupil.
RIGHT: However, by the 19th century, scientists were making progress at gaining views into the eye. In this eye the pupil is widely dilated by using pharmacologic agents termed mydriasis. This eye has an advanced cataract. A clear view behind the iris was made possible by a new invention, the ophthalmoscope, which became available in the 1850s.

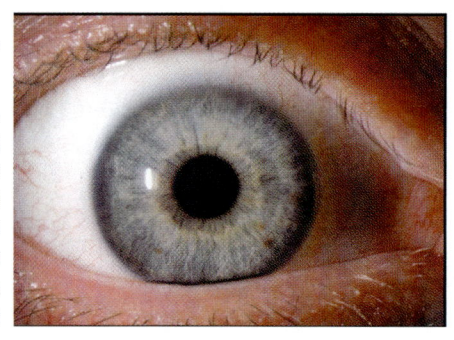

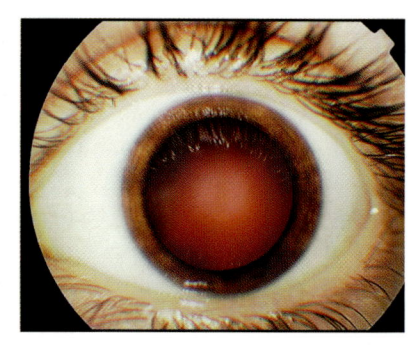

Photographs of the human retina through the magic of the ophthalmoscope. For the first time examiners were able to examine such tissues as the optic nerve and the retinal vessels.
TOP: A clinical photograph of the back of the eye using a "fundus" camera, as the specialized cameras are termed.
BOTTOM: In the 19th century, prior to the invention of the fundus camera, drawings done by very skilled artists were the only means of preserving a given fundus image. Note the optic nerve and the vessels that emanate from it.

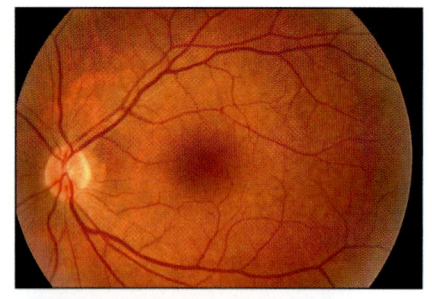

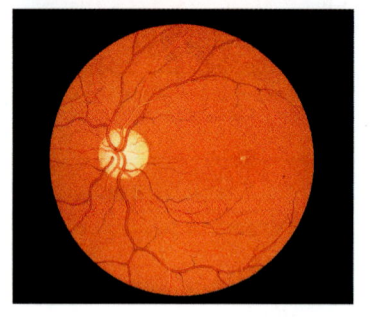

the problems that affected it, greatly enhancing ophthalmologists' ability to accurately diagnose and, therefore, cure a wide variety of diseases, ultimately including cataract.

Even as efforts to improve surgical operations were being made by the 18th and 19th centuries, cataract surgery in the hands of surgeons worldwide remained sometimes dangerous and continued to be an incomplete operation. Even if the diseased lens could be safely extracted from the eye utilizing new technology, the patient's resulting vision was usually very poor. Just as we noted with couching, the problem was as follows: after the cloudy lens was removed, nothing was yet known to be available to adequately replace it. To be sure, even with the imperfect help of thick aphakic glasses, the patient would always suffer from aphakia (having no lens).

As ophthalmology emerged out of its Dark Ages, the stage was set for the final cure to the age-old, very common problem of cataracts, the replacement of the lens—a cure that would become a reality with Harold's operation of November 29, 1949.

At this point in the book we have introduced enough information and terminology, especially in conjunction with the glossary, to include a simple diagram of the basic substructure of the eye. The discoveries by such authorities as Newton, Helmholtz, and many other scientists have made possible the accurate designations of structures, from the very front of the eye, the cornea (left) to the rear passing toward the retina and the optic nerve (right).

The essential chore of an ophthalmologist is to keep the media of his or her patient's eye clear of any obstruction or opacification. The most common sites of blockage are by far, the lens (cataract), and to a lesser extent, the cornea (corneal opacity or keratopathy). Both of these conditions are generally treatable by surgical procedures.

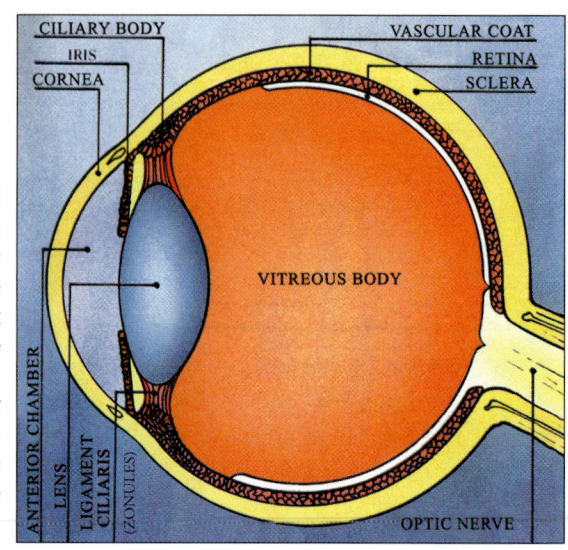

20

FROM DARKNESS TO LIGHT

Cataract—The Most Common Cause of Visual Loss

As we first noted when referring to Monet's eye troubles (see Chapter 1), a cataract is a clouding or opacity of the natural transparent lens of the eye. Normally, the eye's lens is crystal clear; hence, it is termed the "crystalline" lens. The eye's lens functions much as does the lens in a camera, transmitting and focusing light from the outer environment into the receptive part of the eye, the retina, with its photo/light receptors, the rods and cones. An important component of the retina is termed the macula, the site where many light rays converge to allow for central 20/20 (6/6) vision. As a cataract forms—as the lens in the eye turns opaque—it becomes white or otherwise discolored. The most common cause of cataract is long-term exposure to the rays of the sun. Not surprisingly, cataracts are common in sunny, tropical countries and are more common as people age. There are many types or manifestations of this disease. One common symptom relates to night vision. People with cataracts sometimes notice that lights, especially at night, are blurred and appear to have halos around them.

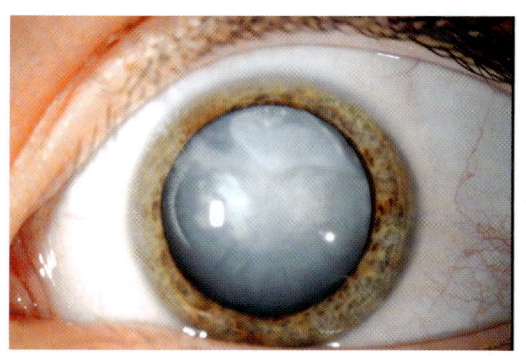

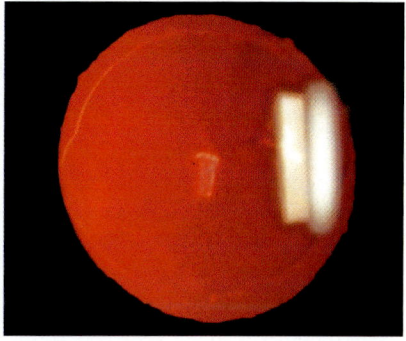

The ability to dilate the pupil with drugs and the special instrumentation now available allows diagnosis at virtually all levels within the eye. LEFT: The camera focus is near the front of the eye, just behind the cornea. There is a dense white opacity of the lens—a cataract. It fills the pupil and is surrounded by the brown iris. Such an opacity totally blocks any view behind it. The typically red fundus color (see figure on the right) that normally emanates from the back of the eye (retina, fundus), is obscured. RIGHT: This is a photograph of an eye into which an IOL had been implanted. The result was excellent and the appearance is such that the surgeon appears to see only a normal fundus or background of the eye. The IOL optic itself is virtually invisible, proving that the IOL is clear and this allows light to finally pass in and out of the eye.

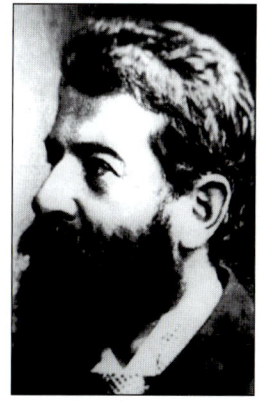

Commensurate with our focus on history in this text, it is of interest to document the individual who is credited with performing the first cornea transplantation. The first penetrating keratoplasty was performed by Dr. Carl Edward Zirm (1863 to 1944) of Innsbruck, Austria.

As we begin a description of cataracts, it is well to remember that corneal opacities are often confused with lens opacities even by some physicians who are not trained in the field of eye diseases. The eye below clarifies the difference between the two.

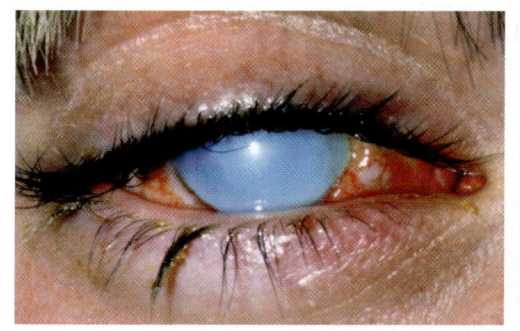

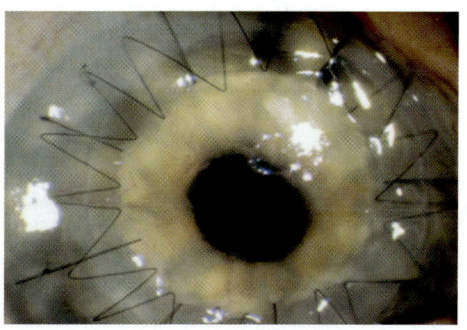

LEFT: This is an opacification of the cornea, the watch glass-like cover over the front of the eye (note diagram on previous page). The cornea has assumed a bluish opacification due to a disease, which could be one of many things ranging from a degeneration, to an infection, to an inflammation, to trauma. RIGHT: The main treatment available now and indeed a successful one with modern techniques is a corneal transplant, officially called a penetrating keratoplasty (kerato = cornea; plasty = greek, plastia, molding, surgical repair [PKP]). A donor cornea from an eye bank is sutured in the place of the removed damaged cornea.

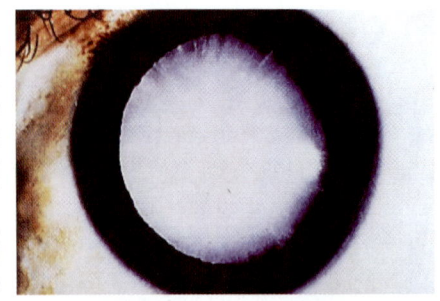

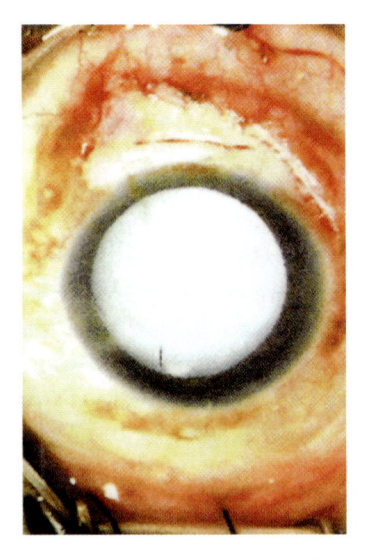

CHAPTER 2

Three examples of human cataracts.

TOP LEFT: This cataract shows areas near the periphery where the opacity is not so dense, a sort of "foamy" appearance—especially at the top of this photograph. The early anatomists thought this had some resemblance to the foam created at the base of a waterfall. Hence the term "cataract" was derived, from the Greek word for waterfall. This is a good example of a clinical name derived from nature, as is not at all unusual (see also the sunflower cataract illustrated later in this chapter).

RIGHT: On the right is another example of an absolutely dense cataract. Sometimes these eyes would appear clinically gray to the observer and the Germans gave these the name "Grauer Star" (gray stare), to signify the appearance of the patient peering through this gray opacification.

LOWER LEFT: This photograph shows an example of the Miyake-Apple posterior photographic/video technique that my colleague, Dr. Miyake in Nagoya, Japan first developed and my team (the Apple Korps), modified and expanded (see Chapter 4). This is an excellent way to provide a view of the interior of the eye in cadaver specimens. (It can even be used clinically in living patients with small fiberoptic cables if indicated.) In this figure we see an intact lens in place viewed from behind. It reveals a gray-yellow discoloration with a focus of white degeneration centrally. In this view one is essentially viewing the anterior (front) segment of the eye, especially the back aspect of the lens. One can imagine that the photographer with his camera is standing on the optic nerve and viewing forward in a direction from the brain. This has been a superb teaching and research tool for almost 25 years, just about the duration of my intraocular lens and biodevice research laboratory.

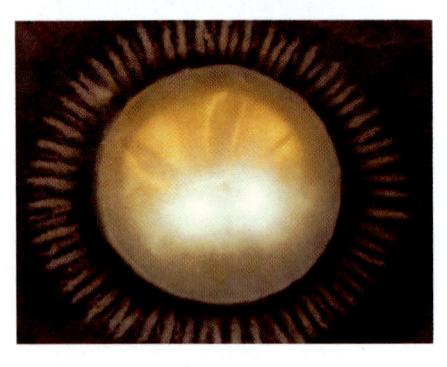

Cataract formation is analogous to the frying of the white of an egg. Initially, a normal lens is clear like the uncooked white part of the egg—the albumin, or protein. Once the egg is placed in a heated skillet, the albumin begins to transform from a clear substance to one that is dense, opaque, and white. This is what happens to the eye's lens after long exposure to the sun's ultraviolet light: it is slowly "fried" as decades pass, and it eventually begins to turn white and opaque. Most of us cannot totally avoid the sun for a lifetime. This helps explain why almost all individuals will develop a clinically significant cataract if they live long enough, particularly those living in climates where the amount of sunshine is great.

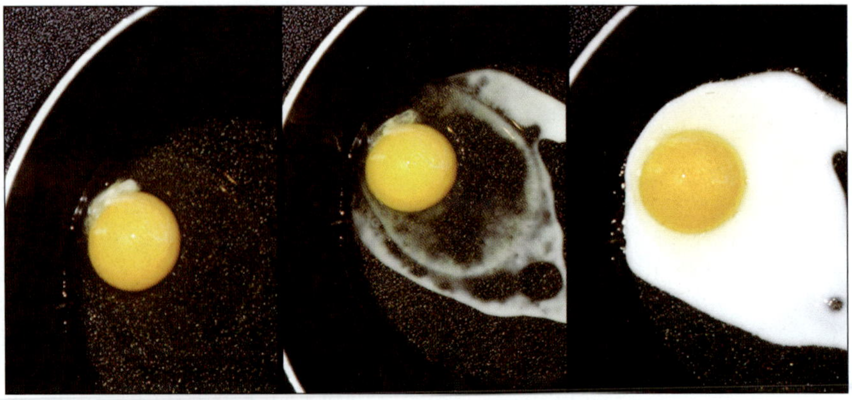

Cataract formation can be likened to slowly "frying" a person's lens for many years, precisely as one would fry an egg. Both the lens and the white (albumin) of an egg are made from protein material.

LEFT: On the left, the egg has just been placed in the skillet and the egg white remains clear.
CENTER: The early mid-stage of whitening is occurring, analogous to formation of early moderate cataract.
RIGHT: The late stage where the entire egg white has been cooked, analogous to advanced cataract formation as we saw in the illustrations at the top of this page.

FROM DARKNESS TO LIGHT

The inevitable result of an untreated cataract is severe visual loss or legal blindness. A common but highly underestimated result of cataracts is a decreased ability to work or even loss of the affected individuals' jobs. This disease, therefore, has very important financial implications for the patient and for the economy. A relatively unusual but very understandable example of this concept relates to an airplane pilot's ability to fly. Prior to Harold's IOL, a pilot was finished as soon as his/her cataract began to form. As will be noted in Chapter 12 by Captain Steven Schallhorn, United States Navy, there are many still-productive pilots and other personnel who owe the continuation of their vocation to Harold's IOL and the operation that many consider a cousin to it—refractive surgery.

Even today, with all of our modern gadgetry and drugs, there are no known alternative treatments for cataract—no medical, pharmacological, herbal, or other nonsurgical treatments. The opaque lens must be removed by the surgeon and its optical (focusing) power must be replaced by some form of appliance. Prior to Harold, the only alternatives were spectacles or contact lenses. By carrying through with his first operation on November 29, 1949, Harold dared to do something virtually unheard of before, namely to insert a foreign plastic device into the eye, which he (correctly) believed would provide a third and far superior alternative for visual rehabilitation—the IOL.

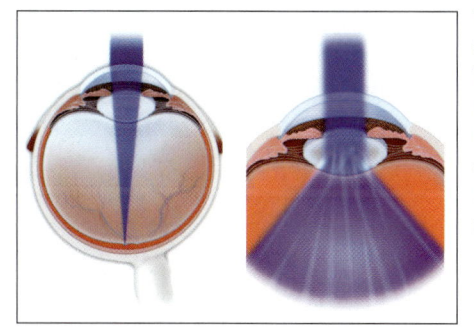

The loss of visual acuity caused by a cataract occurs because light cannot pass through the opacified lens without being dispersed and thrown into disarray with loss of focus. This is illustrated schematically in these two images.
LEFT: Normal entrance of light into an eye with a healthy lens and no cataract. The light rays (blue cone) comes to a focus on the retina (the photoreceptors or rods and cones) (below).
RIGHT: The dense cataract causes a marked dispersion of the rays in a haphazard fashion. Proper focusing is rendered impossible.

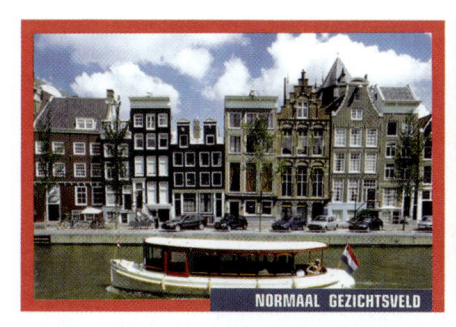

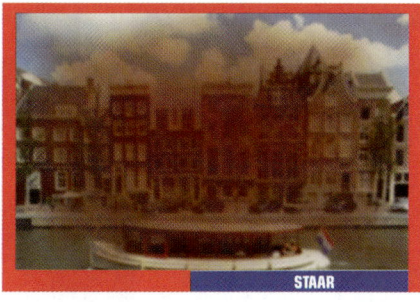

Three pictures of the beautiful canals of Amsterdam illustrate the pattern of visual loss with cataract. In this particular case, the cataract is characterized not only by a simple opacification but to some degree a brownish discoloration, which is not an infrequent occurrence. LEFT: Normal vision with 20/20 visual acuity, no evidence of cataract. CENTER: Beginning haze and brownish discoloration signifying an early to moderate cataract. RIGHT: Advanced cataract approaching blindness.
In the early days of cataract surgery when the operation was often quite dangerous, the surgeon had to wait until the cataract reached this advanced ("ripe") stage in order do an operation. This was based on the theory that one could not make an already blind person any worse if operative failure occurred. This is a concept that has long been discarded by most surgeons because today's operations are much improved.

CHAPTER 2

Cataracts May Cause Morbidity in Addition to Simple Vision Loss

Cataracts are a not only a vision-threatening condition; they may be indirectly contributory or responsible for injuries or even death.

Consider the following: People with cataracts are often elderly. Falling is one of the most common causes of injury and traumatic death in older people, especially those with impaired vision. The loss of vision caused by cataracts has historically been a significant reason why the elderly fall. Death does not always result when one falls, of course, but injuries that result from falls—particularly the all-too-common injuries to the hip, sometimes forcing the patient to a bed-ridden status—are often devastating to people in their later years.

Stairs are a particular danger to people with cataracts. Stairs that are wet and slippery, beautiful spiral staircases where the treads fan out on an angle, and wide staircases where railings may not be at hand pose particular problems.

Thus, cataracts may be, in fact, life threatening and have certainly been a cause of death and suffering through the ages. Not only can cataracts cause injuries and premature death, they can also precipitate severe psychological problems that, in some cases, may lead individuals to the depths of depression or even to early graves. This was particularly common in the distant past when treatment was primitive and often failed, leaving patients with absolutely no hope.

The rich and famous are, of course, not immune to the problems of cataract. Nor are the artists of the world. Both visual and musical artists are, of course, susceptible. Rosalba Carriera (1675-1757) was a Venetian artist who created many wonderful paintings. She was stricken with cataracts in her early sixties. She had couching operations in both eyes. Both were abject failures, and she was permanently blinded. This led to the loss of her livelihood and decreased her will to live. She wrote of her despair not long before she died:

"I am entirely deprived of sight. I do not see any more. I am plunged into the darkness of night."

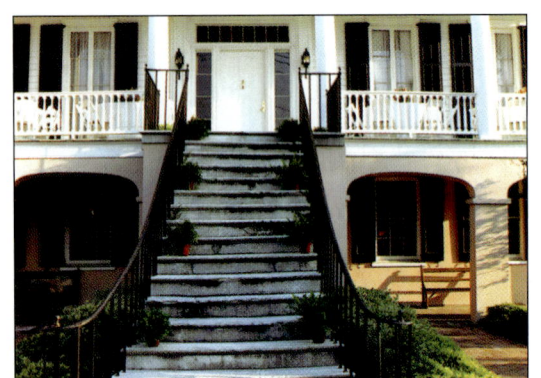

Falling from stairs is an all to frequent occurrence in patients with visual disabilities, especially the elderly. This stair is especially dangerous because it is wide with limited access to the railings if the person has to walk in the center. This home is located in a very humid, rainy area where the steps are often very slippery.

The morbidity of cataracts includes not only visual loss, possible indirect trauma, but also includes the onset or exacerbation of biologic or psychiatric symptoms from the disorders created by dealing with the stress of condemnation to blindness. This often occurred in those early days of bad, failed surgery, often perpetrated by charlatans and quacks. This was often devastating. I believe this is what happened to the great Venetian artist, Rosalba Carriera. She painted beautiful works and was highly respected in her city. By age 65, she developed bilateral cataracts, which impeded her work and required "surgery." The surgery—couching in both eyes—failed. A second operation was required in each eye, also unmitigated failures that forced her to cut back on her beloved work. She died a distressing death "plunged into the darkness of night."
Any chance to enjoy life had been lost. Such a fate should never occur today. Her fate should always remind us to give pause and retain a keen appreciation of the gift of sight.

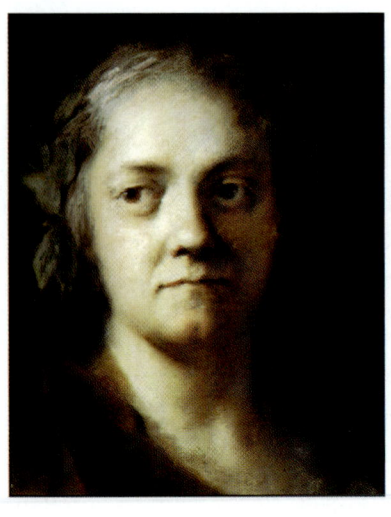

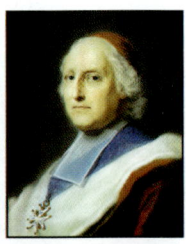

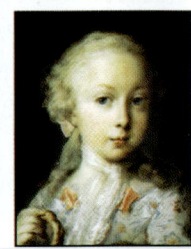

FROM DARKNESS TO LIGHT

The composers Johann Sebastian Bach (1685 to 1751) and George Frederic Handel (1685-1759) were born in the same year—Handel in Halle in Saxony, today's Sachsen-Anhalt, and Bach not far away in Thuringen, another small state in the central eastern part of Germany. Handel resided in England most of his adult life, while Bach remained in Germany with a post at a church with a great musical tradition—the St. Thomas Church in Leipzig. Both composers developed cataracts at approximately the same time: about 1750. Their clinical histories have been researched and reported extensively in numerous works.

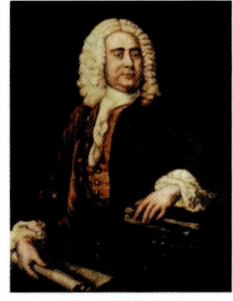

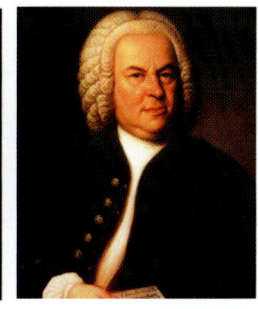

Unfortunately, both were referred to what we would today call a quack or charlatan—a man named John Taylor and nicknamed "Chevalier." To make a long story short, Taylor operated on both within a span of a few years around 1750. Both operations were utter failures. Bach, no doubt suffering serious depression from the condemnation to permanent blindness, died shortly thereafter in 1751. Handel managed to hang on until 1759, although of course not under the best of conditions.

John Taylor was an excellent example of an "operator" in a negative sense of the term—an unscrupulous self-promoter. He had been oculist to George II of England and allegedly to every head of state in Europe. He was famous for his womanizing and for his habit of prefacing all of his operations with a long-winded speech in praise of his own skills. Some of the techniques he used would seem appalling today. For example, his basic operation was the couching technique. It is historically certain that he used this technique on Bach and very likely on Handel as well. He often applied outrageous pretreatments and treatments, such as bloodletting, laxatives, and eye drops made of blood from slaughtered pigeons, pulverized sugar, or baked salt. For all of this, he charged exorbitant fees, and for a time, he prospered. Things must have caught up with him, however, because he died in poverty in 1772. As fate would have it, he also died blind.

The great baroque composers, Johann Sebastian Bach and George Frederick Handel were born in the same year (1685) in adjacent provinces in Germany. After illustrious careers, both developed cataracts late in life. They both were operated upon by the same surgeon, a Mr. John Taylor who apparently turned out to be less than ethical, namely a quack. Both operations were abject failures. They were thus condemned to difficulty in working, while also severely depressed because of the visual problem. Bach died not very long after his surgery, no doubt related to his depression.
LEFT: Johann Sebastian Bach (1685-1751).
RIGHT: Frederick Handel (1685-1759).

COLORS AND THE CATARACTS OF CLAUDE MONET

As first noted in Chapter 1, Claude Monet had lived in London in St. Thomas' Hospital for portions of three years at the beginning of the 20th century. He completed many paintings of the Houses of Parliament and other nearby structures. He of course did not know that this was the hospital in which Harold many years later would perform an operation that would have been a great benefit to him as an artist, especially because of his need for good visual acuity and color perception.

Early 20th century photograph of St. Thomas' Hospital at the approximate time period when Monet would have worked there.

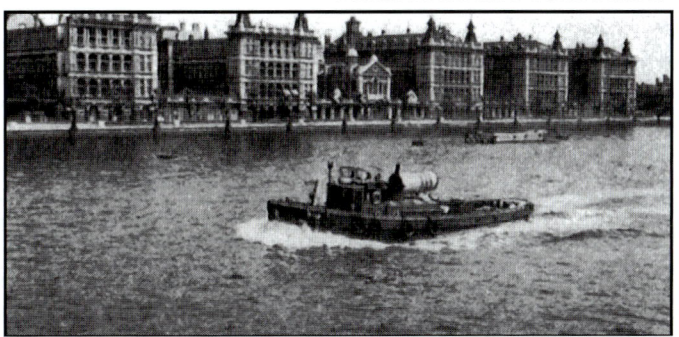

CHAPTER 2

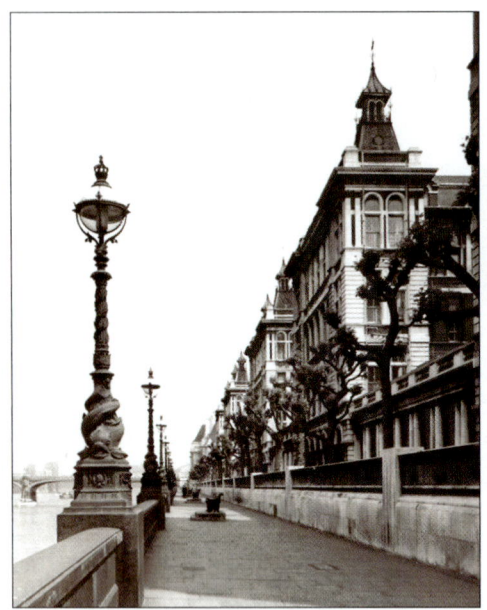

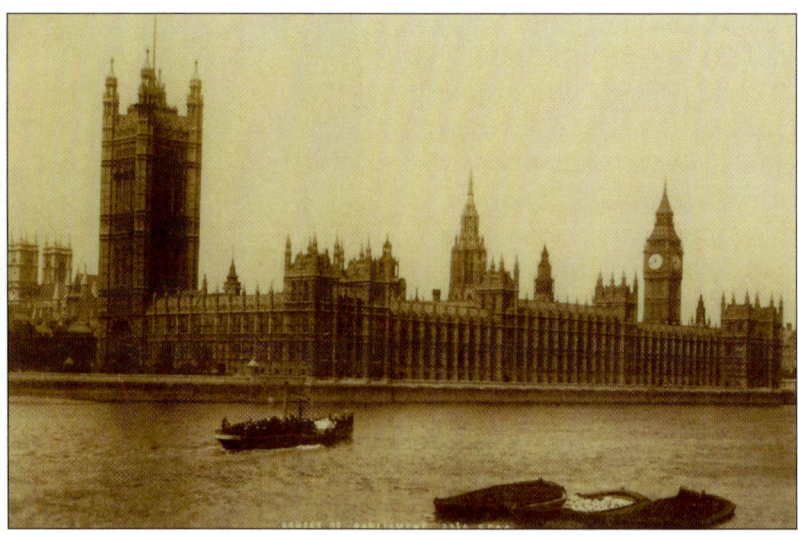

St. Thomas' Hospital.
LEFT: Monet's room was on the third floor of the hospital. The long street below his windows is the Albert Embankment.
RIGHT: Parliament. Almost the precise view that Monet would have had from his studio across the river, ca. 1900.

These are several paintings of Parliament and the nearby structures he completed from his room. He had exquisite views of the towers of the houses of Parliament. The differences in color in these views are not related to his cataracts, since they only became symptomatic about 20 years later. The color differences represent views at different times of day and/or season.
LEFT: Parliament buildings at sunset.
RIGHT: Parliament buildings basking in brilliant yellow light.

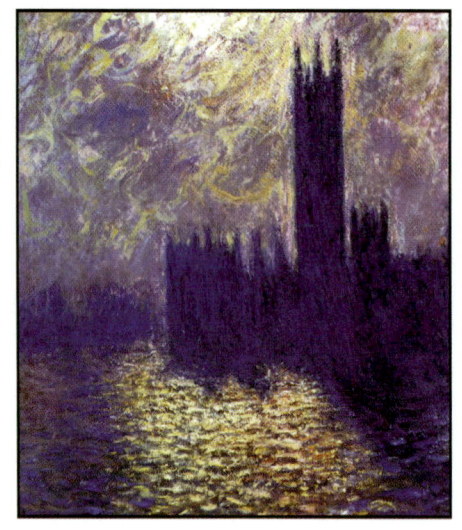

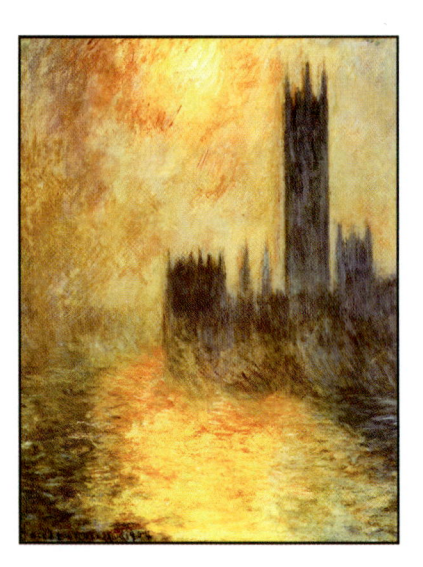

When clear lenses age and become cataractous, they often turn white. However, they frequently undergo a discoloration ranging from gray to brown with many variations in between. This can cause changes in the patient's color perception.

Monet developed his cataracts in the early 1920s. The visual problems that come with these were extremely problematic to him because he depended on good vision and color perception. After he had undergone cataract surgery, he was given the thick aphakic spectacles that were the only alternative during his time. Because of his cataracts, he had become used to seeing colors a certain way. His lens, in effect, had become a light filter, and images appeared more yellow-brown than usual, as incoming light

FROM DARKNESS TO LIGHT

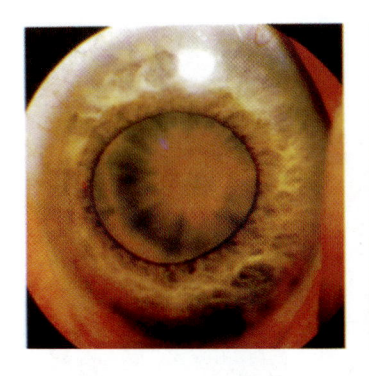

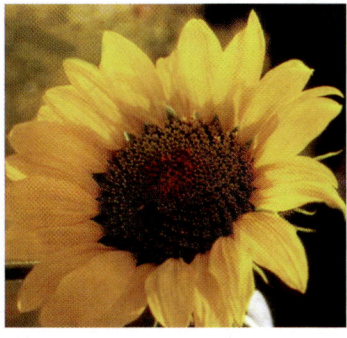

Sunflower cataract.
LEFT: An example of brown (brunescent) lens that derives its name from a product of nature. It is caused by the discoloration that can occur during a cataract's maturation. It is so named because the lens's yellow discoloration associated with the brown streaks within the lens substance that has a resemblance to the flower.
RIGHT: Normal sunflower showing its beautiful flowers.

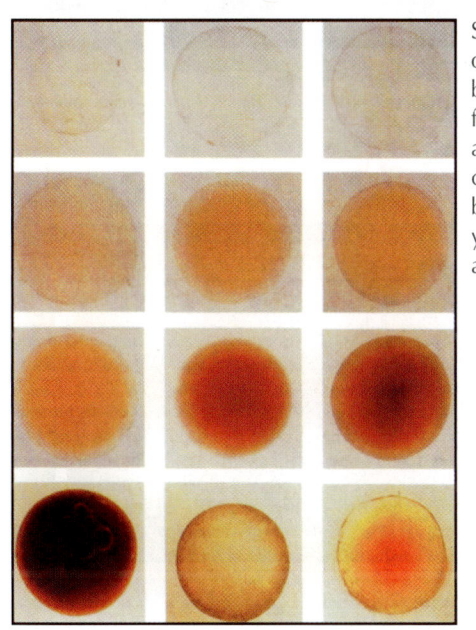

Special research studies have shown that as the human lens ages, varying amounts of pigment infiltrate into the lens substance and cause a discoloration, as well as the basic opacity that of course is the cataract. The study results demonstrated here show, for example, an increased amount of yellow to brown discoloration during the lens's aging process. This is the reason that many cataracts (as they are viewed clinically) can show different colors ranging from white to brown to yellow, to many colors in between. This also causes the patient to see the world differently. The more brown or yellow intensity of the pigment within the lens, the more the patient's environment appears to be that color.

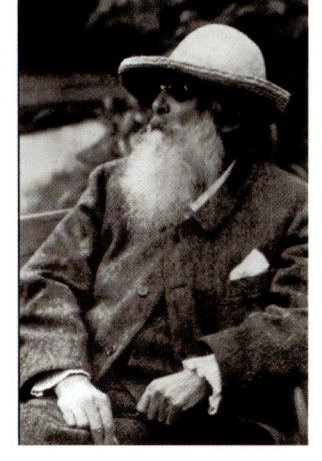

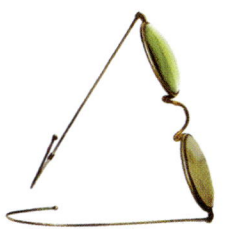

passed through his cataractous lenses that had become slightly yellow-brown. Various "pigments of aging" had penetrated into the substance of his lens; the "filter" thus created a penetration of only selected colors of light. After the surgery, in order to obtain the "normal" color perception that he had become accustomed to prior to the surgery, he tried several glasses that were tinted different colors. He chose spectacles that had a yellow tint; he had apparently gotten used to the image seen through his own discolored lens.

The paintings that he made of the Japanese Bridge at his garden in Giverny provide some of the best examples of how his cataract operations affected his color perception.

LEFT: By the 1920s, Monet had developed cataracts and required surgery. One eye did reasonably well and the other did not. He wore aphakic glasses with thick lenses. In his era these were required to compensate for the surgical removal of his own lens.
ABOVE: He was actually given a choice of colors for his replacement spectacles. He chose yellow lenses. These seemed to be more comfortable and brought back some of the "yellow" that he had lost as his own cataractous and discolored lens was removed.

CHAPTER 2

As most art lovers know, Claude Monet settled in his country residence at Giverny, not far from Paris. The Japanese Bridge still stands above a small stream.
LEFT: A photograph of Monet himself at the bridge, ca. 1920.
RIGHT: The Japanese Bridge today. It retains it basic blue color and is beautifully enclosed by greenery.

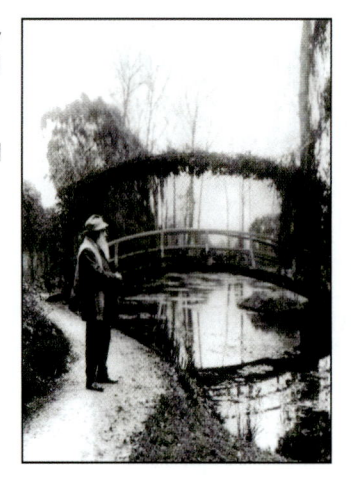

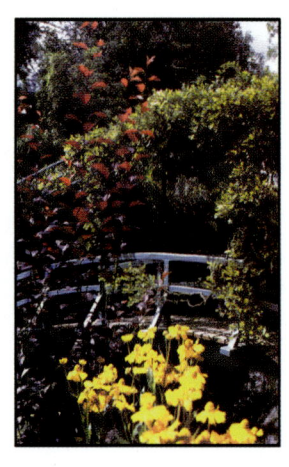

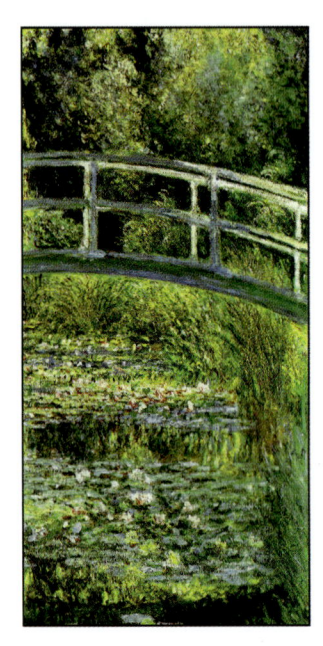

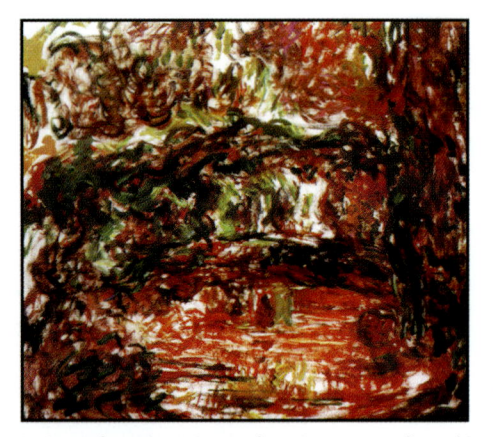

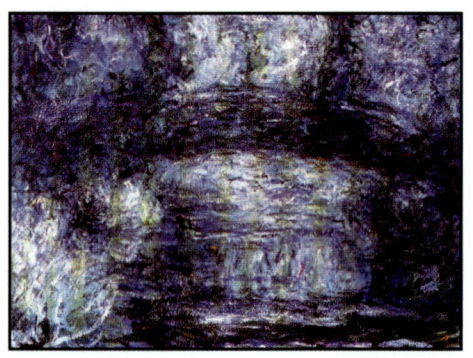

Paintings done by Monet showing examples of how he must have viewed the world, specifically 1) the Japanese Bridge before he had cataracts, 2) then with advanced cataracts in his eyes, and 3) after cataract extraction with removal of the cataractous lens and its yellow-brown pigments.
LEFT: A painting of the bridge by Monet at a time long before his cataract. It appears blue/green, possibly more or less true colors (or as close as one comes to as an impressionist painter). There is no hint of the strong yellow-brown tinting that would indicate the formation and infiltration of aging pigments that accompanied his cataract.
CENTER: The Japanese Bridge, pre-cataract surgery. His cataractous lens must have contained large quantities of yellow-orange-brown aging pigment within the substance of the cataract. the lens therefore imparted those colors to what he visualized. One can still barely see the outlines of the Japanese bridge coursing horizontally.
RIGHT: Same view, painted after removal of the cataract. The entire field now has a blue hue. This is because the yellow-red-brown color imparted by the lens is no longer in existence.

After his cataract operation in 1923/1924 and before he received his yellow spectacles, he told his surgeon, "I only see blue. I not longer see red, yellow, a special green, a certain violet. I no longer see as I once did, and yet I remember well the colors which they gave me."

The Ridley family.
LEFT: Family coat of arms.
RIGHT: Bishop Nicholas Ridley. Born at the beginning of the 16th century, entered Pembroke college in Cambridge in 1518, Fellow 1524. Chaplain to Archbishop Cranmer in 1537, chaplain to King Henry VIII in 1540, Bishop of London in 1550. Excepted from the amnesty by Queen Mary in 1553. Martyred at Oxford on October 16, 1555. He was a collateral relative of the surgeon and main subject of this text, Sir Harold Ridley (1906-2001). (Please refer to the picture of the Ridley Walk later in this chapter.)

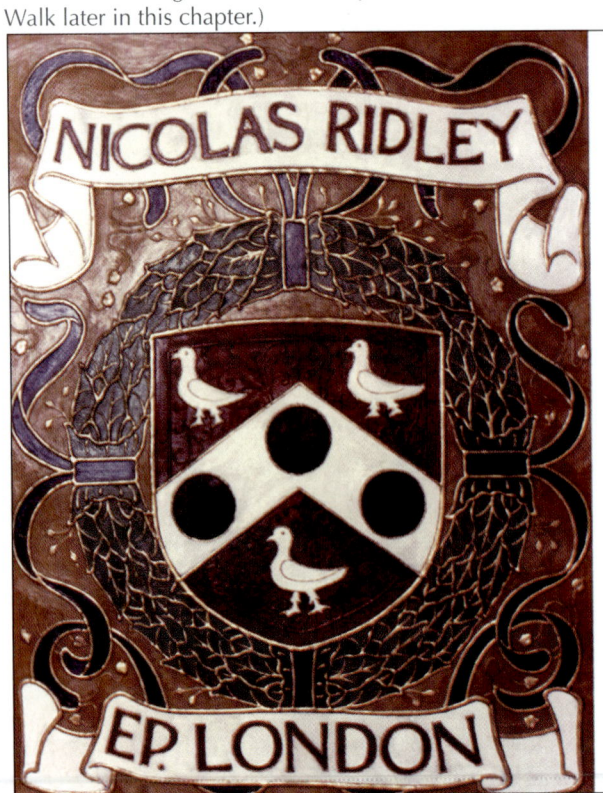

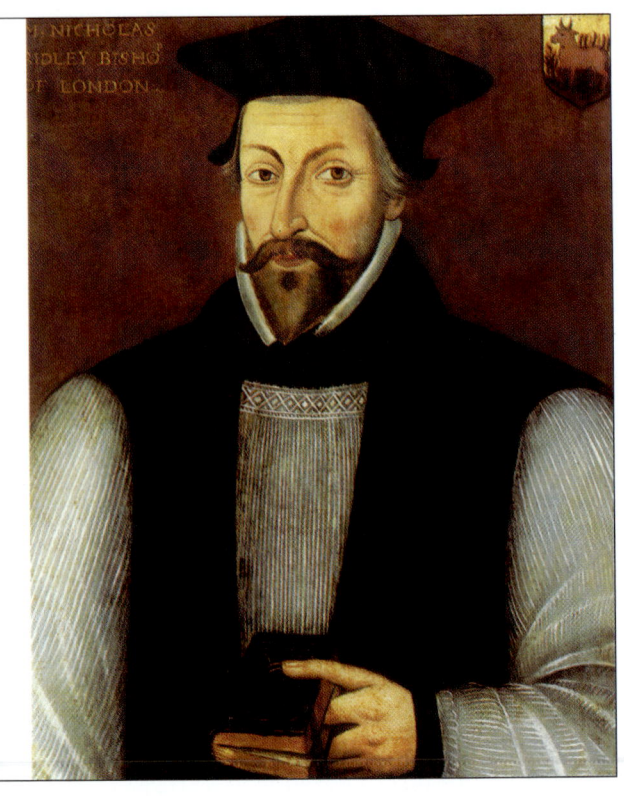

3

Roots of a Modest Giant of Science

"Harold Ridley was a modest giant of science who, despite fierce professional opposition, established one of the greatest milestones in medical history."
Pearce Wright, London Guardian, 2001

"It is great news that Harold Ridley has now been honored in his own country. American eye surgeons are indebted to this man for the great last step he took in daring to invent the implant, this wonderful lens. Tens of millions of Americans would otherwise be living a life of visual impairment caused by the results of cataract treatment without lens implantation. Ridley's invention changed life for the better worldwide—but nowhere more so than here in the US. Deeply felt thanks from your American colleagues and their patients, Sir Harold!"
Charles Letocha, York, Pa, 2003

Dr. Charles Letocha's words were penned in a letter written on behalf of American surgeons. However, it was clearly on behalf of surgeons and their patients "worldwide." This is just one of the many accolades he eventually received. Yet, to look at him and speak with him, casual observers might think of him as a soft-spoken, quiet gentleman and would not realize that the man's inherent modesty hid a world-class innovator who provided a world-changing contribution to medical science.

Unfortunately, most the accolades that came to Ridley did not come until later in his life. For decades, he suffered rejection and scorn, sometimes bordering on a professional excommunication. However, he was not the first Ridley to suffer because of his beliefs.

CHAPTER 3

THE RIDLEYS: 1555

A monument has been recently erected at Cambridge University, Pembroke College. It is designated the *Ridley Walk* (see page 45). It was built to honor two former Cambridge students who, separated by about 400 years, attended that college. We will first mention the former Master of the College, Reverend Nicolas Ridley (birth date unknown, died October 16, 1555). After a few words about Bishop Ridley, I will present an overview of the life of his collateral descendent, the surgeon and benefactor to humanity, Sir Nicholas Harold Lloyd Ridley (1906 to 2002), often affectionately called "HR" or "Harold" by his friends and colleagues. (An explanatory document from Cambridge regarding the monument lists the latter as a collateral descendent.)

I personally did not have the opportunity to trace the family tree for generations past. Tracings have been made by family members, including Harold and his son Nicholas, as well as other family members with records extending back to the 18th century. The original birth certificate from the precincts of his birth is now long lost, but most evidence points to the correctness of this connection.

No one knows exactly when the Reverend Ridley was born. However, the date of his death is very well documented since it is a well-known event in English history. On October 16, 1555, he and two colleagues were burned at the stake.

The Reverend Ridley came from a prominent family of the Northumberland region of England close to the Scottish border. At that time, the region was lawless and unstable. He was raised in the small village of South Tynedale and attended South Tynedale's village church, which had been built in the 11th century in the Norman architectural style. He began his ecclesiastical career path there. Supported by relatives who recognized his intelligence, he continued his education and became a priest in

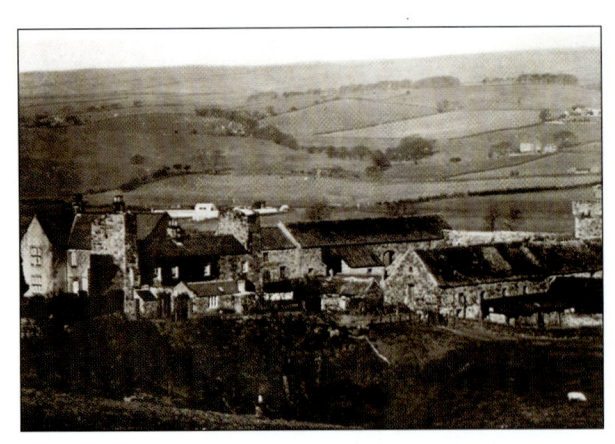

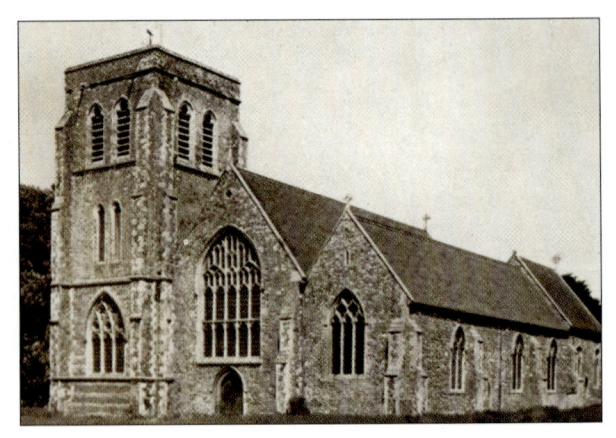

Origins.
LEFT: Nicholas Ridley was born at Willimoneswick, Northumberland and raised in the small village of South Tynedale that is situated at the northern border of England, near the Scottish border. He was from a well-respected family. At that time, this was an unstable and lawless region. The village was anchored by Bostwick Castle (left center).
RIGHT: Nineteenth century photograph of the 11th century church in Tynedale, built in the Norman style of architecture. This is where he was raised and first began his career path in the service of the Church.

Paris at the Sorbonne. He then returned to England in approximately 1529 to become a senior proctor of Cambridge University.

The religious landscape in England at that time was unsettled to say the least. In 1538, Henry VIII began to disband monasteries (the Dissolution) and introduced what is now known as the Church of England or the Anglican Church. This markedly reduced the influence of the Roman Catholic Church in England in favor of Protestant doctrine.

At about the time Ridley became the senior proctor, a heated debate arose regarding the pope's supremacy. Based in part on arguments put forward by Ridley on behalf of Cambridge University, he made the following resolution: "The Bishop of Rome has no more authority and jurisdiction derived to him from God, in this kingdom of England, than any other foreign bishop."

This comment was a very strong questioning and condemnation of the authority of the Catholic Church. In 1540, Ridley was made one of the King's Chaplains and was presented with a Prebendal Stall in Canterbury Cathedral. He succeeded to the office of Bishop of London in 1549/1550 and became a leader in the Reformation. Shortly after coming to office, the new bishop directed that the altars in the churches of his diocese be removed and tables put in their place to celebrate the Lord's Supper. This move was also an anathema to the Catholic hierarchy.

Since the early years of Protestantism—first in Germany in the early 1500s under Martin Luther and then spreading throughout Europe, England, and the New World—conflicts flared between Protestants and Roman Catholic loyalists. When Queen Mary, the daughter of a Roman Catholic, assumed the throne of England in 1553, she immediately ordered a relentless anti-Protestant policy, which included the elimination of those whom she considered to be Protestant "heretics." Her zeal and ruthlessness earned her the nickname "Bloody Mary."

Not surprisingly, after serving in his high position for several years, Ridley came into sharp conflict with this Catholic monarch, whom he considered grossly unfair. Unwilling to agree to adopt the theological principles of the Cthollic Church and to abide by the demands of the Catholic Queen, Bishop Ridley was burned at the stake on Broad Street in Oxford on October 16, 1555. Sharing his fate were two colleagues: Hugh Latimer and Thomas Cranmer.

Reverend Ridley and his colleagues' adherence to their principles and their unwillingness to agree to abide by the demands of the church and the

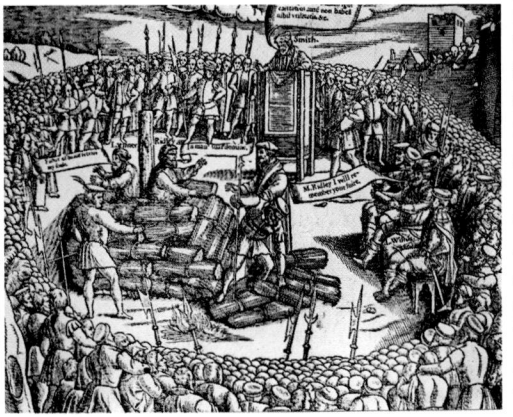

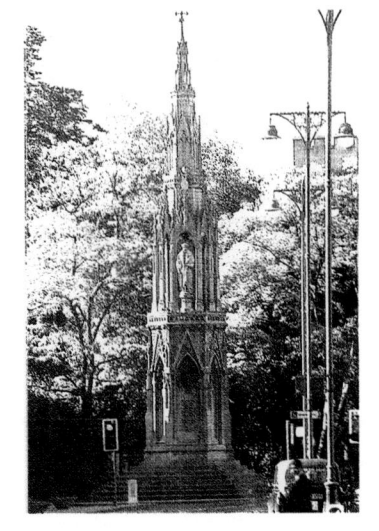

Ever since the beginning of Protestantism, initially in Germany in the early 1500s under Martin Luther, then spreading throughout Europe, England, and the New World, conflicts with Roman Catholic loyalists, including monarchs, ensued. By 1553, Queen Mary I assumed the throne and immediately ordered a relentless anti-Protestant policy.

TOP: Ridley and his colleagues' adherence to their principles led to the sad showdown on October 16, 1555. This woodcut depicts the execution of Ridley and two colleagues: Thomas Cranmer, former Archbishop of Canterbury and Hugh Latimer. They are now known as the three martyrs.

BOTTOM: The three were burned at the stake. This is a photograph of a Victorian neogothic architectural monument dedicated to the martyrs. It is situated a few hundred feet from the site of the execution. Images of the three martyrs are placed in statues on the monument. This architectural style became very popular throughout Victorian England, due to the influence of the royalty and architect Charles Barry, who designed the buildings of Parliament, as well as Queen Victoria and Prince Albert.

CHAPTER 3

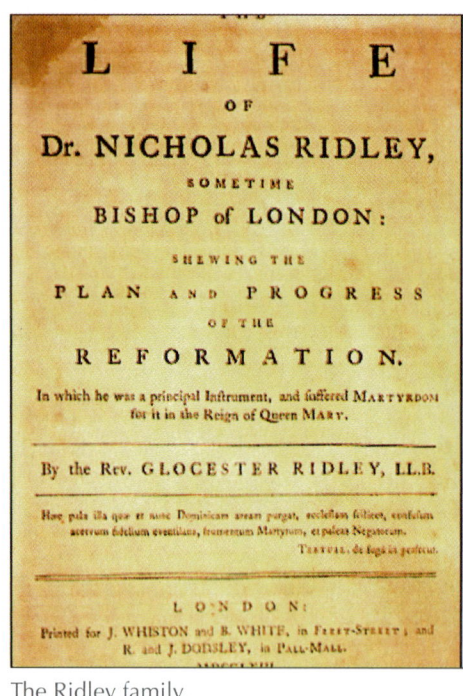

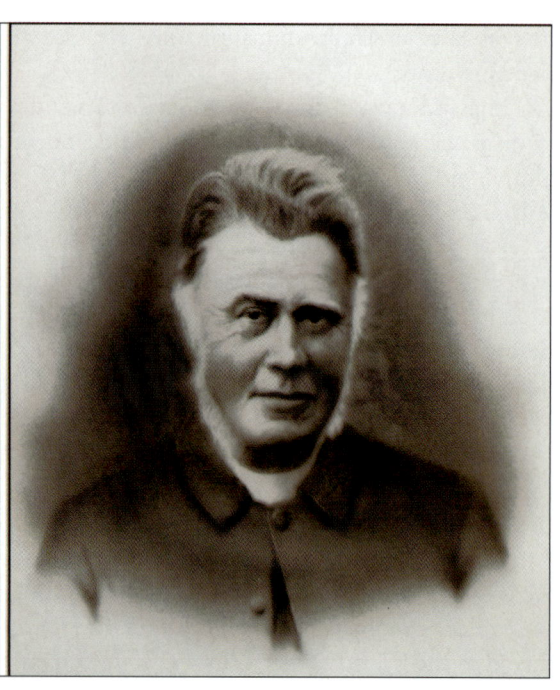

The Ridley family.

LEFT: Front cover of a biography of the martyr Nicholas (Nicolaus) Ridley written by a member of his family line, the Reverend Glocester Ridley, 2 L.B., 1763. This and other writings about the Ridley family line provide an excellent look into the nature of this individual and his beliefs. This Glocester Ridley biography provides a transition from the period of the martyr forward into the 18th century.

RIGHT: Many of Harold's ancestors were involved in the church. His grandfather, Rev. William Charles Ridley, was vicar of the parish of Bratoftal and later of Willoughby, Lincolnshire.

Our story regarding the Ridley family then continues in the late 19th century with the emergence of Harold's father. I have not personally verified the details of the family tree, but Harold throughout his life has maintained the family relationships described here and the martyr and Harold were classified as collateral relatives by Cambridge University at the establishment of the Ridley Walk (page 45).

Catholic Queen led to their sad downfall. The approximate site of the martyrdom is marked by a cross laid out in the cobblestones of the street. In the 19th century, a monument was erected a few feet from the site of the execution. Images of the three martyrs were placed in statues on the monument, which was built in a neogothic architecture style that was popular in 19th century England. This style was strongly supported by Queen Victoria and her husband, Prince Albert, who both popularized a return to gothic architectural roots in England. It was strongly influenced by the architect Charles Barry, best known as the architect of the new houses of Parliament.

THE PARKERS: "DO IT AND IT'S DONE"

Nicholas Harold Lloyd Ridley was born on July 10, 1906, four centuries later. This represented a merger of two very different genetic strains: the Ridleys and the Parkers.

According to Harold, his paternal ancestors—the Ridleys of the Bishop Nicholas Ridley line—were known historically as country gentlefolk (ie, gentry). They helped protect part of Hadrian's Wall along the South Tyne River where Scottish raids and cattle thefts were frequent. Almost all of the male Ridleys were involved in either medicine or the church (see the image on this page). Harold's immediate ancestors followed suit: his father was a physician and his father's father was a schoolmaster before taking holy orders. "Never a Ridley in trade!" was a family dictum.

The Parkers—Harold's maternal line—were known for being practical, hard working, and efficient. Harold classified them as yeoman. The Parker family's ancestral motto was "Do it and it's done." Just as the Ridleys had repelled the Scots along Hadrian's Wall, the Parkers helped control the Welsh who made raids from the west on Cheshire in Southern England.

After studying the characteristics of his mother's family, Harold pointed out the following: "Half the Parkers (including himself) had a particular gene that gave them the tendency to be 'single-minded perfectionists, determined to succeed, quick, efficient, and bluntly honest to the point of tactlessness. In short, they were doers rather than charmers.'"

This set of characteristics, of course, did not always play out well in personal relationships and in social settings. It often made the Parkers who carried this "gene" unpopular and irritating to those of similar intelligence and social status. Nevertheless, they were also known as people who got results. It is said that most of those who worked for or along with the Parkers were happy in their work and even showed great personal affection for them. Harold believed that the other Parkers who did not have the gene were typically more popular but less successful.

One of Harold's uncles, Will Parker, had the gene to "get things done." He was a remarkably successful farmer and landowner. At the peak of his career, he managed 32,000 acres of land in Leicestershire, Norfolk, Scotland, Wales, and elsewhere. King George V, impressed with his managerial skills, sent for Will and ordered him to take over the Sandringham Estates. This property was a royal residence with extensive land holdings where the royal family typically spent some of their holiday periods. Mr. Parker revitalized the property after the king's death, and Will purchased Sandringham from Edward VIII (1894 to 1972). The latter is very well-known to all of us as the King who abdicated the throne in 1936 in order to marry the American socialite and divorcee Mary Wallace Simpson. Many British, including Winston Churchill himself, were unhappy with him not just because of his social behavior, but also because he was perceived to have political leanings toward Nazism. Churchill ordered that he and his wife be transferred far away, to Bermuda. In the meantime, Parker (who had purchased the Sandringham property from him) tore up the contract and conveyed the property back when he learned that the new royal family, George VI, wanted to retain the entire estate.

Another Parker in Harold Ridley's line, named Ted Parker, was a very talented inventor. In World War I he participated in the invention of the Paravane or hydrofoil, a device strung between ships intended to help sweep mines away from ships passing through the minefields.

The World Harold Was Born Into

The world at the time of Harold's birth in 1906—the world that set the stage for his remarkable life—was a smoldering powder keg waiting to be ignited. In England, King Edward VII (1841-1910) had sat on the throne for less than a decade (1901 to 1910). England had been ruled by Edward's mother, Queen Victoria (1819 to 1901), from 1837 when she was crowned until her death in 1901. She presided over the awesome British Empire with her husband, Prince Consort Albert, until his unfortunate death in 1861; her long rule had been very eventful.

Harold was clearly influenced by numerous aspects of the "Victorian" personality, whose vestiges endured during his youth. Britain controlled the seas and therefore, in many ways, she controlled the peace (PAX Britannia). Harold and his peers were products of the ethics and attitudes of both Victorian and Edwardian England. When Edward assumed the throne late in life, after the death of his mother, it became clear that he did not have the keen interest in military matters that many of his contemporary rulers possessed. Nevertheless, England continued a major military buildup that had begun in the 1880s as a response to German militarism, long before his ascension to the throne. It continued through and beyond his reign. In fact, the period between

CHAPTER 3

1880 and World War I was marked by a brisk arms race, primarily between Imperial Germany and England. The period of naval buildup on the English side was termed the "Dreadnaught Era" because of the introduction of huge battleships, called "dreadnaughts." Apparently, the once powerful British Navy had begun to deteriorate, and its armaments had fallen behind under the leadership of a very conservative First Sea Lord, Admiral Arthur Hood (1824 to 1901). He was a descendent of a long line of admirals in existence since the time of Admiral Nelson in the 18th century. It was he who signed the papers in 1889, formalizing Harold's father's commission in the Royal Navy.

Ironically, the buildup on the German side was led by the nephew of Queen Victoria, Kaiser Wilhelm II (1859-1891). Actually, the militaristic buildup on Germany's side had been in full play during the long rule of Wilhelm II's father, Kaiser Wilhelm I. In the mid-19th century, Kaiser Wilhelm I, and his aggressive but highly talented minister, Count Otto von Bismarck, succeeded by both peaceful and duplicitous means in uniting the myriad small German States and principalities that existed at that time, thus creating a powerful Germany—a modern industrial empire. They cre-

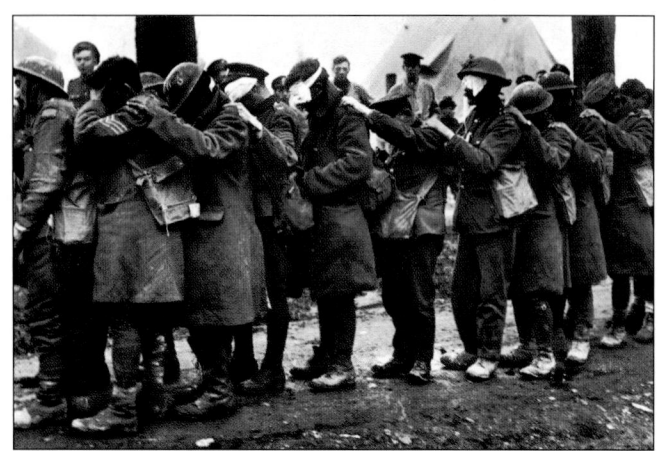

The disaster that was World War I is well known to all. Numerous soldiers in the war were blinded by the use of poison gas. At that time, the world was producing blind people, as well as curing blind people. (Compare with the illustration on the first page of Chapter 2.)

There were extensive geopolitical issues that affected many English families, including the Ridleys during the era of Queen Victoria and her son Edward VII, most especially related to the characteristics of the Victorian/Edwardian eras during which they lived, as well as the two major wars of the 20th century. Many of the factors assimilated by Ridley during his childhood had a great effect on his life and his behavior in terms of dealing with the acceptance or non-acceptance of his future innovations.

As an American, I dare not presume that I can classify a person in terms of issues derived from Britain; I can only limit my comments to what I have learned in reading and discussion with British colleagues, especially contemporaries of Harold—people who themselves were affected by the times.
TOP LEFT: Queen Victoria I (1819-1901),
TOP RIGHT: Victoria's son Edward VII (1841-1910).
BOTTOM: The arms build-up that occurred is sometimes termed the Dreadnaught Era, named after one of the major capital ships in the British Navy that was the premiere navy of the world before World War I.

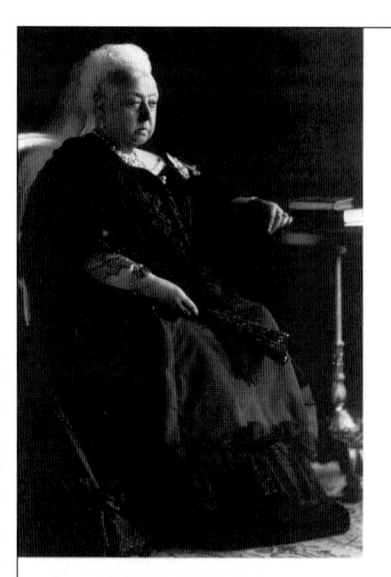

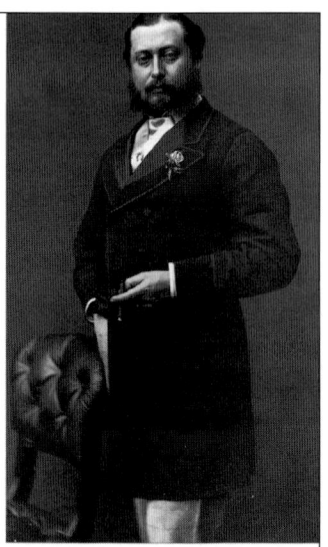

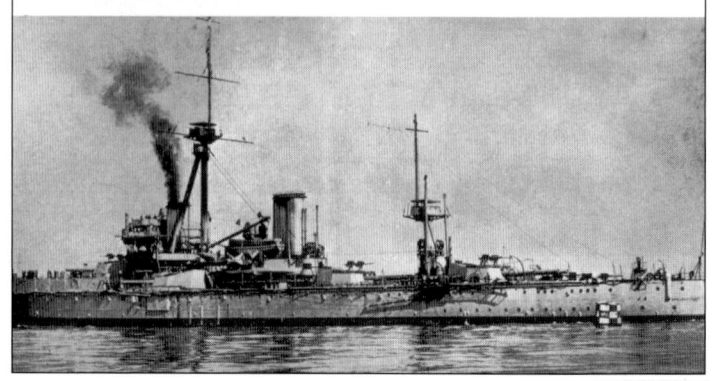

36

ROOTS OF A MODEST GIANT OF SCIENCE

ated a successful and wealthy industrial society where the arts, sciences, and medicine were permitted to flourish in addition to military matters.

Indeed, with regard to ophthalmology, the period between 1871 and 1914—beginning with the conclusion of the Franco-Prussian war and continuing until the start of World War I—could be considered the *First Golden Age in Ophthalmology and the Visual Sciences*. The leading figure in Germany during this era, and arguably one of the greatest, if not the greatest, ophthalmologists in history (most people believe the very best) was Albrecht von Graefe of Berlin. Although he sadly lived a very short life, succumbing early to tuberculosis, he enjoyed a brilliant and illustrious career and developed many important medical and surgical techniques—including several improvements in the cataract operation. It is a credit to him that he was able to flourish even in the shadows of a totalitarian government. His work had a profound influence on Harold as he pondered the IOL (see Chapter 5, page 80). His advances began in Germany and spread throughout Europe and England, rapidly extending to the New World.

One of von Graefe's greatest contemporaries at the time was in England, namely William Bowman (1816-1892). Like myself, Bowman not only practiced clinical ophthalmology, but he also was renown as a anatomist and histologist, using the microscope to study organs and tissues.

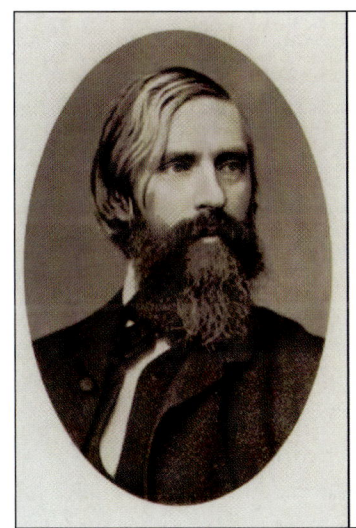

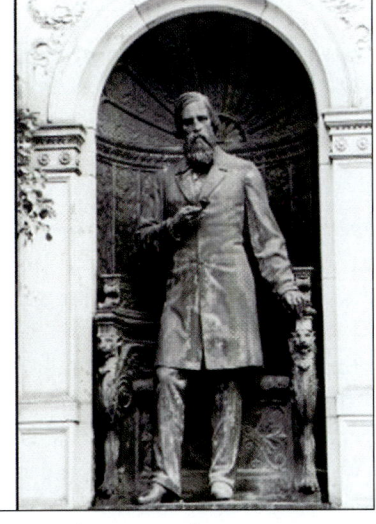

Sadly, this flourishing of arts and sciences began to give way to even more militaristic industrialization as the world was forced to refocus on the Dreadnaught-type arms buildup. The technology formerly used to create instruments of diagnosis and healing—devices as simple as the basic ophthalmoscope—was redirected to produce weapons of mass destruction. As the war began, industrial production turned to guns and powder.

Promising young men left university eye clinics to enter military training camps. By the end of World War I, a horrendous number of these young people had either been killed, wounded, severly disabled, or were missing. Those who survived became members of what was called the "lost generation" —so named because an entire generation of young men was almost wiped out by the carnage of the war. Harold was too

Moving forward to the 19th century, the period between around 1880 up until World War I consisted of an era of arms build-up—an arms race primarily between Imperial Germany and England. The leader on the German side was actually the nephew of Queen Victoria, Kaiser Wilhelm II (1819-1941), and enthusiastic proponent of German militarism. His father, Kaiser Wilhelm I, in association with his minister, Count Otto von Bismarck, succeeded by diplomacy and war to build up a united powerful country in which the arts and sciences actually flourished.

With regard to ophthalmology there is no doubt that a first Golden Age of Ophthalmology and the Visual Sciences occurred between the major wars of the time, beginning in 1871 with the conclusion of the Franco-Prussian War, continuing until the beginning of World War I.

LEFT: The supreme ascendancy of ophthalmology as a specialty was due to the work of many individuals, not the least, Professor Albrecht von Graefe of Berlin—who Harold Ridley greatly admired. He was a contemporary of the great English ophthalmologist William Bowman.

RIGHT: To my knowledge, von Graefe is the only ophthalmologist who is remembered by a life-sized monument that had been erected in Berlin. Unfortunately, he lived a very short life (1828-1870), succumbing early to tuberculosis. He had an absolutely brilliant and illustrious career and developed many important surgical and medical techniques within his specialty—many in the subspecialty of cataract surgery. Many of the successes in ophthalmology that began in Germany spread throughout Europe and also to England and the New World. All seemed to be going well, but unfortunately fate had it that this Golden Age came to an unfortunate end in 1914 as World War I (termed the Great War) began.

CHAPTER 3

Harold was too young to serve in the First World War, but it had an awesome influence on him for his entire life, as is evidenced by his writings and many conversations I had with him. He often spoke of the "lost generation," so named because almost an entire generation of men was wiped out by the carnage of the war. This had a very important and indeed positive effect on his career as he began his ascension in the field of ophthalmology in the 1920s. He advanced rapidly, but he did not savor the reason, namely that there were few doctors left available.

I heard Harold refer to the huge numbers of single women that he knew throughout his entire life—as patients, as friends, or associates. He always brought up the comment something to the effect that "she never married because her potential husband fell in World War I."

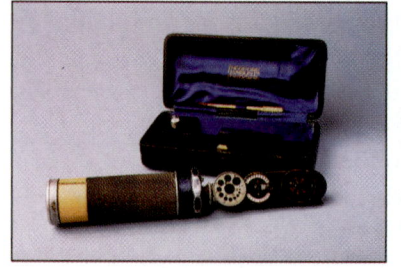

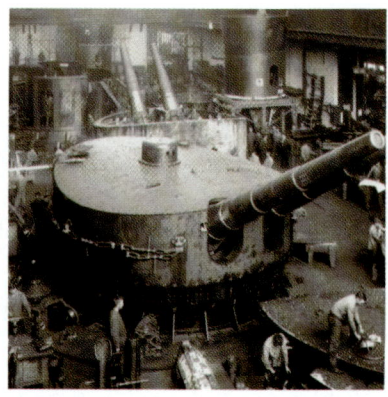

Nations' economies shifted from peaceful endeavors (like ophthalmoscopes) to the creation of weapons of mass destruction.

Several times he used a metaphor that seemed very poignant. He spoke of how the great technology available to the world by the beginning of the 20th century was being twisted and wasted. For example, the technology used to create instruments of diagnosis and healing (ie, the simple ophthalmoscope) was being replaced by weapons of mass destruction (such as the cannon shown here). LEFT: Harold's direct ophthalmoscope. RIGHT: Cannon manufacture prior to World War I.

young for service (age 8 at the start of the hostilities) and had then become a member of this "lost generation" —a very important aspect of his life that later affected his thinking about life in general. For example, after the war, he believed that he was privileged to still be alive after that era of mass carnage. He went out of his way not to take advantage of what was basically his good luck. He was never attracted to financial profit from his work in medicine. He felt that would have been a "slap in the face" to the many war dead forever deprived of such benefits.

During one of our river walks (Chapter 5), Harold and I had a conversation that arose from the fact that I had recently been diagnosed and treated for a throat cancer that required intense treatment with surgery, chemotherapy, and irradiation. This led to a discussion on how this disease had a major effect on the world's welfare during the period prior to World War I.

The course of history is often set by seemingly random events—in this case, the period during which the bloody canvas of World War I was painted. History might have been very different if Frederick Wilhelm (Kaiser Friedrich III, 1831-1888), the eldest son of Kaiser Wilhelm I (1797-1888), and the future Kaiser's father had not been stricken with throat cancer at a relatively young age (precisely the same condition I had, but, of course, without the benefits of modern treatments). He was diagnosed just as he assumed the throne after his father's death in March of 1888.

He was known to be an intelligent, honorable man—as appropriate a leader as might possibly be expected to provide a benevolent rule in the hard Prussian society of the time. However, he died of the disease only 88 days after his father's death. This led to a passing of the baton of leadership on to his eldest son, who became the infamous Kaiser Wilhelm II (1859-1941), under whom so many suffered. Wilhelm II was much less suited for the position and was much more aggressive and disposed to war. Many, if not all, authorities and historians are convinced that a rule of Frederick Wilhelm (who became known as the "88-day Kaiser") would have been far more benevolent and successful. Many believe the war might have been avoided. I wish he could have had the excellent treatment that was available to me.

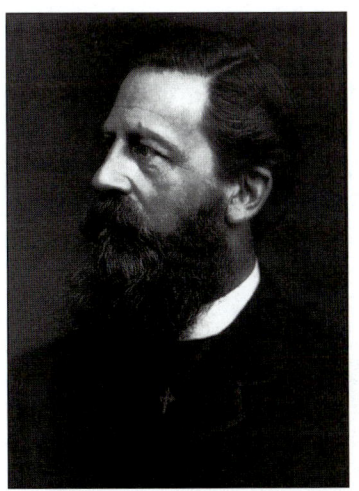

Before leaving the topic of the disruption caused by the arms race, World War I itself, and creation of the "lost generation," I recount a conversation I had with Harold one afternoon when we were actually discussing an illness that I personally had been dealing with, throat cancer diagnosed in 1999.

A Very Sad Stroke of Fate: The 88-Day Kaiser

The man illustrated in this figure, the 88-Day Kaiser Frederick Wilhelm (Kaiser Friedrich III, 1831-1888), was the eldest son of the previously mentioned Kaiser Wilhelm I, who had relatively successfully ruled Germany in the 19th century, albeit with an iron hand. He did, however, preside over the Golden Age as was just mentioned. As the senior Kaiser passed away in March of 1888, his eldest son assumed the throne but remained for only a period of 88 days. Most unfortunately, he also developed a malignant cancer of the throat, which (in contrast to my case) was untreatable. He succumbed, being forever known as the 88-Day Kaiser. Because of this, it allowed his eldest son, Kaiser Wilhelm II to assume power, leading in the horrible direction of World War I. Many, if not most, authorities feel that war could have been averted had the elder brother lived and provided a more reasonable period of rule during this era. The German Imperial family sent Frederick Wilhelm to England to be treated by a famous otolaryngologist named Morel McKinzie. The treatment was obviously unsuccessful. McKinzie, who resided on Harley Street quite near where Harold Ridley was later to take up residence. Noteworthy in the history of medicine is the fact that he is known as one of the first, if not the first, to associate smoking with cancers of the lungs and respiratory tract.

THE EARLY YEARS

Harold's father, Nicholas Ridley, was spared direct involvement in the war, not by choice, but by fate. Born April 6, 1863 in Bratoft in Lincolnshire, he was commissioned in the Royal Navy in 1889. As noted previously, his commission papers were signed by the famous Admiral Arthur Hood (see below right). A tall, impressive, and intelligent man, Nicholas appeared to have a promising career ahead of him. Following his commission, he was sent in the 1880s to serve in the China Station. While performing routine duties there, he developed severe joint hemorrhages, which were found to be the result of hemophilia. This resulted in a mandatory discharge from the Navy for health reasons in 1891—unfortunately, without much of a pension.

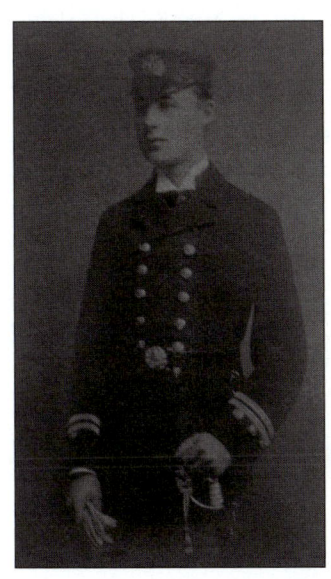

The father of Harold, Nicholas Ridley (1863 to 1937). The elder Ridley was born in Bratoft in Lincolnshire. He entered the Royal Navy and served primarily at the time of the above-mentioned massive arms build up in the late 19th century to 20th century prior to the war. Important for our story, Nicholas Ridley was never forced to enter the combat that had become inevitable. He was assigned to serve in the China station in the 1880s. While performing routine duties, he developed severe joint hemorrhages, which were found to be the result of hemophilia. This dictated that he be discharged from the Navy for health reasons and he retired in 1891, unfortunately without a significant pension. He was forced to continue to work for a livelihood, but because of his health, he was not able to pursue his chosen career as a general surgeon.

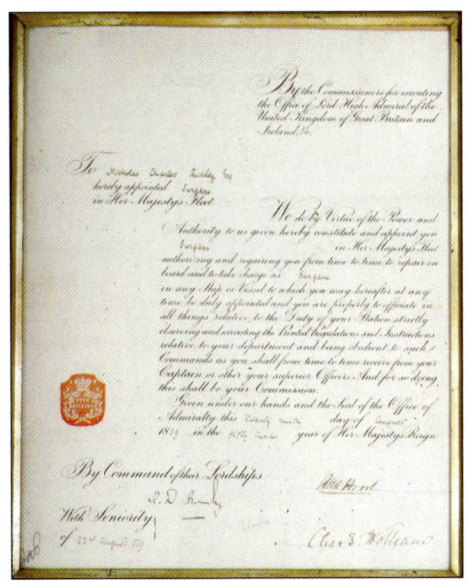

Nicholas Ridley's commission into the British Navy. His commission was signed on August 27, 1889 by the famous Admiral Arthur Hood.

CHAPTER 3

Nicholas was forced to continue to work for a livelihood, but because of his health, he was not able to pursue his chosen career as a general surgeon. This subsequently required a significant amount of physical exertion. He, therefore, chose what he believed to be a less strenuous pathway: a career in ophthalmology, including eye surgery. He obtained training posts at several institutions, including the London Ophthalmic Hospital (later named the Moorfields Eye Hospital). He received a hospital appointment

Having retired, Harold's father, Nicholas (left) chose a career in ophthalmology, which was less arduous. He held training and work posts in several institutions, including the Royal London Ophthalmic Hospital (Moorfields), before receiving a hospital appointment in Leicester in 1896. My wife, Ann and I, with the help of Dr. and Mrs. David Austin had the opportunity to visit and photograph the Leicester Royal Infirmary (right) where he had worked.

His hemophilia-induced arthritis that ensued was so crippling that for many years he was compelled to perform his work, including eye surgery, using crutches—often in considerable pain. Despite his health problems, he had a successful practice. He lived in Oadby, a village near Leicester for many years. He died at home of cerebral hemorrhage in 1937.

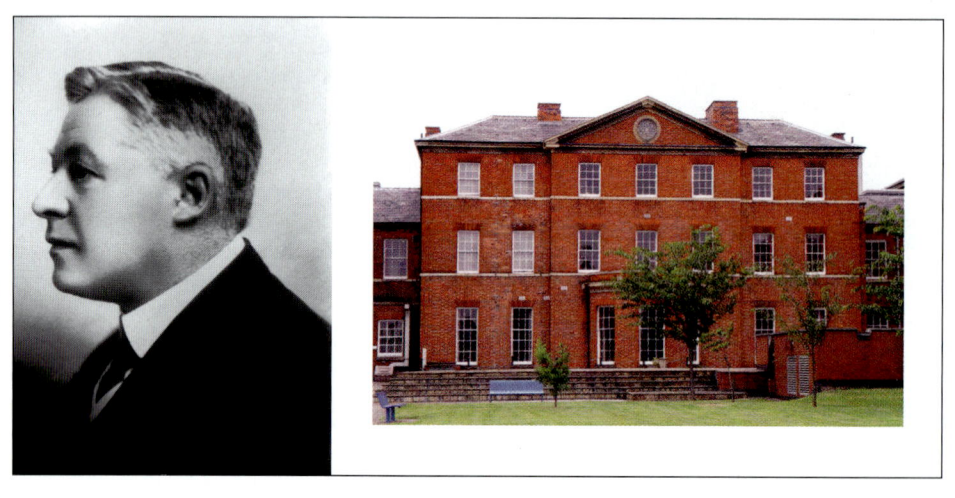

in Leicester in 1896 at the Leicester Royal Infirmary. A hemophilia-induced arthritis ensued, which was so crippling that for many years he was compelled to perform his work, including eye surgery, using crutches and often in considerable pain. Despite his health problems, Nicholas successfully practiced ophthalmology until his death from a cerebral hemorrhage in 1937.

He and his wife Margaret (Parker) had two sons. Nicholas Harold Lloyd Ridley (Harold) was born on July 10, 1906 in a nice, middle-class home, The Gables in Kibworth, Harcourt, a village near Leicester. The home still stands and has been well maintained. He spent some later years of his childhood in nearby Oadby. A few years later, in 1909, Harold's younger brother, Allder, was born.

Several years later, Harold noted the following:

"Sadly my parents, both of whom were hardworking and virtuous, were very dissimilar and quite unsuited to be man and wife. After about five years and shortly after the birth of their second son, a legal separation, which in 1909 was almost as disgraceful as a divorce, was agreed."

Margaret Parker, Harold's mother, in 1905. (Photograph courtesy of Nicholas Ridley, Harold's older son.)

Harold was born to Margaret and Nicholas Ridley on July 10, 1906 in Kibworth, near Leicester.

40

ROOTS OF A MODEST GIANT OF SCIENCE

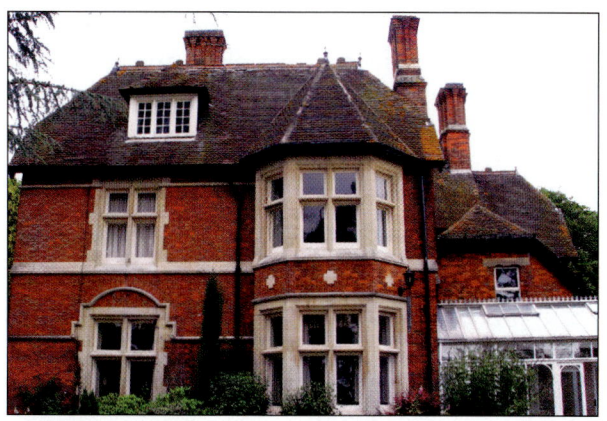

Harold's birthplace is shown in this photograph, a house which has been beautifully maintained over the years (Courtesy of Dr. and Mrs. David Austin, photograph by Ann Apple).

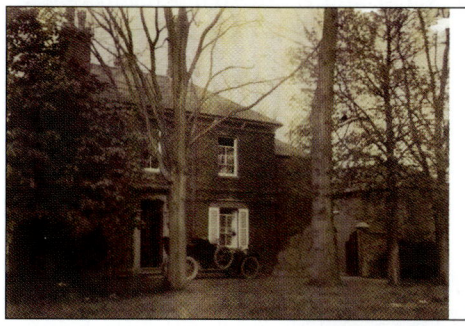

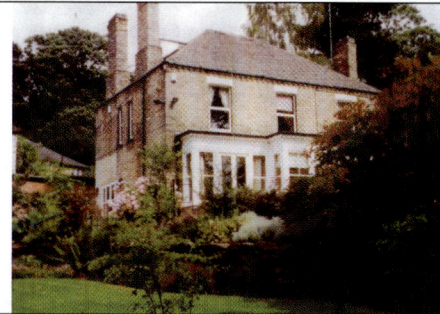

At a young age, the family moved to another house just a few miles away in Oadby.
LEFT: Contemporary photograph showing the first automobile to which Harold was exposed.
RIGHT: Photograph of the house today (courtesy Dr. and Mrs. David Austin).

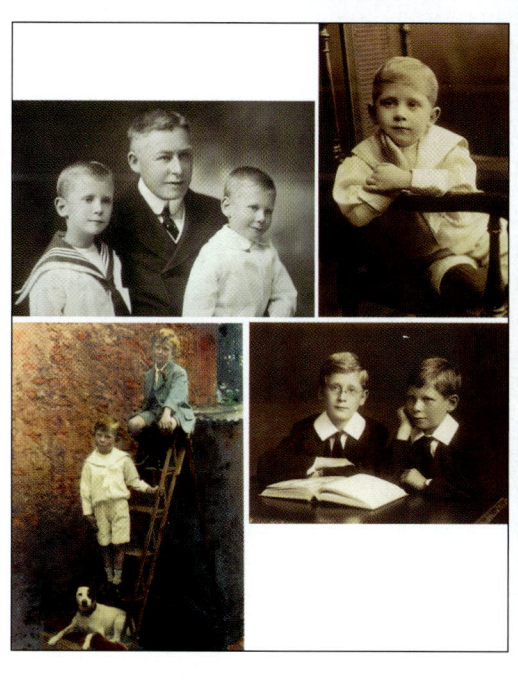

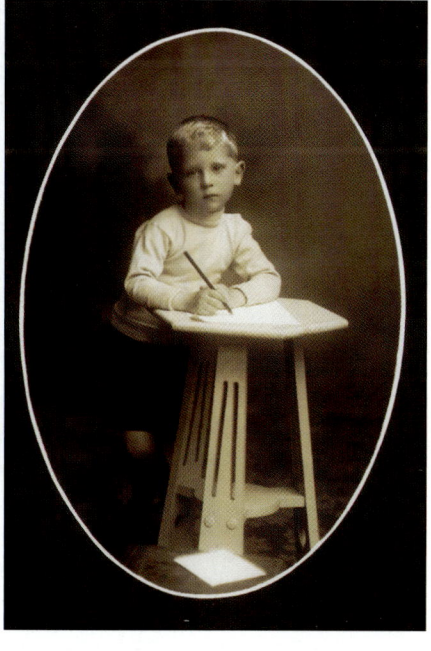

LEFT: A montage of images of Harold, his father, and his brother Allder. Harold Harold can best be identified by observing his round head.
RIGHT: This illustration brilliantly shows the scholarly demeanor that Harold exhibited from his early years, continuing throughout life.

The "disgrace" of his broken home followed him for years. Harold noted that he and his siblings had difficult childhoods. When Harold was 80 years old, shortly prior to the death of his brother Allder, he recalled the trauma:

> "We both seem to have been lucky in marrying loyal and loving women, and this is surely our greatest blessing in these days when so many marriages break up, often it would seem for little reason. We experienced enough of the resulting trauma in our childhoods. How could the personalities of our two parents ever have been compatible?"

CHAPTER 3

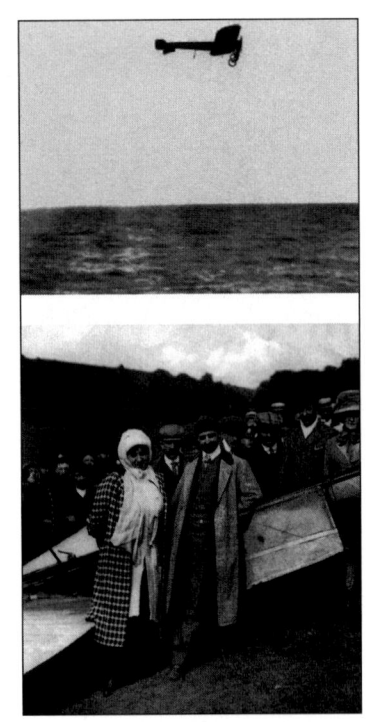

Looking back, Harold said that he and his brother were: "only just able to conceal from our fellows the disgrace of the family breakdown. We had two homes. In each house, only the name of one parent could ever be mentioned. Because of these circumstances, unusual for the times, we led double lives from an early age."

After the separation, the boys spent much of their time with their mother in a flat she had rented in the town of Hove on the south coast. Coincidentally this is the town where Rayner & Keeler, Ltd.'s IOL manufacturing facility is located today. It had gas lighting and only fires for heat. At the age of five, young Harold was taken for a month from his mother and little brother and sent alone to a strange house where only the cook, Sarah, was friendly. He later reported that he soon "became nervous and later stammered unlike anyone else in the family." He then attended an elementary school in Brighton, a seaside resort city next to Hove on the channel—very near where later action in World War II would have so much effect on his life and indeed, subsequently, all of our lives.

When Harold was almost three years old, an event took place that would have far-reaching consequences on the British Isles and, indirectly, on his future career. In 1909, a Frenchman named Louis Blériot became the first man to cross the English Channel in a heavier-than-air aircraft. Harold accompanied his father to the southern coast of England to see this historic event. He was there but, of course, had no memory of it.

The flight, however, was a wake-up call to the English people, who had long relied on the Channel as a defensive barrier against aggressive intruders from Continental Europe. The moment Blériot successfully completed his flight in 1909, the British knew that their home was no longer as isolated and protected as it had formerly been. In a sense,

"Britain was no longer an island."

Another very important event in Harold's life is one that he, of course, does not remember, namely, the occasion of the first flight in the heavier than air airplane over the English Channel by the Frenchman, Louis Blériot (1872-1936). The flight occurred on July 25, 1909. Harold had accompanied his father on a trip to the South English coast to witness the event. It is not clear whether it was at Dover, where he had landed, or elsewhere as Blériot made a "triumphal tour" after the flight.

This flight is not only important in terms of the history of Harold Ridley, but it is of supreme symbolic importance to the history of England. Prior to this time, the British Isles had indeed been an island, separated from the mainland of Europe by the English Channel. It was immediately recognized by men with vision that this was no longer the case—that England could be vulnerable to air attack, which was indeed the case and actually forms a major part of our story (see Chapter 6).

TOP: The Blériot's airplane in flight over the English Channel.
BOTTOM: The end of the successful journey, Blériot poses with his wife, friends, and colleagues, resting adjacent to his flight machine. Never more could Britain be considered an island, at least in terms of potential air invasion was concerned. This lesson was learned over and over almost a half century later in World War II.

This would have dramatic consequences in the coming decades. It can be said, in anticipation of the events of World War II, that the English had adapted to this change very well. In essence, when the foreign invaders arrived by air, the first fighter squadrons of the German Luftwaffe were turned back. Then later, when the time to bomb Germany arrived, bomber forays from Britain onto the Continent became necessary. The British in effect adroitly and successfully turned their island nation into a great stationary "Rock Aircraft Carrier."

At the age of six, Harold had another experience that had a lasting, positive effect on him. He spoke to me often about a visit to see Florence Nightingale. His mother was a close friend of Miss Nightingale (as she preferred to be called), the founder of modern nursing. When Harold was six, he and his mother were guests at the home of a mutual friend who hosted the visit. He was later told that he had an opportunity to sit on the knee of the great lady—a privilege in which he took great pride throughout his life. This was not the last of his connections with Florence Nightingale. Later, he would practice medicine at the same hospital where she had served—a hospital with a special Florence Nightingale wing, where being a "Florence Nightingale Nurse" was and remains an ongoing honor for

ROOTS OF A MODEST GIANT OF SCIENCE

young people entering nursing and throughout their lives. He would also, for a time in later years, live and have his practice just a few doors away from her on Harley Street (pages 49 and 50).

Harold was only eight years old when Britain entered World War I in August of 1914. The fighting stopped with the signing of Armistice on November 11, 1918. He was not yet a teenager when the war started and was too young to have been called to serve as a soldier. However, the turbulence and suffering of the war certainly had its impact on his young mind and heart. The blind individuals in the image on page 36 were not blinded by diseases or accidental injury, as were the individuals pictured in the illustration in Chapter 2 on page 14 that shows a similar pattern of patient movement. The nature and etiology of the blindness that sadly emerged in many devastated soldiers in World War I was vastly different—simply gruesome. We witness here (page 36) the absolute terror of soldiers blinded by poison gas, the folly of war—in stark contrast of that seen in the previous illustration. The effort of symbolism of the "blind leading the blind" had turned in a perverse direction from preempting a blindness that was secondary to disease as opposed to blindness caused by the absolutely mindless destructive processes of armies.

These and innumerable other such images had a profound effect on Harold, as it must have had on most people. In spite of his "stoic" outward appearance, a reading of his memoirs convinced me that he was an extremely sensitive man. It seems that he had very conservative political leanings in the sense of having supported basic party politics; for example, Margaret Thatcher. However, in one focused compartment of his thinking, he was absolutely antiwar. As an adult, he felt that war should be eliminated as quickly as possible. However, while it raged, as it did through the two world wars and several armed conflicts that coincided with his life, he did his best to make whatever positive gains he could from its carnage to the benefit of all of us.

In conversing with Harold, I determined that one of his absolutely proudest moments in life was a moment he of course could not have remembered in 1910. He was only four years old. He and his mother had journeyed to the home of Mrs. Edward Lloyd at Coombe Farm in Shirly Surry in the spring of 1910 to visit the great pioneering nurse, Florence Nightingale. Harold sat on the knee of Miss Nightingale (as she liked to be designated). Florence Nightingale died soon thereafter in December of 1910.
LEFT: Florence Nightingale in later life.
RIGHT: Letter written by Florence Nightingale in the possession of Harold Ridley.

SCHOOL DAYS AND MEDICAL TRAINING

Following his year or so at boarding school in Hove (see below), he attended Charterhouse, a prominent boarding school near Godalming, Surrey. He entered when he was about 14 years old and remained from about 1920 to 1924. "At school I was not the cleverest," he later recalled, "but considered one of the two who would go far." His best marks (grades) at Charterhouse were consistently in scientific subjects, where he was always at or near the top.

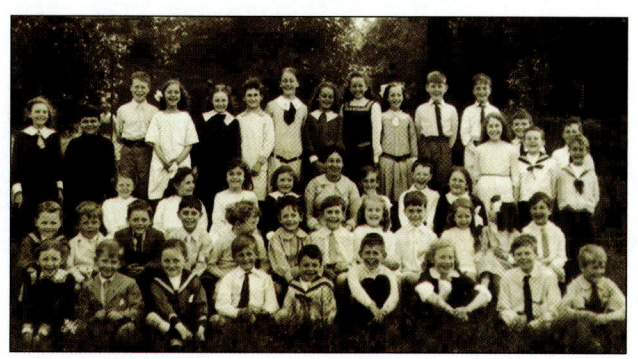

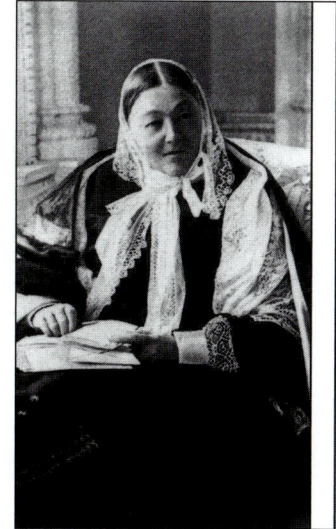

Having spent his early childhood in Kibworth and Oadby, Ridley was sent to a boarding school near Dover on the Southern coast of England, ironically not at all far from 1) the site of major activities in the Battle of Britain, which turned out to be such an important aspect of his life and 2) the site of present day Rayner & Keeler Ltd. (Brighton, Hove). Harold is approximately 14 years old in this photograph and sits in the lower left front row, in the light gray jacket.

43

CHAPTER 3

Following completion of grammar school studies, Harold entered Charterhouse, one of the finest schools of this type for young men in the country. The present infrastructure and buildings stem from the mid-19th century and reveal a very impressive, albeit quite stoic, architecture.

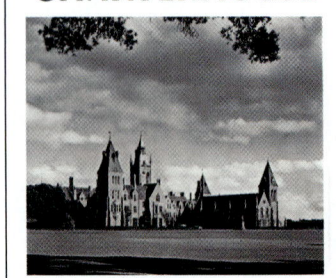

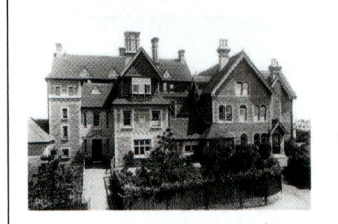

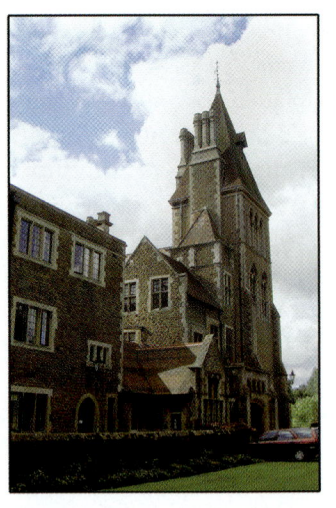

The librarian of Charterhouse School pulled out records that verified that Harold had been there at least two years in the early 1920s. She also fetched his notes from the archives and found that he was a good student overall and indeed had excellent grades in mathematics, science, and the technologies of the time, which as we now know from Harold would be expected. The librarian was extremely kind to my wife Ann, our friend and colleague from Advanced Medical Optics Giulia Newton (who herself had grown up in Goldamming very close by in this region and whose mother was a Florence Nightingale nurse at St. Thomas' Hospital, it is truly a small world), and me.

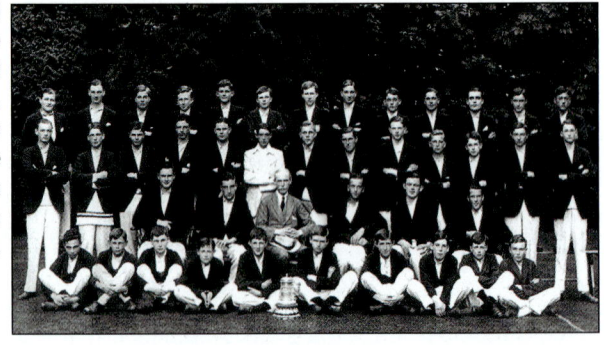

In 1924 Harold began studies at Cambridge University, Pembroke College. The illustrations here show two views, the left showing the archway into the college courtyard, and the picture on the right showing an exterior view of the great chapel designed by Sir Christopher Wren. This of course is where Ridley had studied in his early years. Looking ahead to Chapter 4, Harold's collateral ancestor, Nicholas Ridley the 15th-century martyr, was a master of Pembroke College.

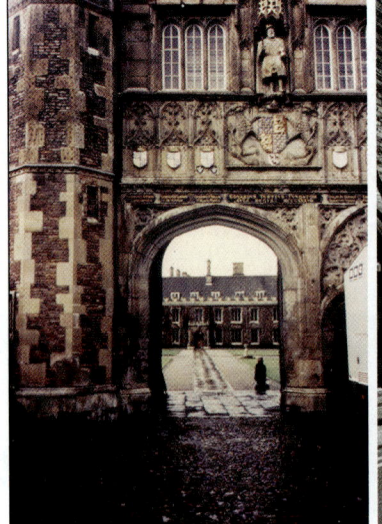

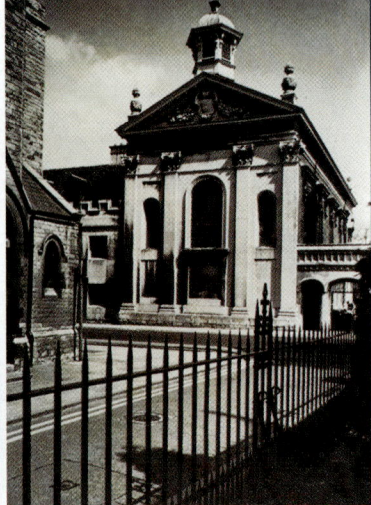

In 1924, he entered Cambridge University, Pembroke College, where his strength was again in the sciences. He completed his studies there in 1927, successfully receiving an honors degree. The "Ridley Walk" is based on his successful years at Cambridge, 1924 to 1927.

In 1927, he began his medical training at St. Thomas' Hospital in London. At this point, he clearly began to excel, and in his second year there, he entered for the "prizes" a year too soon. Despite this, he did remarkably well. He just missed receiving a coveted scholarship, which was won by a student one year more advanced. This unexpected success dramatically boosted his confidence. It also assured him of a house surgeon's position at his teaching hospital—almost essential for those rising to the top.

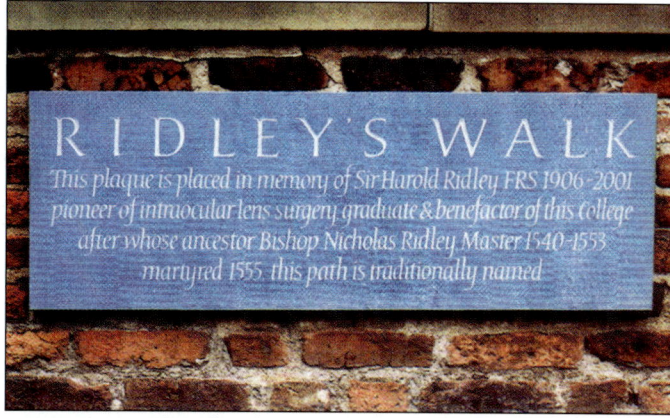

Just a year ago, the officials at Cambridge established a Ridley's Walk in honor of both Harold and his illustrious distant grandfather. This was a very helpful means to help provide recognition to Harold.

During part of his training, Harold worked under Cyril Nitch, a very severe master who broke nearly half his assistants. But Nitch gave him excellent surgical experience and a laudatory testimonial, something never expected from the man.

It was not all work for the young medical student: "I played a lot of tennis, usually for the second six, but very occasionally for the first for which I was not really good enough." In the same self-effacing tone, he also reported that he never won a prize or scholarship. He should have added that he was second on multiple occasions.

Harold completed his basic medical education in 1930. He then spent 6 months as a casualty officer at St. Thomas' Hospital, followed by a year of general surgery at the same location. During this period, he completed a very significant segment of his training, a 6-month sojourn under the legendary Mr. A. Cyril ("Huddy") Hudson. In July of 1932, at the youngest eligible age of 25, he received the FRCS (Fellow Royal College of Surgeons) designation.

Ridley's father influenced him to enter ophthalmology. The first exposure to ophthalmology that is listed in Harold's letters and papers in my possession occurred when he attended the Oxford Ophthalmological Congress in 1930 as his father's guest. This was the same Congress that was the site of his first presentation of his innovation, the IOL, in 1951, which turned out also to be a disastrous rebuff (see page 154), only to later be rectified years later at another event in 1991 at that Congress.

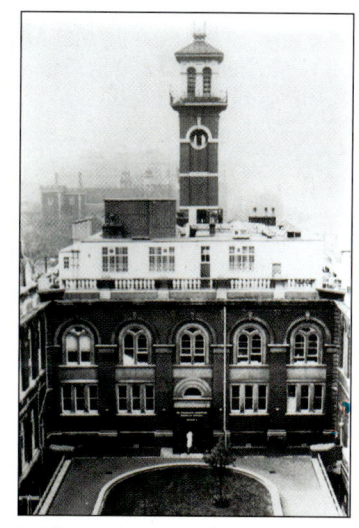

St. Thomas' Hospital is composed of several blocks of buildings seperated by interior courtyards.

The time he spent with Hudson in ophthalmology at St. Thomas' also played a pivotal role in Harold's ophthalmological training. He always regarded "Huddy" as his finest teacher: "He certainly taught me how to do extracapsular extractions (ECCE) and the no-touch technique, and he was far better than anyone else in London."

Mr. Geoffrey Doyne was another surgeon who influenced Ridley during his training years at St. Thomas' Hospital. Doyne's father, Robert, was the discoverer of a retinal disease appropriately termed Doyne's honeycomb retinal dystrophy; he was also the founder of the Oxford Congress. With appointments at both St. Thomas' Hospital and Moorfields Eye Hospital, Geoffrey Doyne had advanced Ridley's career by recommending that he do further training as a registrar at Moorfields.

Consequently, Harold was exposed to the best eye surgeons in London from the beginning, and he learned well from them. Doyne took him in hand and became almost a second father, giving wise advice and encouragement. Harold later acknowledged Doyne's and Huddy's roles:

CHAPTER 3

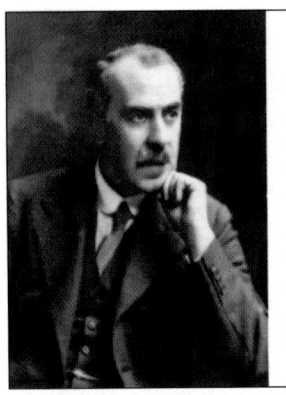

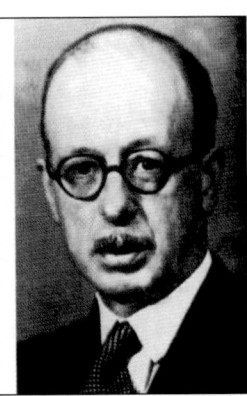

In addition to Huddy (left), he again was "blessed" to have Mr. Geoffrey Doyne (right) as a mentor and advisor. Doyne was the son of the famous Robert Doyne, the discoverer of a significant lesion of the eye "Doyne's honeycomb chorioretinal dystrophy." He was also the founder of the Oxford Ophthalmological Congress.

"I am very conscious of the great dept. I owe to these men who could surely not have had an enemy in the world. My career would have been very different without Doyne and his wise guidance. He was a good ophthalmologist. Though he did not live to see our work fully accepted, I sincerely hope that he derived some pleasure from supporting me in the early stages. How kind God was to give me two such wonderful teachers. Of the two—Huddy was the finest teacher, but I really believe that Geoffrey Doyne gave me the greater help and guidance."

Soon after his qualification and prior to beginning further ophthalmology training in 1935 at Moorfields Eye Hospital, Harold bided his time as a temporary house surgeon and anesthetist at Derby Royal Infirmary. In addition, recalling that "my father had wanted me to see the world before I became too busy," he found various positions as a ship's surgeon in 1933 and 1934. He wrote of that period of his life:

"As soon as I had qualified, I was appointed temporary house surgeon and anesthetist at Derby Royal Infirmary. I was scared stiff to anesthetize miners with chloroform, for they were said to be immune from sleep after ether. However, all went well and I drove home in my very early Morris Minor with £23, one pound daily for my labor, and I was proud of this.

"I had to wait for some weeks before starting in casualty at St. Thomas'*, so I made enquiries and found a small shipping line. The Anglo Baltic sent ships to Riga, Tallin, etc, and they had to carry a doctor if there were passengers. We had an interesting passage through the Kiel Canal.

"Riga remains the only place where I was accosted in a cathedral. One evening I went round the town with the wireless officer. I think he was drunk when we started and so I had one vodka to every two he swallowed, but at the end I was drunk for 10 and a half pence and he was almost sober."

Ridley also served on a four-month voyage to Japan—again reliving an experience of his father, who had worked as a ship's surgeon in Japan in 1884 to 1885.

Following these adventures, he was very keen to find useful work again and, through a recommendation by Doyne, he was offered an 18-month period of ophthalmology residency training at Moorfields Eye Hospital in 1934 to 1935. There, Ridley observed:

"In the early '30s, hospital conditions were little better than a century before, except that local and general anesthesia had become available. There was only one operating table, a masterpiece of carpentry. To readers of this report the theatre must seem unbelievable, but sepsis was uncommon except after orbital trauma. The striking discovery for me was that operative technique was really poor and far below the standard of Huddy at St. Thomas' Hospital. This was because World War I had deprived aspiring surgeons of their proper training. A generation of ophthalmologists, German as well as Allied, had been lost in the war. The next generation therefore was not properly taught. Some men indeed had actually been promoted to staff level when still house surgeons.

---

* According to Harold's written records, a copy of a police report, his first patient as a casualty officer, was a young man who Harold successfully treated for four gunshot wounds.

ROOTS OF A MODEST GIANT OF SCIENCE

"Believe it or not, when I became a Moorfields resident, only two out of twelve full surgeons had ever been 'through the house.' Huddy, had he still been at Moorfields, would have been a third. There was I, the first of a new generation of ophthalmic surgeons given, by God, the chance to pick out the best features from the work of each of my superiors and develop technique up to the standard of the day. I was given much more surgery than any of my predecessors and passed up some suggestions to my seniors."

Ridley performed 109 cataract extractions during 12 months of active time in the operating room. In those days, the average number of cases performed by young residents was 30 to 40.

His first techniques for cataract surgery were influenced by the Viennese School of Ophthalmology. Harold and his father visited Vienna, Budapest, and Munich for about 4 weeks after the completion of training in 1935. Harold was very impressed by the "general excellence of ophthalmology throughout continental Europe." The great Viennese clinician and ocular pathologist, Ernst Fuchs, his successor, Professor Karl Lindner, and their team manned one of the finest eye clinics in the world at that time.

The preferred single technique on the continent and in England during Harold's early years was intracapsular cataract extraction (ICCE). However, even though Harold was not permitted to perform the technique of ECCE until somewhat later. He recognized at this early stage that the ECCE technique was generally safer and preferable to ICCE. Fortuitously, ECCE turned out to be the best technique for use with the IOL—the invention that would later make him a giant of ophthalmology!

In 1938, Harold was appointed full surgeon and permanent consultant at Moorfields Eye Hospital—the youngest person even to receive such an appointment. Ridley wrote:

"In my second year as a resident, my seniors sometimes called me in for second opinions. Three surgeons made me run their practices during their absence on summer holidays. Inevitably, this good fortune brought forth jealousy among my contemporaries, but the staff supported me and made a special vacancy for me to registrar (resident). When staff vacancies arose the following year, I was appointed full surgeon at the very early age of 32 years and 9 days, with all votes save one: the aunt of a rival."

Harold was concerned with more than his own training and advancement. He knew that something had to be done to restore the hospital to the ophthalmic center of excellence it had once been. He wrote:

"I spoke to the chairman of the governors, Mr. Luling, and he immediately promised money to pay the costs of more junior staff if the medical committee so recommended. The duration of a resident's job was increased from one to two years, and soon after to three. Teaching, however, was still to be done entirely by clinicians who were always overburdened with patients who had to be seen. Some of them charged fees to earn the surgeon's meager living.

"I believe that the re-founding of Moorfields as a teaching center was the very best thing that I ever did for British ophthalmology until implants eventually arrived. Within a few years, World War II began and little could be done until peace returned."

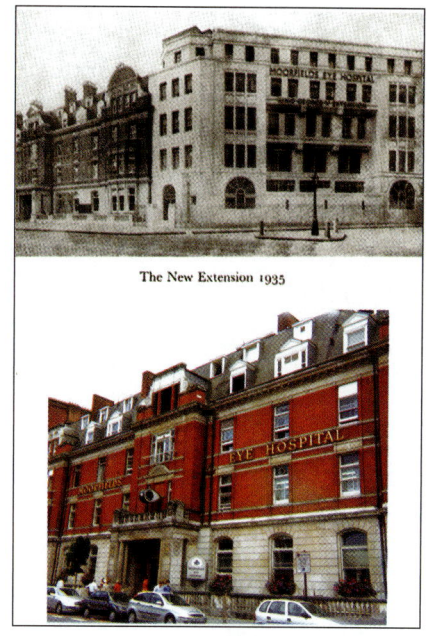

Moorfields Hospital, prior to 1957.
TOP: A new exterior was add in 1925.
BOTTOM: Original building dating form the late 19th century.

CHAPTER 3

As part of the "lost generation," at a time when so many young men had been sacrificed to war, Ridley found himself during those years in a very thin field. This circumstance, combined with his very real talents, set the stage for a rapid climb up the ladder of professional success.

Although Harold's professional growth was rapid, an important event occurred that most certainly had an adverse affect on his later career, when the time came in 1951 to begin his defense of the IOL. It began in 1935 when Sir Stewart Duke-Elder, unfortunately, later to become his archenemy, had written Harold a very positive letter in Harold's behalf (Chapter 9, page 157). Not long thereafter, Harold and Duke-Elder had differences regarding minor clinical issues in the patient examining area in Moorfields Hospital (page 158). Harold himself later recognized that he had not exhibited the necessary "political correctness" regarding the issues in dispute—even though I believe Harold's view in the matter was the correct one. I am sure that the longstanding conflict between the two, the aggression clearly emanating mostly from Duke-Elder's side, began with this small altercation and then grew completely out of proportion. After Duke-Elder learned the details regarding Harold's invention of the IOL (page 158 to 160), his animosity increased. (The details of Harold's professional life will be described later in the chapters that deal with events occurring at the beginning, during, and after the war.)

In May of 1941 Ridley was appointed temporary Major, Royal Army Medical Corps. In that year, he was sent to Ghana in the Gold Coast of west Africa by Sir Stewart Duke-Elder, then the ranking ophthalmic officer in the British Army. Harold notes, "This dis-

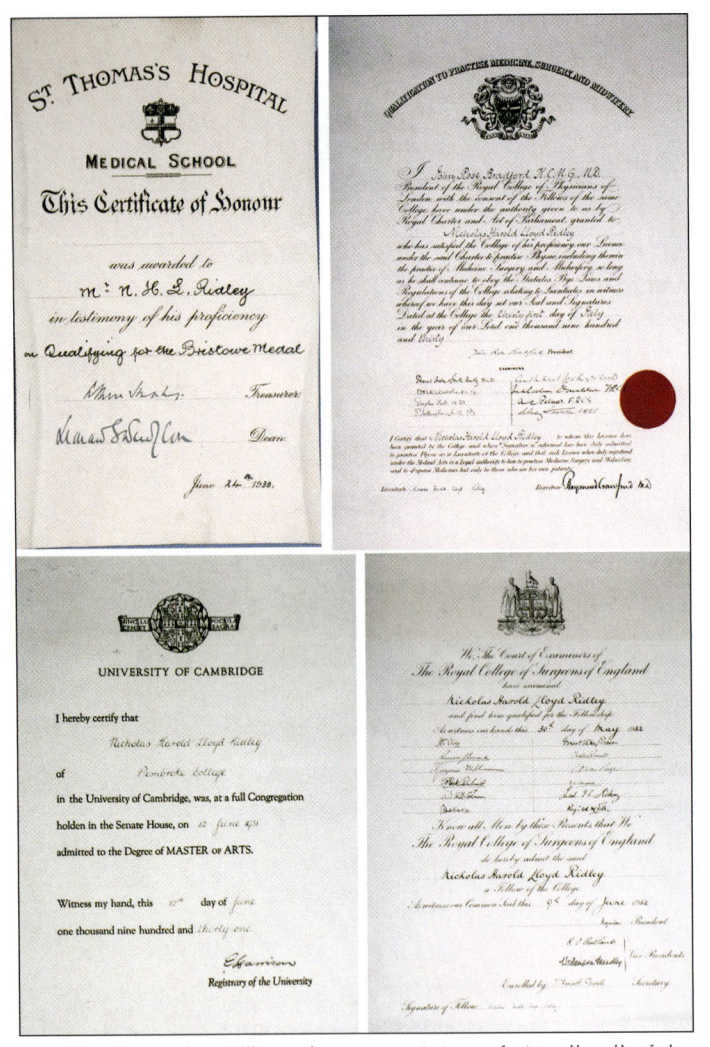

Harold advanced rapidly and was a recipient of virtually all of the relevant honors and certificates that were commonplace in his situation, a small few of which are illustrated in this figure, and many more are resting securely at my home.

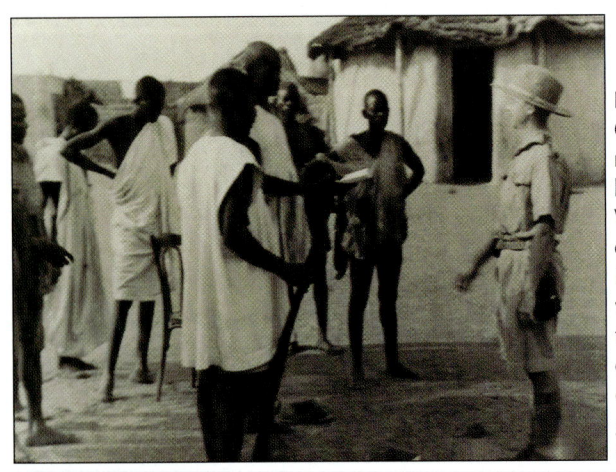

Duke-Elder had Harold Ridley shipped to Ghana on the Northwestern Gold Coast of Africa in order to pursue his medical service among the natives. Ridley did not expect any fighting or any chance to utilize his experience in casualty medicine and indeed there was none. What happened, however, in this period between 1943 and the end of the war, Harold had his opportunity to observe new things, new ideas, and put his fertile mind to bring some more innovations to the world—innovations we still utilize. (This is, of course, in addition to the intraocular lens.) In Chapter 13 we will focus on his work with onchocerciasis. A letter from Sir John Wilson in the text of Chapter 13 clearly emphasizes, from an impeccable source, Ridley's priority as a great worker in the field of tropical medicine and treatment of people in the underprivileged world.

ROOTS OF A MODEST GIANT OF SCIENCE

tressed me, for West Africa was not likely to be a fighting area where surgical experience would be of value."

Harold married his beautiful wife, the former Elisabeth Weatherhill in Surrey on May 10, 1941—during the Blitz while bombs were falling everywhere around them. She had grown up in India where her father was employed.

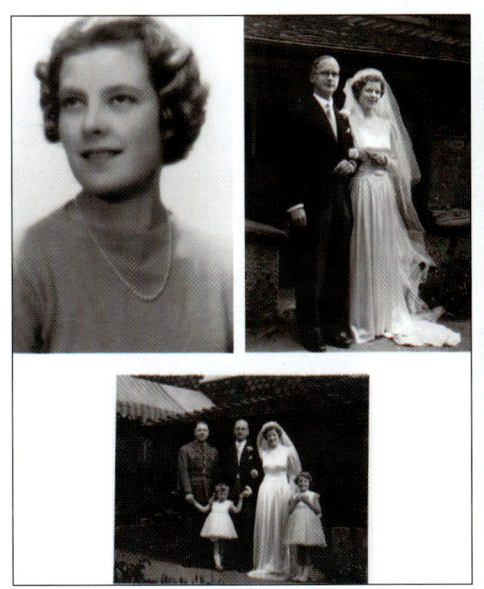

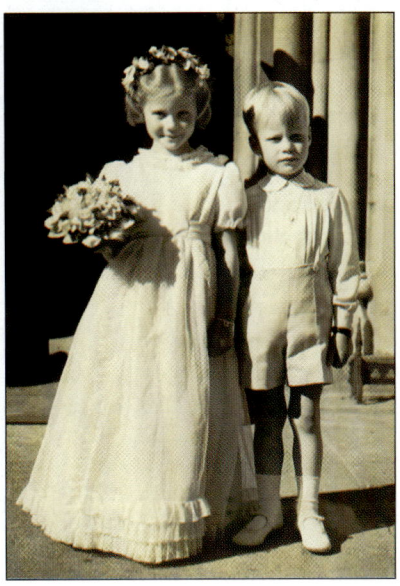

Elizabeth and Harold were married on May 10, 1941, a ceremony that occurred during the Blitz as bombs over London were over the exposed wedding party, but no harm done.

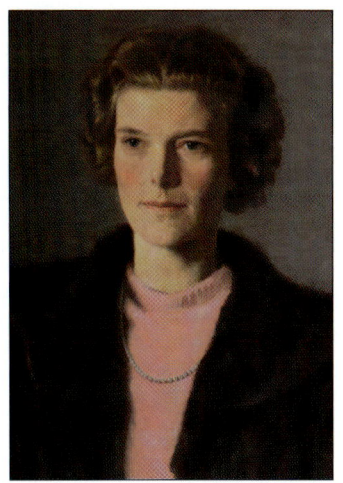

Harold spent his early war years as a civilian and actually, his activities in the famous Battle of Britain were as such as we will see in Chapter 6. He did meet a very wonderful lady who I got to know well for many years, Miss Elisabeth Jane Weatherhill (born August 16, 1916). Elisabeth's parents served in the British Royal Indian service and she was therefore often away in India during her younger years.

Off the scale Harold noted: "She was by training a school teacher, but worked as a Red Cross nurse during wartime. However, ultimately for me she was a secretary, diarist, and general helper in many ways—not at all medical, but an essential part of the team."

Elisabeth and Harold had three children: Margaret (born 1942), Nicholas (born 1943), and David (born 1951).

During the war, the Ridleys purchased a home at 53 Harley Street, which functioned as his ophthalmology practice (rooms) on the ground floor and the family's living quarters in the two overlying floors. He bought the home from Mr. Henry Stallard, an eye surgeon at Moorfields who was famous not only as an outstanding surgeon, author, and consultant at the hospital but also because of his prowess as a long-distance runner. His persona was featured in the film "Chariots of Fire" in which an actor played Stallard, using his actual name in the film. The movie accurately portrayed and showed correctly that Stallard had finished second in the race that was the climax of the film.

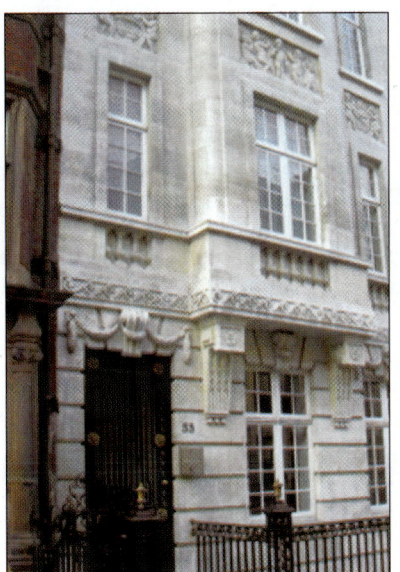

Early in the war, Elisabeth and Harold bought a house on Harley Street from Mr. Henry Stallard, a surgeon also working at Moorfields Hospital. Stallard was extremely well known throughout Britain as a long distance runner and became immortalized in the movie "Chariots of Fire." It turns out he was considered to be an expert in eye surgery at the time and wrote a famous text on this topic. He never did become a real fan of Ridley and the IOL, although in his book he did give honest and adequate time and space to this topic.

It is not known why Stallard left his very pleasant townhouse at 53 Harley Street, but Harold moved in and remained there in this house until his retirement from the hospital and the National Health Service.

CHAPTER 3

Harley Street is well known worldwide as the street where many physicians and other professonials established offices and visiting rooms ("rooms" is the English equivalent as to what we term office in America).

TOP LEFT: Just 10 numbers north of Harold, on the same side of the street is 63 Harley Street, is the former home of Sir Stewart Duke-Elder. He had, many years ago, done extensive renovations on his home, including some use of the art nouveau (deco) style, which was in vogue years ago.

TOP RIGHT: The luminaries on the street included Prime Minister Gladstone.

BOTTOM: Florence Nightingale lived just a few addresses down Harley Street.

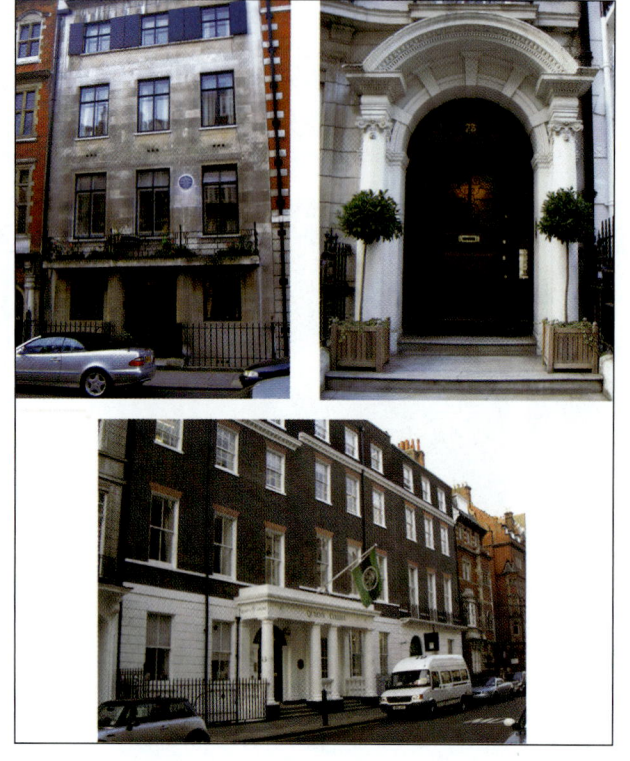

Henry Stallard was not a supporter of Harold's later invention of the IOL, almost surely in part because of his association with Duke-Elder at Moorfields. Several important personages were Harold's neighbors on this street, an address that was renowned because of its being home and rooms of some of the most important figures in London, ranging from numerous physicians' practices to politicians and others.

None were more important in Harold's life than his neighbor at 63 Harley Street, Sir Stewart Duke-Elder (see photo at left). Duke-Elder was a major nemesis of Harold following the invention of the IOL. Another vocal foe was Derrick Vail of Chicago, a close friend of Duke-Elder's—so close that he died in the latter's home during one of his many visits.

Harold retired from Moorfields in 1971—a retirement that was officially prescribed in the medical system in which he worked but was not fully voluntary or very amicable.

The formal photograph recording Harold's retirement from Moorfields Eye Hospital in 1971. Harold sits in the front row, 3rd from the left.

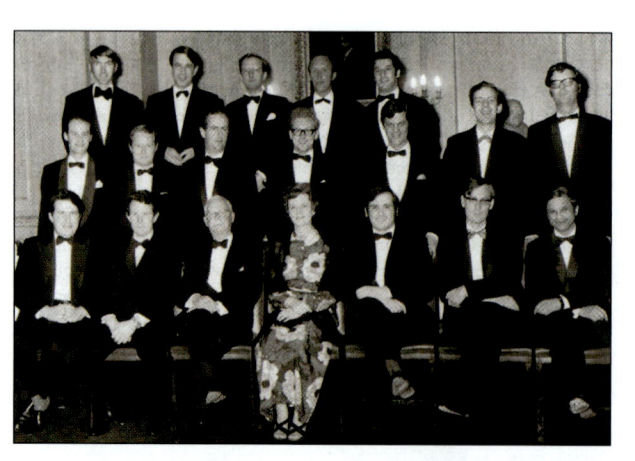

It turned out that following his invention of the IOL, he was not well-accepted by some of his colleagues at Moorfields (or at St. Thomas'), and Harold privately and correctly felt that he was being "put out to pasture"—a belief that he noted in his private papers that I have reviewed.

Thereafter, he sold his home in London and moved his wife to Keeper's Cottage in Stapleford, near Salisbury. By that time, the children were grown. It was in this charming cottage purchased in 1950 to use as weekend lodging and for fishing (angling) that, in 1985, we began our long collaboration and friendship that lasted until his death in 2003. This was the beginning of the period where I devoted a major portion of my professional time to 1) continuous scientific studies and analyses of IOLs that were intended to help avoid complications of implants and 2) to help assure that Harold received appropriate credit for the many things he had done.

ROOTS OF A MODEST GIANT OF SCIENCE

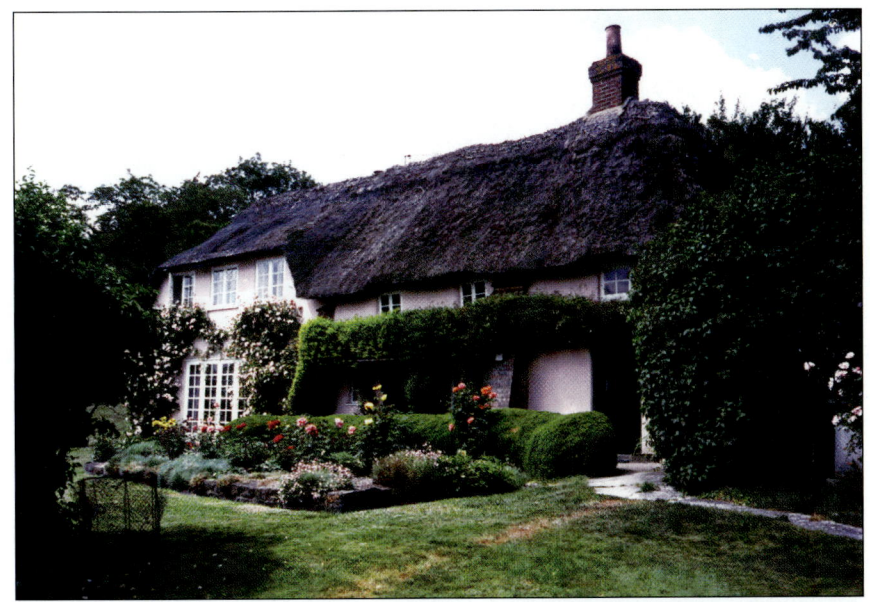

Like so many of us who should retire before we do, it turns out that Harold's retirement was probably a blessing in disguise. It almost forced him to start using the small cottage that he had bought many years ago as a vacation home and site for fishing (angling). Now he had the opportunity to live there full time, which he soon began to savor. These are the years when I really began to know and work with him, and these were the years when I noted the transition in his personality from one requiring antidepressants to a happy, self-fulfilled man.

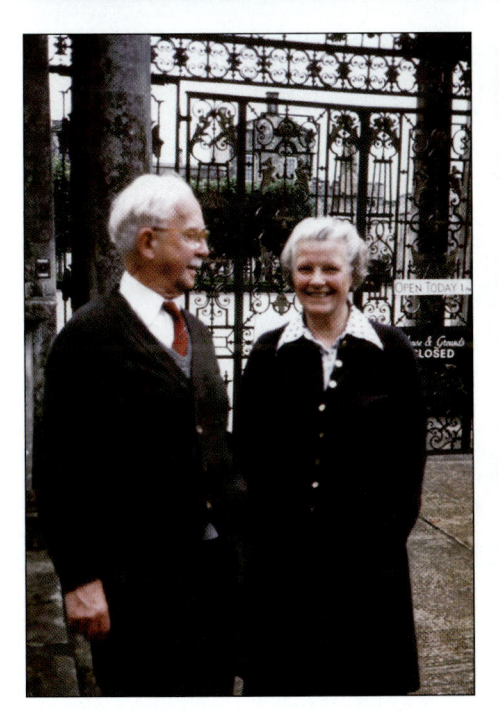

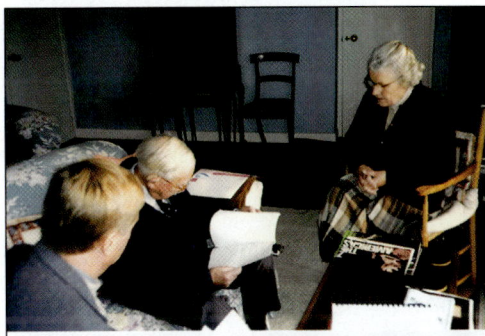

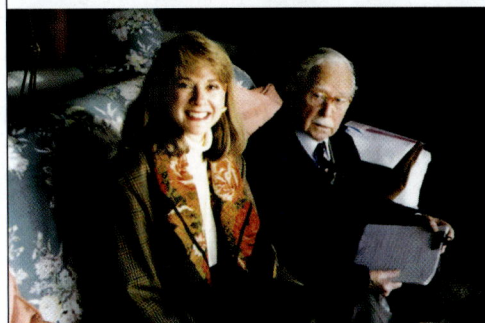

LEFT: The Ridleys' home in Stapleford was very close to one of the famous English majestic homes that we all read about or sometimes have the opportunity to visit—in this case Wilton House, the site where Elisabeth and Harold actually took me during my initial visit to their region near Salisbury.

TOP RIGHT: Harold and I literally spent hours with pages strewn all over his home and furniture. We collected an immense amount of data, especially from our river walks and other chats, that has allowed me to function as his official biographer and to create this text.

BOTTOM RIGHT: Ann joined me on all of my trips to see Harold after our marriage.

Maps of London and England showing important locations from Harold's life can be found in the Appendix of this book.

I was an eight-year-old schoolboy in 1949, when Harold performed his landmark operation.
LEFT: David Apple (born September 14, 1941).
RIGHT: Harold Ridley (born July 10, 1906, died May 25, 2001).

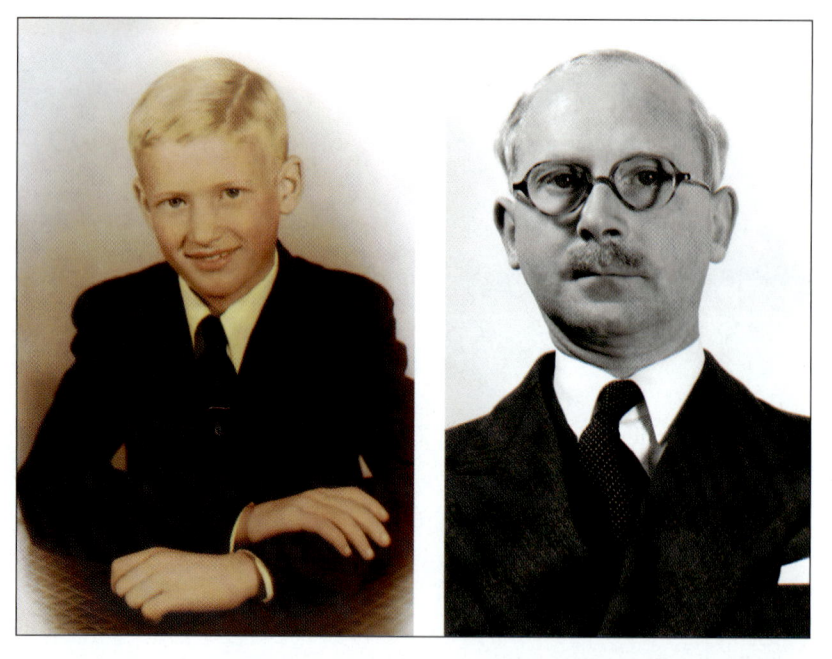

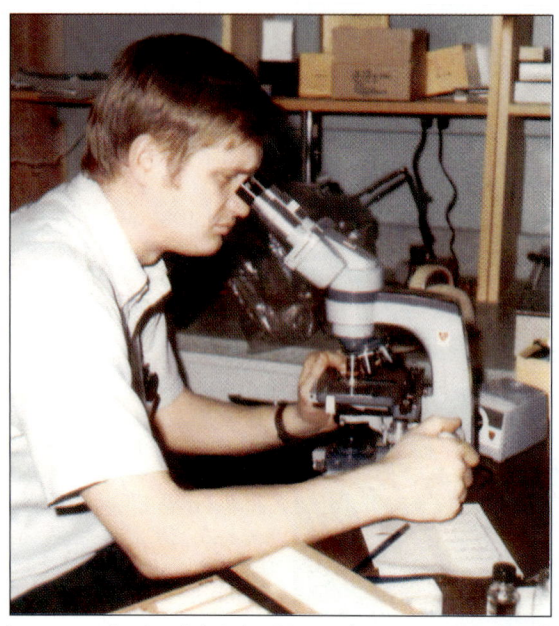

I was recruited to Salt Lake City, to the University of Utah in 1980. It was my goal to establish an ocular pathology laboratory and to set up an eye research facility. Upon my arrival, the laboratory consisted of a small microscope. My past research efforts were in the field of retinal laser photocoagulation (especially treatment of diabetic retinopathy), studies on tumors of the eye, research on congenital malformations affecting the eye, and several other conditions. I had done extensive cataract surgery for a two-year period, just about the time that many surgeons were transitioning from aphakic spectacles to IOLs, but had very little laboratory experience with the IOL. In those days the majority of cataract operations were still accomplished using aphakic (thick) spectacles, and IOLs were just beginning, my timing seemed to be perfect; a new era was about to begin.

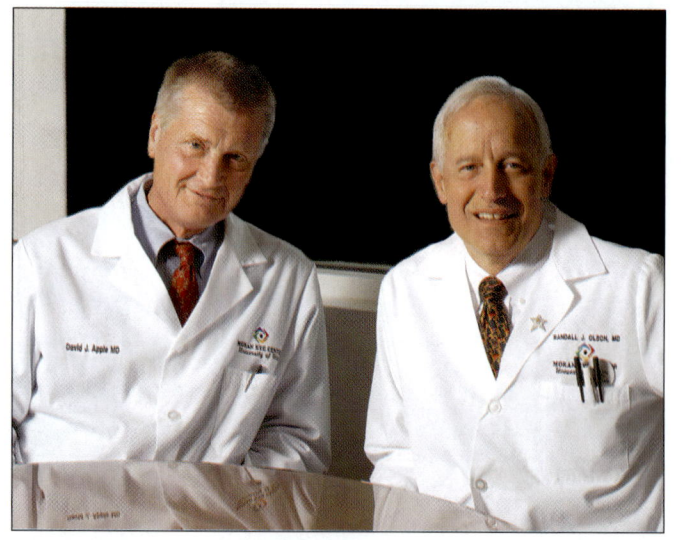

In 1980, Dr. David Apple (left) and Dr. Randall J. Olsen (right) founded the Center for Intraocular Lens Research in Salt Lake City. Dr. Apple moved to South Carolina in 1988 and returned to Utah in 2002 after the onset of an illness in 1996, which began to worsen in 1999. Dr. Randall Olson, a Utah native, had just returned to Salt Lake City from his fellowship training. He had assumed the chairmanship, and I was one of the first faculty members he recruited. He already had some interest in the field of IOL complications.

4

"David, Mr. Ridley Wants to Meet You"

I was an 8-year-old schoolboy when Harold performed his landmark operation in November 1949. Little did I know, of course, that 35 years later I would visit Elisabeth and him and that we would become close friends. As cliché as it may sound, it was not long before I began to regard him as a genuine hero. I couldn't have possibly guessed that I would thereafter dedicate much of my career to researching and helping him advance his innovation in eye surgery.

Why, where, when, and how did I meet the Ridleys? To explain this requires some comments about myself—a mini autobiography. This is difficult for me to write, but as they say, "It ain't bragging if you really done it."

JULY 1980 TO MAY 1989: ARRIVAL TO A NEW JOB

Instead of starting at my birth in 1941 and progressing through my childhood, schooling, and medical training, let us cut to the chase and fast forward to 1980 to some of the events that brought the Ridleys and me together, and initiated the beginning of the "second half" of my medical career.

I was 39 years old and enjoying a successful career as a practicing ophthalmologist and a pathologist—an unusual combination. I specialized in research on eye diseases and had been recruited to Salt Lake City, Utah to work in a very young, embryonic ophthalmology department at the University of Utah. Our working area consisted of 4 or 5 rooms off a hallway in the main university hospital. Dr. Randall Olson had just assumed the chairmanship of the department. The eye pathology laboratory, such as it was, was located in the basement and consisted of an administrative assistant with her telephone and word processor and me with my

CHAPTER 4

microscope. Later, I was able to have a young lady named Tina Yates who did much of the complicated technical work required for the procedures needed to bring specimens to the microscope for analysis. I had learned a long time earlier that the leader of the team, in this case myself as director of the laboratory, is only as good as the workers under his or her leadership. I am forever grateful to all of those colleagues—and I mean colleagues—who have done so much for me since the early days of my career in Chicago in the early 1970s and continuing now in my present situation.

For several months after my arrival, all was quiet. Well, not quite! Two events that were important in the history of medicine at the University of Utah occurred. The university had long been a center of research in the field of biomaterial sciences and devices. This had its origin in part in the work of the Dutch physician, Dr. Willem Kolff (born 1911), the inventor of the artificial kidney. I learned much from his work. By the time I had arrived in Utah, there was a brilliant biomaterials team led by Dr. Joseph Andrade. The cardiovascular surgery team had also been well-established and a world-famous operation from this group, the implantation of the artificial heart—the Jarvik-7, which was designed by Dr. Robert Jarvik and implanted by Dr. William De Vries, was performed on December 1, 1982. Barney Clark, DDS, was a brave volunteer who sadly only lived 112 days with the artificial heart.

My dual specialization came in very handy at that time. Mr. Clark developed postoperative problems and I saw him clinically while he was in the hospital. After he unfortunately passed away, I put on my other hat as a pathologist and had the opportunity to examine tissue from his diseased heart muscle as well as other tissues.

The experience I had working in an environment where people were discussing such things as "artificial devices, various biomaterials such as polyesters, plastics, pumps, donor tissue, etc" provided a new vocabulary and horizon for me and no doubt helped prepare me for new adventures in the nascent field of biomedical engineering. I had no idea that the knowledge gained from these experiences would soon be applied!

After a flurry of activity surrounding the heart operation, it was quiet again and we then focused on outfitting our laboratory. All was tranquil. Then, in the summer of 1981, a specimen was mailed to my laboratory from Eugene, Oregon. It was an explanted (removed) IOL. A surgeon in Oregon had implanted it. Multiple postoperative complications related to the IOL had ensued after the implantation. The eye itself was severely damaged and the patient had lost most of his vision in the eye with the IOL. When the complications first began to affect the patient's vision, he consulted a second surgeon, Dr. John Lyman. Dr. Lyman then discussed the case with Dr. Howard Fine, one of the more prominent eye surgeons in the world and the writer of a Foreword of this book. They both agreed that the IOL needed to be removed. Dr. Lyman did the procedure and, upon Dr. Howard Fine's recommendation, sent the IOL to us in Utah in order to somehow analyze what might have caused all of the problems. I labeled it IOL #1 in my laboratory log book.

I knew little about laboratory analysis of IOLs at that time, so I went to work to learn as much about them as was possible from the scant literature that was available. I spent a lot of time studying the explanted specimen, using my basic microscope and other techniques to which a pathologist normally has access, plus a few that aren't normally used on a day-to-day basis. I was soon able to identify and catalogue several of the complications that had been caused by the IOL and other associated surgical complications in this single case alone. The details of these are far beyond the scope of this text but are described in the original article that we subsequently published in the

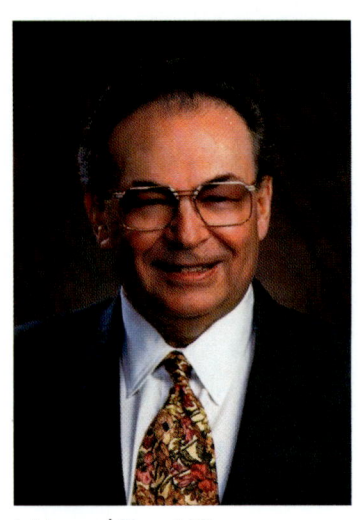

I. Howard Fine, MD.

journal *Ophthalmology* (Vol. 91, pp. 403-419, 1984), which is the official journal of the American Academy of Ophthalmology. In this article, we described the complications and also provided some proposals as to how the surgeon might prevent or manage them in the future. I was very surprised that the journal editors reviewed and accepted the submitted manuscript and photographs with only a few request for revisions, criticisms, or other delays that were usually associated with submissions of this type.

It was almost as if the journal editors were *overly* anxious for the paper to be published. I found out later that they indeed may have been. For the first time, I became aware of the anti-IOL sentiment that Ridley had endured for years and which he and I, as we would soon be working together, would encounter for the next two decades. The two senior editors of the journal, both members of the "academic establishment," were strongly against IOLs. They saw our paper as a golden opportunity to publicize severe and apparently negative findings and illustrate, using the black and white and color photographs we had enclosed, the unpleasant lesions (blood, tissue erosions, destructions, and more) and the litany of complications we had described. There was no collusion intended; they were simply and honestly against IOLs. They had long expected complications to occur with what they and many colleagues believed was a "time bomb." They believed that our report was proof of that. Their intention was to take advantage of our findings to convince their readership that Harold's artificial lenses may not be the way to go. They believed that the publication of such negative images would help drive IOLs off the market.

On the contrary, I believe that our article was an example of what a pathologist should do. A pathologist's duty is to perform a study on tissues or even do autopsies in fatal cases in which it is necessary to understand the cause and effect regarding maladies of any type including the cause of death in fatal cases. What I did was simply an "autopsy of an IOL"—in this case postmortem examination of IOL #1. I have continued to do this over the years with the IOLs the we have acquired in the laboratory. After completing the tissue study, we would report the results to the surgeon who had removed the lens. They were then often able to take corrective measures. This cooperation between the pathologist and the surgeon forms the basis of what we call *"clinicopathological correlation,"* a good technique to provide communication between the specialists.

The IOL #1 article gave the readers of the journal, most of whom were practitioners who did cataract surgery and would like to use IOLs, an opportunity to read and apply our laboratory findings to what they encountered in their operating rooms. It became clear that many of the problems seen were not just related to the IOL, but were also related to variations in the surgical techniques that needed to be modified. Based on the laboratory findings, surgeons were able to reduce the incidence of at least some of

A publication with the very complicated title, as documented here, was one of the first reports regarding complications of IOLs. An explanted (removed) IOL was removed from a patient's eye because of multiple complications, and it was sent to our facility to see if a pathological analysis could elucidate some of the causes. It was obvious, even at first glance, that the implant had become markedly opaque, one of a myriad number of complications we observed and reported. Once this case was published with an explanation of how one might prevent such findings, it was read by many surgeons who benefited greatly and were, therefore, able to enhance the quality of their surgery and achieve better results with their patients.

Without getting too technical, we found that some of the components of the IOL (termed "loop") in this diagram had been misplaced when implanted in the eye and caused excessive pressure on tissues with erosion, which set in place a cycle of adverse complications. It was easy to observe this with the tools of the pathologist, and it soon became obvious that such pathological analyses were very beneficial in helping decrease the incidence of complications of implants, thus opening new possibilities for improved results in cataract surgery. The lens that we described in this photograph and on the previous page was labeled IOL #1, based on the chronology of excision in the laboratory. By the turn of the new millennium, the number of such specimens has increased to over 19,000.

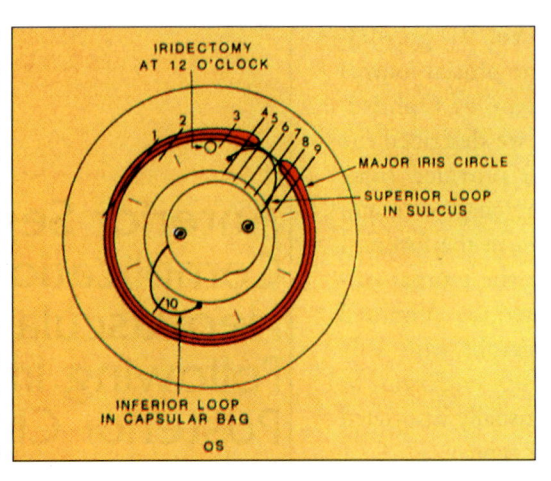

the complications.

The follow-up was gratifying. By this time, much of the "nonmedical, political" opposition to Ridley's IOL by naysayers was being answered. Physicians were beginning to have greater confidence in both the safety and efficacy of IOLs and in their ability to prevent or manage complications that occurred. The number of IOL implants, which had remained abysmally low since Ridley's beginning in 1949, began to skyrocket (see page 11).

By far the most important finding and recommendation that came from our report on IOL #1 was that after the opaque cataractous lens is removed, it is best to place the artificial lens (IOL) back to the site where the crystalline lens had originally been situated. Note in the figure on this page that one supporting "loop" (haptic) has been placed into the "sulcus" and the other "loop" (haptic) has been placed into the "capsular bag." Without explaining the terminology, suffice it to say that the correct way of doing this would have been to place both loops into the "capsular bag." Almost all surgeons accept this method today. However, it was not a forgone conclusion in those early years. The "capsular bag" is that structure that remains after the cataractous lens material is removed. The empty space is surrounded by the residual lens capsule (page 94). Placement of the IOL in the capsular bag is analogous to packing a commercial product into a tight cellophane-like wrapping, a process termed "shrink wrapping" (eg, the sealing of a music CD or DVD in a tight package). By doing so, the complications began to melt away and the number of satisfied patients grew. Each satisfied patient would talk to his or her close relatives, friends, etc, and as they sought treatment, the growth of the IOL procedure increased in an exponential pattern (page 11). Many early pioneers of IOLs had also recommended this type of fixation, including Harold himself and several surgeons from Holland and the surrounding low countries, who turned out to be remarkably advanced with the technique. However, our study on IOL #1 was the first showing that this was the best method. As Jack P. Strong, MD, my professor of pathology in New Orleans, used to say, "One cannot argue with the autopsy findings. They represent the final referee."

My own career was impacted dramatically by IOL #1. Almost immediately, the IOL #1 publication triggered an absolute deluge of submissions of such cases to our laboratory; this became the main focus of my research career. I soon had no time to do anything else. I had to forgo all opportunities to return to clinical practice and doing surgery again. The research and teaching projects that ensued thereafter were simply more important. The focus on research on IOLs has remained the priority, although we have added glaucoma devices, ophthalmic lasers, and other artificial prostheses to our field of study. In 2006, we celebrated the 25th year of service of the "David J. Apple, MD Laboratory," celebrated at a dinner in Chicago at the annual meeting of the American Academy of Ophthalmology. It was organized by one of my loyal Apple Korps team members, Dr. Guy Kleinmann of Tel Aviv, Israel.

After completing the publication of that first IOL case report, my students, colleagues, and I moved quickly to IOL #2 and the many specimens that were beginning to pour in. Our findings from many cases allowed us to more fully catalogue the various IOLs and other complications and to write a monograph on the topic. The monograph, entitled *Complications of IOLs: A Historical and Histopathological Review,* was published in the *Survey of Ophthalmology,* Vol. 29, pp 1-54, 1984. It proved to be even more helpful to the practitioner because it was more comprehensive than the single case reported with IOL #1.

The success of this article turned out to be beyond my wildest dreams. Many of the lens manufacturers purchased it in bulk quantities and distributed it to customers and colleagues. It was one of the most reprinted and read articles in eye literature.

In effect, we had created a new subspecialty in the field of eye research and treatments. More accurately we had made a subspecialty from a subspecialty derived from still another subspecialty. In other words, 1) eye (ocular) pathology is a subspecialty of clinical ophthalmology and 2) IOL *pathology* is a subspecialty of eye pathology. Hyperspecialization has become especially important as other fields of organ/tissue/prosthesis. Transplantations have evolved (eg, heart transplants, kidney transplants, and cardiac pace makers).

Since receiving IOL #1, the laboratory has received over 19,000 IOL-related cases. Many are still waiting additional detailed analysis. The deluge slowed during my illness but has not abated. I look forward to continuing work in the future and my goal is to train young colleagues to move in and take my place after I retire. This is even more important today than in the "old days" because the devices in question are getting more complicated and will require more and more oversight.

As we moved forward in Utah, even with the newfound credibility IOLs were gaining, the antagonism toward them was still strong in some sectors and among some well-placed professionals in our field. We even felt the effects of this antagonism in our laboratory for some time. For example, in 1984 we applied to the federal granting agency that today is known as the *National Eye Institute* for a research grant to help support us during the early phases of our studies on the complications of IOLs. It was a good application that was worthy of funding. Indeed, it was given a positive ranking, but to our surprise and disappointment, it was turned down! Two separate referees made two noteworthy statements as they reviewed our application. These two were no doubt highly reputable and respected members of the "medical establishment." They were critical of our proposal because 1) they felt that we would never have enough specimens to study IOL complications, which obviously was a very erroneous assumption on their part, given the reality of the above-mentioned 11,000 specimens we have received, not to mention experimental animals, and 2) a more damning criticism from the reviewers claimed that there was a strong chance that *IOLs would not be accepted,* that they would not succeed clinically and would not remain a viable, useful means of treatment. This assertion, which seems incredulous and incredible today, was made as late as 1985!

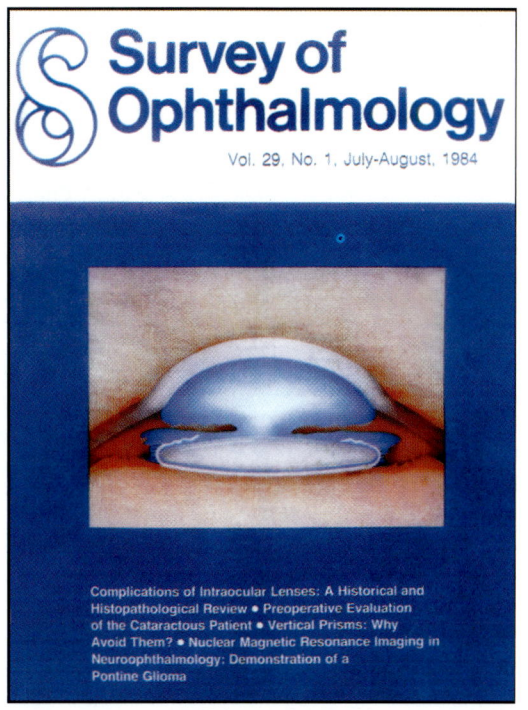

Following the publication of the first IOL (IOL #1), we collected many more cases and were able to put together a monograph that cataloged findings of many clinical cases. These cases allowed us to understand the clinical behavior of this relatively new innovation, and the information contained in the monograph entitled "Complications of Intraocular Lenses" was disseminated widely with very positive results for surgeons and their patients.

CHAPTER 4

In retrospect, the grant rejection turned out to be a blessing in disguise. Left with limited options, we turned to the IOL manufacturers—the companies that fabricated the lenses—to provide funding to continue our work. Some of these companies (listed alphabetically) included Advanced Medical Optics (AMO), Allergen, Bausch and Lomb, Cooper Vision, Hoya, Johnson and Johnson (IOLab), Nestle (Alcon), Pfizer, Pharmacia, Staar Surgical, and Rayner & Keeler, Ltd. The latter company was, of course, the manufacturer of Harold's original IOL. The agreements we made with these and other companies were beneficial to all concerned. The research and IOL analyses helped the companies make better and safer products and that became even more beneficial to patients worldwide as time passed. The companies' support helped us to continue our research. In effect, this type of arrangement represented a type of symbiosis that was mutually beneficial to all parties, thus creating a new model that was not routinely used until that era. Today, such affiliations of researchers and industry are becoming more and more commonplace.

What has all of this to do with the question, "Why, where, when, and how did I meet the Ridleys?" The answer is everything!

SUMMER, 1985: A SUMMONS TO VISIT MR. RIDLEY, THE "BAD BOY WHO DARED PUT FORIEGN BODIES INTO THE EYE"

For my first four years in Utah I was able to enjoy Utah's wonderful environment, a mecca for skiers. I skied 40 or more times each year for the first few years. But, the new efforts with IOLs changed everything; I could no longer spare that much time. Not long after the two previously mentioned publications appeared in early 1985, I received a message from England. It seems that two ophthalmologists who were close friends and professional colleagues of Harold and who obviously knew of the difficulties he was having with many naysayers regarding his ground-breaking work with IOLs had told him about our research and results. I was later informed that his colleagues had told him that there was an "American guy" whose research writings seemed to confirm what he had been trying to tell all who would listen for decades. I was never told who these two individuals were, but my guess is that they may have been John Pearce and Peter Choyce. We will never know for sure since they are both now deceased. Fortunately, based on their recommendations, Harold forwarded me an invitation to visit him during my next trip to England.

I was dumbfounded. After all, I was a relatively young ophthalmologist and researcher living in the mountains and beauty of Utah—ostensibly far removed from the centers of academia that in general seemed to be situated in American's costal regions. To be summoned to visit this man, who by then (in 1985) I had realized from my brief work in the field was destined to become one of the world's greatest innovators of this specialty, was a completely unexpected surprise and honor.

My next planned trip to Europe was set for the summer of 1985 (see Preface). Therefore, after finishing some meetings in Europe, it goes without saying that I made it a point to schedule an additional flight to London. From there, I then transferred and boarded a train to Salisbury, the famous and beautiful old cathedral city in Wiltshire. As I exited the train station in Salisbury, I laid eyes on Harold Ridley for the first time just outside the gate; he was standing alone and had a forlorn appearance about him. He had driven approximately 5 to 6 miles from his cottage in his burgundy-colored auto to fetch me at the station. He had never seen me before (he probably had no photograph), but somehow his recognition of me was immediate. We shook hands and chatted for a few minutes, and I had no doubt whatsoever that we were soon to become friends. However, I also had no doubt that something was wrong. It became clear to me from his visage that he was concerned, if not indeed very depressed. It was during this visit that I vowed to help do something about that.

He drove me to his home at Keeper's Cottage, his 16th-century thatched roof structure situated on the edge of the tiny village of Stapleford, just a few miles north of Salisbury and not far from the world-famous monument of Stonehenge. Elisabeth's and Harold's cottage was named after the person who was assigned by the original landowner(s) to act as the warden or overseer—to watch over or "keep." The "keeper" would have the responsibility of guarding and maintaining the surrounding property, including the adjacent River Wyle and its stock of fish. Harold had purchased it years before his retirement.

As we drove into his driveway, I was amazed by the beauty of this cottage and the adjacent River Wyle (in reality a stream). His wife was in the yard and appeared grateful that I had come. Almost immediately, on a personal level, Harold had become like a father to me and I know that they both had good feelings about me. In my mind, I felt that ours was about to become the type of relationship described in the book *Tuesdays With Morrie* by Mitch Albom.

After that initial visit, I made it a point to visit Harold and Elisabeth at least 3 times a year, alone during the years between 1985 and 1995 and then joined by my wife after our marriage in 1995. These visits occurred consistently with few exceptions until Harold's death in 2003. We remained dear friends until the end. One of my fellows, Dr. John Sims, and his mother Margaret also visited Harold and Elisabeth.

The following letter, written on July 23, 1986, just after his 80th birthday and about a year after I first met him, exemplifies how our relationship grew both on the scientific/clinical level as well as on a more human level. Note in the letter how he looked back to those early years when he was designated as "the bad boy who dared put foreign bodies into the eye." I myself was of course touched anytime he mentioned kind things about my work and how it was so helpful to him.

Keeper's Cottage
Stapleford
Salisbury SP3 4LT
23 July 86

Dear David,

I am quite overwhelmed by your kindness and generosity just in remembering my 80th birthday and then by this morning's post sending more fishing things. I particularly want to thank you not only for all these but for the care which you, almost alone, have taken to read and study my early papers on implants. I am delighted that you understand the honesty of my reports of complications. Implants were a scientific project from the start and none of those who were the pioneers made any money, unlike many of our successors in England and elsewhere. The granting of my FRS (Fellow of the Royal Society) has greatly pleased me for it is not easy to "Advance Natural Knowledge" (1640 terminology) in practical surgery. There are at present only two other British surgeons who are in the Royal Society.

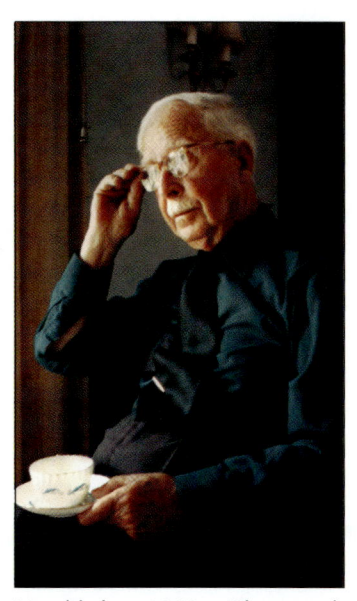

Harold, late 1990s. (Photograph courtesy of Dr. John Sims.)

CHAPTER 4

On July 25, I am to be awarded a gold medal, the Galen Medal for Therapeutics by the Worshipful Society of Apothecaries of London (1614) which is another high honor. Anyway the sentiment for intraocular implants is at last good after many years in which I suffered greatly for being the bad boy who dared to put foreign bodies in the eye. I had 100 wonderful letters about the FRS which have greatly improved my morale at long last.

It will be a great pleasure for both of us if you can come to our little house here again and I look forward to seeing a copy of your book which ought to be really useful to all implant surgeons. It is an honour to me to be a contributor. How I wish all this had happened in my active years when I could have made full use of your work. Anyway it is a joy to us to have a friend in Utah.

With my thanks again to the Apple Korps (author's note: the designation given to the young research students, fellows and colleagues I have worked with over the years, ca. 210 individuals between 1968 and 2006).

With best wishes from Elisabeth and myself to you. Yours ever,
Harold

P.S. What remarkable country you have in Utah. Sincerely, Harold

The book he mentioned was our 1989 text on IOLs that summarized our work up to that time (see page 74). He told me later that this was the book he consulted when choosing an IOL for his own eye.

Professionally, my relationship with Harold allowed me to use the talents I had been given to help stimulate a continuing forward movement of his invention. The most important contributions were to help identify the best means, which thus far had eluded surgeons—including Harold himself—to avoid some of the serious complications of the ever-improving cataract IOL operation that had been plaguing surgeons.

It was during these visits that we put together two handwritten agreements. One was related to the preparation of this book. It stipulated that I would become Harold's official biographer. The other agreement was related to his very sincere and humane desire that I would refrain from publicizing and personalizing the many relentless attacks on his clinical judgment and professional integrity. Though these had been extremely painful for him and had, in fact, led to several episodes of severe depression, he requested that I not make them public, at least while he lived. After his death, he said, I would be free to use my own judgment on these matters. In this latter request, he was giving me a message to not dwell negatively on the past, but to tell his story in a straightforward and positive way.

That is how it began. I was 39 when I came to Utah and was 44 at the time I began meeting with Harold. That marked the turning point in my career, a definite shift of emphasis and direction. It was a shift that I was excited to make because it represented an opportunity to participate in a transition in our specialty that helped usher in what all agree was to become a *second golden age in ophthalmology and the visual sciences* (second to the first golden age that occurred mainly in Europe between 1871 and 1914).

"DAVID, MR. RIDLEY WANTS TO MEET YOU"

From the Old Country to America's Heartland, My Ancestors, Origins, Childhood, and Medical Training (1941–1985)

My mother's ancestors came from Anderbeck, a small village in Germany founded in 1086. The village is situated in the north central region of Germany, in the present state of Sachen-Anhalt, not far from its provincial capital city, Magdeburg, which

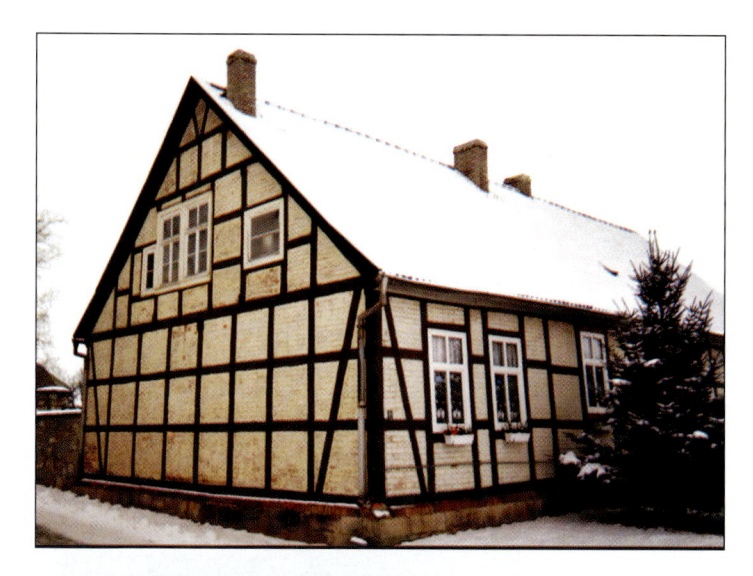

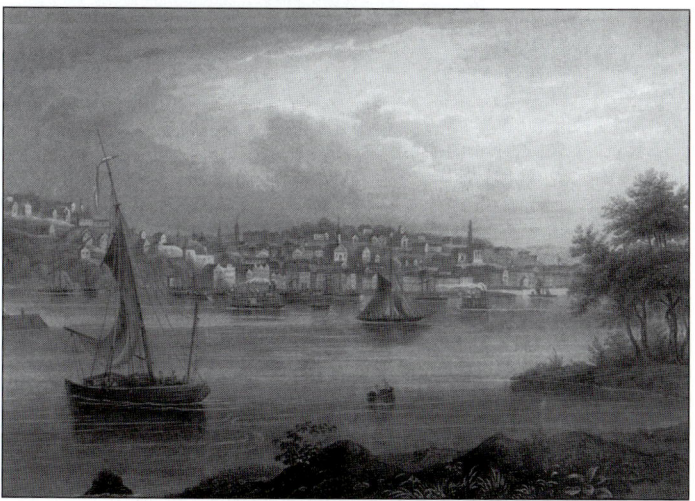

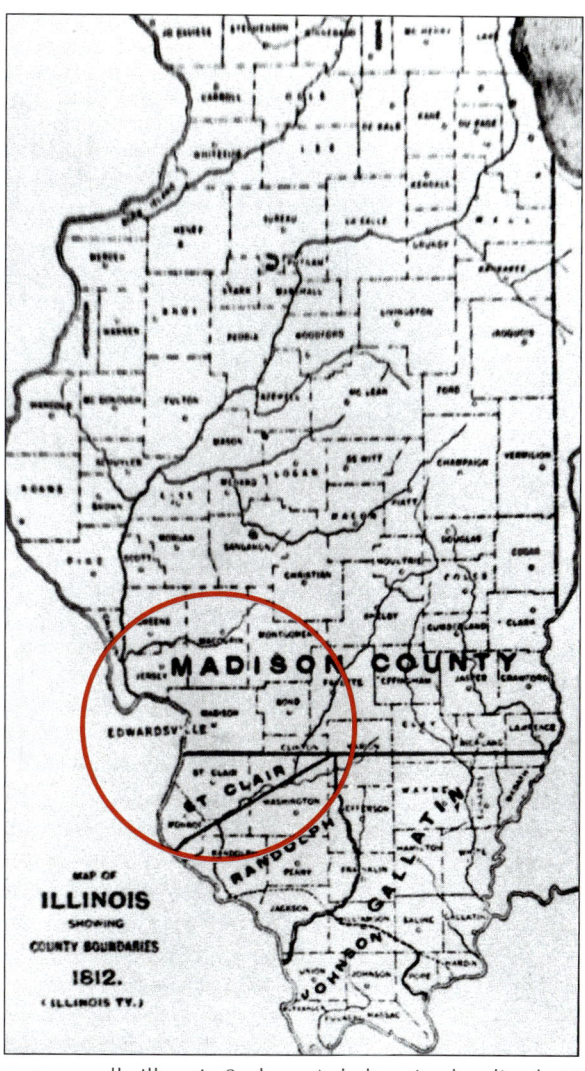

Some of my ancestors were of German origin, and I have traced them to a very small village in Sachsen-Anhalt, a tiny locality that I could not find on most maps and, indeed, was unheard of until the reopening of the Berlin Wall in the 1990s. It was a 1000-year-old village named Anderbeck, located just a few miles west of Berlin. Most of my relatives came to the United States during a period of revolutionary uprisings in 1848 to 1849. Most settled in the midwest because the climate and general conditions were not unlike the old country. LEFT: Typical architecture of the region.
RIGHT: Most of my ancestors from both sides of the family clustered in settlements in Illinois, south of Chicago (red circle) and not far from St. Louis where the Mississippi and Missouri rivers come together. This represented a region that was very rich in American history and, undoubtedly, had a great influence on my being very interested in history.

CHAPTER 4

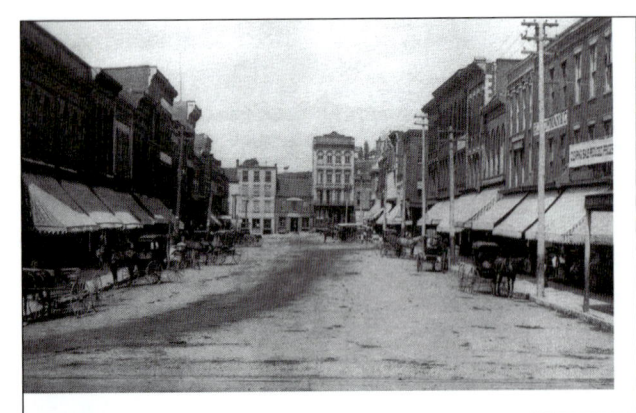

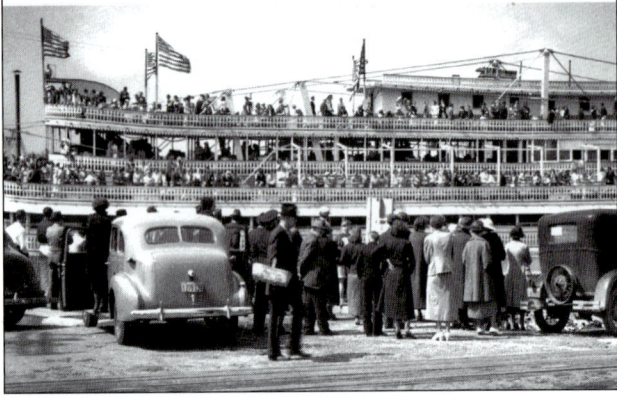

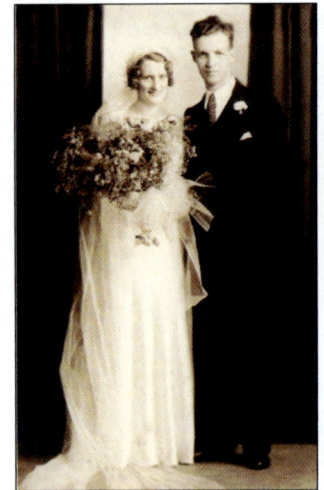

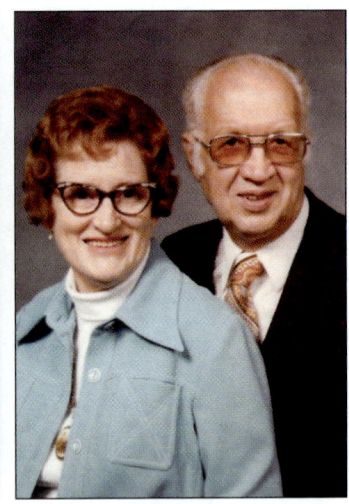

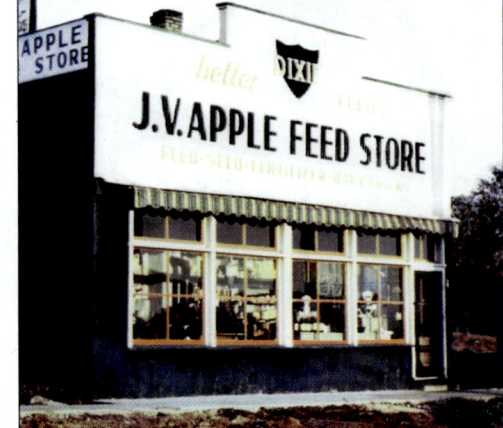

ABOVE: I was born in Alton, Illinois, a small town on the Mississippi River near St. Louis, Missouri that in fact was for a short period in its early history as large as or even larger than St. Louis. It had a beautiful location on the bluffs alongside of the Mississippi River and was the site where Lewis and Clark camped prior to beginning their famous exploration of the West in 1801.

Alton was a typical midwestern river town and was well-known to Samuel Clemens (Mark Twain), who grew up in Hannibal, Missouri, just a few miles up the river, and became famous as a river pilot and as the author of the *Adventures of Huckleberry Finn* and many other great stories.

TOP CENTER: My father, Joseph B. Apple, married my mother, Margaret Bearden in 1934. Both were attending college at a small institution in Alton at the time of their meeting. The parents of the author on their wedding day.

TOP RIGHT: My parents later in life. Their main focus during their later years, especially after my brother had passed away, was to assist me as I made my way through life and entered medicine.

BOTTOM RIGHT: I worked at my father's feed store for many years.

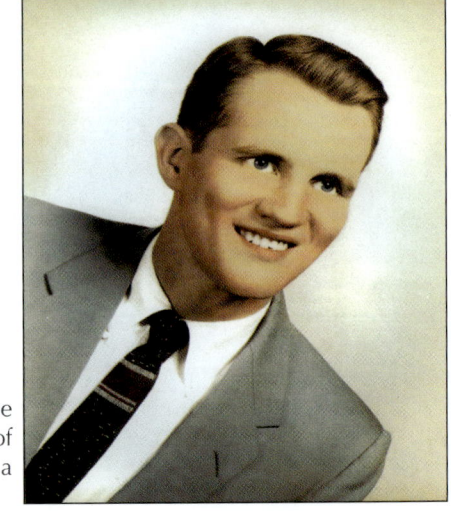

My brother, Bob, passed away from heart problems at the young age of 57. He was a graduate of the University of California at Berkeley and worked most of his adult life as a social worker.

in turn is not far from Berlin. Most members of the German line of my family were driven from Europe during the widespread outbreaks of revolution that occurred in 1848–1849. Other ancestral family members came from England and Scotland. They virtually all settled in the Midwest of the United States. Most of the male members of these families fought on the Northern (Union) side in the American Civil War (see page 64).

I was born in Alton, IL, on September 14, 1941, the second son of Margaret Josephine Bearden and Joseph Bernard Apple. My middle name "Joseph" was derived from portions of both of their names. My parents had grown up during the sad years of the depression of the 1930s. My older brother Robert was born in May 1937. My parents were capable, honest people who had a marked influence on my life. My father owned a feed store. He was actually rejected from military service in World War II because his job was deemed to be of strategic importance in feeding the nation. I worked in the store in my childhood, starting with no pay, then gradually increasing to 15¢ per hour, then 25¢ per hour. I owe my strong work ethic to my father. My mother, a schoolteacher, and my brother introduced me to books and the arts, especially music (see photo at right). My mother was also clearly the major influence in my decision to go into medicine. She and her family were also responsible for planting and nurturing in me an intense love of music, which has continued on throughout my life.

My brother Bob, a social worker, had attended the University of Kentucky and the University of California at Berkeley. He was a very intelligent and cultured man who taught me an immense amount about life and I will forever be grateful to him for all that he had done for me. Sadly, he died of a cardiomyopathy at the relatively young age of 57. In the United States, this condition is well-known as a malady that occasionally afflicts otherwise "healthy" individuals (eg, some otherwise healthy athletes such as basketball players. Several have been known to collapse and die while playing on the court).

History and Heroes

Some friends questioned me as to why I was writing about heroes who are, at first glance, seemingly unrelated to Harold Ridley. I was also asked what Abraham Lincoln had to do with an eye doctor, apart from the fact that Lincoln indeed had a disease that not infrequently effected the eyes, Marfan's syndrome. Actually, I believe these connections are very important. Without the images and insights gathered during the early years of my life in this region of the American midwest, a land area no greater than perhaps 90 miles by 90 miles, I would not have developed the insight to have had the strong admiration of Harold that I did. I saw him not just as a doctor, but also as a genuine hero. This caused me to connect with him and to provide all in my power and mind that I could to help ensure the positive outcomes described in this book.

I grew up at the confluence of the Mississippi and Missouri rivers, scarcely 2 miles from their junction. The region where Illinois borders Missouri is rich in American history. Undoubtedly, my passion for history and my love of great heroes stems from having grown up in such a region; a fact that may help explain my later intense admiration for Harold.

Abraham Lincoln lived in and around Springfield, IL, just 90 miles away from where I grew up. General Ulysses S. Grant was stationed in St. Louis, less than a few

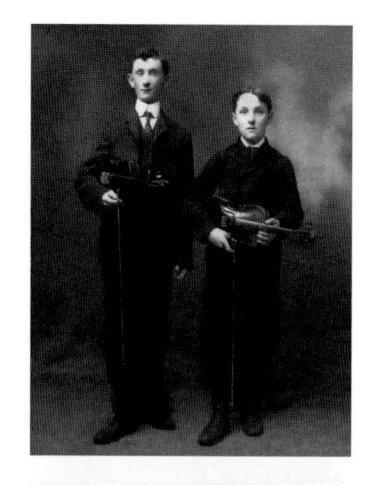

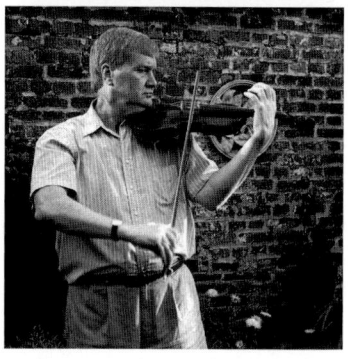

Both my mother and members of her side of the family as well as my brother had a strong influence on my love of classical music, which remains ingrained in me today.
TOP: My mother's father (my grandfather Bearden) and her younger brother John were excellent string players.
BOTTOM: I also was and am a string player, no doubt not so excellent.

CHAPTER 4

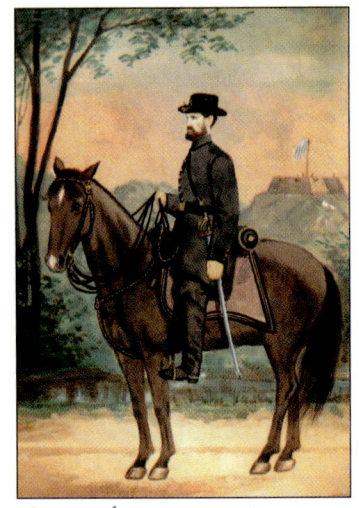

Many of my ancestors were engaged in the American Civil War and fought on the Northern side under Lincoln and his military protégé, Ulysses Grant. My great, great, great grandfather, shown here, died at age 22 in the Battle of Shiloh. Throughout my entire childhood, I heard tales of all of these people who had done so much to settle our country, and it is no doubt they developed from day one a marked sense and understanding of history. This certainly has carried on to the present in my great feelings about Harold, who in his own way represents as much of a hero as the great national figures such as Lincoln, Grant, and many others.

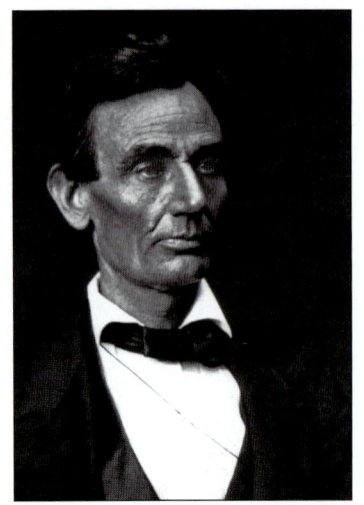

This region was indeed the "Land of Lincoln," and Alton was noteworthy in hosting the last of the famous Lincoln-Douglas debates of 1858, which indirectly ensured that he became President of the United States a few years later. The painting shown in this figure became the property of the local Alton newspaper after his election; it was done by Alexander Halder in Chicago in 1860. I purchased it from the local newspaper, and it now sits in my living room as a cherished possession (see below).

dozen miles away. It was there that he met and married his wife. Many of my direct ancestors played a role directly under Grant in the great American Civil War. Some made the ultimate sacrifice during that brutal conflict.

Literally, just behind the property line of the backyard of the home where we lived is a small tributary of the great Mississippi called Wood River Creek. This is the site where Lewis and Clark encamped both at the beginning of their epic voyage to the Northwest in 1801 and again on their return. Many institutions in the region today are named after Lewis and Clark or the Wood River Creek (eg, my high school, East Alton-Wood River Community High School).

I can still remember as a child seeing steamboats on the river, steamboats not unlike those piloted a century earlier by Samuel Clemens (ie, Mark Twain) who himself was born and raised in Hannibal not far up the same river.

A very famous and supremely important event in American history occurred in Alton in 1858, the final Lincoln-Douglas debate. It is no exaggeration to assert that this planned political encounter played a major role in assuring Lincoln's later election to the presidency in 1860. The debates occurred just a hundred yards from the street shown in the illustration on page 62. I still have in my possession an original oil painting of Lincoln rendered in Chicago during his campaign. After his victory, Lincoln gifted the portrait to the *Alton Evening Telegraph*, my hometown newspaper, which had supported Lincoln. One hundred years later, I purchased the portrait after the death of the publisher. It now hangs in the living room of my house in Charleston (see below).

In my opinion, my intense respect and the very high-esteem in which I hold Harold are based on numerous childhood images and influences. Sometimes I feel that the world today does not have the same type of respect for genuinely great individuals as was the case in the 1940s, the very early formative years of my life—when a very serious war was raging. We were not distracted by much of the clutter of modern marketing. I personally derived my concepts of history from books and from actual experiences and observations, not the television set. In my opinion, this is what prepared my mind to recognize the special nature of

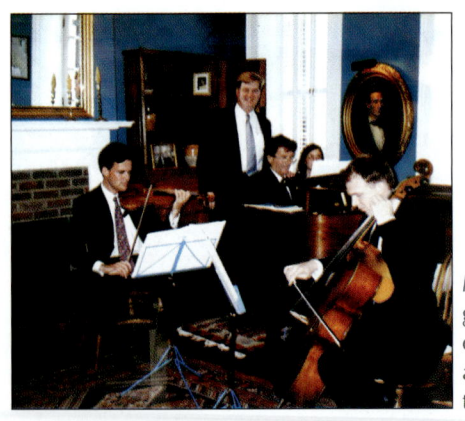

My style of leadership had been relatively low-key, and I particularly enjoyed get-togethers for musical evenings. The group in my house is a team of young ophthalmologists from Munich, Germany, led by the group's "father", Peter Clemente, a close friend of our German colleague in ophthalmology, Dr. Thomas Neuhann. Note that on the wall to my left is the portrait of Abraham Lincoln that is shown above.

this man almost 30 years later. Harold is not the usual hero in terms of being the great athlete, war hero, or show business figure. He is a hero in terms of the genuine and lasting contributions he has made to medicine and especially to the field of eye care.

ENTERING THE FIELD OF MEDICINE— THE EYES HAVE IT

After graduating from high school in 1959, I attended Northwestern University in Evanston, IL for two and one-half years. We playfully considered ourselves the "Harvard of the Midwest." I started out as an engineering major, but I transferred to pre-med and in 1962, I gained early entrance to the University of Illinois in Chicago. I developed a firm interest in ophthalmology in the second year of my medical studies. I had a few rotations through ophthalmology and also met a fine role model, the Professor and Chairman of the Department of Ophthalmology at the University of Illinois Eye and Ear Infirmary, Peter C. Kronfeld, MD. He was a graduate of the great pre-World War II Department of Ophthalmology in Vienna. A refugee from the war, he settled in Chicago and was an expert in the field of glaucoma.

I completed two specialty residencies after graduating from medical school in 1966, and they formed the foundation of my career in eye research. The first of these was a residency in pathology at Charity Hospital in New Orleans, LA with one year of extra training in studying eye pathology at the Armed Forces Institute of Pathology at Walter Reed Hospital in Washington, DC. I received a specialty certification by passing the board examinations given by the American Board of Pathology in 1971.

Although growing weary of training, I then continued on to complete a clinical ophthalmology residency at the University of Iowa in Iowa City, IA (board certified, 1975). This was a fine department that was also chaired by several World War II refugees from Vienna, Austria, led by Professor Frederick Blodi. His wife was a nurse in the American army when Fred finally freed himself from the German (Austrian) army. The two met and he became the "war bride." Fred was from the same institution in Vienna in which Fuchs, Lindner, and Kronfeld had served—the Department visited by Harold and his father in 1935. Harold, like Winston Churchill, deduced that war was not far away. All of these European-trained eye surgeons had a great influence on me, and this prepared me for a career that combined the two subspecialties of ophthalmology and pathology. The combination was extremely helpful in studying diseases of the eye and their causes and treatments. I am sure that my daily learning experiences and the wisdom conferred to me from those Austro-German pillars of wisdom prepared me for future periods of sabbatical research in Germany.

It was always my intent to study an important and timely topic, regardless of where I was working. In retrospect, it has become clear that my career was based on this concept. For example, during my early years while working in Chicago and Iowa, there was a major worldwide concern about two pharmacological agents, lysergic acid dehydrogenase (LSD) and thalidomide. I did work on the embryopathy (congenital malformations) that apparently sometimes accompanied these various agents and others. Soon thereafter, when lasers appeared, I focused my research on laser treatment of retinal diseases such as diabetic retinopathy and age-related macular degeneration.

CHAPTER 4

My first full-time official academic faculty appointment was at the University of Illinois Eye and Ear Infirmary also at the University of Illinois, Chicago. My "boss," Dr. Morton Goldberg (subsequently the well-respected chairman for many years at the Wilmer Eye Institute, Johns Hopkins Medical School, Baltimore, MD), accepted me as an assistant professor and I was soon thereafter promoted to associate professor. In retrospect, as I look back on the time of that appointment, I recollect that IOLs were not implanted and rarely, if ever, mentioned at the Infirmary. It was the 1970s and still too early. My focus during those years remained on laser retinal photocoagulation. One important finding we noted after doing electron microscopy of laser-treated eyes was that the usual treatments were often too strong or powerful. Sometimes the surgeon would accidentally destroy healthy retina or optic nerve tissue instead of properly selected diseased tissue and vessels. Therefore, one had to adjust treatment parameters and doses very carefully. As mentioned above, treatment of retinal diseases was a major priority, especially with the new lasers that had become available in the 1970s. I owe much to Dr. Goldberg, who taught me many skills, including some research techniques and also methods for fundraising—methods used to build and maintain an eye department. These came in very handy when I was the chairman of the department in South Carolina. These years in Chicago represented a wonderful experience, but still no exposure to IOLs. I vaguely heard about one colleague in practice in Chicago who did implants, a certain Dr. Parrott, who I recall was also an early user of the newly developed operating microscopes. I believe that Dr. Manus Kraff, another colleague, was at the beginning of a illustrious career with IOLs.

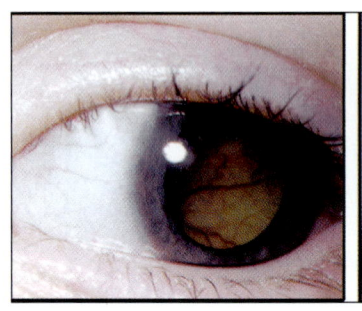

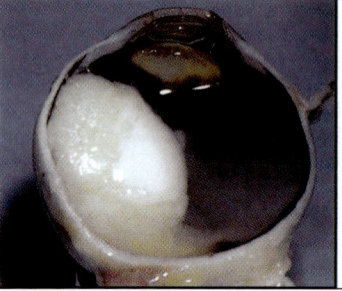

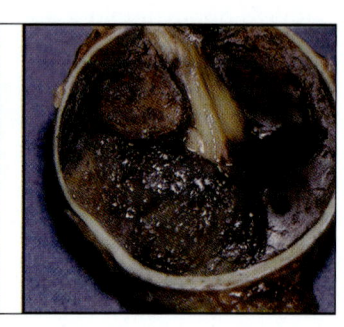

This essence of pathology is the understanding and diagnosis of tissue changes as seen pathologically or under a microscope followed by clinically useful correlation of the findings. The three images shown here are examples of potentially deadly diseases that may affect the eye.
LEFT: Clinical photograph of a retinal tumor (retinoblastoma).
MIDDLE: Gross photograph of a retinoblastoma invading the middle of an eye.
RIGHT: Gross photograph of an eye containing a metastatic cancer that spread from the breast to the eye. It was discovered after a surgeon mistakenly attempted cataract-IOL surgery on this diseased eye.

It was while working in Chicago in the early 1970s that I had made my definitive decision to concentrate on the subspecialty to which I already alluded—a relatively obscure field, namely ocular (ophthalmic) pathology. My friends often joked about me entering a laboratory career in addition to the clinical/surgical pathway of pure ophthalmology. They sometimes declared that I was making a pathologic decision to enter the field of ophthalmologic pathology.

In actuality, a pathologist works with all types of tissue (eg, surgical, such as a frozen section of a breast biopsy). The old fashioned stereotype of a pathologist working with a microscope in a dark corner of a morgue is no longer a reality. Bridging both specialties was the best professional decision that I ever made. I was able to apply findings from the laboratory to clinical/surgical situations that were ultimately helpful to patients.

Although ophthalmologic pathology was a very *small* subspecialty, it was an old and venerable one. Very few people worked in this very narrow subspecialty of pathology, which included the field of ophthalmic prosthetics (artificial biodevices). I entered the field almost by total serendipity on that day in 1985 when IOL #1 arrived.

Harold revealed a superb understanding of the need to apply pathology research to clinical ophthalmology, including his IOL. One of his best professional friends in London, Mr. Norman Ashton, was a superb eye pathologist (see pages 156, 246, and 247). He worked at the famous Institute of Ophthalmology with Sir Stewart Duke-Elder. It is ironic that in many ways, Mr. Ashton was more receptive to Harold and his IOLs than many of his clinical colleagues in Britain who came out against Ridley. He actually, and perhaps bravely, nominated Harold for membership in the Royal Society (see Chapter 17).

Harold's opinion of ocular pathology is summarized as follows:

> *Our interest and attention must be directed toward the relatively small proportion of patients whose results are less perfect than expected. Evaluation of these patients marks the stepping stones to prevention of their complications. It is clear that for future developments, we must move from the operating room, which has so interested us all, to the pathology laboratory.*

He also wrote, "I was a great admirer of Ramon y Cajal, Nobel Laureate, who did splendid work on the structure of the retina. He was a histologist and not an ophthalmologist."

Together with my dear friend and colleague, the late Maurice Rabb, I coauthored a book on eye pathology that is now in its fifth edition. Professor G. O. H. Naumann and I also coauthored a very successful book on pathology of the eye written in the German language, which had its origin in two separate year-long research sabbaticals I completed in Germany. The sabbaticals were sponsored by the Alexander von Humboldt Foundation, the first in 1971 in the small but renowned university town of Tuebingen and four years later, one year split in the cities of Bonn and Munich. I translated this text from German into English. My friend from Japan, Dr. O. Nishi, translated it into Japanese.

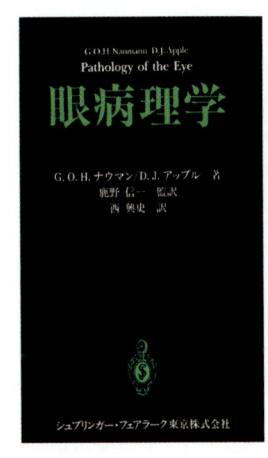

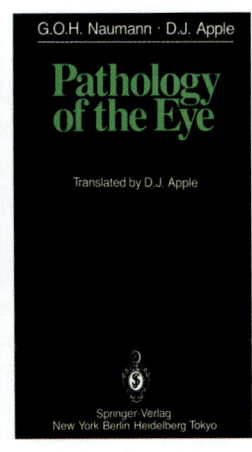

CHARLESTON AND THE APPLE KORPS

After the first meeting with Harold in 1985 described earlier in this chapter, I spent the next four years building the IOL/Biodevice Research Center at the University of Utah. During those years the fellows who worked with me were affectionately referred to as the **Apple Korps**. The German spelling was in honor of several young Research Fellows from Germany who were working with me in the laboratory, chosen to resemble the designation of the German soldiers under General Rommel—the Afrika Korps. (This had *nothing* to with our political preferences.)

We also finished our 1989 book of the *Pathology of IOLs* during this period (the era of rigid IOLs) (page 74). One of the most positive comments I had on that publication was actually provided by an attorney who was working on an IOL-related case with Dr. Eric Arnott of London. One day the attorney spoke with Dr. Arnott, who is himself the author of a text that covered his experiences during the early years of the IOL and is entitled *A New Beginning in Sight*.

For the first 12 to 15 years of my medical career, I focused on general pathology of the eye and published two textbooks, including the one noted here, written in German with my colleague, Dr. G. O. H. Naumann in 1975.
This book was translated into foreign languages, including Japanese. It is now in its second edition.
TOP LEFT: Japanese translation.
TOP RIGHT: English translation.
BOTTOM: Title page of the original German text.

CHAPTER 4

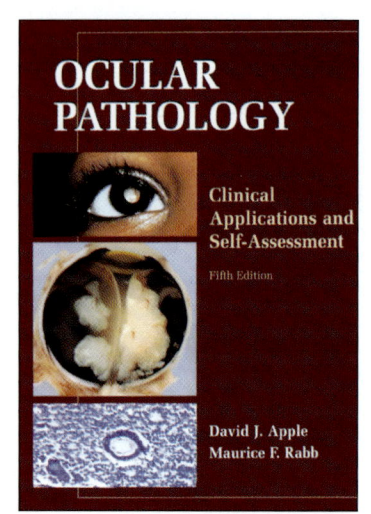

My first major publication in the field of ocular pathology occurred prior to my sojourn in Germany. This book, entitled *Ocular Pathology* (co-authored by the late Dr. Maurice Rabb and myself), is now in its fifth edition and covers all aspects of diseases affecting the eye. The period of emphasis on general ocular pathology lasted until the early 1980s, when my career changed critically as I moved into the field of IOLs.

Referring to the attorney, Arnott noted that:

"He was a brilliant attorney. He devoted most of his previous five years entirely to my case. Added to his sincerity and belief in our case, was his compulsiveness for detail and a deep knowledge. He had read David Apple's text 'IOLs, Evolution, Designs, Complications and Pathology', 1989, over 500 pages long from cover to cover, therefore, knew more about lens implantation than most eye surgeons."

Our department was in a building-mode construction. During that time, I participated in the application process for our first Research to Prevent Blindness (RPB) grant, which was successful. I had done the same in Chicago and also did it one more time later in Charleston, so I felt a great deal of satisfaction of helping build up young departments where I worked. We were also planning for the next stage of the department's growth: the construction of the Moran Eye Center.

Another opportunity came my way in 1989, one that was very tempting to a relatively young academic faculty member. I was offered a position as a chairman or department head. I had just completed a few days of guest lecturing on a tour boat to Bermuda sponsored by the Storm Eye Institute of the Medical University of South Carolina in Charleston. My host was Dr. William Vallaton. Having gotten to know him on the ship, it was clear that he was aging, not in good health, and would soon be retiring. He decided on the spot that he wanted me to assume the chair position. He himself had done great work for the state of South Carolina, being the first to introduce phacoemulsification and the IOL as well as laser technology and other modern techniques to that state. In addition, he had obtained funding from a grateful patient, a certain Mr. Storm, to construct an eye institute. The first institute was a five-story unit that was built in the mid-1960s.

Dr. Vallaton was a very fine man with a very independent streak. I recall that he had a very, very effective way to force people who did not take their eye drops in proper compliance. If, for example, a glaucoma patient did not take his or her drops regularly, the glaucoma could progress to almost *total blindness*. When he encountered a "guilty" obviously noncompliant patient during an office visits—and if he realized the care was positively hopeless—he would do the following. He would lock the patient in a totally dark (black) room next to the clinic for up to 1 hour and would not let him or her out, showing him or her what would happen if he or she didn't take his or her medicine or

After I made my way through medical school, I made the decision to enter ophthalmology after having studied engineering and premedical studies at Northwestern University. Very early in medical school, I decided on ophthalmology and had a strong interest in research on the eye. I found that the study of pathology (examination of tissues) provided a good means of doing basic and applied research on the eye. By 1980, after I had developed the interest in IOLs I have already described, I constantly used a technique pioneered by my good friend, Dr. Miyake in Japan, as shown here. This shows a means of looking at a cadaver eye from behind after it has been cut open in order to view structures within the eye and in this case, an IOL. The lens is visible in this photograph as consisting of a central round lens, or optical component, and two yellow "loops," or "haptics," that help hold the lens in position. Much more about these is discussed later on.

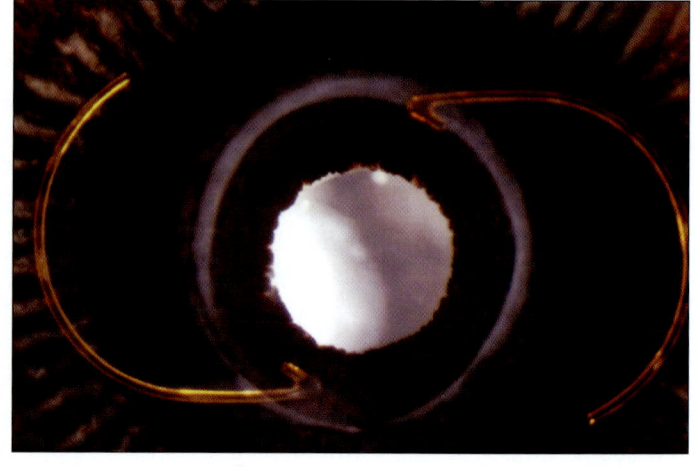

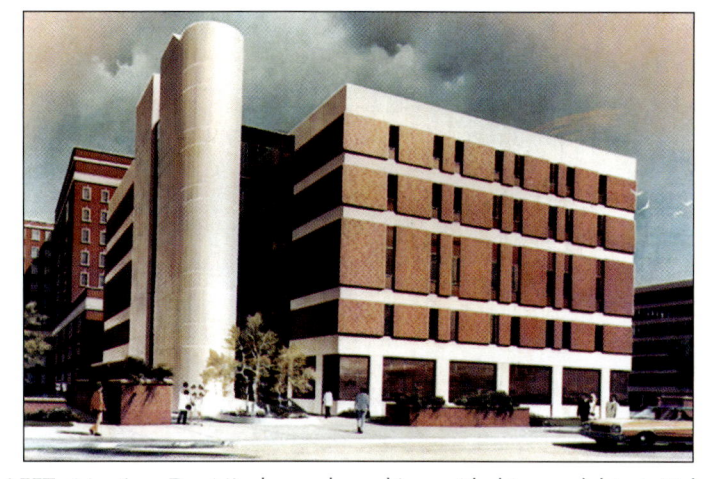

LEFT: Meeting Dr. Miyake and working with him and his initial innovation of the technique (now called the Miyake-Apple technique) has been a joy. In this photograph, we together have received honorary recognition from one of the large IOL companies for our research endeavors.

RIGHT: I had been recruited to Charleston in 1989 to become the Chairman of the Department of Ophthalmology at the Storm Eye Institute. At that time, the building was a five-story square block that was showing signs of aging, especially since the previous chairman had become ill. It was my goal to help rebuild the department and improve the status of clinical treatment and research as well as to continue with my IOL research begun in Utah in 1980.

A photograph of the modernized building seen here is where Harold visited each time that he came to Charleston and visited us in the Department of Ophthalmology.

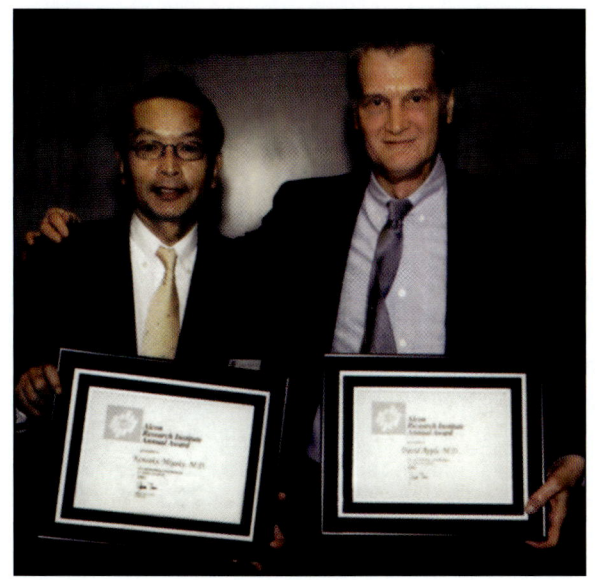

therapeutic drops. He was correct! Most patients responded well to this "treatment."

Dr. Vallaton worked for many years building a good department. I decided to take the South Carolina challenge.

By the time I arrived on the scene, Dr. Vallaton had retired because of severe health problems and the building was in dire need of repairs and expansion because of his illnesses. An expansion represented an attractive opportunity for me to improve on the institute and thus provide a service for the citizens of that state. In addition, an opportunity existed to continue the legacy and expand the research center. My IOL/Biodevice Research Center and Miyake Laboratory (named after our wonderful benefactor and founder Dr. Kensaku Miyake [seen above on this page and page 86]).

We also built a laser center, the Arthur and Holly McGill Center for Vision Correction. It was underwritten and founded in 1997 by a generous donation from a wealthy industrialist from Greenville, SC (in earlier years, he manufactured the famous line of Her Majesty ladies' and childrens' clothing) and his wife Holly. Unfortunately, both Holly and Arthur, both wonderful friends of Ann and myself, have passed away.

The expansion benefited greatly by the generosity of Dr. Miyake. He was the first doctor to utilize the posterior video/photographic technique for the study of cataract surgery and IOLs, a technique we have modified and improved over the years. He contributed a large amount of funding for this endeavor, and it flourished.

As I had hoped and anticipated, the biodevice laboratory did flourish in Charleston. Our first book on cataract-IOL surgery was published in 1989. This covered the field up to the end of the era of rigid PMMA (polymethyl methacrylate) lenses. The later books covered the field after 1989 (page 74), the era of modern phacoemulsification and small incision surgery.

CHAPTER 4

Dr. Charles Kelman, Dr. Miyake, and I had the honor of receiving both the Binkhorst Medal and the Innovators Award from the American Society of Cataract and Refractive Surgery. The latter award is now designated as the Kelman Medal Lecture Award. I am very pleased that I have given six Ridley Medal Lectures throughout the world.

My hope was that the entire vision center and its components could be modeled after the center that had been built in Salt Lake City, with contributions from foundations, industry, and private corporations. I had roots working in the field, first in Nigeria, later in the Center for Developing World Ophthalmology in Charleston, and then with the Collaborating Center with the World Health Organization, the latter two I founded in Charleston, a time prior to when my illness slowed me down.

The laboratory grew as time passed. We had many visitors, not only for the purpose of training, but also for professional consultations. Our Center worked with the International Lions Clubs and World Health Organization for our work in this endeavor.

Our main function in this initiative was to improve the quality of surgery and lenses available for distribution to underprivileged countries. This included bringing surgeons in from numerous countries to our facility or making trips to their countries. In 1990 there was a serious question as to whether IOLs should be introduced to the developing world at all. We, of course, advocated doing so, and judging from the centers that have sprung up worldwide with this goal in mind, I believe now that our efforts paid off. I am very proud that the models we helped set up worldwide in the early years (Nigeria, 1977, Project Focus; Madurai, India, 1980; and others under the umbrella of our Center for Developing World Ophthalmology) have functioned as good models for later clinics established in other locales such as Ethiopia and Nepal.

As this work was going on, Charleston became very special not only to me, but also to Harold and Elisabeth. They visited us two times while I lived there. The Ridleys also developed a close and affectionate friendship with my mother, who had been widowed since 1972.

I am pleased that during that period I was able to see to it that Harold received an honorary doctor's degree from our department in 1989 (see Chapter 17). It was very difficult to successfully push it through the university's bureaucracy, but thanks to a very enlightened president, Dr. James Edwards, we were able to do so. It was the first academic award from a university that Harold received.

Harold truly enjoyed Charleston. In addition to the academic accolades he received here and the opportunity to visit the facility that was one of the first to recognize his efforts, he loved the fact that Charleston had many features similar to England. Indeed, the area was settled in the 17th century by the English and was governed by England until the time of the American Revolution. While in Charleston, Harold and Elisabeth particularly enjoyed St. Michael's Church, which was built with the same architectural plans as St. Martin's in the Field in London.

Harold also very much enjoyed the row houses along the waterfront, which of course were very English in nature. However, he was pleasantly amused by the fact that the houses had been painted multiple colors in the 1920s and 1930s, mimicking the Caribbean style of architecture. I was in the process of remodeling one of these homes at the time of his first visit, and he seemed to enjoy the remodeling process.

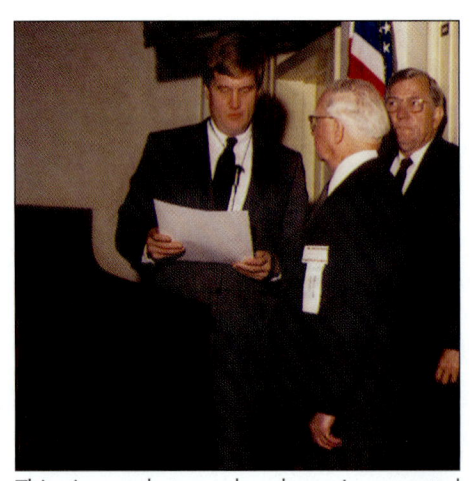

This is a photograph where I presented Harold with an honorary doctor's degree from my department, presented in 1989. This was the first honorary degree presented to him by a medical school, and he very much appreciated this. At that time, he was just beginning to come out from the doldrums, having very importantly just received in 1986 a membership in England's very prestigious Royal Society.

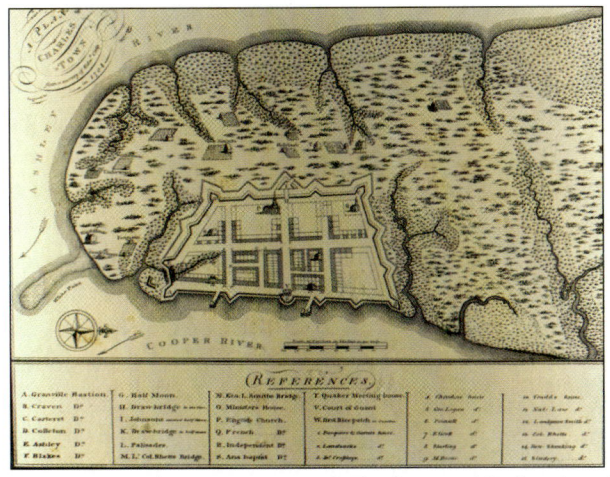

TOP LEFT: 18th century map of Charleston, SC showing the layout of the early settlement. The street along the bottom faces the harbor of the Atlantic Ocean, where the early homes were built.
TOP RIGHT: Harold and Elisabeth very much enjoyed seeing Charleston and noted the similarity between the row houses there and back home in the United Kingdom. These are row houses before renovation along East Bay Street in the 1920s.
BOTTOM: This is East Bay Street after renovation using different colors, creating Rainbow Row. Ann and I live in the yellow house on the left. This is the longest group of intact row houses remaining in the United States.

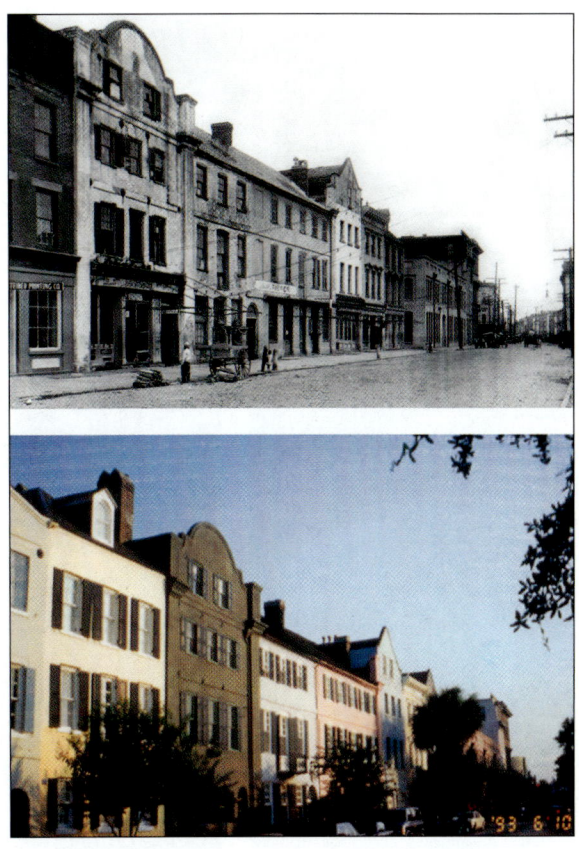

Not only was the street view interesting, but the back gardens of the homes along "Rainbow Row" were used as the model for the stage setting of George Gershwin's opera, *Porgy and Bess*. I personally had another wonderful feeling about the garden because that was the site of my marriage to Ann Addlestone in 1995. Harold and Elisabeth visited the garden twice during their visits.

Harold also became very close to my group of researchers, the equivalent group to the "Apple Korps" that had been named in Utah.

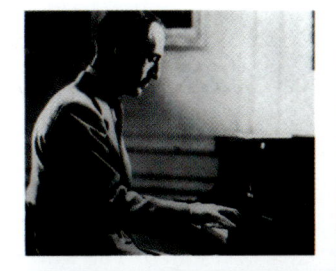

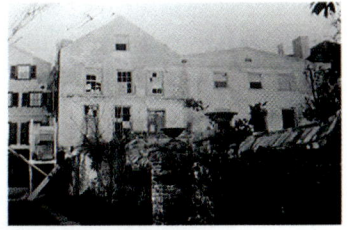

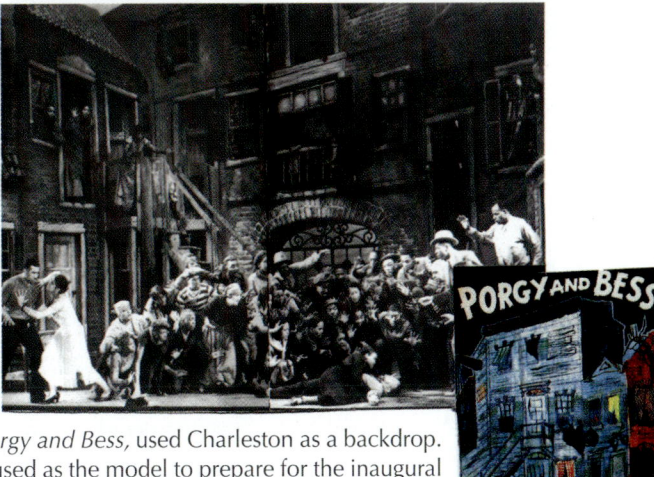

George Gershwin's great opera, *Porgy and Bess*, used Charleston as a backdrop. The rear garden of our house was used as the model to prepare for the inaugural performances in the 1930s and is still used today.

CHAPTER 4

TRIUMPHS AND TRAGEDIES: 1989–PRESENT

By the late 1990s, we had completed most of my goals for the center, including a $10 million fundraising project to remodel and enlarge the institute from the original 5 floors to the present 10 floors. The fundraising was successful, even though it was done at a difficult time when the stock market was down and funds were scarce. Unfortunately, I will not be able to enjoy it in the future. I felt very good about having achieved my objectives. The wall behind my desk was full (see page 75); I had no lack of honors.

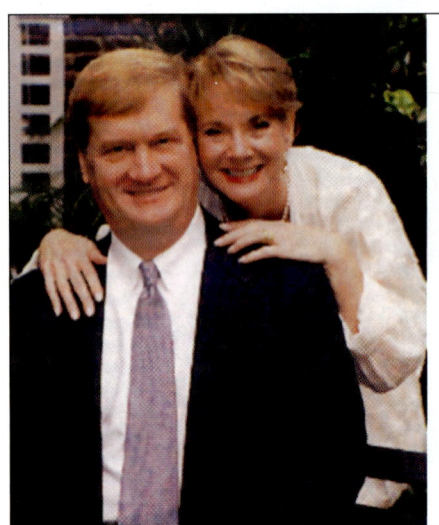

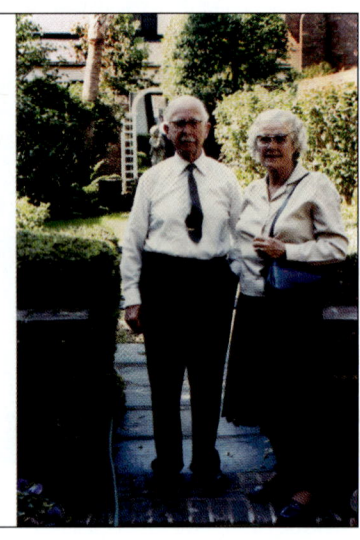

LEFT: Ann and I were married in 1995 in the garden of 93 East Bay. RIGHT: Harold and Elisabeth enjoying the relaxation of the same garden a few years later during one of their visits to Charleston.

The one thing that could have slowed me down in my career at that point was a serious illness. Unfortunately, that's exactly what hit me. I began to notice certain symptoms such as fatigue in 1997, but didn't realize what they were. Then in 1999, I felt a swollen lymph node on my neck and diagnosed myself with a metastatic cancer, which a biopsy of the neck confirmed. Subsequent small biopsies in the oral cavity showed a primary cancer at the base of the tongue. It was confirmed as an advanced stage III lesion.

I considered retiring or at least cutting back my efforts. But as fate would have it, I ran into my friend and former colleague, Dr. Randall Olson, and once again my plans changed. Upon his invitation, I returned to Salt Lake City in the year 2000 where we have just finished completing a celebration of the 25th anniversary of our Center.

After we moved to Deer Valley (Park City), I had much difficulty breathing in the high altitude range of 7000 to 9000 feet above sea level. My health problems were complicated a few years later by a cerebral vascular stroke resulting from radiation therapy. In spite of my health challenges, I am doing my best to push ahead in my area of research. The work seems to be even more important now than before because numerous new lenses and devices are appearing on the market almost every week and there is a marked lack of oversight in evaluating these from the clinical pathologic perspective.

Indeed, the future study of pathology of devices, especially implantable prostheses, is becoming more and more endangered as time passes. I am concerned as to what might happen after my retirement. The autopsy study has begun to languish. Our best option will be to recruit some very smart young men and women to keep this work going. Otherwise there will be insufficient oversight of new products. Perhaps the last tangible goal I have is to participate in the dedication of the new Moran Eye Center facility in Salt Lake City. I am deeply honored that our cataract/IOL/biodevices research group will be named the David J. Apple, MD Laboratories for Ophthalmic Devices Research.

Specific details regarding the various types of scientific and analytic work we have done are beyond the scope of this chapter. Perhaps the best way to describe my efforts is to equate them to a consumer advocate in which I search for potential or real complications of the cataract-IOL operation and then attempt to reconstruct the problem and suggest means to treat them. I will provide a few examples of a few of the parameters in Chapter 11.

Summary

We achieved our goals in Charleston as is summarized in this closing group of illustrations.

The funding for the renovation and rebuilding of the Storm Eye Center was successful and we are appreciative for what the South Carolina Lions Clubs did in supporting our 14 year tenure.

Thanks to Dr. Miyake's generosity, the pathology and IOL laboratory (Miyake-Apple Laboratory) peaked in its productivity during these years.

The efforts of our Center for Developing World Ophthalmology and the World Health Organization Collaborating Centre for Prevention of Blindness, again with the help of the Lion's Clubs, in association with Christoffel Blindenmission (CBM) grew and evolved over the 14-year period that I worked in Charleston. Similar organizations are now functioning throughout the world, including in Africa, Nepal, and elsewhere.

We celebrated the 25th anniversary of our David Apple Center (Salt Lake/Charleston) in Chicago at the American Academy of Ophthalmology in 2005. My personal goal is to continue our work (health willing) in Salt Lake City training new individuals to carry on for another 25 years.

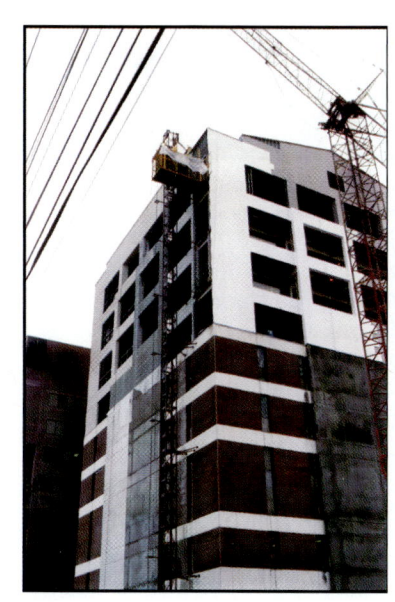

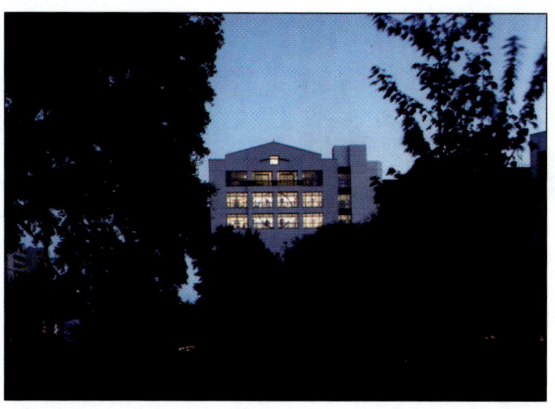

LEFT: Construction underway to modernize and increase the size of the original Storm Eye Institute (see page 69).
RIGHT: The Storm Eye Institute at night.

CHAPTER 4

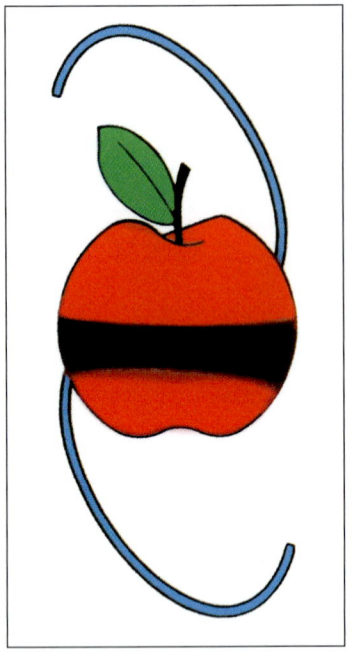

Apple Korps logo.

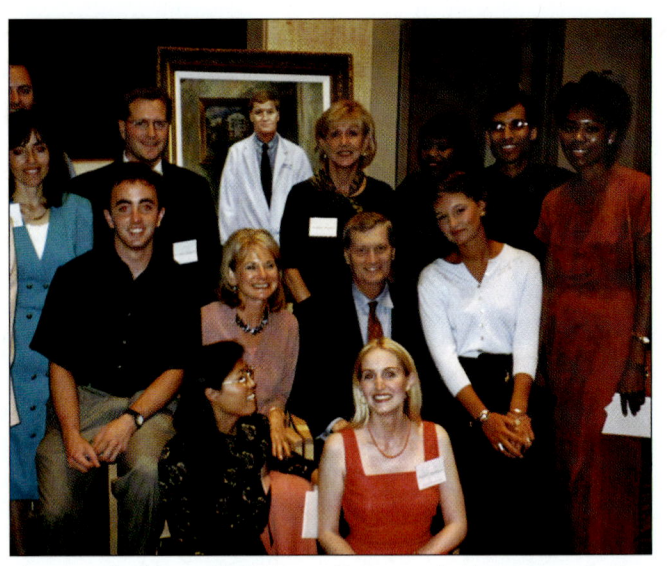

Photograph of my wife and myself surrounded by many members of the Apple Korps, 1999. This was the year I developed my illness and retired from the Medical University. I have learned that the best way to get the University to make your poster is to have an illness.

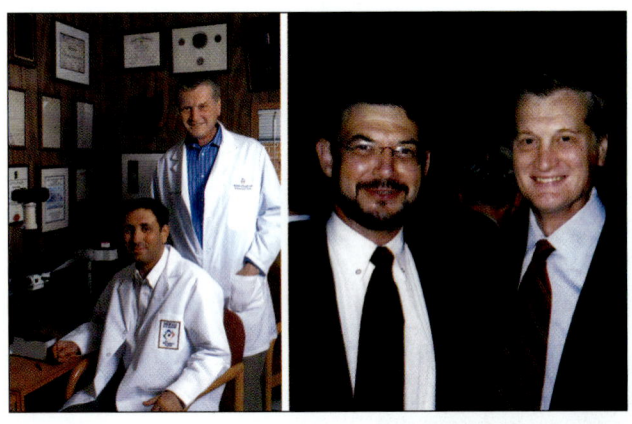

Our Apple Korps team is now entering a second generation. These are two of my fine former fellows from Israel. Both of these fellows were from Tele Aviv.
LEFT: Dr. Guy Kleinmann and myself.
RIGHT: Dr. Ehud Assia and myself.

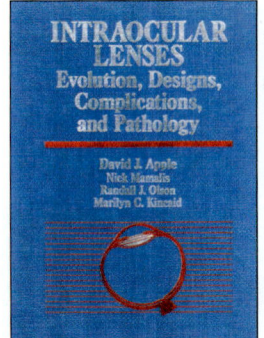

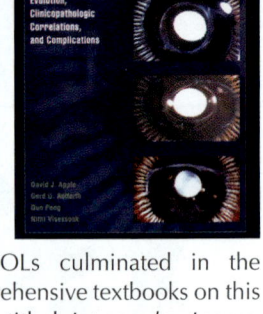

LEFT: Our work on IOLs culminated in the publication of two comprehensive textbooks on this subject. The first text entitled *Intraocular Lenses,* shown here, was published in 1989 and represented what was know in this specialty through the era of the rigid (PMMA) IOLs, before the era of foldable lenses came into being.

RIGHT: Ten years later, the era of foldable lenses had come into prominence, and that coincided with the publication of our second major text, *Foldable Intraocular Lenses.*

"DAVID, MR. RIDLEY WANTS TO MEET YOU"

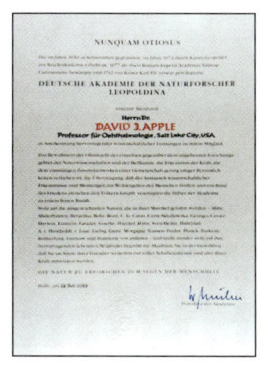

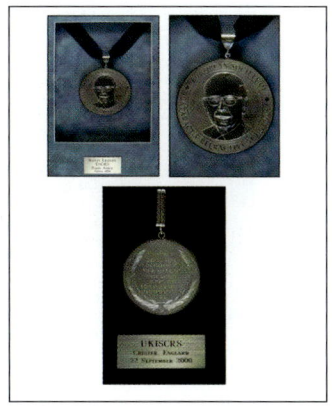

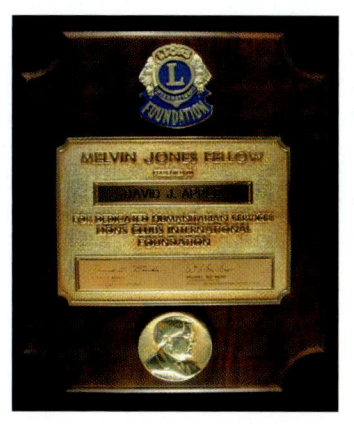

LEFT: Certification of election into the German Academy of Natural Sciences.
CENTER: Three of the Ridley medals received by the Author.
RIGHT: Medal from the Lion's Club International designating membership in the Melvin Jones Fellow.

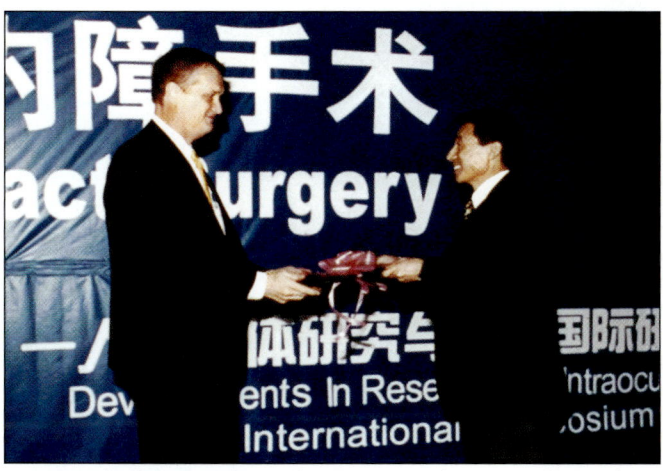

In 1996 I had the privilege of receiving an honorary degree from Beijing, People's Republic of China.

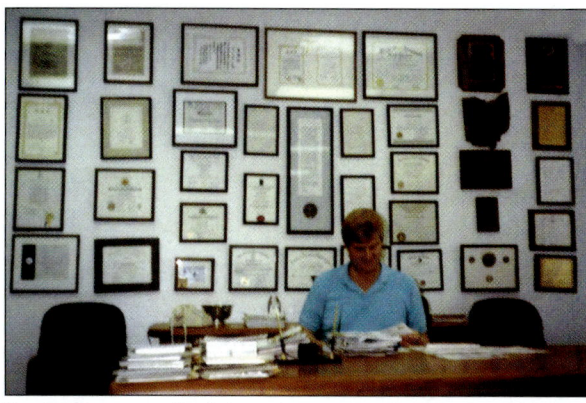

By 1999, my walls did not have room for more certificates and my illness had become very serious. It was time and I felt like making a move.

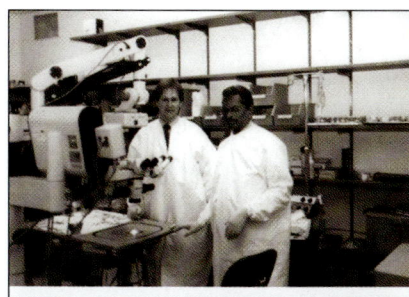

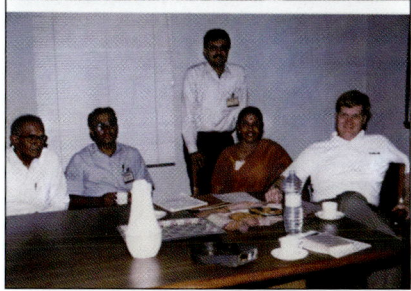

It has always been my impression that the best way to influence young doctors beginning eye surgery is to teach them in wet labs or using the Miyake-Apple technique.
These are photographs showing two groups of doctors from underprivileged countries visiting our Miyake-Apple laboratory.

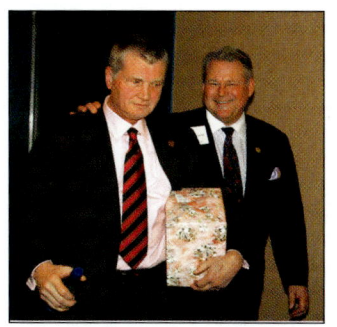

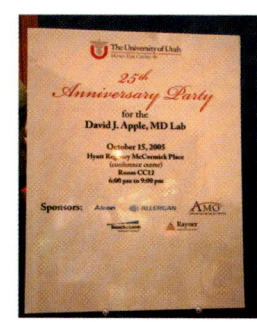

A surprise party for the 25th anniversary of the Apple laboratory was celebrated while attending the annual meeting of the American Academy of Ophthalmology in Chicago. I was indeed, so surprised, that Dr. Dick Lindstrom brought me into the door in hopes that I would not collapse and fall.

75

CHAPTER 4

Architect's drawing of the new Moran Eye Center in Salt Lake City. This is the third structure I have had the privilege of working in at the University of Utah, having started my career in the hospital in the 1980s.

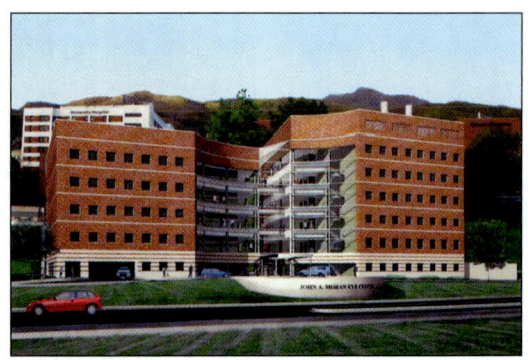

Wiltshire.

TOP: Harold had an original 16th century map of the region in which he lived. His cottage was in Stapleford (arrow), just a few miles northwest of Salisbury, in Wiltshire, about 90 miles west of London. The River Wyle flowed from Salisbury past Harold's home. This is where we began our walks. Stonehenge (circled) is just a few miles from Ridley's home.

BOTTOM: The beauty of the River Wyle in front of Harold's home.

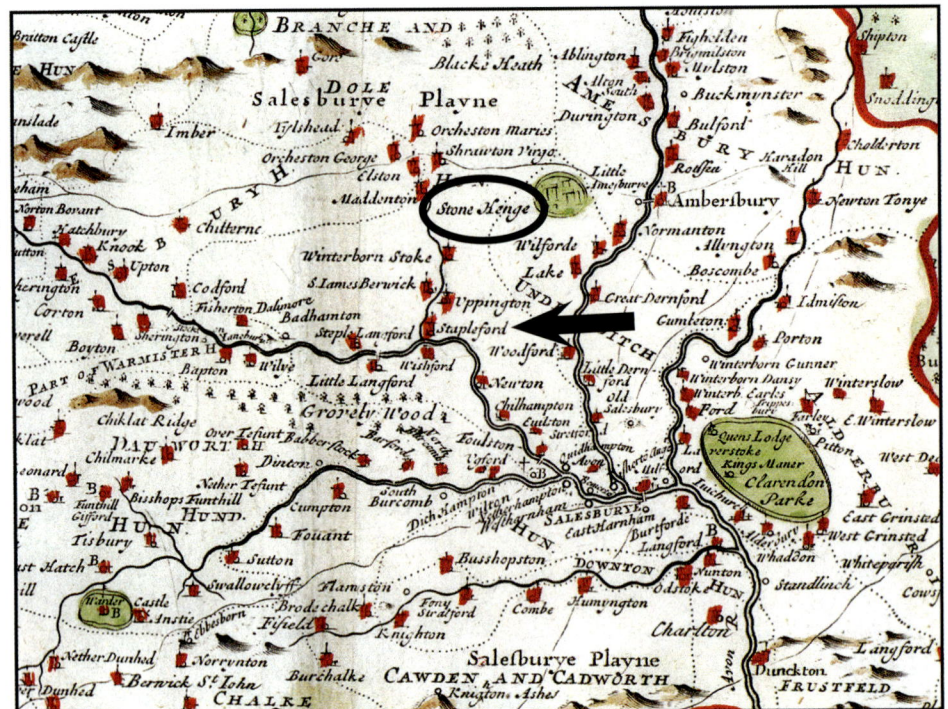

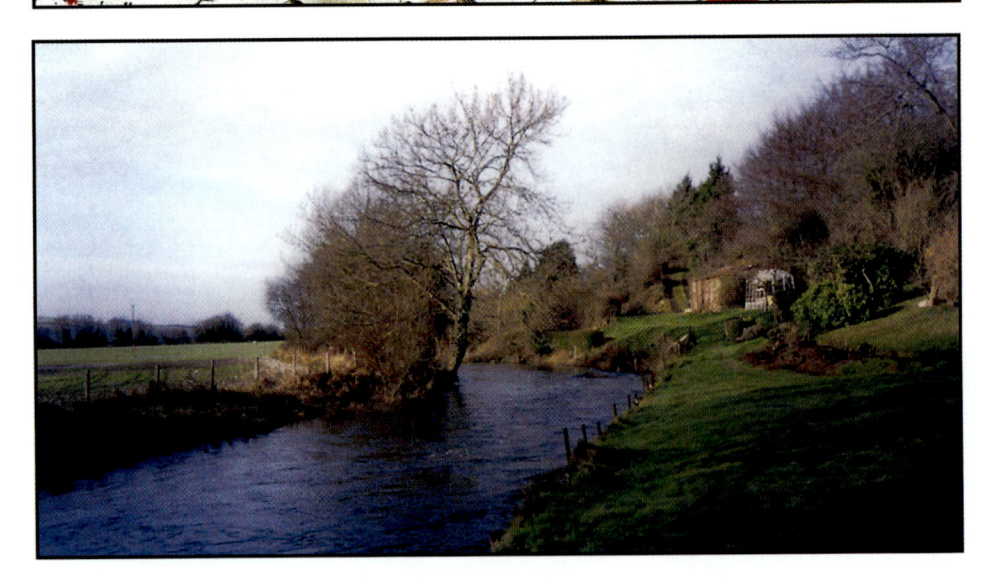

River walks. LEFT: Harold and I beginning a walk along the stream adjacent to his cottage, ca. 1990.
RIGHT: When the weather was inclement, we would carry out our discussions in his comfortable living room.

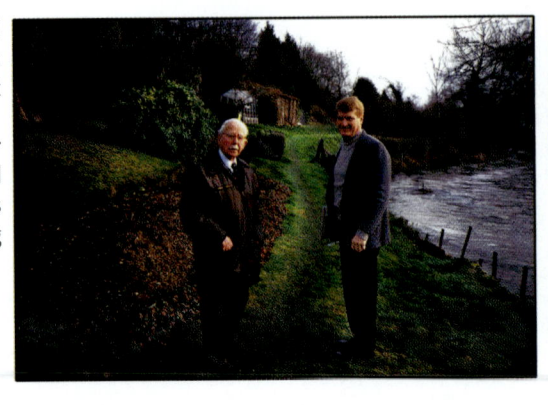

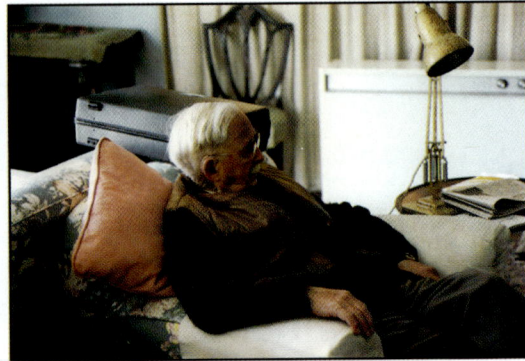

5

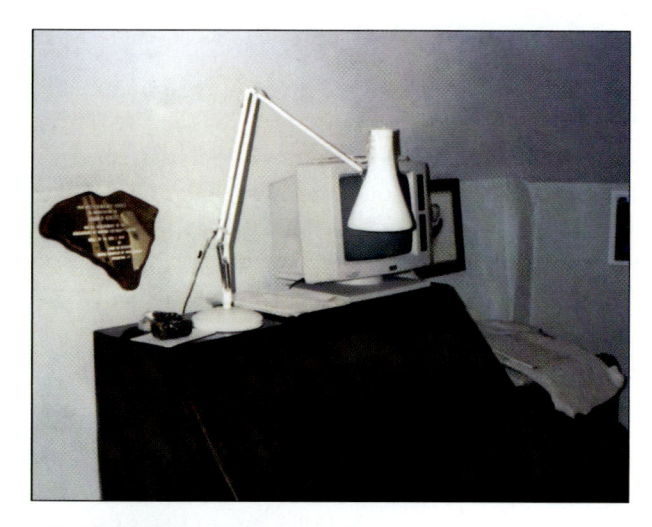

"The best crystal ball is a rearview mirror."

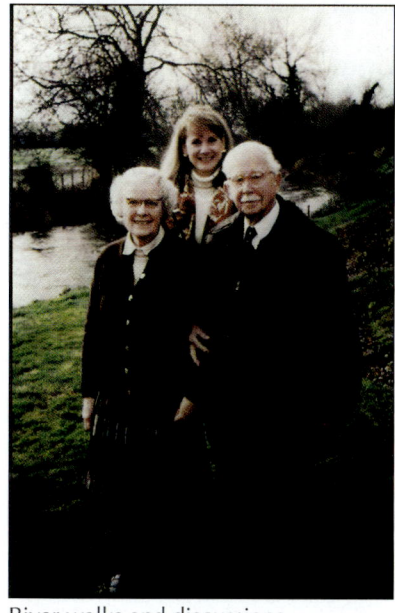

River walks and discussions.
TOP: Photograph of Harold's study just up the stairs from his living room. It was a very important room to him. It was at this desk in this modest room that he typed literally scores of pages of documents regarding his invention and other matters. Harold would type a few new ones on each visit and hand me even more to take back home. I was always flattered that he kept one prominent wall plaque hanging in the study, which can be seen here on the left. It is a plaque that I gave him during one of his trips to South Carolina. It is shaped like a map of the state of South Carolina.
BOTTOM: After our marriage in 1995, my wife, Ann, joined me for many trips to England. Here, Harold and his wife, Elisabeth, pose with Ann.

River Walks

THE QUEST FOR A COMPLETE CATARACT OPERATION
STEP 1: DIAGNOSIS AND SURGICAL REMOVAL OF THE CATARACT

After our initial meeting in 1985, I visited Elisabeth and Harold 2 or 3 times a year, alone in the early years, and together with Ann after our marriage in 1995. This pattern remained consistent until Harold's death in 2003.

Harold and I spent many enlightening hours together exchanging ideas. These talks often took place as we walked along the beautiful River Wyle that flowed behind his 16th-century thatched roof cottage. When the weather was inclement (as it frequently was), we chatted in the comfortable living room in his home.

I came to treasure these interchanges. He spoke often about the information that he had accumulated that helped him proceed with his planning for the IOL. He applied knowledge from several sources, including studies in the history of ophthalmology, peering as far back as antiquity.

After we finished our discussions, Harold would usually climb the stairs quickly to his second floor study and type out on his tiny word processor whatever came to his or my mind on that given occasion. I now have most of these documents in my possession. I have used them, along with many letters and other documents he sent or gave to me, to compile the chapters for this book. He was also generous in sharing with me his memories of the history and practices of ophthalmology both prior to and during his lifetime, from the ancients to the doyens of the 18th and 19th centuries, including his own mentors in ophthalmology in London.

CHAPTER 5

In the 1930s and 1940s, there was almost no organized protocol regarding a complete cataract operation; it didn't exist at that time. Harold organized the "steps" that would be required to achieve a *complete* cataract IOL operation. He described his thoughts to me; I recorded and updated these based on his ideas at that time (1930 to 1940s) into what I have recorded as List 5-1. The contents of this list appear quite obvious to today's surgeon, but not so in the early to mid-20th century. It will serve as an outline as we proceed to describe the evolution of the IOL in subsequent chapters.

CLINICAL DIAGNOSIS OF CATARACT

Ridley had little appreciation for music but loved fine art and considered the many early drawings of eyes as such.

These images are drawings and sketches by Leonardo DaVinci showing amazing foresight in outlining the anatomy of the eye and the nerve tracks that connect the eye to the brain.

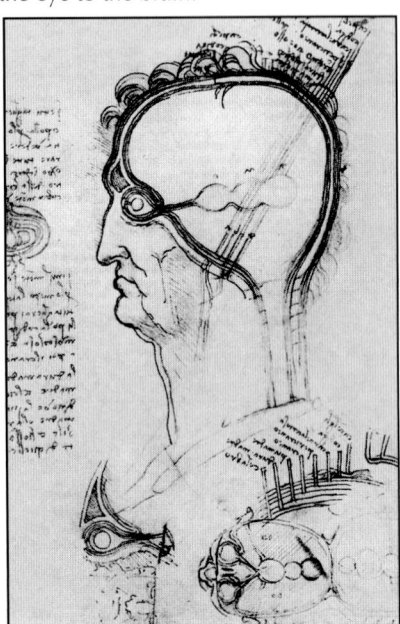

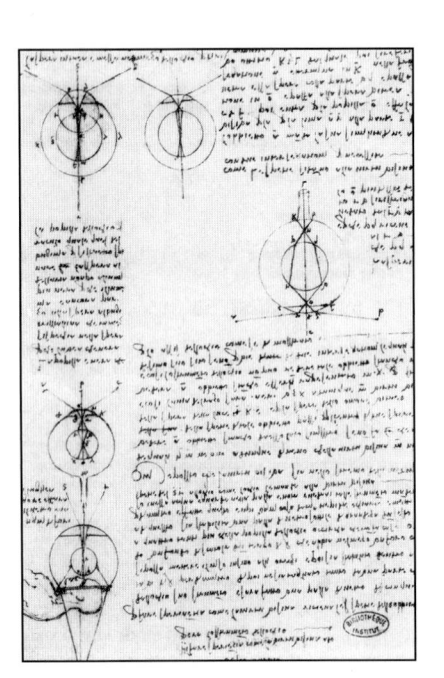

In this chapter, we will focus on a very brief overview of step 1, the *clinical diagnosis* of the cataract and its *surgical removal*. During our walks, Harold and I singled out several individuals—giants in the history of our specialty—who handed down the wealth of knowledge that was essential to Harold as he moved forward. He singled out several ancient thinkers as well as more recent groundbreakers, including Newton, Helmholtz, von Graefe, Bowman, Gullstrand, and other important figures.

This chapter, with a brief mini-history of the basic surgical techniques that evolved as a basic means of finishing step 1 of the cataract removal will set the stage for Harold's breakthrough to finally achieving a completion of step 2—to use his terminology, the "cure of aphakia"—outlined in Chapters 6 to 12.

Harold had great respect for the ancients. He and I shared a passion for studying early documents and discovering how ophthalmology progressed and how early mistakes were eventually corrected. We both enjoyed a very important book from the 16th century. A German layman with no formal education, Georg Bartisch, wrote the first and what some consider to be one of the most important ophthalmology books ever written. Bartisch lived and worked in Dresden, Saxony in Germany. His comprehensive illustrated text was called *Ophthalmoduelia*, or *Augendienst* (published in Dresden in 1983). It was one of the first ophthalmological texts published in the German vernacular—a departure from the usual Latin texts. His extensive descriptions of surgical procedures and the beautiful drawings have led many historians to call him the father of modern ophthalmic publishing. Many also credit him as the first to use the term *ophthalmology*. He describes and illustrates couching, the only cataract operation in existence at his time. One could appreciate how gruesome this procedure might be just from his pictures alone.

> **List 5-1**
>
> # THE TWO STEPS OF THE COMPLETE CATARACT OPERATION
>
> **Step 1.** Clinical diagnosis and removal of the cataractous (cloudy or opaque) lens
> After the patient's cataract is diagnosed, the first requirement is to remove it, namely the opaque lens material that is situated within the interior of the lens inside the surrounding capsule. If we consider the basic structure of the lens as being similar to an M&M candy (Mars Incorporated, Reston, VA), the cataract would be analogous to the soft chocolate material within the outer shell or capsule, except of course for the color. That central material must be removed or sucked out by whatever method the surgeon decides is appropriate for his or her surgical technique.
> This step is a prerequisite that must be accomplished to permit complete unimpaired or unfettered entrance of light and visual images into and out of the eye. It is necessary that the incoming light image pass first through the outer (watch glass-like) cornea and then through the crystalline lens in order to reach the retina and the optic nerve. The visual impulse then passes to the visual cortex of the brain.
> Removal of the light-obstructing lens or lens material (ie, the fried egg white or albumin that we compare to in Chapter 2) can be accomplished by:
>
> a) Couching (a now discredited 6,000 year old procedure).
> b) ICCE, which is removal of the entire lens, both the outer membrane or cellophane-like capsule as well as the inner material, which is termed collectively as the nucleus and cortex.
> c) The ECCE procedure includes the technique of phacoemulsification, which is now the most common and popular procedure.
>
> ECCE is the procedure that Harold himself used during his period of active surgery in the years just prior to the invention of the phacoemulsification machine. ECCE, using either manual or automated lens removal, and especially phacoemulsification, based on technology borrowed from our dentist friends, turned out to be an almost perfect operation for use with IOLs. The opaque cataractous lens substance in the interior of the lens is removed by a process of dissolving or emulsification, leaving almost intact the entire surrounding capsule except for the small orifice (the capsulorrhexis [CCC]) that is cut into the front of the capsule in order to gain entrance to the interior of the lens.
>
> **Step 2.** Visual rehabilitation with a device or appliance. (It is at this stage of the operation that Harold's invention of the IOL gained acceptance and became indispensable.)
> As Harold himself stated many times, step 1 alone is only half an operation. After the cataractous lens is removed but before the application of an optical appliance, the eye is "aphakic" (without a lens).
> The human lens normally has significant focusing or light-gathering power. This is analogous to that seen with manmade lenses needed for many applications (eg, a camera). For the cataract operation to be completely successful, a replacement lens must be provided to the patient. This is the visual rehabilitation component of the surgery.
>
> The 3 choices for this are as follows:
> a. Thick aphakic spectacles, first used after cataract surgery in the early 17th century. The optical quality of these is mediocre at best. Furthermore, if they are broken or lost and not replaced, the individual's vision is often worse than when the cataract was present.
> b. Contact lenses. The optical quality is better than thick spectacles, but they can be difficult to wear and maintain.
> c. Ridley's IOL. This provides the best longevity and is, by far, the best choice.

The works of Sir Isaac Newton and his contemporaries, as well as those of Hermann von Helmholtz, the inventor of the ophthalmoscope, were held in high esteem by Harold. Being British, Harold would always vehemently, but correctly, assert that his fellow countryman Charles Babbage should share the credit for the invention of the ophthalmoscope. Babbage is also credited as one of the pioneers of the computer. The ophthalmoscope helped deliver ophthalmology from the dark ages. Albrecht von Graefe of Berlin (see Chapter 3) and William Bowman, Harold's countryman, took advantage of this discovery in their clinical practices. They were each recognized as one of the—if not the—greatest ophthalmologist of their respective countries.

CHAPTER 5

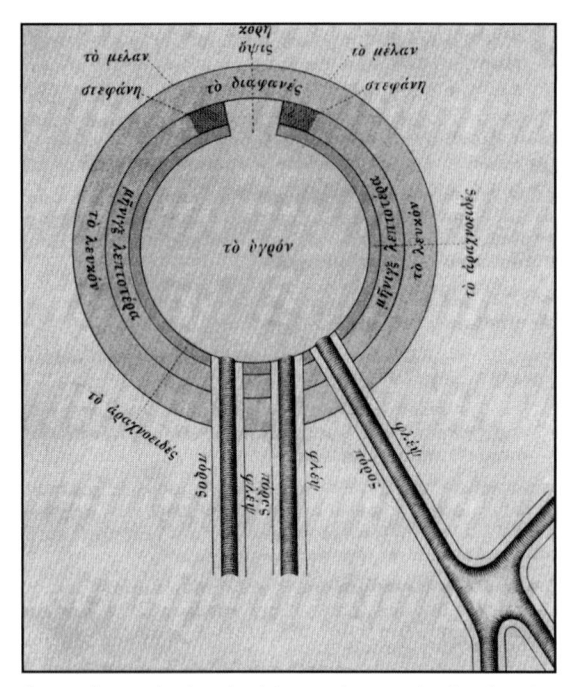

Copy of an early sketch of the eye from antiquity showing the researcher's concept of the multiple layers of the eye and the various connections emanating from the back of the eye toward the brain. By far, the best summation of early work of the history of ophthalmology, beginning in antiquity, has been provided by Sir Stewart Duke-Elder in his *System of Ophthalmology*.

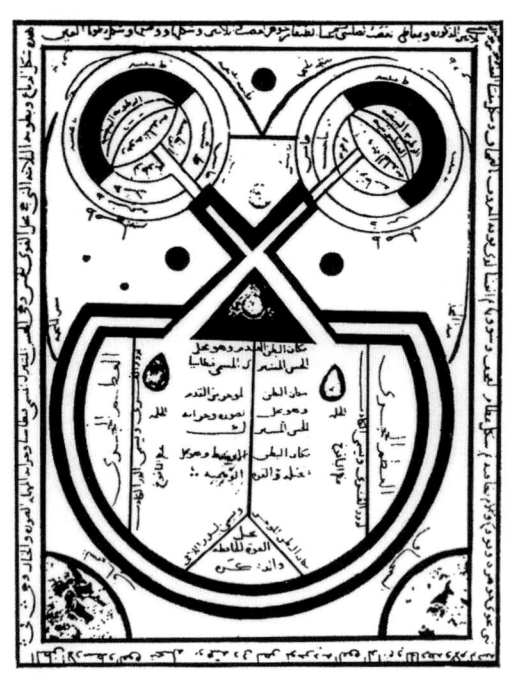

Early Arabian work showing, possibly for the first time, the crossover of connections between the eyes and the brain. Clearly marked on this sketch is the optic chiasm, where the nerve fibers from each eye cross and continue into the brain. This helps explain why the patient often has "left-sided" or "right-sided" lesions when certain diseases or trauma affect the visual system.

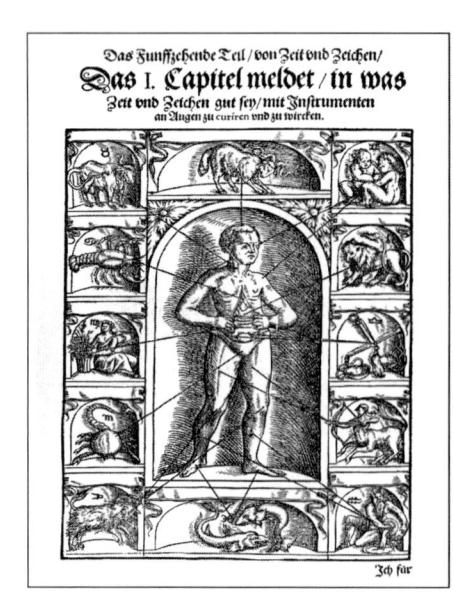

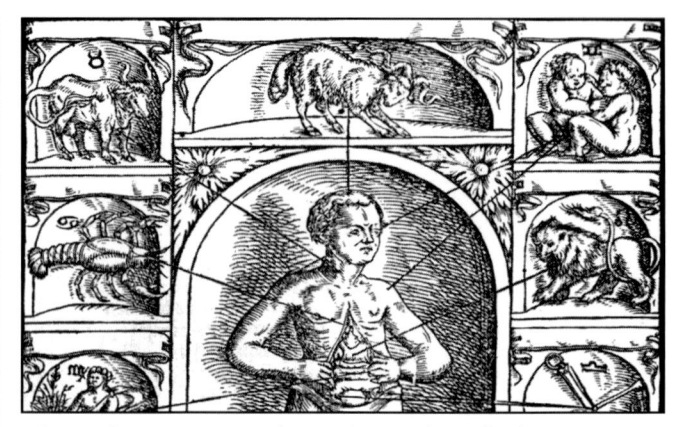

As late as the 1500s—even beyond—astrologic thinking sometimes dominated scientific thinking.
LEFT: A page from the classic textbook of Bartisch showing various figures from astrology and corresponding body parts.
RIGHT: The small figure at the upper right of this drawing relates to the eye.

RIVER WALKS

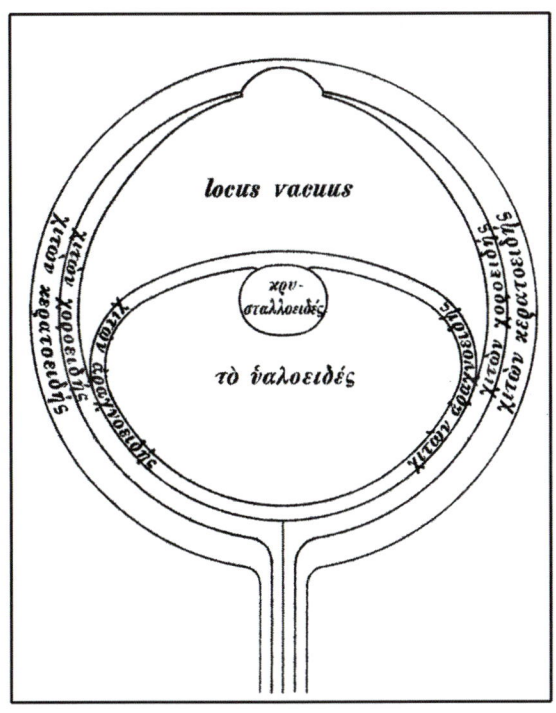

The location of the lens. Even into the Middle Ages and early Renaissance, many authorities believed that the lens was in middle of the eye, much further back than it really is.

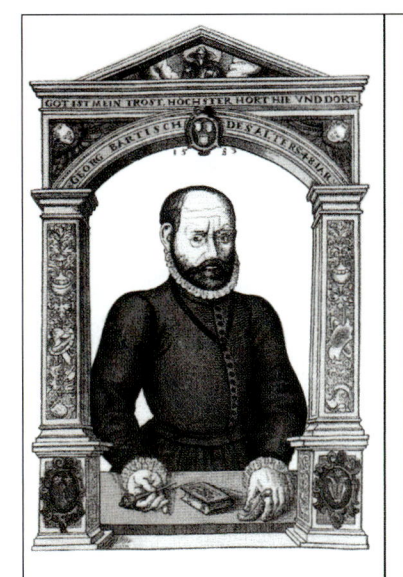

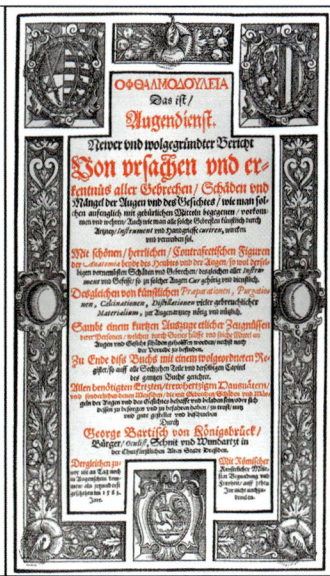

One of the greatest comprehensive books on ophthalmology of the renaissance was written by Georg Bartisch of Dresden, Germany.
LEFT: An image of Bartisch in the front material of that text.
RIGHT: The title page. The book is titled *Das ist Augendienst,* loosely translated as *Ophthalmology* (service to the eye).

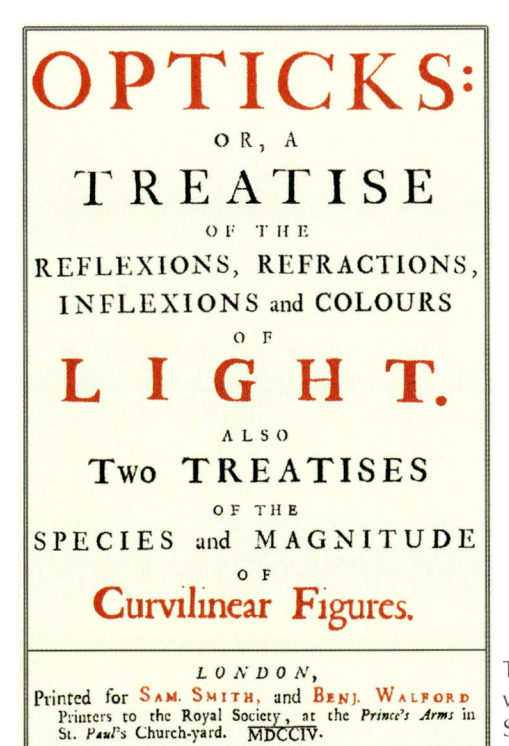

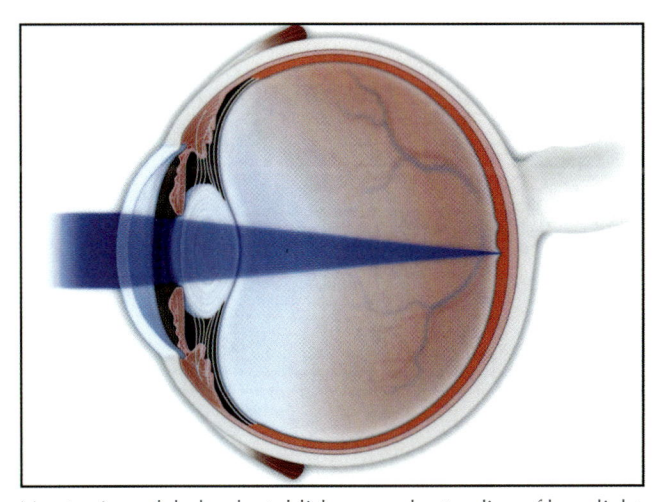

Newton's work helped establish our understanding of how light rays enter the eye and helps us understand the field termed "refraction": for example, the study of near- and farsightedness and astigmatism.
A diagram of how the external rays enter the eye through the cornea, anterior chamber, and lens and are focused onto the retina (right in this diagram).

Title page of the great treatise on optics written by Sir Isaac Newton, 1705. This text was translated into multiple languages and became the Bible in the field of optics. Some of Newton's work is considered controversial today, but most of it still applies in clinical practice.

CHAPTER 5

Newton's work helped clarify the anomalies termed farsightedness (including presbyopia or vision of old age) and nearsightedness (myopia). We can thank Newton and his colleagues for our understanding of these problems, often termed "errors of refraction."
TOP LEFT: This diagram shows the problem of farsightedness (hyperopia) in which the focus of the cornea and lens does not bring the rays onto the retina.
BOTTOM LEFT: The figure shows how a so-called plus or biconvex lens is necessary to bring the rays to focus on the retina.
TOP RIGHT: This diagram shows the problem of nearsightedness (myopia). The focusing power of the lens and cornea does not bring the rays to focus on the retina; rather they converge in the center of the eye (arrow).
BOTTOM RIGHT: Nearsightedness can be corrected by a so-called minus or a concave lens. This latter lens is seen in spectacles of thousands of people who classically "have problems seeing the blackboard at school."

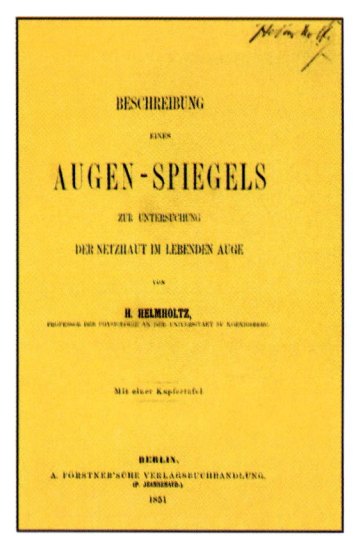

Title page of Helmholtz's description of the ophthalmoscope. Literally translated, the term "augen-spiegel" means *eye mirror*.

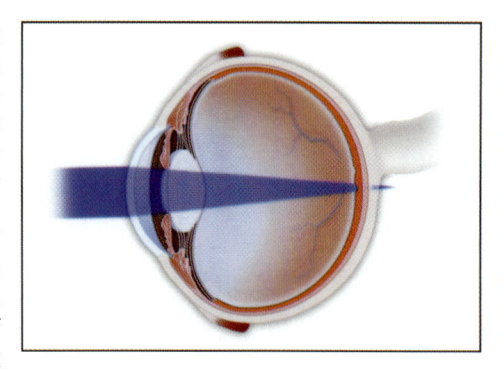

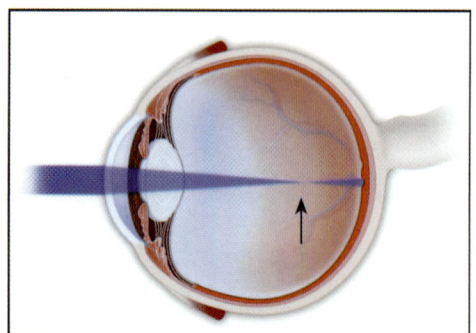

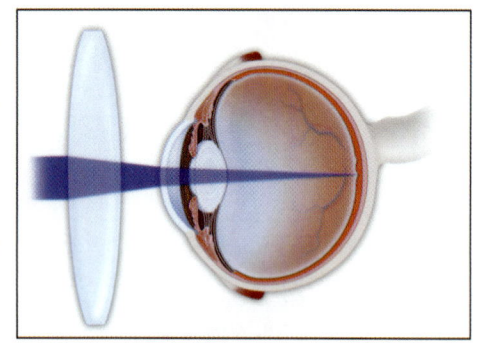

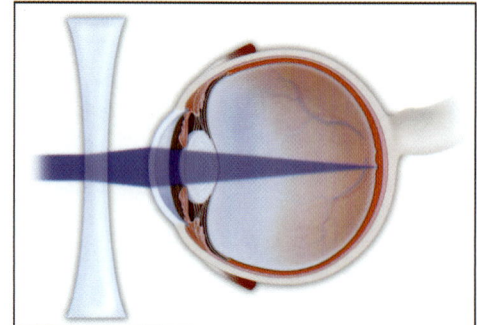

Harold paid a special tribute to the Swedish ophthalmologist, Alvar Gullstrand (1862 to 1930). Just a few decades prior to Harold's first IOL implantation, Gullstrand was actively studying the optics of the visual system and laid out the principles that led to his invention of the biomicroscope or slit lamp. This is the instrument that revolutionized our ability to examine and hence diagnose diseases of the anterior segment of the eye, especially the cornea and the lens. Gullstrand is one of only a few ophthalmologists who have received the Nobel Prize.

The great eye pathologists of the 19th and 20th centuries had a strong importance for Harold. He learned about the anatomy of the eye from them and about the causes of various eye diseases, cataracts. Ernest Fuchs of Vienna (whose clinic Harold visited in the 1930s) and John Parsons of London were among the most important pathologists of the late 19th and 20th centuries.

Our conversations were not solely focused on historical events and advances, of course, but we also talked about current trends, practices, and innovations. Although Harold had no special training in ocular pathology, he enjoyed discussing various aspects of this field with me. He had a great respect for his English colleague, Dr. Norman Ashton, and he of course eventually savored my studies on the histology and pathology of the IOL. We also discussed our common friend and professional colleague, Dr. Kensaku Miyake of Nagoya, Japan. Dr. Miyake had developed his posterior viewing technique so that ophthalmologists could study the interior of cadaver eyes from behind. My team and I modified and improved it, thereby developing the procedure that Miyake named the Miyake-Apple posterior video/photographic technique, an excellent tool for research and teaching.

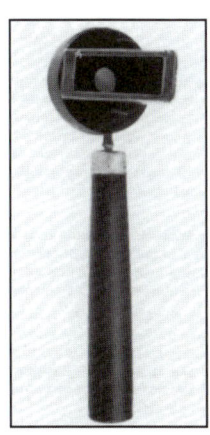

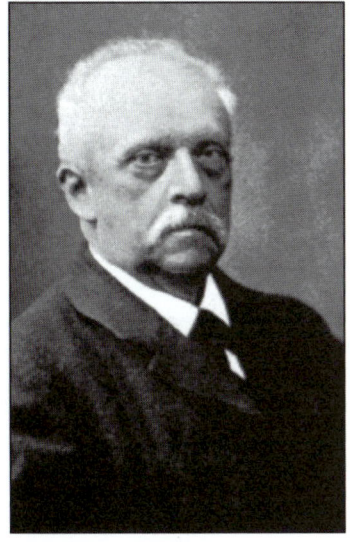

The invention of the ophthalmoscope. LEFT: The original ophthalmoscope was a very simple device with an appropriate lens that allowed light to enter the patient's eye and then be reflected back into the eye of the examiner, creating the needed image for examination. RIGHT: Photograph of Hermann von Helmholtz, Professor in Berlin. He was both a trained physicist and ophthalmologist.

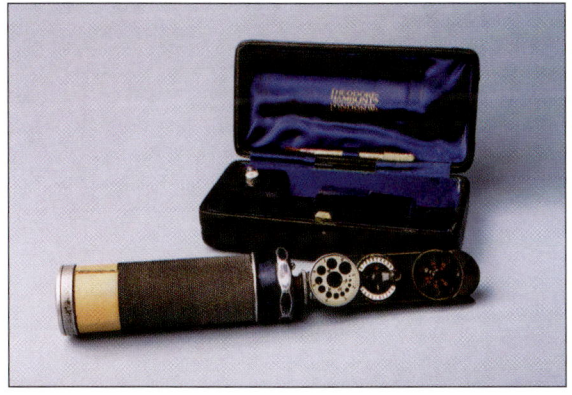

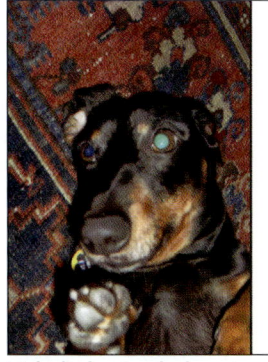

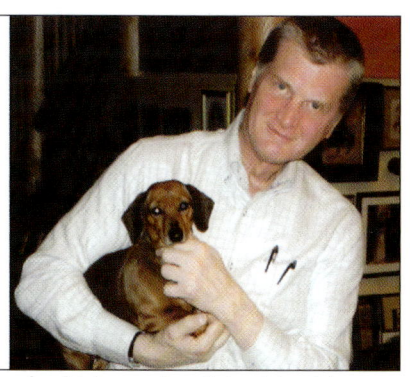

Helmholtz (and almost everybody) knew that light shined into an animal's eye at night would present a glow. This is a photograph of such a "glow" from my dogs
LEFT: The conditions are right—the location of the camera and the direction of view of the dog—to allow for this bright reflex.
RIGHT: There is minimal reflex in the other dog's eye because the rays of light are not directed as needed. Helmholtz and Babbage were able to harness this in order to create a clinically useful instrument.

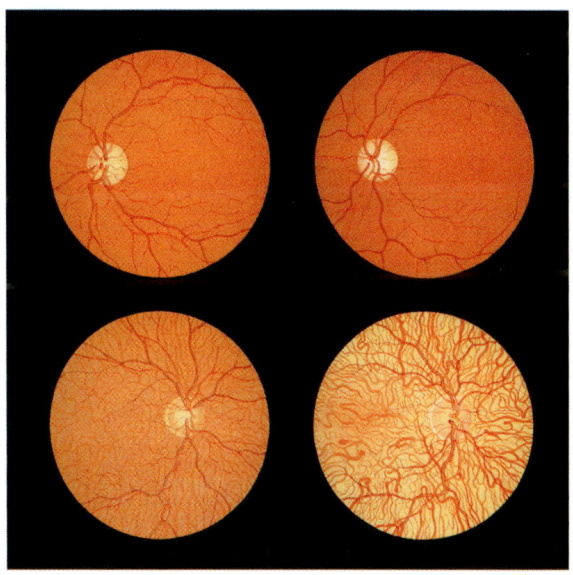

More advanced ophthalmoscope with several dials that provide different functions; owned by Harold Ridley.

Early artist's drawings showing four different eyes and revealing how the vessels in the eye may assume different patterns. Some authorities have actually attempted to utilize various vascular patterns in the eye to function as "fingerprints" in criminal investigations.

CHAPTER 5

The great Swedish ophthalmologist Gullstrand did brilliant work in several fields, including optics. He is credited as the inventor of the slit lamp, on which every patient who visits an eye care professional places his or her chin and is viewed by the light of the examiner. He is one of the few ophthalmologists in history to receive the Nobel Prize.

Gullstrand's work was closely examined by Harold Ridley and his colleague from Rayner & Keeler, Ltd., Mr. John Pike, as they made calculations in the development of the IOL.

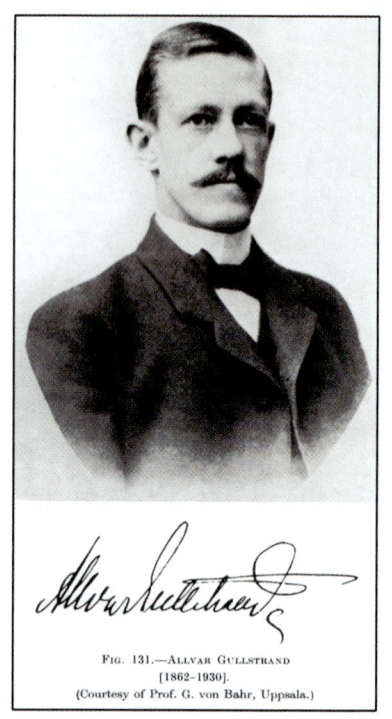

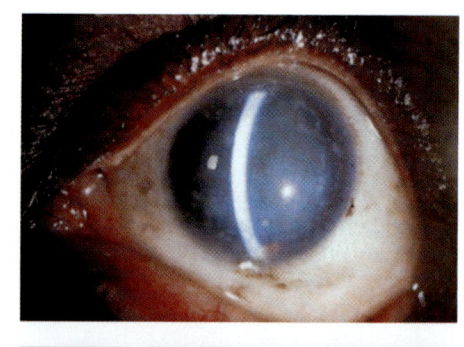

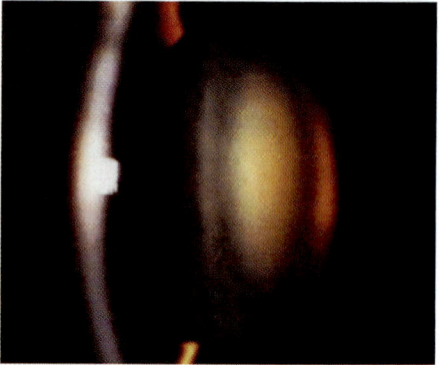

Fig. 131.—ALLVAR GULLSTRAND [1862-1930]. (Courtesy of Prof. G. von Bahr, Uppsala.)

The slit lamp allows a view of the eye structures almost at the level of a microscope. It is sometimes termed "biomicroscopy." The term slit lamp was coined because a slit of light is directed onto the eye, and the level of disease can therefore be documented.
TOP: The slit of light is focused on the surface of the eye, connoting corneal disease.
BOTTOM: The slit of light on the cornea is relatively normal, but the massive white opacity behind it connotes a cataract.

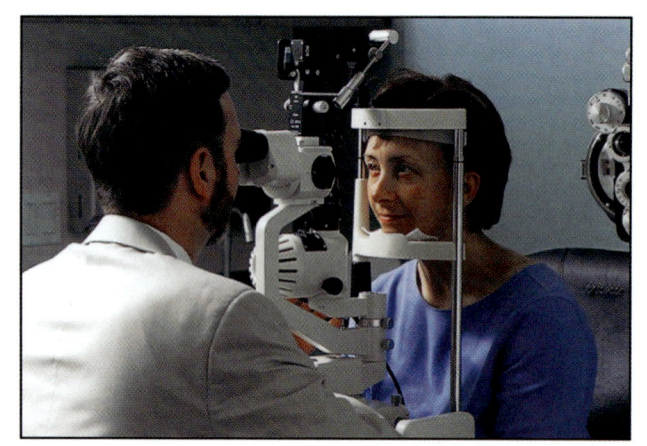

A modern slit lamp. All of us who appear for eye examinations appreciate this. Now we know that we can thank Professor Gullstrand for this invention.

An important modification of pathologic techniques was introduced by Dr. Kensaku Miyake in Japan, shown in this photograph. He was the first to photograph an IOL in an eye obtained postmortem, viewed from behind. This was a technique used by myself and my colleagues in our laboratory. We modified and improved it, and it is now termed the Miyake-Apple posterior video/photographic technique.

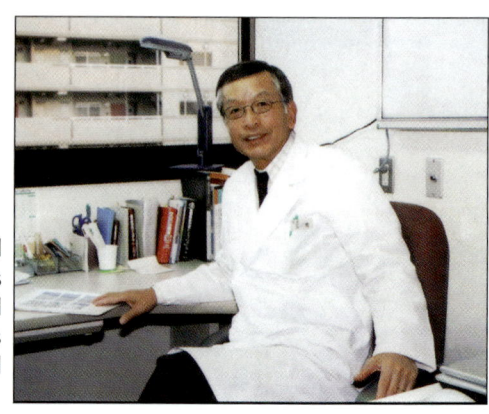

RIVER WALKS

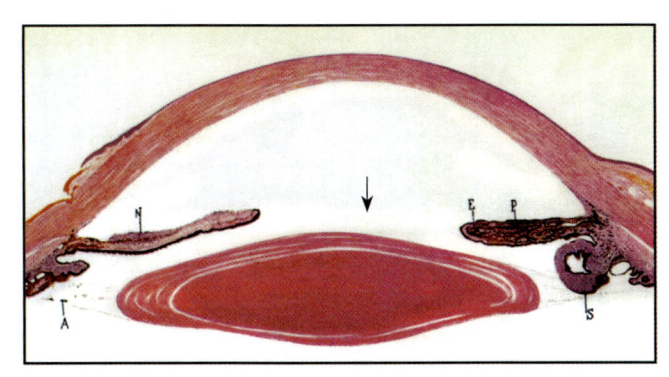

A high-power photomicrograph (picture taken through the lens of a microscope) from the early 20th century. Note the details. At the top is the cornea, analogous to the cover of a watch crystal. At the bottom center is the lens: the space between the cornea and lens is termed the anterior chamber. Note the two leaves of the iris, which terminate just in front of the lens, leaving the open space (arrow), which is the pupil.

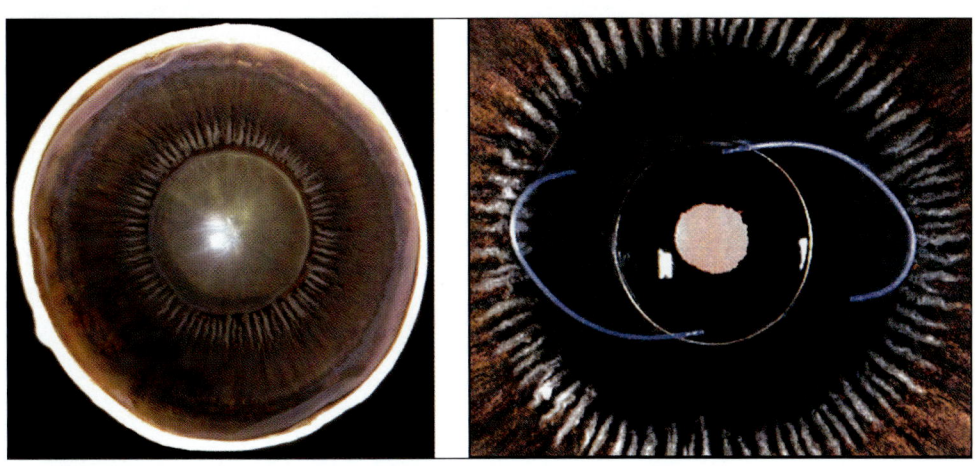

The Miyake-Apple technique, what it shows.
LEFT: A cadaver eye viewed from behind (looking from the brain), showing an intact lens that has a cataract, as evidenced by the discoloration and haze that is visible.
RIGHT: A different cadaver eye. The Miyake-Apple technique is used to show an IOL in place. This IOL has been placed within the residual capsule (almost invisible in this photograph) after ECCE. The lens is beautifully centered, and the optic is clear. The lens is held in place by the two blue loops, or haptics. Views such as this have provided magnificent opportunities for teaching and research since their first use in the mid-1980s.

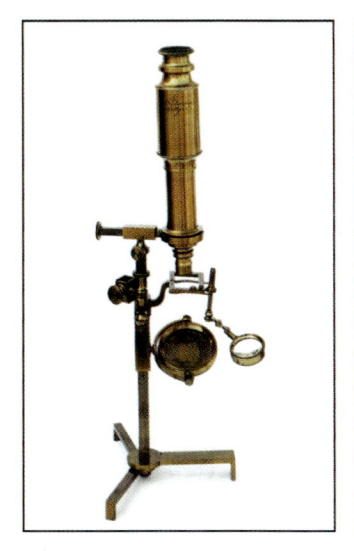

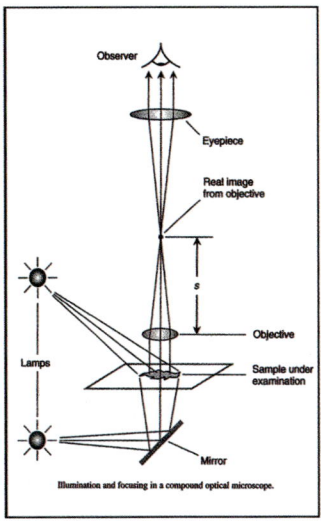

A haberdasher in Holland named Leuvenhoeck invented the microscope. For the first time, tissues could be examined at very high power, and from that time on, we could begin to understand diseases and, therefore, learn to treat them.
LEFT: An early 16th century microscope.
RIGHT: A diagram showing the path of light rays in a standard microscope.

CHAPTER 5

This photograph shows a montage of several possible views with different lens styles and surgical techniques—applications with modifications of the original Miyake-Apple technique. Note that the lens can be viewed from the side, obliquely, or from above. The lens at the upper left is actually being inserted into the eye, an image taken from a video. This technique has been applied to video cinematography, and actual movements that occur in surgical techniques can be recorded.

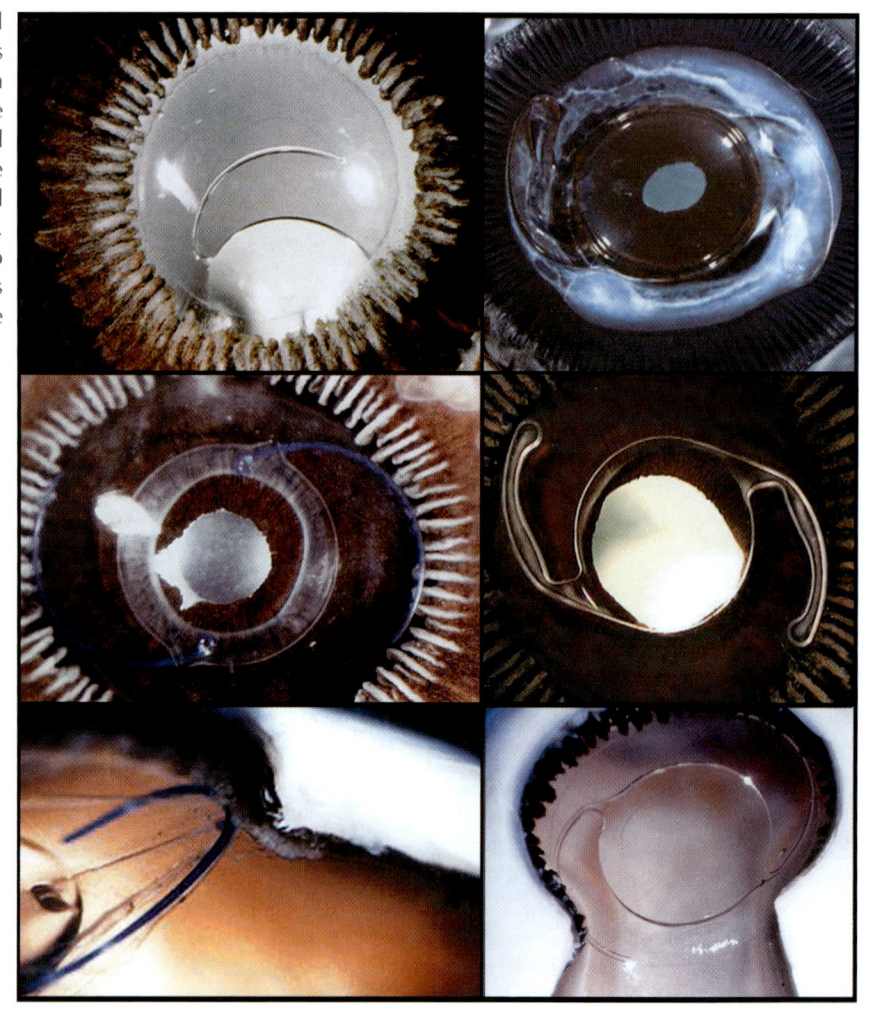

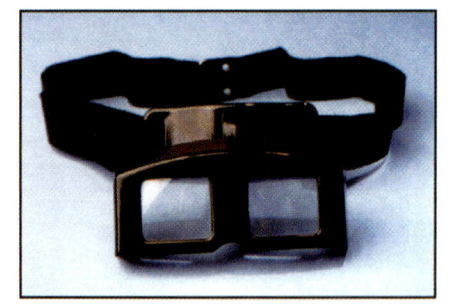

Optical aids used by Harold. Loupes that provided magnification of the operative field at surgery. This was the best option available before the invention of the operating microscope.

Recall Ms. Clarke's assigned job in the operating room at St. Thomas' Hospital on that fateful day in 1949 when the implant procedure was born (see Chapter 1). She was to manage the flashlight (torch) according to the surgeon's instructions. This of course underscores the fact that there were no self-illuminating operating microscopes at that time. Harold himself had attempted to fabricate one using discarded metal tubes, illuminators, etc, but the lighting he generated was less than he could depend on with his loupes and the flashlight.

As we discussed the topic of surgical field illumination, I told Harold about a one-year sabbatical postdoctoral fellowship I completed at the Eye Clinic of the University of Tübingen, Germany, in 1972. This had been one of the stellar departments in Europe since the mid-19th century and it has remained so. I mention this now because, in many ways, Tübingen and various sites in the surrounding region can lay claim to being the birthplace of the operating microscope. Professor Heinrich Harms and Professor Gunther Mackensen are credited as codevelopers of today's operating microscope along with others, including Dr. Richard Troutman in New York. Without this invention, today's modern small incision phacoemulsification surgery with IOLs would be possible.

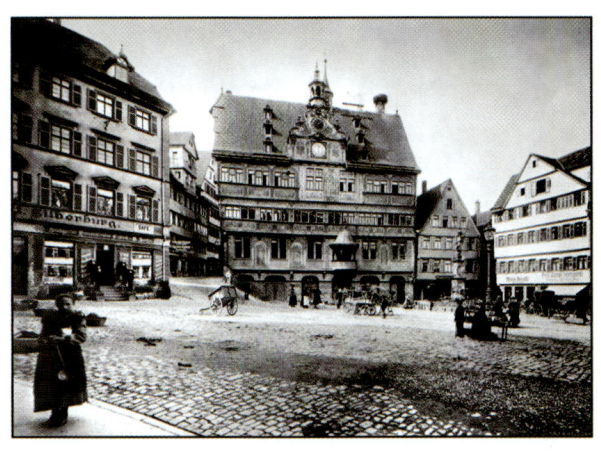

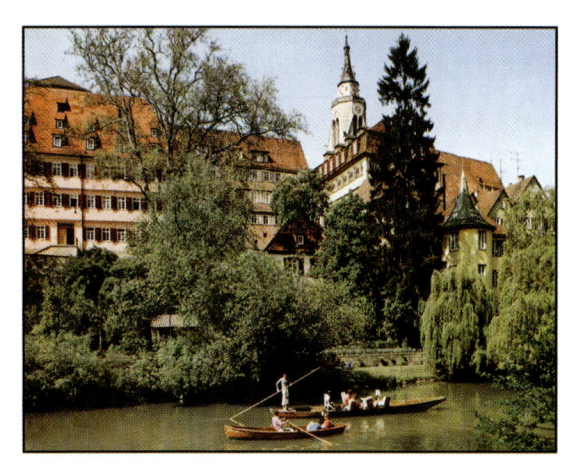

The university town of Tübingen. LEFT: Nineteenth century view of the Central Square. RIGHT: Twentieth century view of the waterfront. Being a university-oriented town, students would often congregate along this waterfront. This river is the Neckar, which flows into another great university town, Heidelberg.

The German colleagues were fortunate that in the closing days of World War II, a truck carrying refugee scientists and technicians from the world famous Zeiss factory in Jena of the former East Germany, formerly termed the "German Democratic Republic," escaped westward. The story is that they ran out of gas at a small town that was called Oberkochen, quite close to Tübingen. This became home of the new West German Zeiss facility and, therefore, provided the expertise and access to technology that continues to provide all sorts of optical instruments today. These were the individuals who helped fabricate the operating microscope.

The Eye Clinic at the University of Tübingen was a leader in the field of operating microscopes and microsurgery and was also a leader in other fields that proved necessary for modern cataract surgery. These included anterior segment microsurgery (chaired by Professor G. O. H. Naumann, with whom I coauthored a book in German on ocular pathology, see Chapter 4), retinal fluorescein angiography (Prof. A. Wessing), and a new technique for measuring visual fields, which was critical in diagnosing glaucoma (Prof. A. Aulhorn).

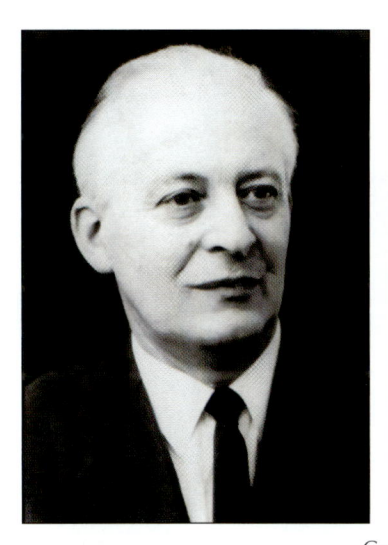

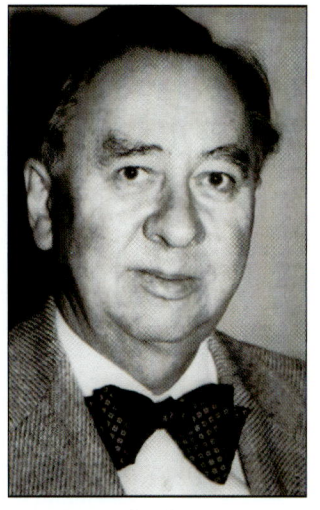

Coinventors of the operating microscope, the instrument that has made possible modern cataract surgery through small incisions. LEFT: Professor Heinrich Harms. RIGHT: Professor Gunther MacKensen.

However, pondering that year (1972), with hindsight over 20 years after the invention of the IOL, I do not believe that the term *intraocular lens* was ever mentioned in that institution, not in the hallways, clinics, or operating suites. No one spoke for or against the IOL; it somehow seemed to be a nonissue. This further symbolized the still-ongoing difficulties that Harold had in gaining acceptance.

CHAPTER 5

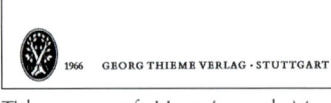

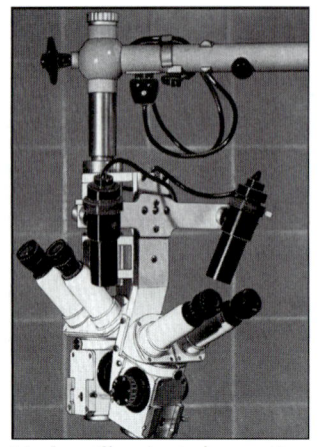

Title page of Harm's and MacKensen's classic book on *Eye Operations Using the Microscope*.

Modern illuminated operating microscope. These devices were initially manufactured by Carl Zeiss, Inc but are now manufactured by many firms.

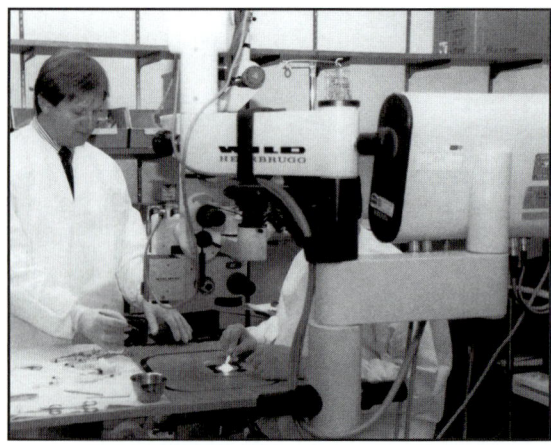

A modern illuminated operating microscope, manufactured by Wild, used for experimental surgery in my laboratory. Note that the young surgeon has placed a portion of the cadaver eye on the wooden operating table and is now able to do experimental and teaching operations through this microscope.

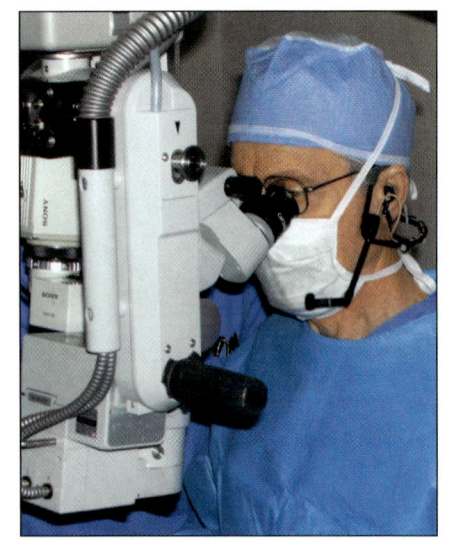

Microscopic procedure performed by Dr. Howard Gimbel of Calgary, Canada. Dr. Gimbel, who works with Dr. Thomas Naumann of Munich, introduced the continuous circular capsulorrhexis (CCC) technique, which helped revolutionize modern cataract surgery. As he began his career in cataract-IOL surgery, he visited the great Dutch pioneer Cornelius Binkhorst, who was one of the early advocates of ECCE.

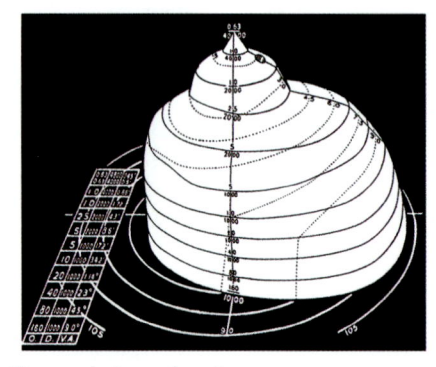

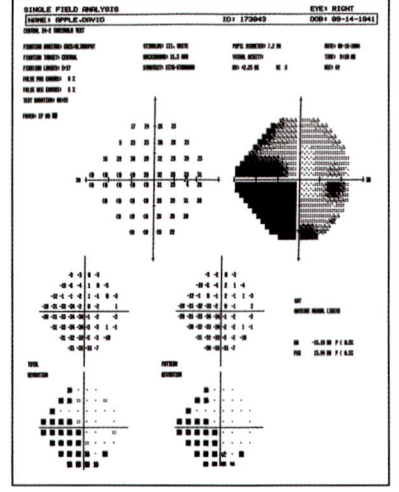

The evolution of perimetry.
LEFT: Our visual field is like an island in a sea of darkness. Our best vision is when we look straight ahead, the mountain peak on this island, and it tapers down as we move toward the periphery. In early times, this was directly measured by shining a light on a wall and asking the patient to respond regarding the visibility.
RIGHT: The great contribution of the group at Tübingen, directed by Professor Aulhorn, was to introduce what is called static perimetry, which now is used as a form of digitalized perimetry and analysis of the visual fields. This is a visual field taken on the author, who had some vascular problems. Note that the lower left quadrant is black, representing a focal loss of vision in that quadrant of the eye.

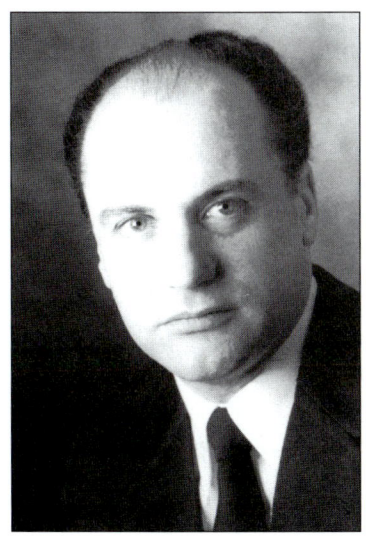

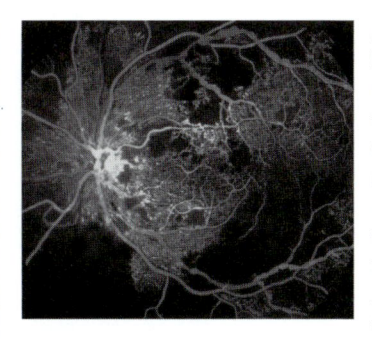

Major contributions to fluorescein angiography were made by a professor in Tübingen.

LEFT: Dr. Achin Wessing, who began his career with the great Professor Gerd Meyer-Schwickerath in Essen, Germany, worked in Tübingen and advanced knowledge regarding the technique of retinal fluorescein angiography. Ridley knew Meyer-Schwickerath very well because the former was the inventor of photocoagulation, which is now the procedure used for laser therapy of retinal diseases. Angiography, first proposed by some medical students in the United States, is now an advanced procedure helping in the diagnosis of such diseases as diabetes and macular degeneration.

RIGHT: Fluorescein angiogram, a form of x-ray of the blood vessels. This shows a patient with diabetes and large clusters of abnormal vessels that have a potential to bleed and scar and, thus, lead to blindness.

THREE SURGICAL METHODS TO REMOVE A CATARACT

Harold indeed realized that "the best crystal ball is a rear view mirror." The accumulation and assimilation of knowledge, data, and techniques advanced over the years by the above mentioned researchers and many others had helped grow the field of surgical ophthalmology, so that by Harold's time, he had gained confidence in his ability to proceed with his experiments on the IOL. After all, the placement of an IOL depended on applying most of the previous techniques learned in the past in order to get the faulty lens out of the eye and then prepare a "field" for the implant.

List 5-1 summarizes the three major possibilities that Harold had for lens removal. Before he settled on one as his favorite, he studied all three.

Like most surgeons, he rejected couching. Not only was it dangerous, but as he began thinking about the IOL, it was impossible to imagine having 2 lenses in a single operated eye—the "couched lens" displaced and floating somewhere in the bottom of the globe and the IOL itself.

Harold did not strongly object to ICCE, the operation in which the entire lens is removed in-toto, capsule and all. This is probably very surprising to today's young surgeons who have never done an ICCE. Harold told me that most of what he knew about the ICCE operation he had learned on a tour of the European continent he had made with his father in the 1930s, particularly in Vienna in the great eye clinic chaired by Professor Ernst Fuchs and his successor, Karl Lindner. Harold felt that the choice of the procedure was an individual one. ICCE worked very well in specific situations in which ECCE was unusually difficult or impossible, especially in the underprivileged world.

I actually began my career in surgical ophthalmology in the early 1970s. My first 10 cases were done with ICCE with no problem. For several reasons, including the introduction of high quality IOLs designed for placement in the posterior chamber in the capsular bag, the third alternative, ECCE (C in List 5-1), became the preferred choice.

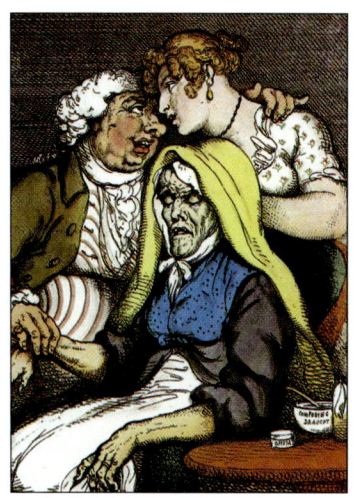

Eye surgery was sometimes a primitive and barbaric procedure. In some cases, families would take advantage of their local eye surgeon to actually eliminate elderly members of the family. In this illustration, the daughter is conversing with the surgeon with the intention of "killing two birds."

CHAPTER 5

An illustration showing unique Roman couching instruments excavated from an ancient camp situated near Mainz on the Rhine, Germany.
LEFT: Five individual instruments were found in this container. They are noteworthy for their skillful decoration.
RIGHT: These instruments were x-rayed, and it was discovered that several were more than simple needles. A careful study revealed that some of the needles were hollow, containing an interior needle that could be withdrawn. The purpose of these needles was to remove the cataract by a suction technique. The needle was inserted into the cataractous lens, the central portion withdrawn, and the surgeon literally sucked through the hollow tube in an attempt to extract some of the lens material. This form of couching was indeed revolutionary since it was in effect the forerunner of modern extracapsular surgery, which also has the purpose of extracting lens material with suction.

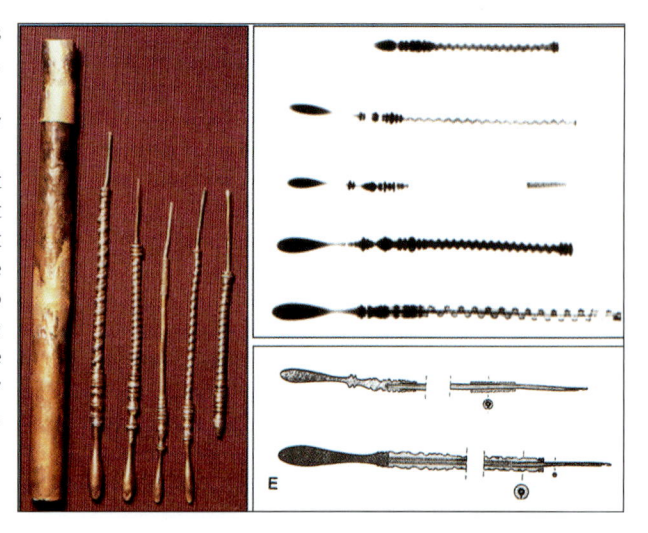

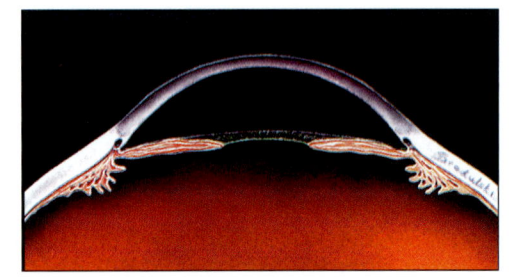

Schematic illustration of an eye showing the result of an ICCE. Note that no lens is present. It has been removed in its entirety from the eye. The result here is actually no different from that which occurs with couching. One negative feature of both couching and ICCE is that by removing the lens in its entirety, including both the interior material and the surrounding capsule, there is no scaffolding left to fixate an IOL to in this space, as is required for a modern posterior chamber lens—the type that Ridley invented and advocated.

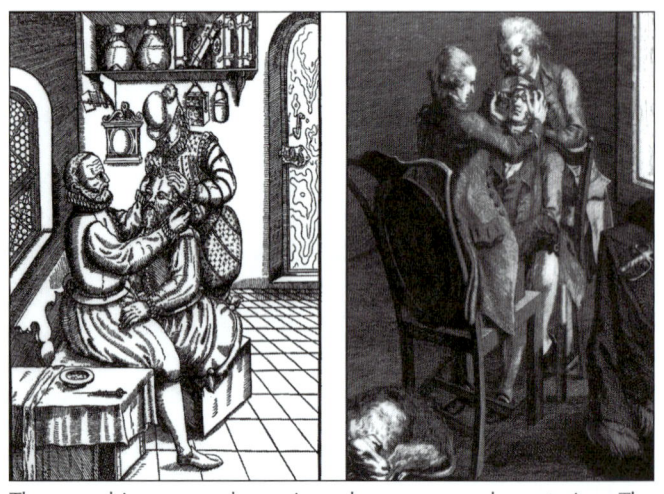

The couching procedure viewed over several centuries. The procedure remained the same: in general, a gruesome and futile attempt to dislodge the lens without complications. Only the dress of the doctor and patient changed. LEFT: Sixteenth century. RIGHT: Eighteenth century.

By the beginning of the 20th century, the ICCE technique came to prominence. This is the technique where the surgeon removes the entire lens by pulling it away from its surrounding zonules. This was commonly performed in the underprivileged world where rapid and effective surgery was required for large populations.
LEFT: Colonel Henry Smith who worked for the British Colonial Medical Service, resided in India and over his lifetime performed thousands of cataract procedures, all of the ICCE type.
RIGHT: A photograph of Colonel Smith examining a patient. He almost always had a cigar in his mouth, even during surgery.

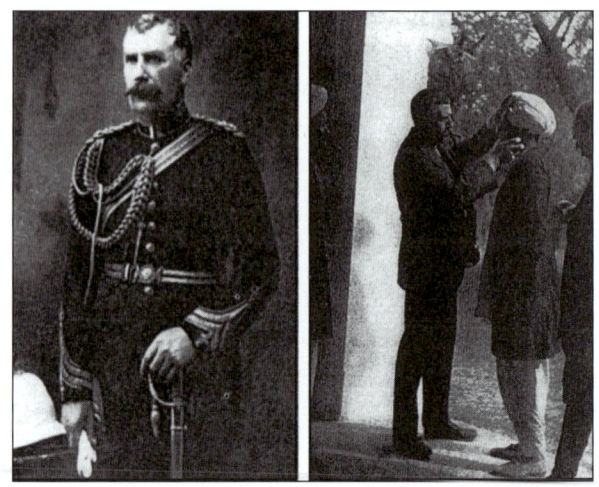

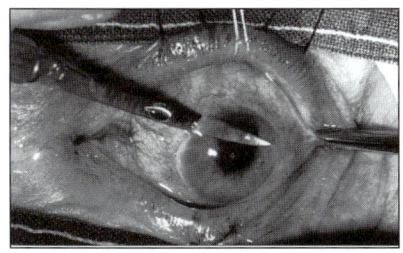

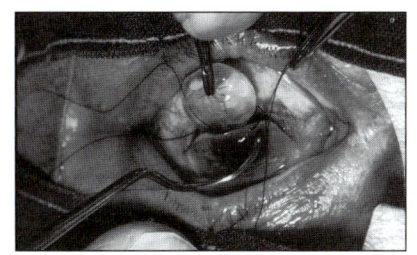

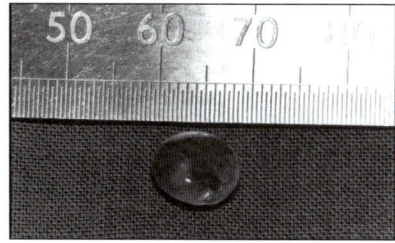

The essence of the ICCE procedure is shown in these photographs, courtesy of Peter Choyce, MD, UK.
LEFT: Entrance into the eye with a knife.
MIDDLE: The removal of the entire lens through the large corneal incision that was made.
RIGHT: A photograph of the intact extracted capsular bag.

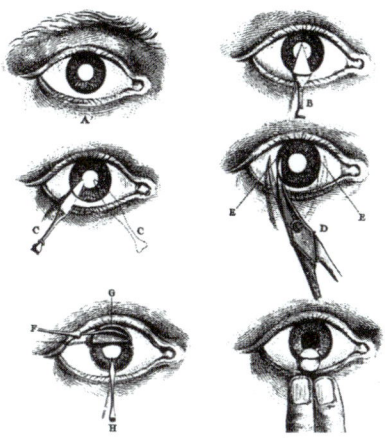

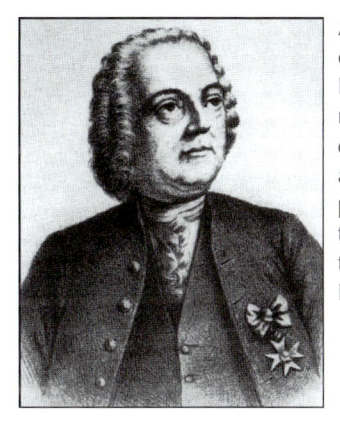

A drawing of Jacques Daviel, who revolutionized cataract surgery, as reported in an article in 1744. He devised what is now termed the ECCE. This represented one of the first attempts to actually *extract* cataractous lens material from the eye, as opposed to, for example, the classic couching procedure, where the lens was simply *pushed* into the bottom of the eye. This was a major advance that Ridley was able to apply as he developed the IOL.

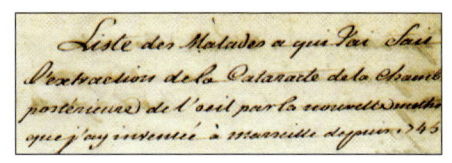

A diagram from Daviel's original article showing the steps of his technique of cataract removal.
TOP LEFT: The original cataract.
BOTTOM RIGHT: The final removal of the cataractous lens material.

A photograph of a small segment from Daviel's original surgical notes, the first description of what is modern ECCE.

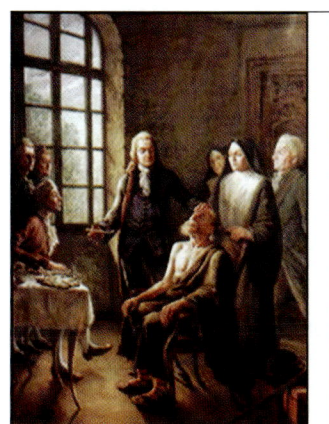

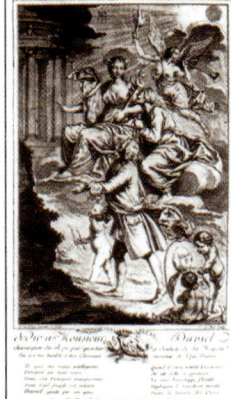

Daviel's procedure was so successful that he was revered and feted, treated by many almost as a god.
LEFT: An idealized painting showing Daviel conversing with a patient.
RIGHT: A sketch showing Daviel surrounded by heavenly figures.

CHAPTER 5

Harold quickly concluded that the ECCE was his preferred procedure, not only because this was a safe operation as he was able to do it but also because it was best suited to his concept for fixation of his planned IOL within the eye.

He was very fortunate that his teachers Hudson and Doyne at St. Thomas' Hospital had taught him to perform a very high quality ECCE that he himself was able to continuously improve. This of course was the procedure that Daviel had introduced to the world and represented the first attempt to *extract* the lens out of the eye, as opposed to *pushing* the lens further into the eye, as was the case with the couching operation. This was important because the latter operation with IOLs, which he eventually invented and advocated, required the presence of a capsule so that the IOL could be held in good position. We have not yet differentiated between the 3 basic IOL types; that will come later. For now, suffice it to say that the Ridley IOL and most IOLs studied are posterior chamber IOLs that require ECCE. Had Harold been focused on ICCE, it is possible that he would have had difficulty in making the proper transition that would have been necessary to accommodate his own invention.

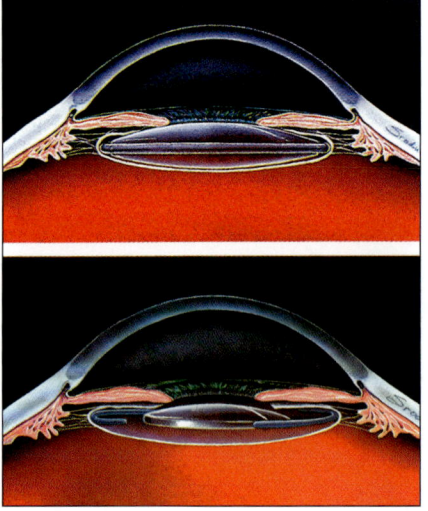

Finally, it is beyond the scope of this book to detail the fine work of Charles

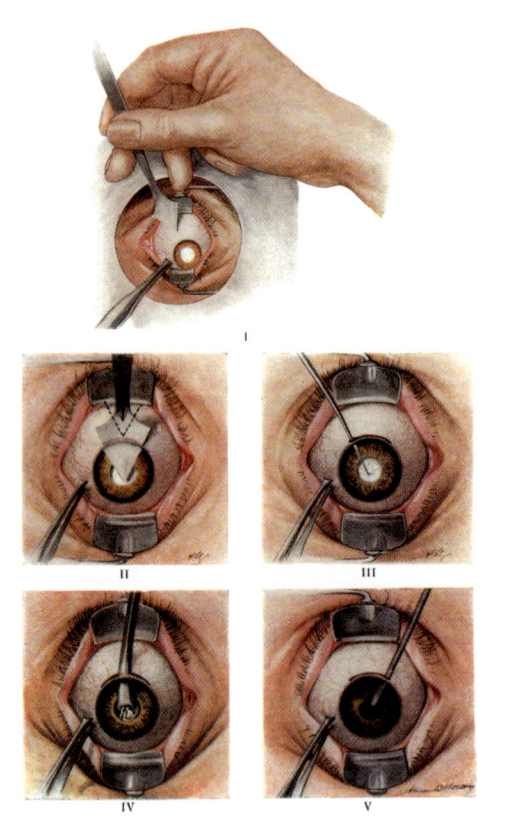

A series of paintings from a 19th century textbook showing the steps of the ECCE procedure.
The cataract (top, figure I) is removed by opening the capsule and expressing and washing the material out of the lens interior (figure IV). All that remains in the eye is the clear posterior capsule, which does not interfere with passage of light to the visual axis (figure V).

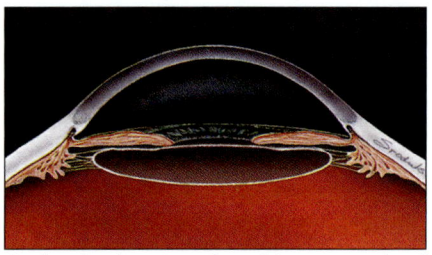

A sketch showing the ultimate result of an ECCE. Notice that the lens capsule is present except for a small region in front, within the realm of the pupil where it had been cut into in order to gain surgical axis to the interior of the lens. The residual empty lens, as seen here, is called the lens capsular bag. The lens capsular bag is Harold's preferred site and the preferred site that surgeons use today for placement of modern posterior chamber IOLs.

Two sketches showing the placement of IOLs into the lens capsular bag, which had been previously evacuated by the surgeon. TOP: Placement of a Ridley-type IOL into the capsular bag. We will see later that Ridley intended for lens placement into the bag as illustrated here, but because of limited surgical technique available at the time, it was not always possible for him to achieve this goal. Many times the lens would be placed outside of the capsular bag, but if secured well next to the iris, it would remain in place. BOTTOM: An idealized drawing of the preferred placement of modern posterior chamber IOLs that have supporting elements (haptics, or loops). The loops are blue in the image.
With today's modern operating microscopes and surgical techniques, it is possible in almost all cases to implant a lens securely in the bag, as seen here.

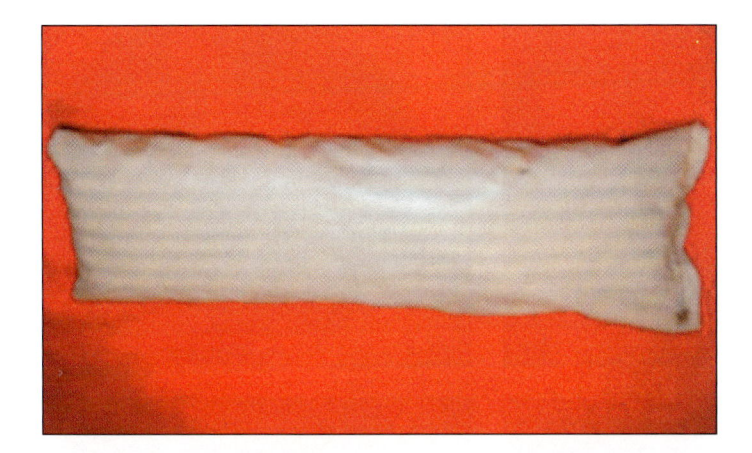

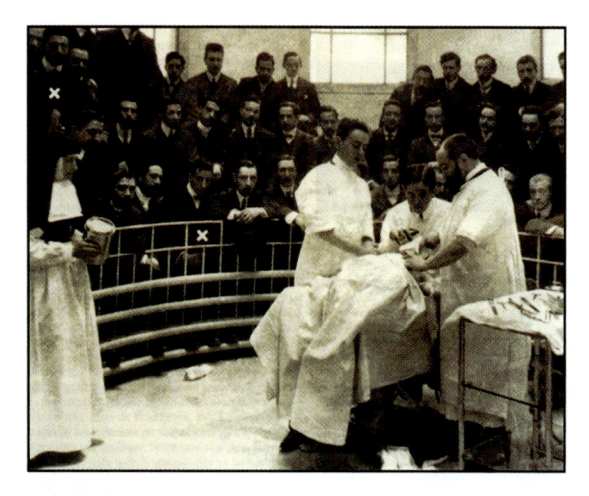

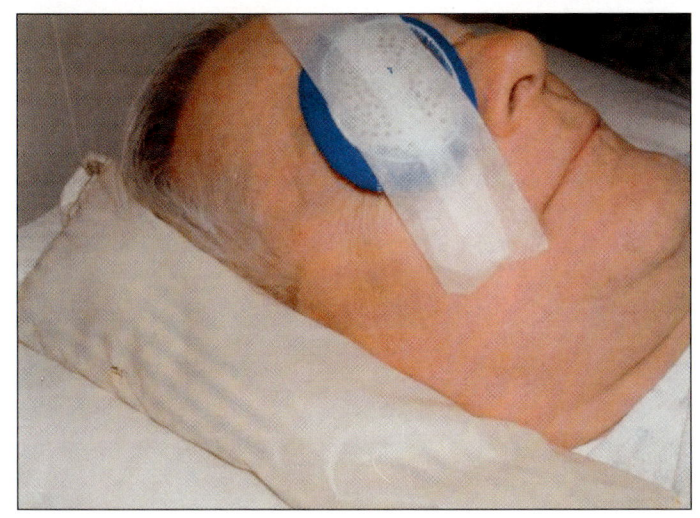

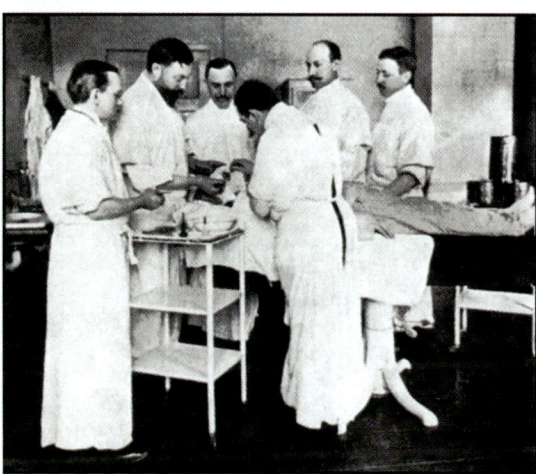

Even at a late date, all aspects of cataract surgery were not rosy. TOP and BOTTOM: Patients were required to lay very still for several days after cataract surgery. I can still remember this practice when I started my career in the 1970s. To keep them from moving, sandbags were often positioned around their head and neck—a very unpleasant feeling. Today the typical IOL patient stands up smiling and is home in a few hours, perhaps even on the golf course.
(Sandbag photographs courtesy of Dr. Charles Letocha.)

By late in the 19th century, the surgical techniques were continuously improved as well as the overall handling and treatment of the patient as a whole. Notice here the operations taking place in relatively clean conditions with the patient lying prone, as opposed to earlier times when the patient was generally sitting up.
TOP: A famous eye clinic in Spain, the Barraquer Dynasty of Barcelona was and remains world famous. Numerous observers are seated within the amphitheater around the patient
BOTTOM: As the operation evolved more attention was given to sterile conditions, as evidenced by the participants' gowns. The patient is in a closed operating room.

Kelman who delivered phacoemulsification to our repertoire. This procedure (inspired by observation of dentists as they utilized the process of emulsification with ultrasonic probes for work in the oral cavity) when applied to eye surgery as a means to emulsify and remove cataractous lens material, allowed surgeons to perform even better operations—to successfully pursue today's modern techniques—foldable IOL insertion through small incisions (a form of arthroscopy). This also helps us use today's specialized IOLs (eg, the advanced multifocal designs shown in Chapter 1 and others [Chapter 11]). Harold never had the opportunity to use phacoemulsification. It arrived too late. An appropriate honor to Kelman would also require an entire book. I hope that one will be written soon.

Now that Harold had established that ECCE and eventually phacoemulsification were most appropriate for his step 1, and having discussed it in this chapter, we can now move to Chapter 6, the beginnings of step 2, the bone-fide complete cataract IOL operation to *modern visual rehabilitation*.

CHAPTER 5

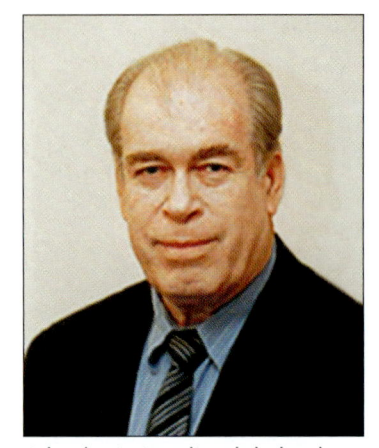

A leader in Israeli ophthalmology, Professor Michael Blumenthal, among many his accomplishments, developed techniques for the application of ECCE throughout the underprivileged world; earlier, at the time of Colonel Smith, only ICCE was possible.

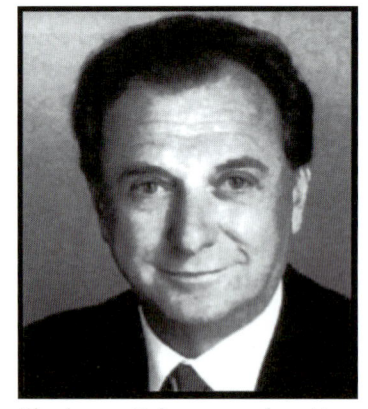

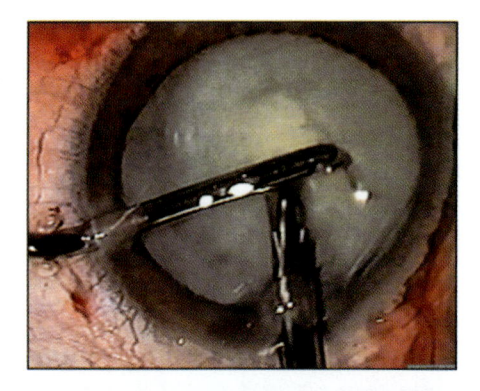

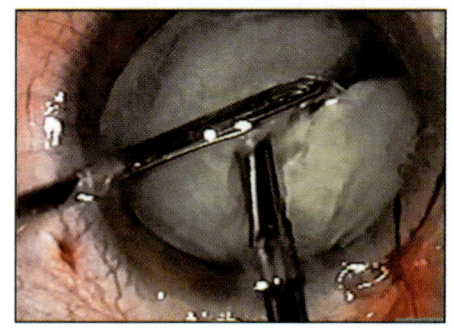

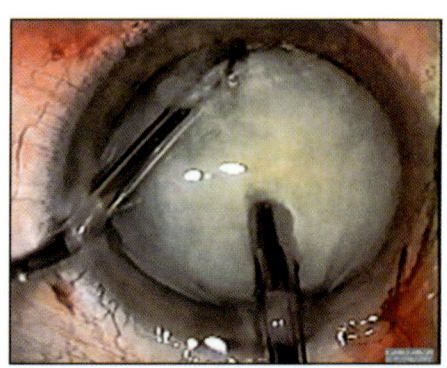

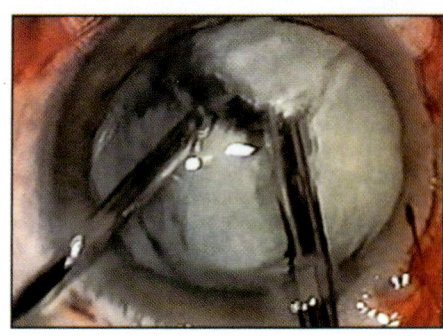

A montage of four illustrations showing the concept of preparing the lens for removal via phacoemulsification. The surgeon enters the lens and divides it into segments, rendering it susceptible for emulsifying or dissolving and then aspirating with the phacoemulsification apparatus.

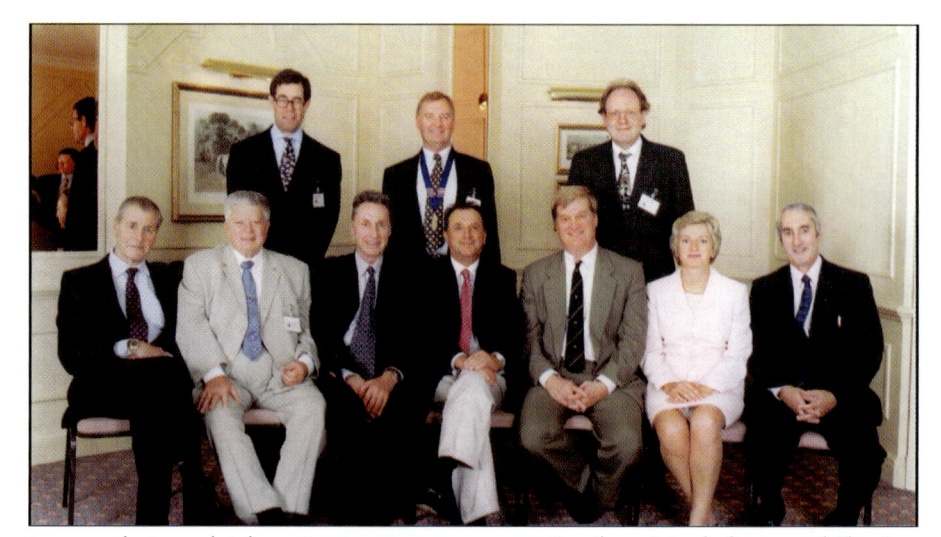

Charles Kelman of New York was the inventor of phacoemulsification, which for the first time allowed surgeons to, in effect, do an advanced form of ECCE in a fashion that allowed modern small incision surgery with foldable IOLs.

A group photograph taken at a meeting commemorating the original phacoemulsification procedure performed in Europe by Dr. Eric Arnott. Several pioneers of phacoemulsification and IOL research are pictured at this gala occasion which occurred in Chester, UK in 2003.
Participants included from front row left: Prof. Eric Arnott; Dr. Fyodorov, Soviet Union; Dr. Robert Sinsky, Santa Monica, Calif; Dr. Charles Kelman, New York City; Dr. David Apple, Charleston, SC/Salt Lake City, Utah; Dr. Helen Seward, London; and Dr. Patty Condon, Waterford, Ireland. In the back row are Dr. Richard Packard, UK; a representative of the Alcon Corp, UK; and Dr. Hans Reinhard Koch, Bonn, Germany.

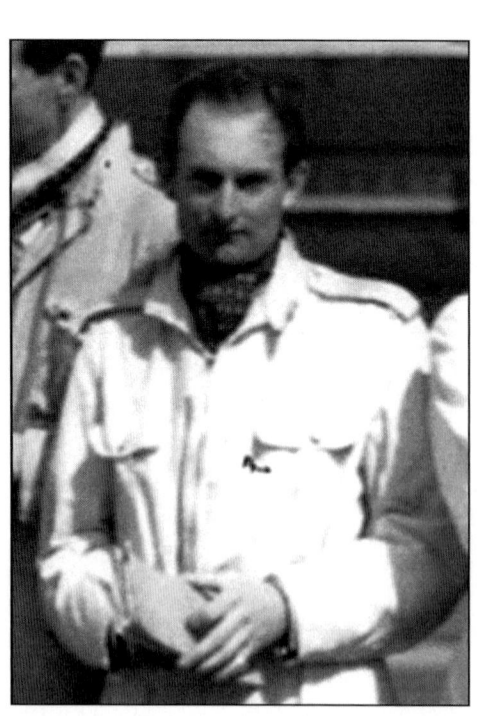

Flight Lieutenant Gordon "Mouse" Cleaver would soon, without realizing it, play a major role in launching one of eye surgery's major advancements. Harold saw several pilots with the same type of injury crucial to the invention of the IOL. Cleaver is the only pilot where records are available.

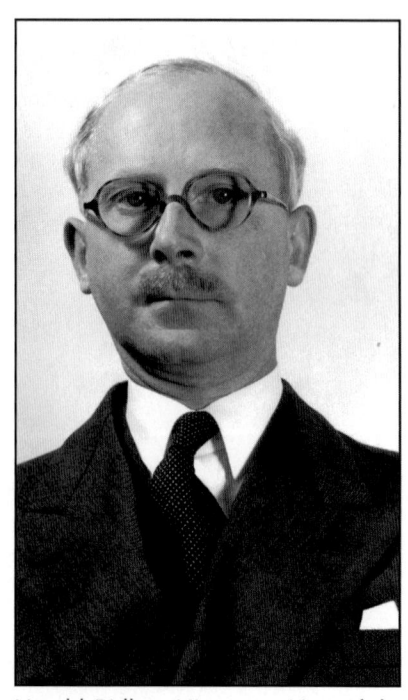

Harold Ridley: His recognition of the significance of Cleaver's injuries with respect to his idea of an IOL would begin the count down that would culminate in the invention of the IOL.

6

Adlertag:
The Quest for a *Complete* Cataract Operation, Step 2: Visual Rehabilitation with the IOL

"A pre-clinical/clinical study is performed on an invention that has not yet been invented."

David J. Apple, 2006

"Unless a sharp edge of the plastic material rests in contact with sensitive and mobile portion of the eye, the tissue reaction is insignificant."

Harold Ridley, 1951

"Everyone is aware by now of Mr. Harold Ridley's recognition of the discovery that fragments of Perspex in the eyes of service personnel appeared not to cause an inflammatory condition and, in most cases, could be left alone as harmless intraocular foreign bodies. As far as I know, service personnel are still walking about with these fragments inside their eyes, and I have not heard any case in which they had to be removed because of chemical reaction. It appears, therefore, that the original form of Perspex has at least 20 years history of inertness, if I may coin such a word, when placed inside the eye."

Mr. John Caudell, Rayner & Keeler, Ltd.

In Chapter 5, Table 5-1, I tabulated, based on our discussions during our river walks, the steps that Harold deemed necessary to ensure a *complete* cataract operation. Step 1 is the diagnosis of the cataract and actual surgical *removal of the obstructing cataractous lens material*. Step 2 is the *visual rehabilitation* with the *IOL*. In this chapter, I will begin the complex story of the origin of the IOL.

CHAPTER 6

Cataract removal began with couching (hammer blow) over 6000 years ago, and by the 20th century, progressed finally to the present modern ECCE/phacoemulsification procedures (see List 5-1, page 81). By the time Harold entered the scene in the late 1930s and 1940s, the basic ECCE procedure had advanced sufficiently, and he deemed the time ready for commencement of experimentation on his new idea of implanting an IOL. The technique of phacoemulsification was popularized long after Harold's first operation, and it came on the scene and was popularized about the time he retired. He, therefore, had no experience with it. From what I know about Harold, he would have been quick to latch onto phacoemulsification. He was a superior surgeon, and he knew it (in a modest way). His technique was so good that he had excellent results with basic ECCE. However, being an extremely forward-thinking person, he would have immediately latched onto the many clear-cut advantages of modern phacoemulsification (eg, the modern small incision foldable IOL techniques).

Harold described the sequence of events from antiquity to the 1940s, as he entered the scene, as follows:

First, he described the evolution of Step 1:

"For centuries, cataracts must have been recognized as the most common cause of blindness in old age; for even in the absence of examination instruments, the change in color of the pupil would have indicated that the lens was abnormal. It is said that an illustration on a stone from a pyramid suggests that treatment by couching was being performed in prehistoric times, but the birth of cataract surgery as we know it dates from 1748 when Daviel described removal of the opaque lens, less its capsule incision."

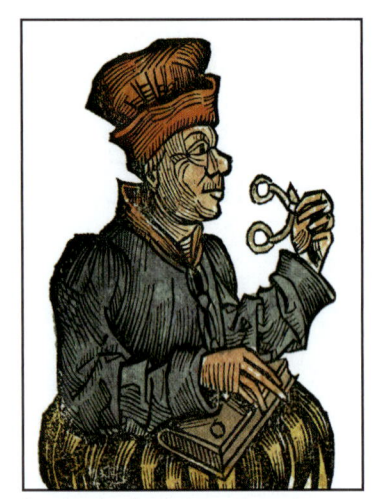

Spectacles have been in existence for centuries, as this illustration from the middle ages exemplifies.

Harold then proceeded to the issue of Step 2:

"This open surgery (ECCE) was surely more reliable and effective than dislocation of the cataract by external hammer blow. However, the sight, even with the aid of powerful spectacle lenses, was found to be far from normal. Within half a century, attempts were made, according to Casanova, by Tadini and others to replace the missing cataractous lens with a lenticulus composed of glass. Their results, however, were immediate failures, for the new lens immediately dislocated into the vitreous, and further attempts to replace a defective lens were abandoned until the time was ripe, which involved a delay of no less than 150 years.

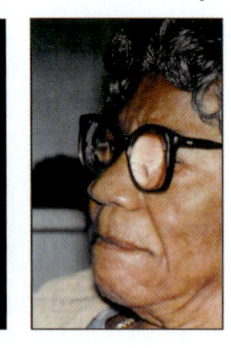

Thick aphakic spectacles, given to patients after cataract removal. These were commonly used for visual rehabilitation of the IOL before Harold's invention.
LEFT: If broken or lost, as often occurs in underprivileged communities, they are usually irreplaceable and the patient is often as blind or blinder than prior to the surgery.
RIGHT: The thick "coke bottle" lenses in aphakic spectacles cause terrible visual aberrations.

"Many primitive eye surgeons must surely have thought that a new lens for old would appear one day when science was suitably advanced, and I was one of the many hundreds who considered but abandoned that possibility before the 1939-45 war. I talked to my father and my great teacher, AC Hudson, about a skilled man whose career had been ruined by a small intraocular foreign body, which had produced a cataract in one eye. Each of his two eyes could read 6/6, but they would not work together. Surely the time would come for someone to attempt the cure of Aphakia."

Stage 1 was discussed in Chapter 5. In this and the upcoming chapters (6 to 12), we will focus on Step 2, the evolution of the implantable device that finally brought to fruition Ridley's goal to cure aphakia (aphakia = absence of the lens). This step (List 5-1, page 81) provides the visual rehabilitation made possible by the IOL.

Regarding the inventor of the IOL, there are only *two* known possible sources that are documented in writing. First, there is a cluster of stories that began with writings by Casanova that I termed the "Casanova stories." Most agree that many if not all of the "Casanova stories" are suspect or apocryphal. Harold was not aware of these before he did his first operations. However, as he learned about these years later, he believed that they were informative in that they helped to confirm his presumption that surgeons and other interested individuals, including both legitimate physicians and charlatans and dreamers, had for centuries thought about the idea of placing an appliance in the eye that would function as an artificial lens: "a new lens for old," as he termed it. "Many others had considered but abandoned this possibility." Harold had discussions with his father and with "Huddy" showing that he had considered this at least as early as the mid-1930s, and throughout the second World War, he obviously *did not* abandon the idea.

Secondly is a tale that I always believed was too good to be true, the "airplane story." We now know it was *not* a tale. There are no other claimants to the throne of being the inventor of the IOLs, and no one doubts that it was Harold. I always found it difficult to believe what I thought to be a fantasy about the gallant pilots and "spitfires." However, the fact is that truth is sometimes stranger than fiction.

Few of the millions of patients worldwide who now enjoy the benefits of the modern cataract-IOL operations are aware of the origin of this innovation. Indeed, few eye-care professionals—even ophthalmic surgeons who implant them almost daily—are aware of the origin of the IOL: the invention that, as Harold Ridley himself liked to say, "cured aphakia." Considering the importance of the IOL and the fact that it brings sight and a higher quality of life to more than 10 million patients worldwide each year, it seems incredible that the evolution of the IOL remains so obscure.

Harold's IOL was made possible in part by observations of downed pilots during the war; this made the cataract operation complete, both quantitatively and qualitatively. It provided for the first time a proper replacement for the ineffective, thick, aphakic spectacles that had been in use for so many years: since the early 17th century, if not earlier. In other words, he broke the huge barrier to achieving Step 2 complete visual rehabilitation. Though Harold treated several pilots who had suffered eye injuries, the actions of only one pilot, Flight Lieutenant "Mouse" Cleaver, who inadvertently became an important player in the history of lens implantation, are fully documented medical records that have become available to us and, thus, allow us to tell his story.

Harold had become an almost forgotten footnote in history. I hope to change that. My research began almost immediately after my first meeting with Harold and his wife Elisabeth in 1985. At first, this was a slow process. I found a scrap of evidence here, another piece of information there, and was eventually able to solve the puzzle and elucidate a fairly complete picture of how the IOL evolved.

CHAPTER 6

Casanova, Quacks, Progressives, and Prophets

At least five different accounts regarding the IOL have circulated over the past 400 hundred years. Most (but not all) were apocryphal, having little or no credibility. Listed chronologically, they involve the experiences of four separate surgeons from the 18th century until the 1940s: Tadini, Casamata, Mikhailov, and Cavka. Finally, Foster, a surgeon from Leeds, wrote a humorous short story that turned out to be prophetic. With the possible exception of the Cavka story, these provide little scientific information but are interesting.

The first surgeon, a *Dr. Tadini*, has been brought to our attention by some research done by Dr. Paul Fechner in Germany. Apparently, Tadini was an itinerate Italian oculist of the 18th century, roaming about south-central and western Europe performing eye operations. He placed advertisements regarding his prowess in the local newspapers of each of the cities he visited.

Tadini met Casanova, the famous Venetian adventurer, in Warsaw in 1766. He showed Casanova a box of glass beads, claiming he could insert them under patients' corneas to replace their eyes' natural lenses after cataract removals. He made this claim in the presence of a local German professor who ridiculed him. Tadini is said to have reacted violently to this demand, threatening to attack the professor with his sword. As the word spread, the Warsaw clinical medical faculty demanded that Tadini pass an examination on the anatomy of the eye if he wished to practice in that city. An impossible task for him, he departed from the city shortly thereafter.

After Tadini departed from Warsaw, he did not see Casanova for years. He continued traveling, performing eye surgery, exhibiting his glass bead "lenses," and explaining to anyone who would listen that he could use them to restore sight to people with cataracts. Then he reached Spain and discovered that the authorities there were not good listeners. They rejected his claims, and in lieu of throwing him into jail, as was the custom at that time for unsubstantiated claims or quackery, he was drafted into the Spanish army.

Shortly after this, Tadini and Casanova had an almost unbelievable re-acquaintance, as described by Casanova in volume 11 of his memoirs. The great lover had recently gotten himself into trouble again (undoubtedly for his serial misbehavior with the local female population) and was serving a short jail sentence in Madrid. This was not an infrequent occurrence for Casanova, due to his tendency to chase down members of the female population in whatever area he lived or visited.

What *was* unusual, was the fact that Tadini—the same eye doctor whom Casanova had met in Warsaw several years earlier—was now standing guard on his prison cell! They spoke through the bars of the prison door. Standing there with his rifle with fixed bayonet, Tadini confided to Casanova that since their meeting in Warsaw years earlier, he had only talked about his small package of lenses and had never actually implanted one. He did state, however, that he felt certain they would have worked if he had been given the chance to perform his experiments. Thereafter, Casanova lost track of him and lamented that he "never learned what had become of the poor fellow, Tadini."

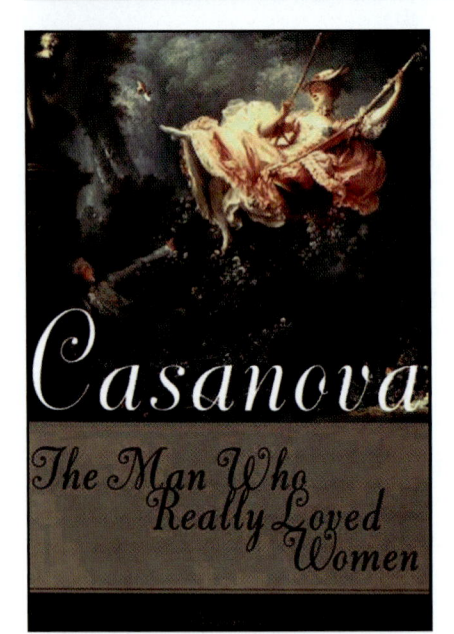

Giacomo Casanova (1725-1798) was a soldier, spy, diplomat, writer, and adventurer, and is chiefly remembered because of his adventures with women. In Chapter 11 of his memoirs he described a meeting with an itinerate surgeon, Tadini, who spoke of his desires to implant an artificial lens.
TOP: Dr. Tadini really existed. This image is an advertisement he placed in a German newspaper extolling his expertise as an eye surgeon.
BOTTOM: A focus on his amorous activities.

The second surgeon whose name has become associated with implants was also an itinerate Italian practitioner: a certain *Dr. Casamata,* the court oculist in Dresden, Germany, the sparkling baroque city sometimes termed "the Venice of the North." He was a contemporary of Tadini, and it is quite possible that these two surgeons and even Casanova may have crossed paths during their sojourns in Dresden, which was the capital of Saxony and a center of high culture. A large Italian colony existed in Dresden; it housed the numerous artists and craftsmen who were involved in helping create the city's great monuments, many of which were tragically destroyed near the end of World War II then rebuilt as faithfully as possible afterward. Casanova often visited Dresden during the short period when both surgeons were there, although those were very often cut short by pursuing husbands and police because of his restless behavior.

While there is no proof that would verify that Casamata was involved with implants, word has come down through an obscure text by a Mr. Schiferli (cited by a Dr. Munchow) that Casamata attempted to introduce a glass lens into a patient's eye through a cut in the cornea. He found, however, that the glass lens was not an adequate substitute for the natural one—at least with his surgical technique. He did not have the means of fixation, such as suturing the lens into the eye. Consequently, when he tried to carry out the procedure, the glass immediately fell down into the rear (bottom) of the eye.

Closer to modern times, another surgeon is said to have attempted to work with artificial lenses. *Dr. Mikhailov,* from the provincial city of Sukmumi in the former Soviet Union, had been doing investigations on corrections with IOLs. He reportedly made an oral report regarding his experiments to a meeting of the Rostov Ophthalmological Society, but the records were burned during World War II, and Dr. Mikhailov did not return to his experiments after the war; he died in 1958.

The next known attempt to replace a cataractous lens with an artificial lens is perhaps the most credible and scientific of all. Surprisingly, it had remained virtually hidden in medical literature since 1954. *Dr. V. Cavka* was a surgeon from Yugoslavia. He had been called upon to treat the severe eye injuries that a 32-year-old man sustained during a bombing attack in World War II. The young man had been successfully treated with corneal transplants in both eyes.

Dr. Cavka then described how he obtained a cadaver's eye and attempted to use the lens from that eye as a replacement for the damaged natural lens of the patient's left eye, which had been rendered totally occluded by the bomb injury. Dr. Cavka clearly described in an article, accompanied by photographs, how he performed a standard ECCE and then teased the cadaver lens into the patient's eye through a corneal incision. The implanted lens came to rest in its location in the posterior chamber, where the natural lens normally rests. Cavka did not mention any special attempt to provide a stable fixation for the lens, such as with sutures. He simply closed the eye, watched, and waited.

According to Cavka's article, he examined the cadaver lens in his patient's eye for a full six months and observed that the lens, amazingly, remained clear. Nothing more was ever heard of the results of Cavka's experiment, and no pictures were ever offered to substantiate anything resembling an acceptable permanent result. Although the attempt was made using what for Dr. Cavka must have been the best clinical and scientific methods of the time, we must assume that the lens had to have eventually clouded over, bringing the experiment to a failed conclusion. Our knowledge of the anatomy and physiology of the human crystalline lens and its cellular structure tells us that a transplant of this type was doomed to fail. This is because the metabolism of the lens would have been destroyed by two factors: first, the death of the original donor, and second, the trauma of the transfer of the lens into the living patient.

Taking himself less seriously than the three aforementioned aspirants to invent the IOL was a fifth surgeon whose name is forever linked to IOLs, Mr. John Foster of Leeds, England. He wrote a small vignette for the *Leeds Medical Society Magazine* in 1940. The article was not meant to be a serious treatise on the possibility of creating an IOL but to provide his local medical society colleagues with a little humor. Although the article was written solely for the purpose of entertainment, it turned out to be highly prophetic, with uncanny timing! Later, at the infamous 1951 meeting of the Oxford Ophthalmological Society (Chapter 9), hearing of Ridley's invention, he reawakened his article, which spoke of an intraocular glass lens that could replace a cataract, as follows:

> "American enthusiasm and the spirit of inquiry has in addition been a tremendous stimulus to all of us," he wrote. "If, for instance, an Englishman woke up one morning and thought it was a good idea to see if an intraocular glass lens could replace a cataract, he would possibly make inquiries and, having found that it had never been considered at Moorfields, and that the boy's school bill was due next week, he would give up the idea. His American homologue, McClusky, on the other hand, would get hold of two bright spirits with similar ideas, approach the Wilber G. Poluker Foundation for a $50,000 research grant and would then disappear under the surface for a couple of years. At the end of that time, a paper by McClusky, Zinzinheimer, and O'Hara would appear, showing that, except for a limited period, the idea was impracticable—negative evidence, of course, but nevertheless of interest. Meanwhile, the paper would reveal three or perhaps four important new physiological or surgical facts, and so the system would go on. A great deal of waste and with a tremendous dynamism, but always advancing!"
>
> *John Foster, 1940*

After hearing of Harold's accomplishment in curing aphakia, Mr. Foster remarked that it was a source of real pride to him that this invention, which might, he said, be one of the most significant advances in the ophthalmic surgical field, had been made by a "Britisher." When Harold heard about Mr. Foster's 1940 article and its connection to his innovation, he was very amused and pleased.

THE "AIRPLANE STORY" UNFOLDS: "A STORY TOO GOOD TO BE TRUE"

Very few of the ideas or attempts of the above-mentioned individuals appeared to advance the theory or development of the IOLs in any serious way. That task would await Harold and the "airplane story."

Although I do not believe that Harold talked publicly about the IOL prior to the time of its invention, he stated many times in his private papers that he discussed this topic in the 1930s, most notably with his father and with his beloved professor, Mr. Hudson (Huddy). Huddy was one of his favorite professors, and Harold considered him to be one of the finest surgeons in London. "Huddy" was, however, extremely conservative in his clinical decisions and always spoke, albeit mildly, against the implant. Neither did Harold's father, Nicholas, provide Harold any encouragement about the IOL. He did not hold discussions regarding this but clearly kept these in mind.

As I carried on discussions with Harold in his later years, I pried for information to verify stories I had heard about the World War II *Spitfire* pilots who had had plastic from their cockpit canopies blown into their eyes during aerial combat. According to many sources, Harold had gotten his idea for a plastic IOL from treating these flyers, observing that their eyes did not reject the plastic even after many years.

This seemed like a wonderful story to me but perhaps one that was *too good to be true*! Whenever I asked Harold about the Spitfire pilot stories during our river walks, he always terminated the conversation. Indeed, he rarely talked or wrote about the connection except in the most general terms, often referring vaguely to the "biomaterial" or the "injuries." Consequently, even though I interviewed him many times, I remained in the dark on this issue for several years.

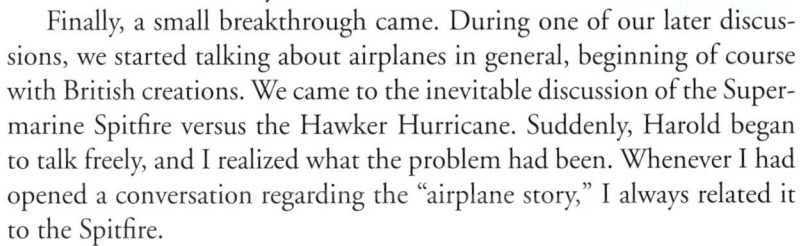

Finally, a small breakthrough came. During one of our later discussions, we started talking about airplanes in general, beginning of course with British creations. We came to the inevitable discussion of the Supermarine Spitfire versus the Hawker Hurricane. Suddenly, Harold began to talk freely, and I realized what the problem had been. Whenever I had opened a conversation regarding the "airplane story," I always related it to the Spitfire.

Apparently, many English people from that era had varying degrees of fondness for the different planes, and some then and even now are very adamant as to which they felt was superior. Harold was a Hurricane fan. Our subsequent conversations made it clear that he felt that the bulk of the work in the Battle of Britain was carried out by the Hurricanes, although the Spitfires sometimes got more publicity bordering on adoration by many. As soon as I recognized that Harold harbored a distinct preference for Hurricanes, I was better able to communicate with him on the subject that had previously been all but closed to me. Even then, in his unique way, he downplayed the importance of the connection. In his private papers, he wrote: "The story of the airplane is true, but overplayed as a good item for the press. However, these observations did provide an opportunity for a good *pre-clinical study*." (author's emphasis).

However, the more he told me, the more doors opened up before me, offering new avenues for inquiry and research. The deeper I dug, the richer the story became. Several individuals generously provided insight, documentation, and photographs that helped confirm the story. I am especially grateful to Professor Eric Arnott, Jack Riddle, Reggie Spooner, Jane Adams, Ian Collins of Rayner & Keeler, Ltd., the museum staff at RAF Tangmere, and the Ridley family for their cooperation in helping

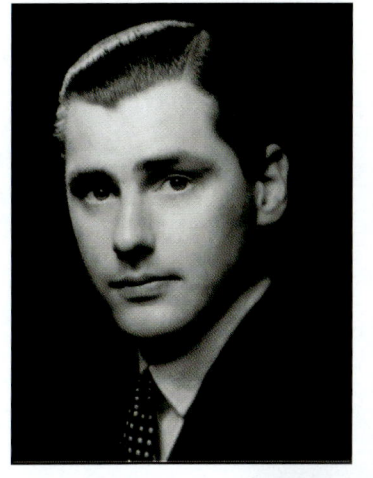

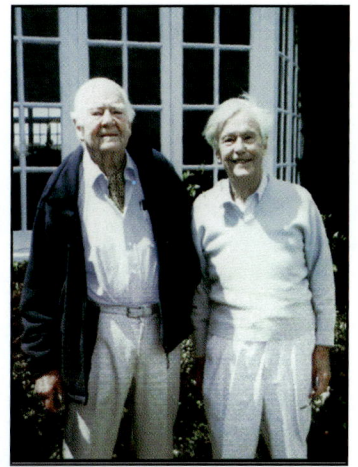

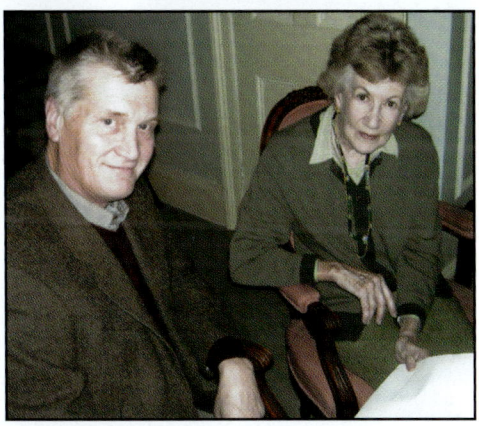

I am grateful to the following for information regarding "the airplane story."
TOP LEFT: Professor Eric Arnott, London, the first surgeon to perform phacoemulsification in England and the surgeon who years after the injury, implanted an IOL in "Mouse" Cleaver. He provided valuable information regarding Harold's role in the events of 1940.
TOP RIGHT: Jack Riddle, age 92 (left) and his 601 squadron adjutant, Reggie Spooner (right) during a visit I made to Riddle's home in June 2005, in Chichester, UK.
BOTTOM: I interviewed Mrs. Jane Adams, sister-in-law to Gordon "Mouse" Cleaver. She provided valuable information and photographs regarding Cleaver's role in the Battle of Britain and his subsequent clinical course after his battle injuries.

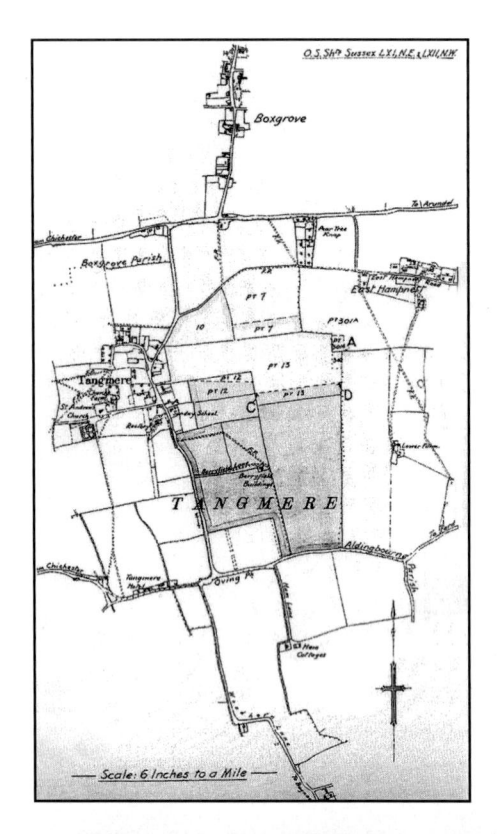

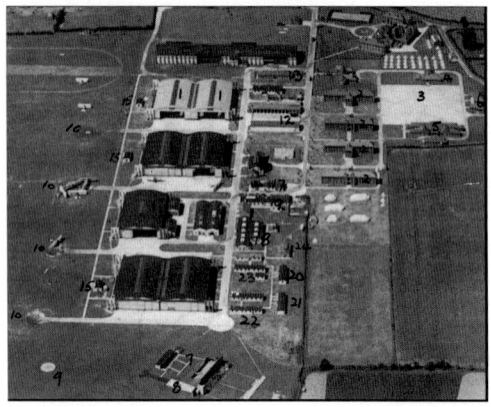

CHAPTER 6

clarify many details of this story. So here it is—this is the story of one of the injured airplane pilots, Flight Lieutenant Gordon "Mouse" Cleaver—a man who was somewhat renowned as a skier though unknown until now in the field of ophthalmology. His story is one that I have always believed was too good to be true—too cute. But it is true, and Flight Lieutenant Cleaver's injuries were connected with Harold's invention of the IOL. Remembering this, we must keep in mind the other young pilots who had similar injuries, but whose records are not available or are long lost. They would also have a nice "airplane story" to tell. We will begin with the story of an airport.

The Setting: Royal Air Force Tangmere and Surrounding Hospitals

The long and complex story regarding the invention of the IOL begins with an airport. For centuries, the English Channel had served as an important defensive barrier for Britain, providing an effective buffer against attacks, both small and large scale. However, as the French aviator Louis Bleriot became the first man to cross the English Channel in a heavier-than-air aircraft in 1909 (an event Harold as a young child attended with his father but obviously did not perceive [see Chapter 3]), that barrier began to crumble. By the time World War I broke out, just 5 years later, the concept that Britain was "no longer an island" was a grim reality. Fortunately, time would show that the British cleverly compensated for this new reality in World War II, both in their defensive strategy in the Battle of Britain and later in their and the American Air Force's bombing strategies in the war.

In the 1920s, Bayly's Farm, in the small community of Tangmere not more than 20 miles from the channel, was quiet and serene. Soon, this was destined to change. A pilot delivering mail crash-landed in the cultivated fields there. He was not injured. While waiting to be picked up by his colleagues and returned to his base, he viewed the surrounding property and quickly concluded that this would be an excellent location for an airport (aerodrome). His superiors eventually concurred, thus setting in motion the construction of what would turn out to be an important military airport: the Royal Air Force (RAF) Tangmere. This was a true godsend because it was destined to cause havoc to the over-flying Luftwaffe, the German Airforce, as they later attacked England in the Battle of Britain at the beginning of World War II.

Indeed, by the time the threat of World War II became a probability, the machines of aerial warfare had been developed to such a point that England was fully vulnerable to fighter attacks and massive bombing raids from across the Channel.

Furthermore, RAF Tangmere was perfectly situated for defense against these aerial invasions. Its construction represented a fine example of good military planning. It grew rapidly in the late 1930s as the government came to realize that a second war with Germany was inevitable. It was readied just in time. Not long after the completion of the major phases of its construction, RAF Tangmere was called upon to play what turned out to be an enormous role in combating the 1940 German invasion from France over the English Channel. At that time, however, very few could have imagined the severity

Bayly's Farm.
TOP: This is the region of flatlands, very close to the English Channel, that is home to the future Royal Air Force (RAF) Tangmere, the airport (aerodrome) that assumed great importance in the Battle of Britain and the invention of the IOL.
BOTTOM: By the 1930s the airport had grown considerably, fortunately just in time for the impending war.

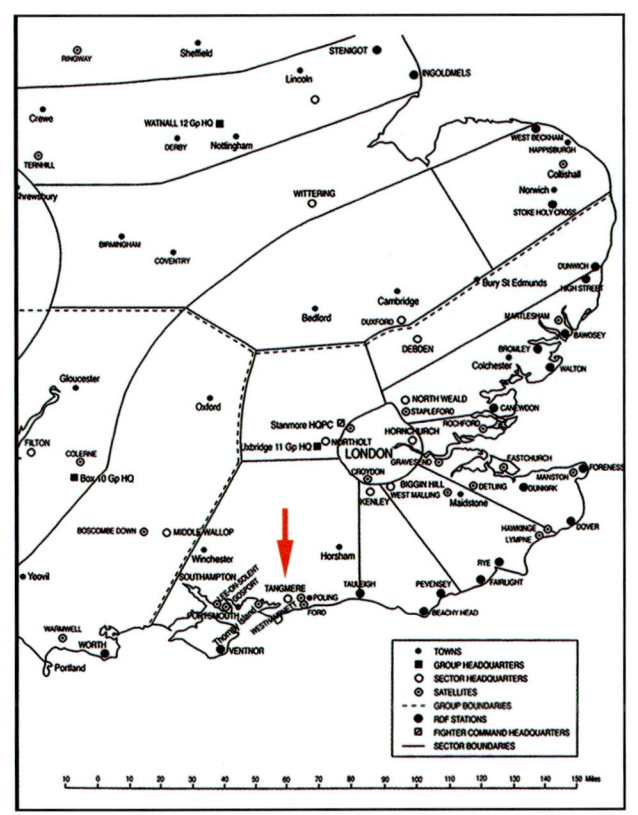

ADLERTAG: THE QUEST FOR A COMPLETE CATARACT OPERATION

1940 Map of British Air Defenses (RAF) Tangmere (arrow) at the bottom center of the map facing the English Channel (below). It was directly one of the lines of the German air invasion from France.

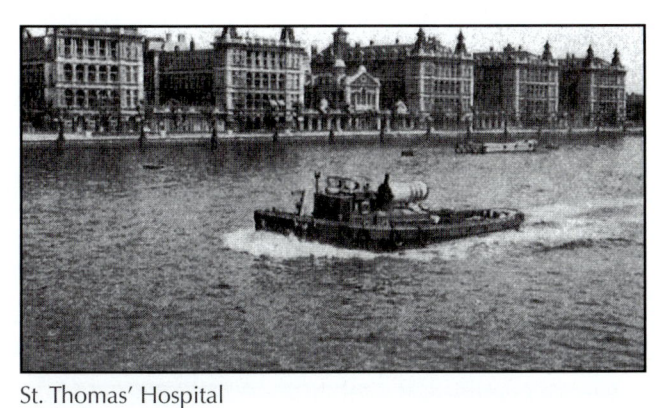

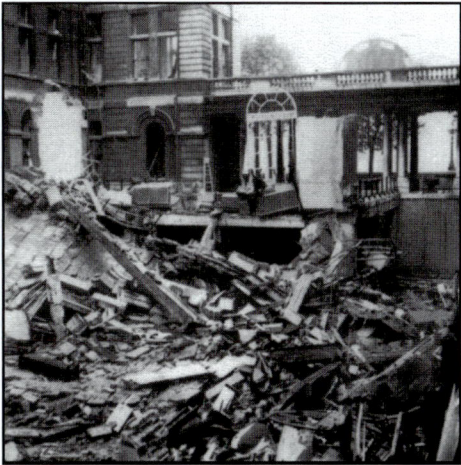

The authorities correctly predicted that St. Thomas' would be attacked and evacuations were ordered. Indeed much was destroyed in bomb raids including the ophthalmology ward and operating theatres. Many of the St. Thomas' hospitalized patients were, by necessity, transferred to outlying regions, including the region in southern England and RAF Tangmere where many battles occurred.

Although a civilian until called into the military in 1943, Harold performed extensive casualty surgery on pilots and soldiers between 1940 and 1943.

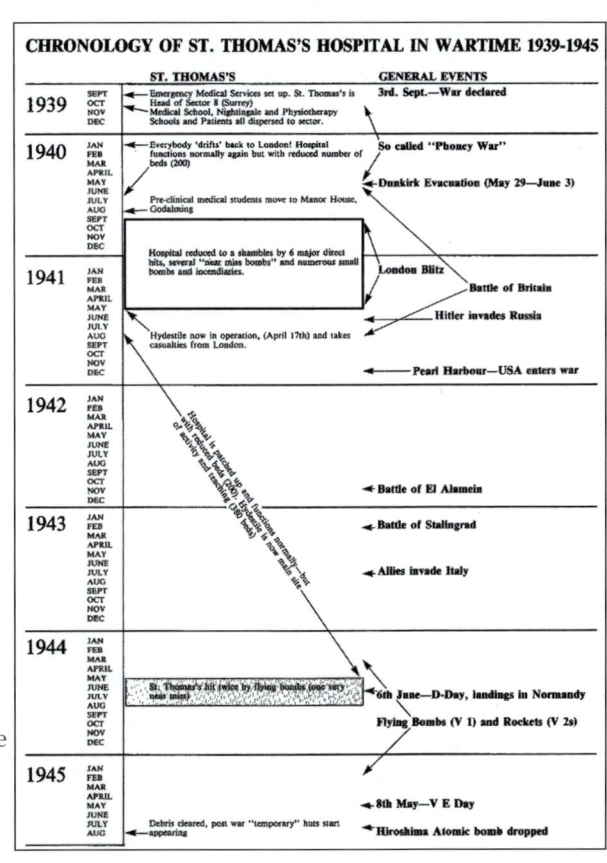

St. Thomas' Hospital
LEFT: Pre-war photo.
RIGHT: Chronology of the hospital in wartime. It suffered multiple "hits" during the Blitz.

CHAPTER 6

The Manor House, near Godalming, Surrey (near RAF Tangmere). It was utilized by St. Thomas' Hospital as a satellite facility.
LEFT: During wartime.
RIGHT: 2005, during a visit by Ann and myself.

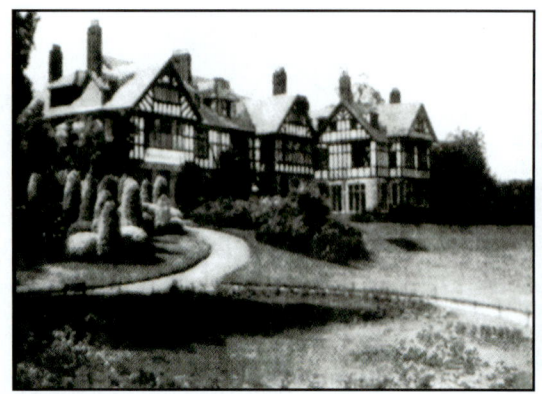

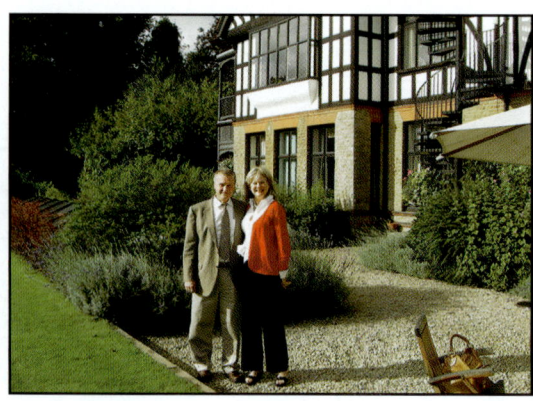

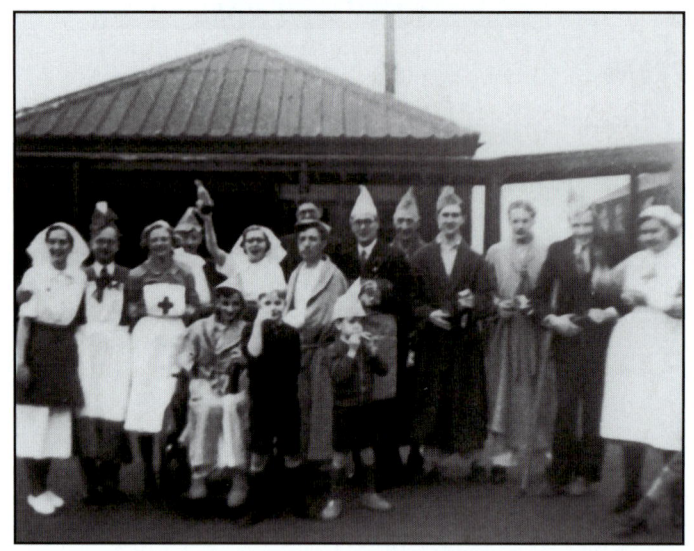

There has been some confusion regarding Harold's role in treating pilots and, indeed, even his whereabouts during the period of 1940-1943. This question has been settled now by several new pieces of evidence, including this photograph showing him at a hospital function at Saint Luke's Hospital in Guildford, one of the hospitals around RAF Tangmere where he worked at that time.

Further proof as to the time and location of Harold's service during the early 1940s is provided in this letter. It documents his termination of his civilian duties and entrance into the military in 1943. This was the beginning of his period in Ghana, Africa (see Chapter 13).

of the coming onslaught, when wave after wave of Nazi aircraft would fly from France across the English Channel to strike at England's heart. Fortunately, very important leaders were among the "very few," including Winston Churchill.

World War II actually began in September of 1939, shortly after Harold's appointment as permanent consultant at Moorfields Eye Hospital. I, of course, was not yet born, so the entire story as presented here is based on historical accounts of the actual occurrences and, most especially, the statements of contemporary witnesses.

Harold expected to be immediately inducted into the Royal Army Medical Corps. However, as soon as the Germans consolidated their gains in Poland, Belgium, Holland, and elsewhere, they halted, and an easy year passed with little active conflict. This was termed the "sitting" war (Sitekrieg) by the Germans and was designated the "phony war" by the English speaking. The paucity of military actions between England and the Axis powers meant that physicians on active military service had little to do.

Harold was not called for service during this period but was much busier as a civilian than he would have been as a military medical officer on active duty.

As time passed, it became clear that the "phony" war would eventually turn brutally hostile. The British authorities decided that St. Thomas' Hospital in London, one site where Harold trained and one of his places of employment thereafter, was a likely prime target of Nazi bombing raids or, at the very least, would be in the path of destruction. After all, it was a venerable and important part of Britain's health care establishment and was located just across the River Thames from the Houses of Parliament.

They were proven correct. Much of St. Thomas' was, in fact, damaged by German bombs throughout the war. Most important to our narrative, many segments of the hospital were evacuated to satellite medical facilities to the south, and some of these satellites were grouped around and within a few miles of a centrally located airport: RAF Tangmere.

Harold apparently did work at several facilities in the region around RAF Tangmere, including a St. Thomas' satellite near Godalming in Surrey, the Emergency Medical Service at St. Lukes' Hospital in Guilford, and the Royal Buckinghamshire Hospital near Aylesbury. He remained in this region until conscripted into the regular army as a brevet major (temporary) in 1943.

Because of a mixture of good luck and good planning, RAF Tangmere was located near satellite facilities of St. Thomas' as well as being situated at a site destined to be in the middle of the upcoming battle. The authorities, military, and civilians in these medical facilities around RAF Tangmere expected heavy casualties if and when real hostilities began. This occurred on May 10, 1940 as the Germans turned the "phony war" into a real war. One of the squadrons "manning" RAF Tangmere was the 601—a squadron flying exclusively Hurricanes, not Spitfires.

The Players

The 601 (County of London, "Playboy," or "Millionaires") Squadron; The Complex Series of Events That Culminated in Bringing the Right Man to the Right Place—Under the Care of Harold Ridley

The 601 Squadron of RAF fighter pilots, nicknamed the "Millionaires' Squadron" was stationed at Tangmere. Several friends and two pilots from the squadron who were in critical air battles in 1940 have generously provided extensive information regarding this unit. This chapter tells some of their story.

The 601 Squadron was founded by a veteran airman of World War I, Lord Edward Grosvenor, a man whose unique background and personality allowed him to put his stamp on this unique group of men. His influence continued long after his premature death in the 1920s. He influenced not only his contemporaries but also many younger members who served in the squadron well into World War II—including Flight Lieutenant Gordon "Mouse" Cleaver, the lead character of this "airplane story." Even though many of these younger men did not meet Grosvenor personally, his stamp and his modus operandi were clearly a major influence to all.

Born in 1892 and the son of a duke, Grosvenor was clearly a restless type—not satisfied to stay home and spend the family fortune. He was richly endowed with the spirit of adventure; among other things, he served in the French Foreign Legion.

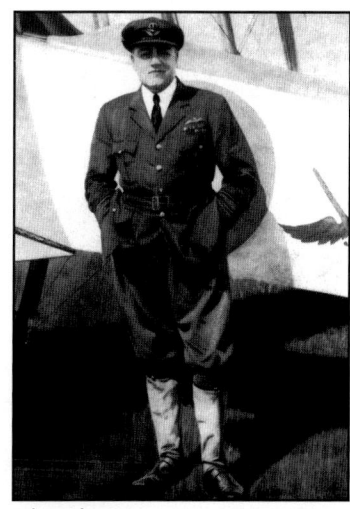

Edward Grosvenor (1892-1920s) Founder of 601 Squadron.

CHAPTER 6

Grosvenor's main interest and goal in life after World War I was to form an air squadron. This desire was based on the fact that after World War I, the British government and military hierarchy had decreased the arms budget for all the services. He, therefore, felt that the air defenses of Britain were severely lacking. At that time, it was possible for someone to form what one might consider to be a "civilian air force," loosely analogous to a reserve unit in the United States. This would be an air group outside of the realm of the official RAF. By 1924, having hounded seemingly every authority in London, Grosvenor succeeded in his endeavor.

The roots of the squadron were established at a famous and, of course, exclusive men's club in London, White's Club, where Grosvenor was always a welcome guest. The squadron's goal was to enlist members of the social and financial classes similar to that which Grosvenor belonged to, namely, the wealthier classes. It was officially called the 601 Squadron. It was designated the "County of London Squadron," another group having already absconded with the socially more exclusive name of "City of London Squadron." The 601 was also referred to as the "Playboy" or "Millionaires' Squadron" based on the wealth and active lives of the members.

Many of the young recruits to the squadron had learned to fly by taking private lessons. This included the above-mentioned Cleaver. Many were well-known throughout London—even prior to the war—because of their charisma, soldier-of-fortune-like status, as well as their accomplishments in the worlds of business, law, sports, and other endeavors. They would soon prove that they were much more than millionaire playboys.

The 601 Squadron was eventually accepted into the RAF as a regular unit, and just before the war, they were assigned one of the two excellent fighter planes available to the RAF at that time: the Hawker Hurricane. While the other plane, the Supermarine Spitfire, was and remains better known in the popular media and literature, the well-armed and durable Hurricane played an equally important—some feel even greater—role in halting the German onslaught. It was the first fighter monoplane to join the RAF and the first combat aircraft adopted by the military that was capable of exceeding 300 mph in level flight.

Many British, including Harold, felt that the Hurricane had been underrated in favor of the Spitfire and that indeed the Hurricane had shouldered the lion's share of Britain's defense. It was designed by Mr. Sydney Camm beginning in 1934, and it entered service in December 1937.

One of my friends and colleagues, Professor Eric Arnott has told me an interesting story about the Hurricane that occurred in the late 1930s, prior to the onset of the war. He noted the following:

> *"Thomas Sopwith, the Director of the Hurricane Company at that time, went to Germany to the Messerschmitt Company in 1938 in order to observe and perhaps purchase some engines for his yacht, a trip that apparently had nothing to do with airplanes. After the visit was completed, Sopwith and some Messerschmitt executives and technical officials went for dinner and drinks. After having extensive amounts of the latter, his German hosts requested that he come and look at something very interesting in one of the company warehouses. They went to the Messerschmitt campus, and as the door of the warehouse, actually a hanger, was opened, Sopwith was amazed in seeing numerous advanced Messerschmitt fighter plane engines and chasses in the process of being built and assembled. At that point, he immediately knew that mobilization for war was not that far away.*

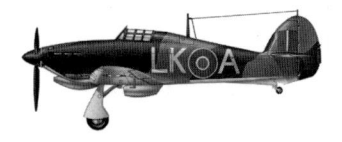

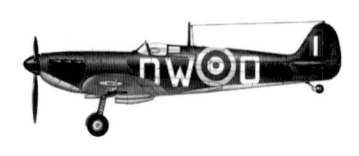

The two most important fighter planes accessible to the RAF during the Battle of Britain were the Hawker Hurricane, assigned to the 601 Squadron, and the Spitfire manufactured by the Supermarine Corporation.
TOP: Hurricane.
BOTTOM: Spitfire.

ADLERTAG: THE QUEST FOR A COMPLETE CATARACT OPERATION

"He took this information back to England and sped up the development of his Hurricanes, which had evolved from previous Hawker models. By doing this, Sopwith had gained a huge start on the Supermarine Spitfire—hence, more Hawker planes were available to respond in the Battle of Britain."

According to Arnott, Sopwith's visit to Messerschmitt may have helped save Britain. "One would need to have prayed for the Messerschmitt tour givers that night if Herr Hitler had gotten wind of this." By the time of the first German aggressions on September 3, 1939, (action for Britain did not occur till later, since this was still the phony war), almost 500 Hurricanes had been delivered and 18 Hurricane squadrons had been equipped, including those of the 601 Squadron.

"MOUSE" CLEAVER AND THE PILOTS OF THE 601 SQUADRON

The photograph of the squadron on this page, courtesy of Mrs. Jane Adams, "Mouse" Cleaver's sister-in-law, is to my knowledge the only known existing image of most of the members of the squadron as it existed in 1938. Mrs. Adams not only gave me this very important photograph, she also provided several other photographs and documentation, for which I am extremely grateful. The Cleaver family had apparently given the collection to her after his death in 1997. This image was made at the time that the British Prime Minister Neville Chamberlain was negotiating with Hitler over Czechoslovakia. The young men in this picture were not sure whether they were going to war or not; in retrospect, we know what happened. I have had contact with two pilots from 601 Squadron who are alive and well; one is Jack Riddle. Reggie Spooner, one of Riddle's best friends, joined the squadron later as Adjutant. These gentlemen have been very helpful in filling in many gaps in the story.

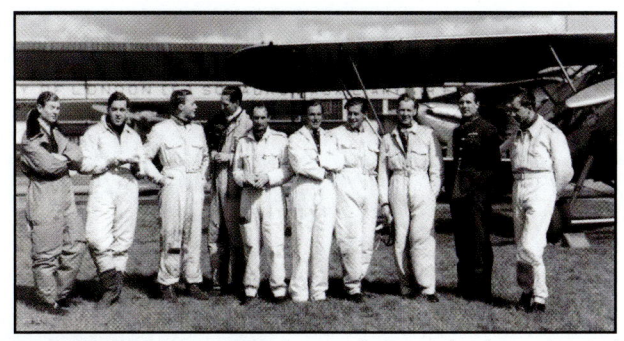

A rare photograph of members of the 601 Squadron, 1937—taken during the period when Prime Minister Neville Chamberlain and Adolph Hitler were meeting at the infamous Munich Conference.
TOP: Jack Riddle is at the far left. "Mouse" Cleaver (fifth from left) would soon, without realizing it, play a major role in launching one of eye surgery's major advancements.
To his immediate left is Sir Archibald Hope, the Squadron's Commander. To Hope's immediate left is Roger Bushell, who later became prominent as a leader of the prisoners who attempted the "great escape" from German captivity. His exploits were recounted in the film of the same name, starring Steve McQueen and Richard Attenbourough.
ABOVE LEFT: Insignia of the 601, County of London, "Millionaire" Squadron.

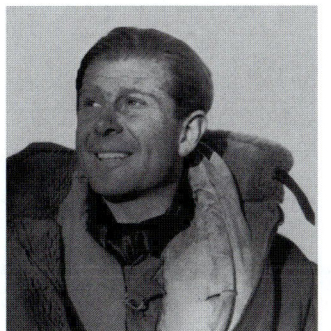

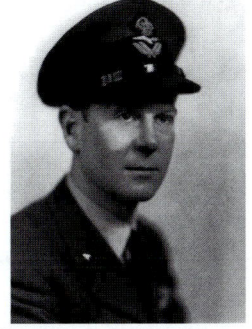

Wartime photographs of Jack Riddle, 601 Squadron, 1940; one of the last surviving pilots from the Battle of Britain.

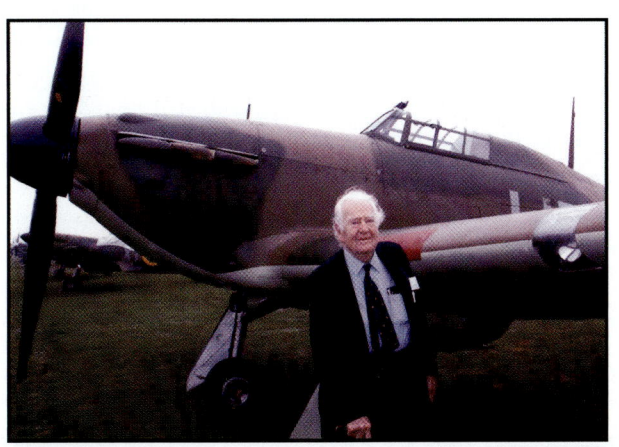

Jack Riddle, age 92. He served in 601 Squadron. This Hawker Hurricane, flown by a friend of his in a different squadron based at RAF Tangmere, is one of the few remaining planes from the era.

111

CHAPTER 6

Enlargement of the photo found on the previous page, highlighting Flight Lieutenant Gordon "Mouse" Cleaver. The official record of his activities in the Battle of France and the Battle of Britain show that he was officially considered an "Ace" based on the number of "kills" documented.

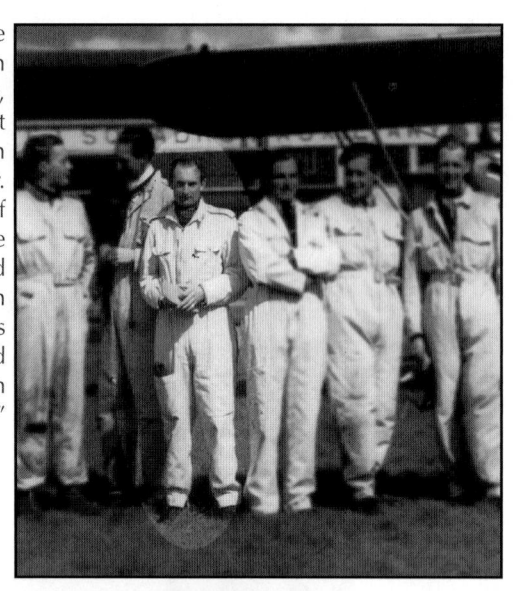

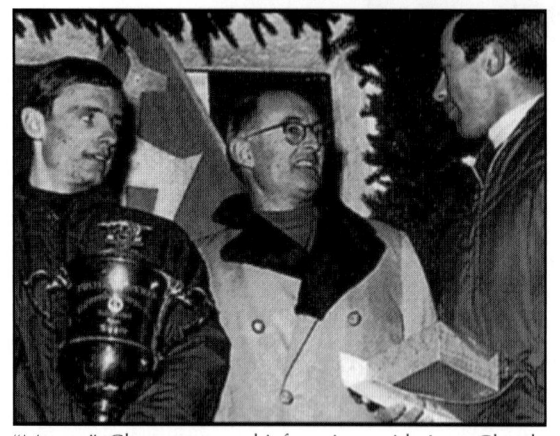

"Mouse" Cleaver at a ski function with Jean-Claude Killy (left) and Karl Schranz (right). Cleaver had received a major ski award, the Hahenkamm Cup in Austria before the war and was honored to present this same award to these two men a years later. Killy was the winner in 1967; Schranz was in 1969.

Jack Riddle was especially helpful in clarifying many of the occurrences of the August 14 and 15, 1940 Adlertag battle that was decisive in helping Britain win the battle and in helping Harold Ridley produce his IOL. Jack, who visited Cleaver later in the hospital after his now famous injury, was greeted by Cleaver with a legendary statement that will be told later.

The illustration on the bottom of the previous page is an acquired photograph of Jack Riddle with an original World War II Hurricane used in and around Tangmere.

"Mouse" Cleaver joined the 601 Squadron in 1937. He was a brilliant, restless young man and an excellent skier. Coming from a country that is not known for its output of Olympic-class skiers (there are few high skiable mountains in Britain to practice on), he was the first British citizen to win the coveted Hahenkamm Cup, a ski race in Austria and one of the toughest races of its kind in the world. The cup is presented in Austria every 25 years. He received it prior to World War II and was present after the war when it was presented to Jean Claude Killy and Karl Schranz some years later. It was announced later in 2006 by the British press that one important subcategory of the Hahenkamm Medal would be designated the Gordon "Mouse" Cleaver Cup. Athletic prowess was one of the characteristics shared by many members of the squadron.

Even though Cleaver was a great flyer and qualified as an ACE, he is still better remembered by the British public for his skiing ability than for this IOL story. We hope that we can change this with this book.

One of the first references to Cleaver as a pilot surfaced in 1939, when his 601 Squadron had the honor of probably being the first of the allied air forces to fly into German territory at the very start of the conflict. This was a little-remembered flight into a city called Borken—a raid that was intended to attack a seaplane base. The mission was accomplished, but soon thereafter, the allies' ventures onto the continent were blocked by the Nazis. Hitler called for the surrender of French and English troops within his sight, that phase ending at Dunkirk.

A second event occurred in May of 1940, just before the Battle of Britain was to heat up. This event is described in a book on the history of the 601 Squadron; Cleaver described the event as follows:

> *"In May of 1940, we were assigned to fly in an escort squadron to escort a VIP to a conference with the French government in Villacoublay near Paris. That VIP turned out to be the new Prime Minister, Sir Winston Churchill. The mission was duly accomplished, and the pilots were ready to return in the evening, but Churchill decided to postpone their departure until the next morning even though the enemy was in striking distance of Paris and the city was experiencing its final days of free-*

dom. Since Churchill remained, we of course all had to remain and wait for him until the next morning.

> "We were told we could go into town and that we would take off the next day at 8:00; Archie (Archibald Hope) managed to borrow quite a lot of money from a pal in the embassy, and we set off for Lust and Laughter. The next day, there assembled at Villacoublay just about as hung-over a crew of dirty, smelly, unshaven, unwashed fighter pilots as I doubt has ever been seen. Willy (Rhodes-Morehouse), if I remember right, was being sick behind his airplane when the great man arrived and expressed a great desire to meet his escort. We must have appeared vaguely human at least, as he seemed to accept our appearance without comment, and we took off for England."

It is difficult to imagine the events of this time as Churchill asked to meet with these young pilots. The pressures of the world were on his shoulders. The battle of France had barely begun a few days earlier, May 10, 1940. He realized that it was hopeless. Indeed, France was to fall on June 22, not long after he departed France for a final time. The entrapment at Dunkirk was soon to follow by the end of June.

Cleaver's experience with the 601 Squadron made him an independent, courageous, capable pilot and individual—characteristics that would later help him survive and overcome the challenges of the eye injuries he would endure over the next several years. The following is an abbreviated military record of "Mouse." Based on the number of "kills," he was a bone-fide "ACE."

FLIGHT LIEUTENANT GORDON NEIL SPENCER CLEAVER

91035   FO   Pilot   British   601 Squadron

Cleaver, who was born in Stanmore, Middlesex, joined 601 Squadron, AuxAF in 1937 and was commissioned in April. He skied for Britain in the years before the war.

Mobilized on November 24, 1939, Cleaver went to Merville, France with 'A' Flight on May 16, 1940. On the 27th, he destroyed a Bf 109 and claimed two other victories before the flight was withdrawn at the end of May.

Cleaver claimed a Ju 87 and a probable He 111 destroyed on July 11, a probable Bf 109 on 26th, two Bf 110s on August 11 and another on the 13th. Two days later, he was shot down in combat over Winchester. When his hood was shattered by a cannon shell, Cleaver's eyes were filled with perspex splinters. He managed to return to Tangmere and was rushed to hospital, where his sight was partially saved, but his operational flying days were over. Cleaver was awarded the DFC (Distinguished Flying Cross) (13.9.40).

In 1941, he transferred to the Administrative Branch and was released from the RAF in late 1943, as a Squadron Leader.

PO (AuxAF) 8.4.37   FO(AuxAF) 8.10/38   FO 24.11.39
FL 24.11.40 SL 1.3.42

Cleaver was one of the "few," as later designated by Churchill, who helped Britain to this eventual victory. Churchill's statement, "Never have so few done so much for so many," was an inspiration stated at the time and is now regarded as a classic example of a great war story. In his late twenties, Mouse was considered rather elderly to be a fighter pilot. Having been brought up with planes on an estate, it was only natural that he would join the elite 601 County of London Squadron.

CHAPTER 6

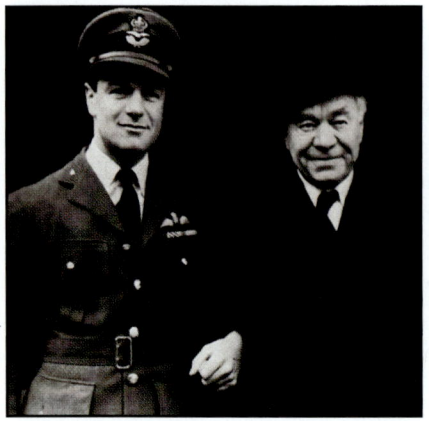

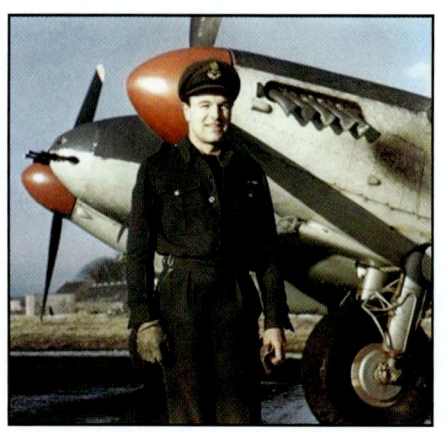

Max Aitken (1910-1985) a prominent member of 601 Squadron.
LEFT: During the Battle of Britain he was of the 601 Squadron. He is pictured here next to his father Max Aitken, Sr. (1879-1964), Lord Beaverbrook. Churchill named the latter the Minister of War Production. It is generally agreed that he did an outstanding job at rapid mobilization in one short period.
RIGHT: Max Aitken in flight attire.

This squadron contained several other illustrious individuals. Max Aitken was the highly respected squadron leader for a period of time during the various battles over southern England. His father, Max Aitken, Sr., Lord Beaverbrook, was a prominent businessman and a close friend of Prime Minister Churchill. Churchill gave Lord Beaverbrook the awesome job of organizing the manufacture, supply, and distribution of all military hardware—in effect, arming the entire British military. He was indeed very successful with his job once he got up and running. It is probable that his son's 601 Squadron never had a huge lack of quality armaments.

Many of the British military squadrons had civilians, often females, who performed various odd jobs that were vital to the war effort. The 601 Squadron was no exception. Ms. Primula Rollo, a beautiful young lady who was well liked by all the pilots and their wives, was one of them. She performed odd jobs such as folding the pilots' parachutes.

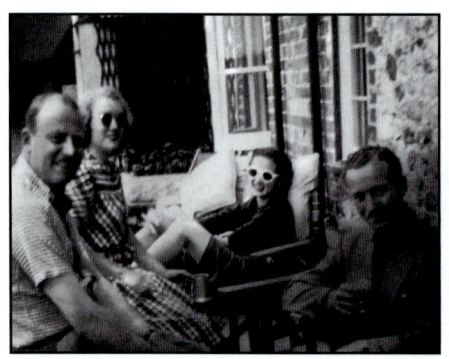

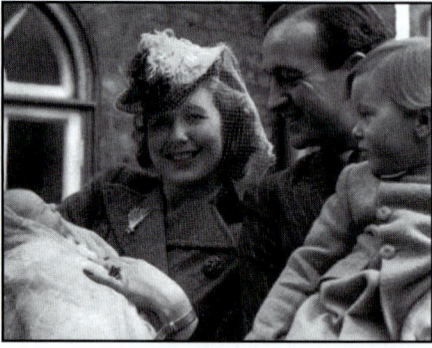

The great film actor, David Niven, served in the army but had connections to the 601 Squadron. He married Ms. Primula Rollo, who had been assigned to the 601 Squadron to do various duties, including folding parachutes. Their courtship was only 17 days, not uncommon during wartime.
LEFT: Niven (far right) and his wife (right center) with members of 601 Squadron
RIGHT: The Nivens with their young children. Unfortunately, she died an accidental death shortly after the war.

In 1940, the famous British movie star David Niven was serving in the British army. He was stationed west of London in the Salisbury plain. He was in a commando unit; one of his jobs was to carry out raids not unlike those seen in one of his famous movies, *Guns of Navarone*. He had several friends in the 601 Squadron. One day while visiting them, he met Ms. Rollo. It was love at first sight, and they were married 17 days later.

Their marriage turned out to be a very happy one, but sadly a short one. Not long after the end of the war, the Nivens moved to Los Angeles as he continued his illustrious movie career. One evening they attended a party at the home of the actor Paul Muni. While playing the game of hide-and-seek within the home, Ms. Rollo opened a door she thought was the closet, but it was actually the stairs leading to the basement. She tumbled and fell, suffering injuries that caused her death. David Niven would later remarry, but those who knew him said he was never the same. She was indeed his true love. Jack Riddle remembers both of them very well.

Roger Bushell was another pilot in the 601 Squadron. Like most members of the squadron, he had special talents. He had a very successful vocation as an attorney or advocate, and he was an excellent athlete, sharing with Cleaver an expertise in skiing. A daring pilot, he flew many sorties, and he was shot down at least three times. Each

ADLERTAG: THE QUEST FOR A COMPLETE CATARACT OPERATION

time, he managed to parachute to safety, but each time, he fell into the hands of the enemy.

Bushell proved to be a great escape artist. Twice, he was able to break out and return to his squadron. Following an unprecedented third capture, he was interned in Stalag III Prison, and his capturers gave him orders not to attempt another escape—that he then would be executed if he did. He could not resist. His desire to get back into action forced him to try another escape. This time, he became the leader of a large group of comrades who began the process of tunneling out of the prison.

Bushell and his cohorts' daring escape attempt was immortalized in the famous film, *The Great Escape*. The leading characters were played by Steve McQueen and Richard Atenbourgh. Reality was not as kind as the film, however. In real life, Bushell was recaptured in southern Germany. He and 49 colleagues were executed on the direct orders of Hitler. The Germans had been very frustrated by having to divert so many troops to round up the prisoners. As Jack Riddle and I discussed the last days of Roger Bushell, his lips tensed up with a firm expression of anger—65 years after the event. His comment: "Hitler killed him" was short, direct, and clear—associated with many tears.

A young American joined the squadron just in time to take part in the intense fighting of the Battle of Britain. Born in Brooklyn, William "Billy" Meade Lindsley Fiske, a young adventurer from a well-established and wealthy family, joined the RAF in September 1939. He arrived in England in July 1940 and was credited with having shot down an enemy JU-88 on August 16, 1940 during the Adlertag battle.

Sadly, his Hurricane was badly damaged and caught fire during landing after the combat that day. He was taken to the West Sussex Hospital in Chichester, but died 48 hours later from his burns and shock. He was 29 years old. It is very unfortunate that he died so rapidly; had he lived somewhat longer, he could have been taken just a few miles to East Grinstead to what was at that time probably the most accomplished and finest burn center in the world directed by the eminent plastic surgeon, Dr. McIndoe. He, in turn, worked in conjunction with the well-known ophthalmologist Dr. Sunderland. They had extensive experience in treating injured servicemen with severe burns. If more pilots burned at RAF Tangmere could have had their eye wounds treated by the East

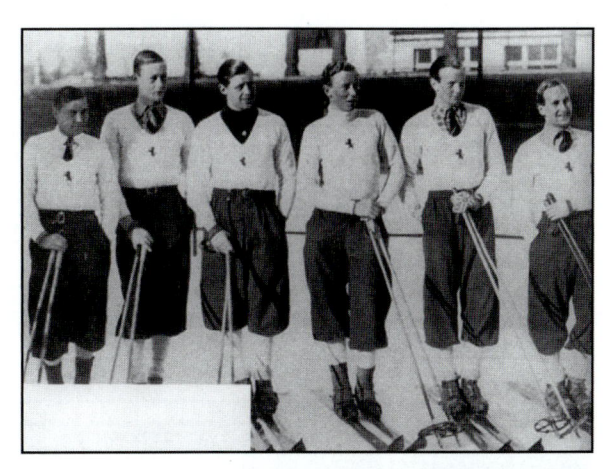

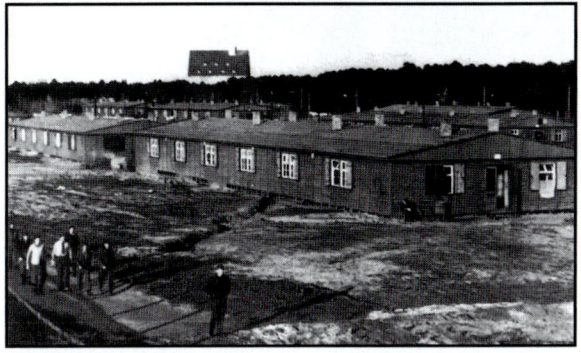

Roger Bushell (1910-1944).
TOP: Squadron Leader Bushell (third from the left) in this photograph with his Cambridge University Ski Team during the 1930s. Not surprisingly, as an excellent architect and prominent attorney, he was a member of the 601 Squadron.
Shot down over enemy territory, he later became prominent as a leader of the prisoners who attempted the "Great Escape" from German captivity. In the film of the same name (starring Steve McQueen and Richard Atenbourgh), he escaped. However, in 1943 Hitler tragically ordered him executed along with 49 other prisoners.
BOTTOM: German prison camp POW Stalag Luft III where Bushell was held.

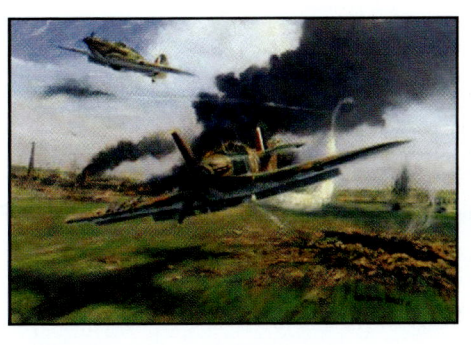

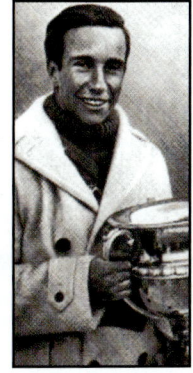

William "Billy" Fiske, (1911-1940) an American in the 601 Saudron.
LEFT: Artist's rendition of his fatal injury on August 16, 1940 while serving in the 601 Squadron.
RIGHT: Born in Brooklyn, he became renown because of his victories in winter sports events prior to joining the RAF. He won Olympic gold medals in bobsledding in 1928 and 1932, the first team to win a gold medal in this event.

115

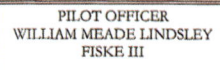

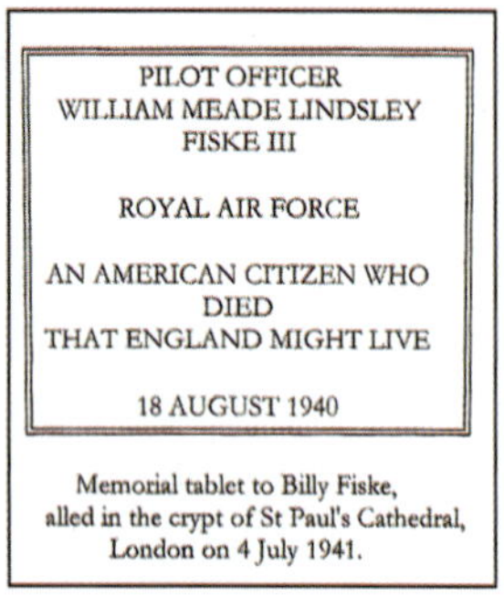

CHAPTER 6

"Billy" Fiske was buried in Boxgrove Cemetery in Sussex, near the RAF Tangmere Airfield. TOP LEFT Boxgrove Church. TOP RIGHT: Fiske's grave. BOTTOM LEFT: His friend Jack Riddle at the entrance to Boxgrove Church and cemetery. BOTTOM RIGHT: Memorial tablet to Billy Fiske, placed in the crypt of St. Paul's Cathedral, London on 4 July 1941.

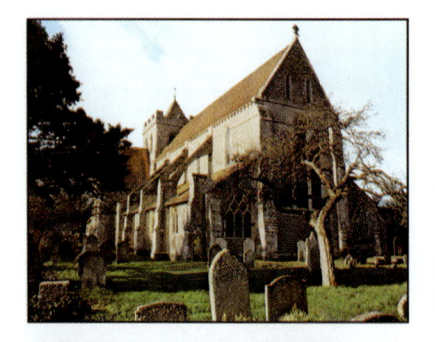

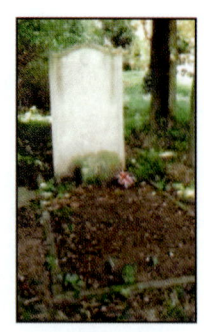

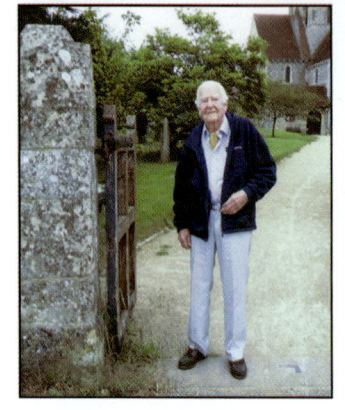

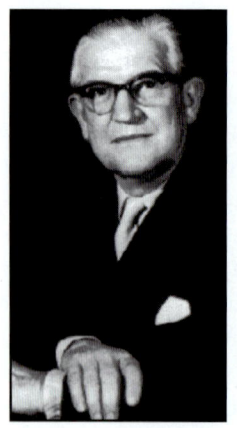

PILOT OFFICER
WILLIAM MEADE LINDSLEY
FISKE III

ROYAL AIR FORCE

AN AMERICAN CITIZEN WHO
DIED
THAT ENGLAND MIGHT LIVE

18 AUGUST 1940

Memorial tablet to Billy Fiske,
alled in the crypt of St Paul's Cathedral,
London on 4 July 1941.

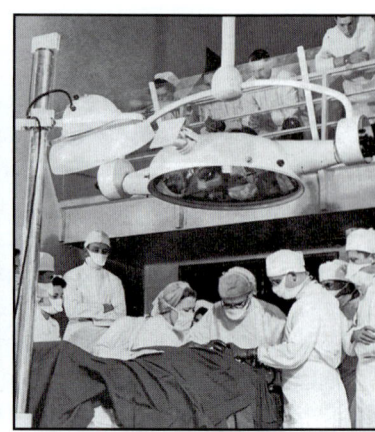

Sir Archibald McIndoe.
LEFT: McIndoe was the director of a world-renown burn-plastic surgery unit in nearby East Grimstead.
RIGHT: Burned pilots were treated there. Perhaps Fiske may have been saved, since his cause of death was shock secondary to his burns.

Grimsted team under Dr. McIndoe, it is probable that more would have survived, including Fiske.

Fiske was one of the first to have died in the service of the King. Churchill learned of this and wanted to use his name as an incentive to help persuade President Franklin Roosevelt to enter the war to help Britain. They tried, but of course, it did not happen. Only when Pearl Harbor was attacked over a year later on December 7, 1941 did America enter the war.

A memorial tablet to Fiske was laid in a crypt of St. Paul's Cathedral in July 1941. He remains an icon even today. In fact, Fiske's story was told in detail in a biographical sketch on the History Channel, and a Hollywood producer is planning a full-length film of his exploits during the war starring Tom Cruise (possibly a *Top Gun II*?).

Fellow pilot Jack Riddle also knew Fiske well. In an interview, he pointed out that he was a "very nice young" man. The Squadron considered his death a real tragedy. That interview was, incidentally, one of two times during my interview with Riddle where I saw tears running from his eyes. The other time was when we spoke of Hitler's murder of Roger Bushell and the 49 other prisoners.

FURY ACROSS EUROPE

By the spring of 1940, Hitler's forces had run up a series of victories that were unprecedented in modern history. Following the initial 1939 invasion of Poland and the period of the phony war (German = *Sitzkrieg*), he had much of Europe in his pocket, including Poland, Austria, and Czechoslovakia.

The attack resumed on the morning of May 10, 1940. The greatest concentration of tanks and heavy armor ever assembled crossed the frontiers of the low lands of France. They used the same technique they had used earlier in Poland: the *Blitzkrieg* (lightening war). "Mouse" Cleaver was assigned to help the French, but the small numbers of planes and pilots available were hopelessly outnumbered, and they had to be withdrawn

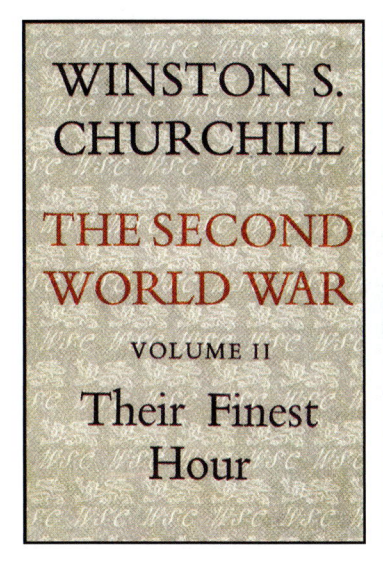

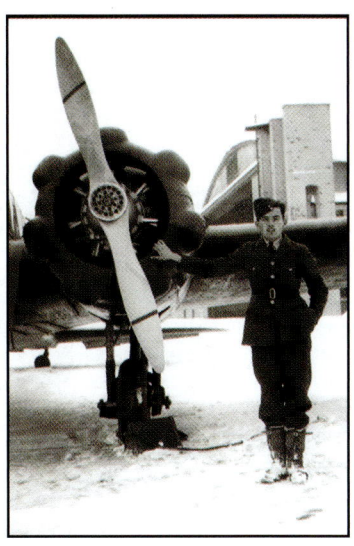

ADLERTAG: THE QUEST FOR A COMPLETE CATARACT OPERATION

The Battle of Britain.
LEFT: Cover of Volume II, titled "Their Finest Hour," of Winston Churchill's book, *The Second World War*. This volume dealt with the Battle of Britain.
RIGHT: RAF Tangmere's hangers in the background. Sadly, this young airman, about 20 years old, statistically stood little chance of surviving the war—statistics made worse by the habit of many pilots flying without goggles. Ridley documented over 200 such cases.

into England. The RAF leader, Air Marshall Dowding, correctly concluded that these planes had to be saved for what he considered an inevitable future invasion of England by the Germans, and the forthcoming Battle of Britain was to prove that he was correct in this judgment.

On June 22, 1940, France was forced to surrender, signing an armistice in the same railroad car in Compiegne where the defeated Germans had signed the armistice of World War I in 1918. More than 300,000 Allied soldiers had been pushed into a bottleneck at Dunkirk, trapped between the waters of the English Channel on the north and the advancing German army on the south. It appeared that they would have been unable to escape; fortunately, thanks to an inexplicable German hesitation and the mobilization of numerous British crafts (some of the small boats and yachts manned by civilians).

With Hitler in control of continental Europe, just as Air Marshall Dowding had predicted, he looked to Britain as his next conquest. Hitler had wanted England to sign a treaty with him—in effect surrender, but Churchill of course summarily rejected that. Therefore, Hitler set in motion a plan to send in massive air strikes across the Channel in order to destroy England's air defenses. These would be followed by an overwhelming invasion of ground troops, which could be ferried across the Channel without fear of attacks from the sky. The German code name of his planned attack was "Operation Sea Lion" (Seeloewe). With the Germans poised to bring the war to a devastating end, the British knew how desperate their situation was.

Winston Churchill had just assumed office as Prime Minister in early May. His words heralded the transition from the campaign on the continent of Europe to the air battle above England: "The battle of France is over," he said. "The Battle of Britain is about to begin."

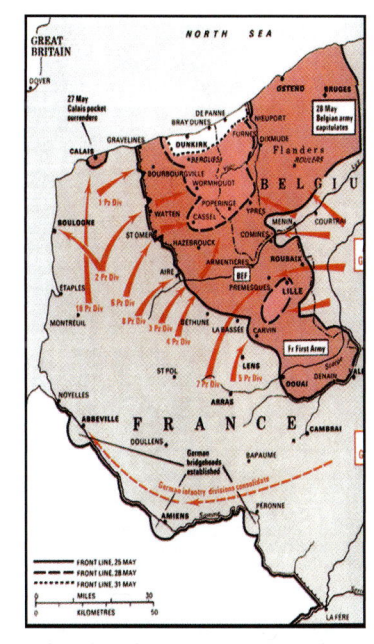

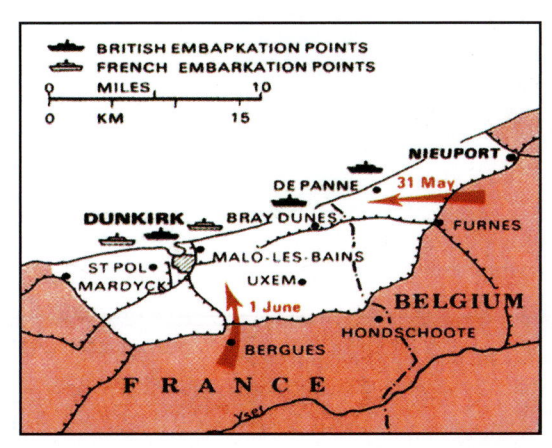

After the Phony War, the Battle of France began in earnest on May 10, 1940.
TOP: The Germans overwhelmed France and the French capitulated on June 22, 1940. The Germans had continuously driven the allies backwards (north) toward the English Channel.
LEFT: Over 330,000 allied soldiers were trapped in a pocket around Dunkirk on the Cannel coast. Fortunately, they escaped during the battle which lasted between May 26 to June 4.

117

CHAPTER 6

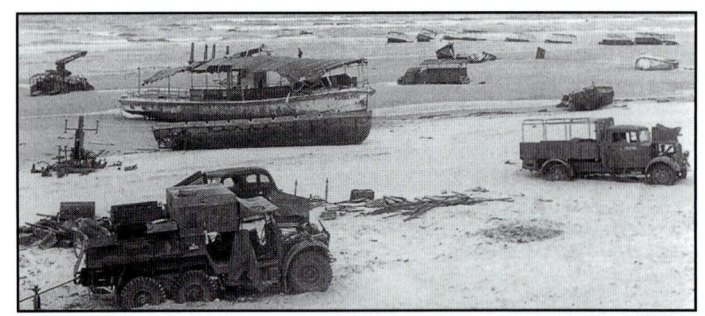

The Battle of Dunkirk May 26 to June 4, 1940.
TOP: 330,000 allied troupes managed to escape from the Germans by using all available ships and small boats. They retreated across the English Channel at Dunkirk.
RIGHT: The successful evacuation of troops from Dunkirk ended the first phase in the Battle of France. It provided a great boost to British morale, but left the French to stand alone against the Germans'. German troops entered Paris on June 14 and accepted the surrender of France on June 22. The stage was soon set for the Battle of Britain.

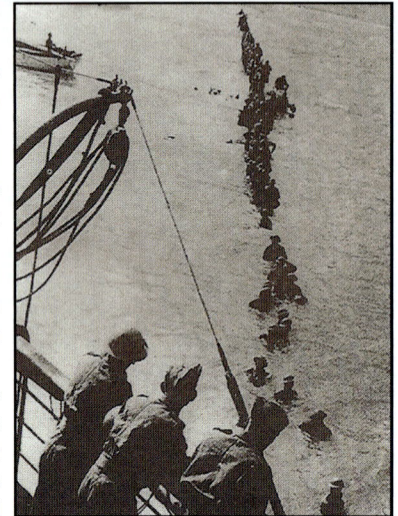

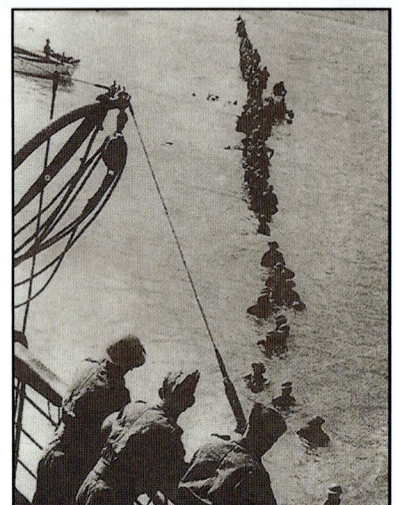

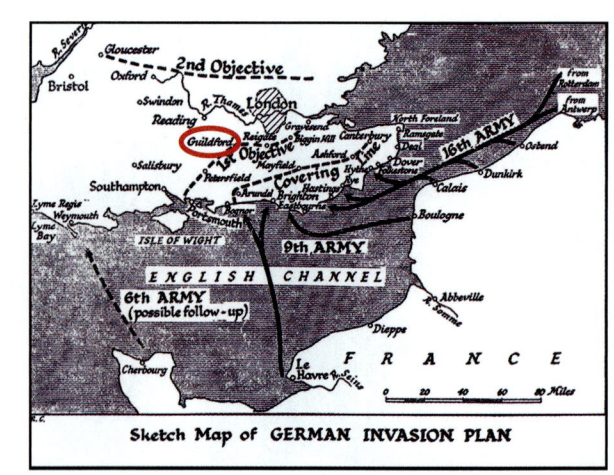

After retreating from Dunkirk, the British had to prepare for an air attack. They had brought home all of their aircraft from France, including Flight Lieutenant "Mouse" Cleaver's 601 Squadron. The air battle began on July 10, 1940 and continued until October 31, 1940. Had the Germans won the Battle of Britain in 1940, they planned to invade England in "Operation Sea Lion." Note on this map from Winston Churchill's *History of the Second World War*, that the center point of the invasion was the city of Guildford (red circle), precisely in the region where Harold Ridley was doing extensive casualty duties.

ADLERTAG: "YOU WILL WIPE THE BRITISH AIR FORCE FROM THE SKY"

The stage was set for what was to become one of the most fierce and heroic struggles in the history of aerial warfare: the Battle of Britain. It began in the summer of 1940 and lasted 4 brutal months through September. Fewer than 3,000 Allied pilots—mostly British—pitted themselves against the German Luftwaffe in a courageous stand. Although one author now contends that Britain could have been defended by the sheer power of her navy alone, the overwhelming majority of historians agree that the role of the air force was critical. The pilots themselves strongly believe that if they had failed, the British Isles would have been overrun and Hitler's onslaught may never have been stopped. The "Millionaire Playboy" pilots of the 601 Squadron were among those who were ready to fight

Although the British air defenses were seriously outnumbered by the Luftwaffe aircraft, taking advantage of their radar warning system, they tenaciously held their own. By the middle of August, a climactic battle plan

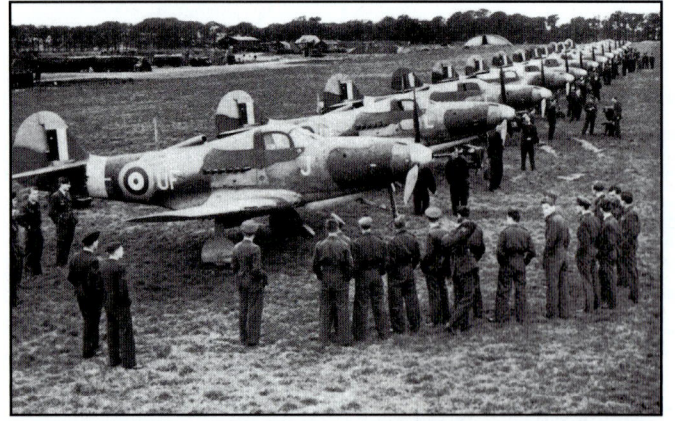

Battle of Britain, July 10, 1940 to October 31, 1940. This is a photograph taken at RAF Tangmere, the home base of Cleaver's 601 Squadron just as the war began.
"The Few" were 2353 men from Great Britain and 574 from overseas, pilots and other aircrew, who are officially recognized as having taken part in the Battle of Britain. 544 lost their lives during the period of the Battle.

ADLERTAG: THE QUEST FOR A COMPLETE CATARACT OPERATION

was organized by the German Luftwaffe. It was called "Eagle Attack" (*Adlereingriff*) on what they designated as the Day of the Eagle (*Adlertag*).

The infamous Herman Goering was the overall head of the German Air Force and his orders were as follows:

Eagle Day
(13 to 14 August)

FROM REICHS MARSHALL GOERING:
TO ALL UNITS OF AIR FLEETS 2, 3, AND 5.

OPERATION EAGLE.

WITHIN A SHORT PERIOD YOU WILL WIPE THE BRITISH AIR FORCE FROM THE SKY.

HEIL HITLER

H. Goering 1940

The operation—the air battle in which Billy Fiske was to die, but in which the British set the stage for final victory that would eventually lead to a subsequent driving of the Germans from England—began on August 13, 1940. On the morning of August 14, "Mouse" Cleaver flew the Hurricane that was normally assigned to him into battle. After take-off, the pilots would typically fly several miles to a location, Goodwood Park, West Sussex, directly on the Channel coast, where they could be positioned at the closest possible distance from the attackers so that they could quickly intercept them. The British had two major advantages on their side: their radar and their tactics.

Cleaver survived the morning foray and returned by noon. He had hardly settled in after the mission and was entering the officers' mess for refreshments when he was immediately called back for another "scramble." The highly sophisticated radar system the British had installed around their coastline made it possible for them to detect

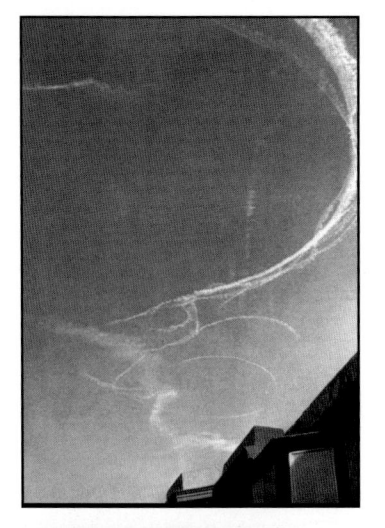

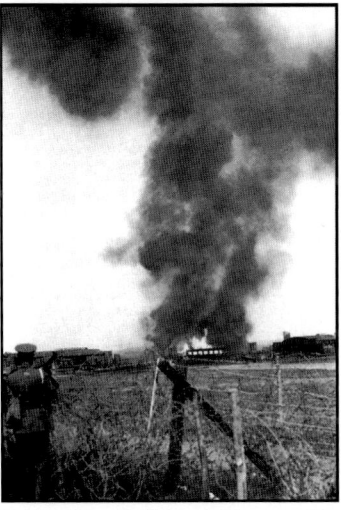

Eagle Day (Adlertag). August 13-15, 1940. This Battle was the fateful day in which the British began to turn around the Battle in their favor. "Mouse" Cleaver sustained his eye injuries. Billy Fiske was also killed in this battle.
TOP: Dogfights over RAF Tangmere.
BOTTOM: Adlertag battle at RAF Tangmere. Flight Lieutenant Cleaver was shot down on the afternoon of August 14, 1940.

Flight Lieutenant "Mouse" Cleaver's Hurricane. He flew this plane on the morning of the fateful August 14th. He was quickly assigned another plane for an emergency afternoon flight. Rushing to the plane, he forgot his goggles. He then crashed, sustaining injuries to both eyes, with numerous plastic fragments from the cockpit canopy embedded in each eye. He was barely able to parachute to safety.

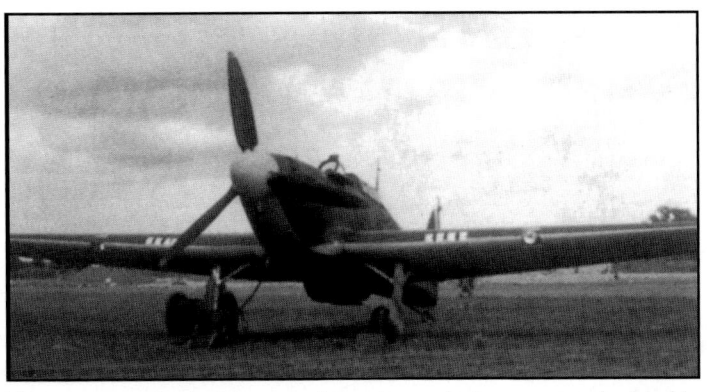

CHAPTER 6

the enemy's approach, and the system warned that another wave of enemy planes was approaching.

The Hurricane Cleaver normally flew was not yet ready to fly again. The engines at that time required that their choke have some time to warm, so his commander, Sir Archibald Hope, assigned a brand new Hurricane to him. In his rush to return to combat in the new plane, Cleaver neglected to bring his flying goggles.

He completed the basic assigned mission without incident, but as he was flying back to the base late that afternoon, he was ambushed, and his plane was hit by bursts of fire from some enemy fighter planes that were escorting bombers returning to their base in northern France. The encounter had caught Cleaver by surprise. A bullet smashed through the plastic plexiglas acrylic that formed the sidewalls of his cockpit. Without the protection of his goggles, he was suddenly blinded by multiple fragments of plastic from the cracked cockpit canopy; the plastic shards penetrated and became embedded under his eyes.

Surprisingly and most fortunately, Cleaver was able to maintain control of his aircraft long enough to turn it upside down, positioning it so he could parachute out by simply letting himself fall out. His parachute brought him to a safe landing over the flatlands. At first, the local farmers came with their pitch forks to be sure that he was not an enemy pilot. He was quickly whisked away to the Salisbury infirmary for emergency treatment. He was never to fly again.

The 601 Squadron and the other brave Allied pilots would go on to win the Adlertag battle and the Battle of Britain, thus preventing the Nazis from overrunning the British Isles. The invasion we refer to as the Battle of Britain was summarily canceled by a frustrated Hitler in September. Since then, the British have celebrated the Battle of Britain Day on September 18 of each year. Hitler could not break the fighter pilots of the RAF and, therefore, could not achieve dominance. He felt that he had to abandon his plans for an invasion of England. Operation Sea Lion was canceled, and Hitler immediately turned his attention to an invasion of the Soviet Union. An estimated 544 Allied airmen lost their lives during the 4-month Battle of Britain, and many more like Cleaver suffered permanent injuries.

A grateful world paid these brave aviators their highest respects, but perhaps Churchill himself said it best when he stated, "Never have so few done so much for so many."

COMING FULL CIRCLE: ONE PIECE OF PLASTIC IS REPLACED WITH ANOTHER

For "Mouse" Cleaver, the "Adlertag" battle marked the end of the combative phase of the war. However, another battle had begun for him: the fight for his sight. In this new war, Cleaver had the best possible care: England's best hospitals and eye doctors.

The pieces of plastic shrapnel that had been blown into his eyes had blinded his right eye completely and had seriously reduced the vision in his left eye. A cataract caused by the traumatic injury to his lens formed when numerous splinters smashed into and embedded themselves in his lens. One week after the injury, Jack Riddle visited Cleaver in the hospital. Cleaver, although totally blind at that point, heard him

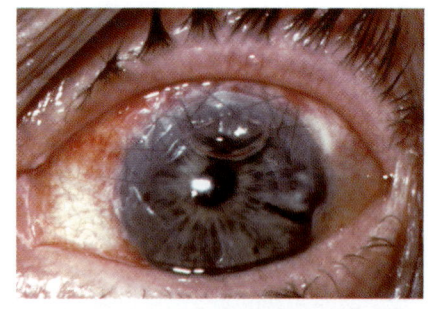

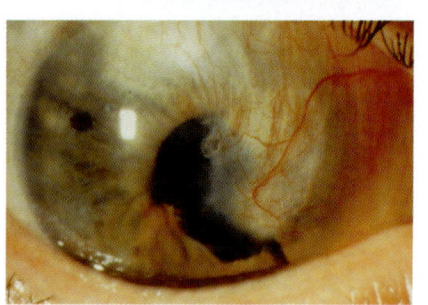

Clinical photographs of Cleaver's injured eyes several months after the crash. Both eyes contained numerous fragments of plastic from the cockpit canopies. One eye was totally blind, but one eye retained a potential for vision. He had 18 eye operations, some performed by Harold himself.

speak as he walked thought the door in his room. The first thing he shouted was "Jack, tell them all to wear their goggles."

The previously mentioned Dr. McIndoe, who treated many pilots with burns, had also addressed that theme. He lamented in a publication that many of the pilots often did not wear their goggles. He had seen over 250 such cases.

Cleaver's right eye was permanently blind, and there was little chance for a successful operation that could restore any vision. The better eye had a cataract secondary to the trauma in that eye. An opportunity to remove that cataract would come much later.

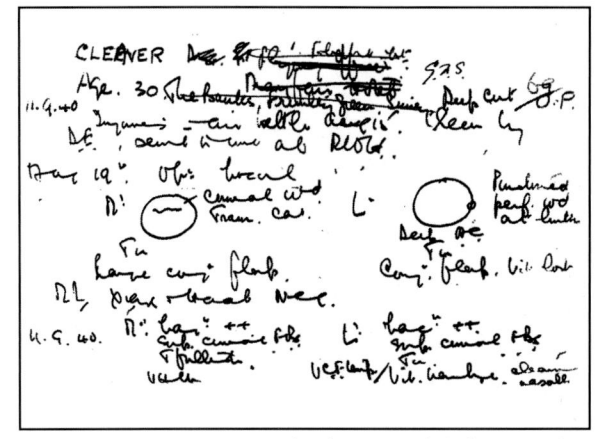

Cleaver was first seen in the acute stages by military surgeons. He was sent to Moorfields Eye Hospital (called the Royal London Ophthalmic Hospital [RLOH]). It is not clear when Harold first saw him. It could have been while pilots and doctors were in the South around Tangmere; it could have been later after Cleaver had been sent to Moorfields.

Medical notes, dated September 11, 1940, that briefly describe Cleaver's eye injuries.

It is known that he had 18 operations on his eye and face to try to preserve some vision and make plastic surgical repairs on his face. I did not have the opportunity to review Cleaver's hospital records myself, but according to two sources, Harold himself performed several of Cleaver's eye operations over the next several years at Moorfields. Some of these operations consisted of removing pieces or portions of the plastic fragments embedded in the coats surrounding his eyes or within the eyes.

Following his eventual discharge from Moorfields, he was followed long-term by Mr. Edgar King, a physician in private practice on Harley Street. He was then transferred to Mr. Eric Arnott in 1975. By the mid-1980s, Arnott felt that he was ready for removal of his cataract and that the technology would allow the implantation of an IOL—clearly unbeknownst to him, the product had been researched in the Lieutenant's own eye since 1940. The right eye never saw again, but the left eye was salvaged, and he could see out of this eye. Cleaver was able to return to normal civilian life. His one seeing eye had a small scar on the cornea and a hole in the iris through which a small piece of plastic had passed before entering the lens. Almost 50 years later, a traumatic cataract had developed in this eye and a cataract operation was performed, replacing one piece of plastic with another! This was successfully accomplished by Mr. Eric Arnott in 1987. Things had come full circle.

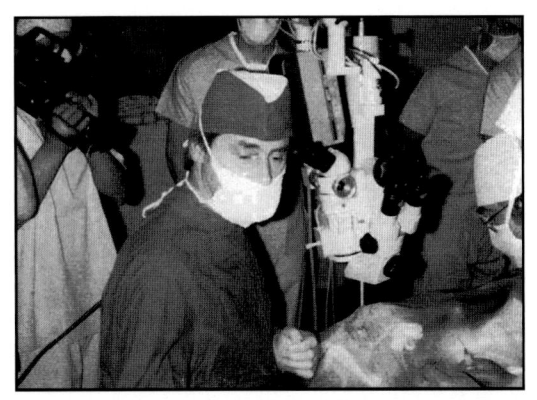

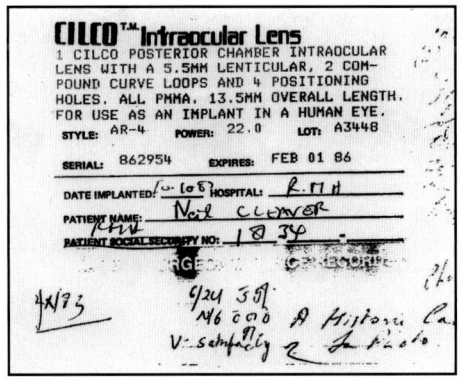

The sight in Cleaver's eye was eventually restored thanks to the IOL implant. Ironically, the artificial lens that restored his vision was made of almost the same material that years before had robbed him of it.

Having received wounds that eventually helped facilitate a study that would help lead to the invention of the IOL, Cleaver himself received an IOL over 46 years later.
LEFT: A successful IOL implant procedure was performed by Professor Eric Arnott.
RIGHT: Details regarding the IOL, the date of implantation and type are documented on this manufacturer's list of specifications.

CHAPTER 6

What Was Flight Lieutenant Cleaver's Precise Role in the Development of the IOL?

He in Essence Served as the Subject of a Pre-Clinical Study of an Invention That Had Not Yet Been Invented*

Harold did not need a test tube study; he did not need explanted rabbits. He had the best of all possible study specimens—a human being.

For many years, based on some lack of hard evidence, I considered the "airplane story" to be very suspect—"too good to be true." However, as I began to accumulate letters, documents, and photographs, it became clear that it was not a myth.

One example of an important document was written by Mr. J. M. J. Estevez, an I.C.I. chemist who worked closely with Dr. John Holt, Harold's original coworker (see Chapter 7), to provide input into the composition of the IOL. In an article published in the July 1966 issue of the *American Journal of Ophthalmology*, Mr. Estevez wrote (courtesy of Mr. Ian Collins, Rayner & Keeler, Ltd.):

> *"As the last war was drawing to a close, H. Ridley made the observation that splinters from the transparent canopies of fighter planes were acceptable within the eye. This was communicated to the manufacturers of the material that was used to make these canopies, and an understanding was given that the material of this quality would be made available to ophthalmologists. The material was poly (methyl) methacrylate. Ridley's main interest at the time was the design and fabrication of artificial crystalline lenses; the assumption was made that poly (methyl) methacrylate was suitable for intraocular lenses. It had already been shown that it was suitable for prostheses such as contact lenses, tear ducts, etc. This impression has been justified over the years."*

Mr. Peter Caudell, who worked for Rayner & Keeler, Ltd. (the company that made the first IOLs) at the time of the first implant, made the following comment in a company document:

> *"Everyone is aware by now of Mr. Harold Ridley's recognition that this material in the eye of service personnel appeared to cause no inflammatory condition, and in most cases, could be left alone as harmless intraocular foreign bodies. As far as I know, these service personnel are still walking about with these fragments inside their eyes. I am not aware of any case in which they had to be removed because of a chemical or other type of reaction."*

Harold had cut through the devastation and wreckage of the war and had found something good for society—an advance that would ultimately improve the lives of far more people than the war had so wantonly and sadly destroyed.

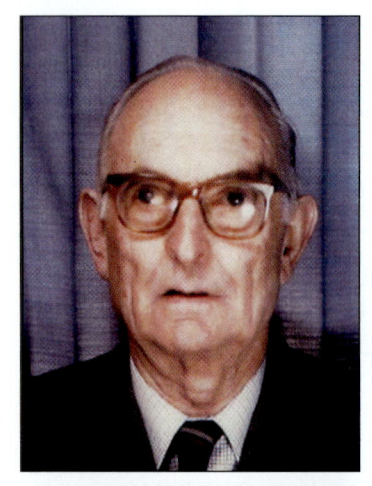

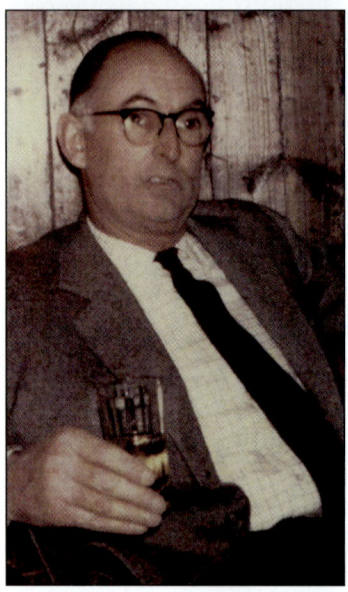

Two views of "Mouse" Cleaver in the 1970s and 1980s (at first unknowingly) a genuine pioneer of implant surgery. Considering the extent of his injuries, his face and eyes appear remarkably well.

---

*A clear review of a few of the terms used by various oversight organizations, such as the FDA, will help clarify Flight Lieutenant Cleaver's role in the invention of the IOL.

The usual procedure that is followed when a device or material is submitted for ultimate approval for use in patients is as follows:

1) A pre-clinical study, generally done in-vitro (in test tubes) or in experimental animals.
2) A clinical study, preformed in humans on a controlled basis.
3) Various levels of approval of a successful product with permission for general marketing and sales.

The study of Cleaver's eyes provided a unique opportunity to do both a "pre-clinical and clinical" study on the best possible model—a human being.

The "airplane story," as detailed here, occurred within the framework of a specific group of pilots, the RAF 601 Squadron. I have told their story in some detail since it represents a complex series of events that eventuated in a study of a single person in that squadron who was at the right place at the right time. It was not only serendipity. We are fortunate that Cleaver, after his training for military service as well as his own personality traits, became an excellent (although unknowing) participant in a long, arduous study.

Flight Lieutenant Cleaver's strength of character and his unflinching reliability during the decade of the 1940s, as his eyes were being followed by the hospital staff members, helped make the necessary follow up and evaluation possible. This, in turn, made possible an incredible sequence of events that is perhaps unique in medicine. By being the subject in a study of a new invention, it helped open the way for Harold to proceed.

THE INVENTION OF THE IOL: THE ACTUAL SEQUENCE OF EVENTS, CA 1935 TO 1951

It is often assumed that Harold simply looked at an injured pilot, a stroke of genius immediately ensued, and the IOL was born. It was much more complicated than that. I have described the sequence of events into seven categories as follows.

1. Mid-1930s: Conversations. The sequence of events began in the mid-1930s when Harold had conversations with his professor "Huddy" and his father regarding the IOL. They did not encourage him. To my knowledge, he wrote very little about the IOL in the 1930s and 1940s, until 1948.

2. August 15, 1940: The Injury. Cleaver was injured and followed by many surgeons at Moorfields and in private practice. Sir Stewart Duke-Elder saw him at least once shortly after the injury (see Chapter 9).

3. 1940 to 1948: The Pre-Clinical Study. During most of the 1940s, the concept of "a new lens for the old" remained in limbo. I doubt that it was ever far from his mind.

4. 1948: The Student. Next, the famous encounter with *the* medical student occurred in 1948. Harold made several references to the student, Mr. Stephen Perry, in many of his papers. There is no doubt that it had a profound impact on him. I will discuss it in some detail in Chapter 7, but I will offer one example of his statements regarding the student at this juncture:

> "One day a student who had never before been into the eye department saw a cataract extracted by the then fashionable intracapsular method and asked if it was intended to put a new lens in the eye. I replied that this was not usual but I began to think that since even students were then discussing the possibility, the time had surely come for a courageous and enterprising surgeon who had achieved all necessary appointments to face the inevitable opposition which would result from a revolutionary operation which offered a 'new lens for old.' It was not until some years later that I learned that the student who had stimulated action was named Stephen Perry."

It is clear from Ridley's reaction and response that the student did not surprise him with a "new" idea. The student had stated a fact that would be obvious to any

CHAPTER 6

thoughtful cataract surgeon. Rather, Mr. Perry's question offered a challenge to him and, most importantly, helped conjure up the courage to proceed forward with the IOL implant—the November 1949 operation.

5. 1948 through 1949: Mobilization. The formal planning began after Harold's encounter with the student—the mobilization of forces. He contacted the various colleagues who would be necessary to form the team he deemed mandatory to design and manufacture an implantable IOL.

In no way was the period that encompassed almost the entire decade of the 1940s wasted. The real, tangible clinical experiment that Harold would need to proceed became a reality.

As noted previously when discussing Flight Lieutenant Cleaver, Harold did not, as is sometimes written, suddenly come up with the idea of an IOL when speaking with the student (just as he had not suddenly seen a "flash of genius" while observing a wounded pilot). The idea was long etched in his mind before he met both Flight Lieutenant Cleaver and/or Mr. Perry. Likewise, the student Mr. Perry did not give Ridley the idea. Perry's achievement was that he gave Harold the *courage* to proceed.

6. 1940 to 1949: The Biocompatibility Study. To reiterate, what occurred after that battle over the shores of England during the "Adlerangriff" (Eagle's attack) in August 1940 was the beginning of the biocompatibility study required to be sure that the material used to make an IOL would be tolerated by the pilot's eye and, subsequently, the eyes' of patients. Companies today would have to pay millions of dollars to carry out such studies within the parameters of the modern FDA.

Harold's role in this compatibility study was to follow the patient and provide therapeutic treatment and surgery on the unfortunate pilot. This was invaluable because an expectation of a safe operation and good long-term clinical success with his future IOL could not be assumed and assured until the prosthetic material was proven safe.

The point in time when Harold made the important connection between the pilot's injury and the idea of an IOL is not known with certainty. This is the moment that, if known, might best serve as the birthday of the IOL. That time would certainly represent the stroke of genius.

Harold's involvement with Cleaver and, no doubt, other pilots with the same type of injuries were crucial to his invention of the IOL. As Harold himself said, Cleaver was a ready-made clinical study. He provided the perfect opportunity to observe the eye's reaction to the biomaterial that would eventually become the material of which IOLs were made. Many opponents later criticized Harold for not doing animal studies with IOLs. They were wrong. He actually had the ultimate study—a human being!

7. November 29, 1949: The First Operation. This operation was possible because of the willingness of Lieutenant Cleaver to allow completion of the pre-clinical study that was thrust on his shoulders after his injury.

Harold's true genius rests with his amazing ability to not only see this wounded pilot as a patient, but to seize the opportunity to do what he did. He recognized what he needed to do and did it. Others at or near that battle were given the same opportunity. Fortunately for the world, Harold's perception was unique!

ADLERTAG: THE QUEST FOR A COMPLETE CATARACT OPERATION

Epilogue: It's Plastic!

LEFT and RIGHT: Damage to airplane wind screen and cockpit canopies were common in World War II air battles.

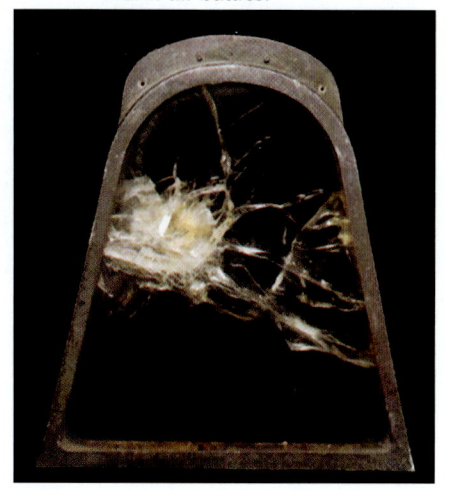

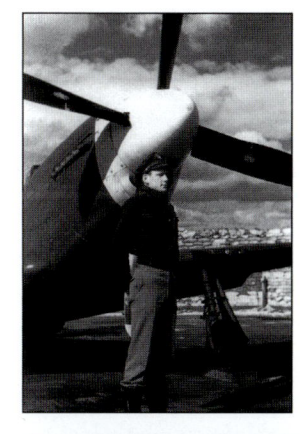

Many of us movie aficionados remember Anne Bancroft and Dustin Hoffman in the film *The Graduate*. The young college graduate was clearly advised that plastics would be a hot item for the future. He was right—and he probably was not even aware of IOLs. Flight Lieutenant Cleaver helped Harold prove that at least one plastic formulation (PMMA) was inert in the eye (ie, it was biocompatible).

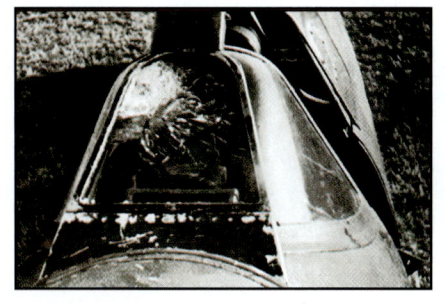

As I did research for this book over the years, I wished to determine whether breakage of the cockpit canopies, as occurred with Cleaver, was a common occurrence. I interviewed several pilots. It did not take long to determine that it was. The injuries were common because many pilots failed or refused to wear their goggles, as was lamented by McIndoe previously, and there were always thousands of bullets flying past during the typical fighter plane battle. It was an awesome privilege to meet the men I interviewed—all between 85 and 95 years old. They had many stories to tell. One pilot, Joe Thompson, now living in Nashville, Tennessee, was a reconnaissance pilot. After we discussed the question regarding the plastic, he kindly showed me a few extra pictures from his collection that he thought might be interesting (eg, the unique images shown below— a unique aerial photo of Hitler's headquarters and Ike and Churchill together smiling after D-Day).

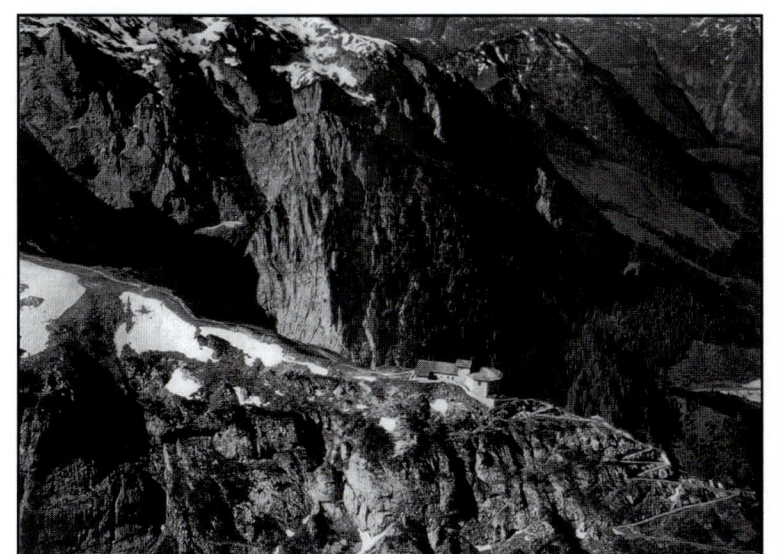

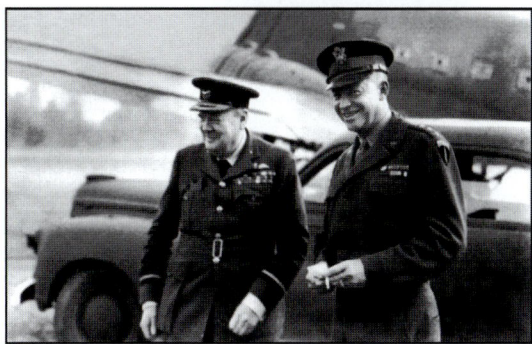

Some important photographs obtained while on the interview circuit. I interviewed Mr. Joe Thompson, shown at TOP RIGHT in a ca. 1944 photograph. He was an expert in aerial photography during the war and advised me regarding eye injuries suffered by pilots. He also gave me some interesting negatives.
LEFT: Mr. Thompson provided this image of Eagle's Nest, the mountain retreat of Adolph Hitler.
BOTTOM RIGHT: Photograph of General Dwight Eisenhower and Prime Minister Winston Churchill, both smiling and celebrating the victory after D-Day, June 1944.

CHAPTER 6

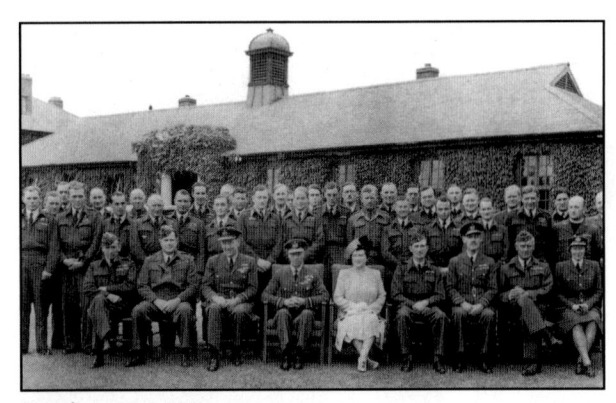

Royal visit to RAF Tangmere, 1944, an expression of gratitude to the many who served in this region during the invasion. King George IV and his Queen are in the front row.

Elizabeth Bowes-Lyon, August 4, 1900-March 30, 2002. Queen Consort to George IV until 1952, the Queen Mother until 2002. She had a cataract-IOL operation shortly prior to her death at age 101.

The British High Command, including the royalty, was well aware of the sacrifices made by pilots throughout the country, including Tangmere of course, and King George VI and his wife visited Tangmere in 1944 to thank the servicemen for the sacrifices they had made.

The Queen Mother lived to age 101 and was very popular. Her daughter is the present Queen Elizabeth II. The Queen Mother had a cataract that arose at age 99. Dr. John Pearce successfully operated on her with excellent results. She greatly appreciated this and had accepted an invitation to a Rayner & Keeler, Ltd. celebration of the 50th year of the IOL in 1949. I was to chair it, but could not because of illness. Unfortunately, the Queen was also quite ill and had to cancel, and she died not long after. However, all of us were gratified that she had a brief enjoyment of Harold's invention.

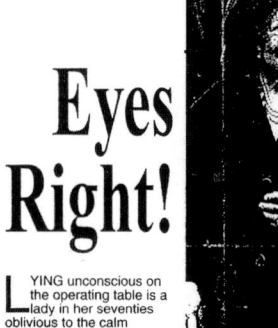

Eyes Right!

Even the Queen Mum has benefitted from lens replacement surgery.

LYING unconscious on the operating table is a lady in her seventies oblivious to the calm ministrations of the handful of theatre staff about her.

She is one of over five million people worldwide who undergo lens replacement surgery as a treatment for cataracts.

This year marks the fiftieth anniversary of the operation that has changed so many people's lives for the better. It takes just 12-15 minutes to perform – a far cry from the the early days, 50 years ago, when British surgeon Harold Ridley became the first person to implant an artificial intraocular lens (IOL) after a cataract was removed.

Until 1949, if you suffered from cataracts, you'd little choice but to lose your lens, and with it, one third of your eye's ability to focus, your peripheral vision and any way of judging distances.

Not only were sufferers unable to see properly, but the thick bottle-bottom spectacles they had to wear afterwards stigmatised them as different or even "disabled".

RIDLEY set about designing a replacement lens with the help of the Rayner Optical Company. He used a type of ICI Perspex, a material he knew to be inert through his experience of treating fighter pilots with eye injuries during the war.

Ridley's pioneering work is still carried on by surgeons like John Pearce, who provides specialist expertise to Rayner Intraocular Lenses, the company which made that first lens back in 1949 and which is the only UK manufacturer in its field.

The work now benefits everyone from the Queen Mother to 74-year-old Dolly Games, a grandmother from Oakamoor who has just had her second cataract operation at North Staffordshire Hospital, and for whom it apparently held no terrors.

"I felt that I was well looked after," she said, "so I wasn't particularly apprehensive about the operation. Though I had mine under local anaesthetic, there was a nurse there to hold my hand, which was very comforting.

"My husband took me home and I went back to the consultant the next morning. When he removed the patch there was a big improvement in the clarity of my vision."

A patient is referred to a consultant via their GP, sometimes following an examination by an optician. The consultant gauges the visual sharpness of the eye, measures the length and curvature of the eye using ultrasound, and uses the results to calculate the size and required focal length of the lens, correcting for long and short-sightedness at the same time.

After the operation, the patient may wear a shield to prevent them rubbing the eye, and will take anti-inflammatory drops for a few weeks.

Mr Pearce warns that though it is a highly successful operation, not every implant is successful. However, developments are constantly ongoing, many concerned with minimising the intrusive nature of the operation.

Meanwhile, Harold Ridley has been honoured at the conference of the American Society of Cataract and Refractive Surgery. Among those who paid him tribute were Cherie Blair and Hilary Clinton.

Though much may have changed in 50 years, the world owes a lot to this early pioneer ■

by Roland Curtis

Finally, we would be remiss if we left Flight Lieutenant "Mouse" Cleaver without one more mention of him, but this time of his skiing prowess, which until now has been his main claim to fame. The figure on this page shows a group of skiers, published in a London newspaper in the early spring of 2006. Note that our friend, Flight Lieutenant Cleaver, is standing front and center (fourth from the left). This, of course, is an early pre-war picture and recalls of his great pre-war victory of a Hahenkamm prize. He has been posthumously honored by naming this cup given to the highest British entrant into this world famous contest after him. We should all appreciate him for both his skiing ability and for the wonderful clinical study he was that allowed the invention of the IOL.

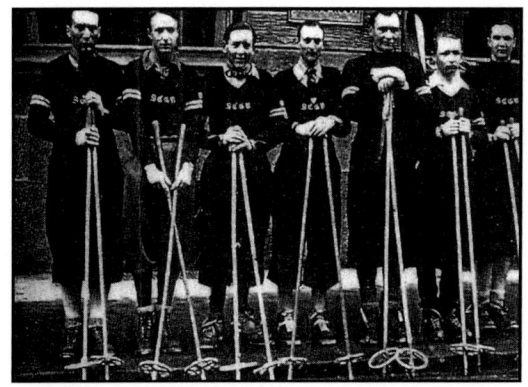

"Mouse" Cleaver's picture appeared in a London newspaper just a few months before this book went to press. It is an old pre-war photo, but it reminds us of his fame as a skier! He had won the prestigious Hahnenkamm (Kitzbuehl, Austria) cup years ago before the war. A Cleaver award has recently been approved to honor the first place British skier in the contest. He is not yet famous in the realm of the IOL, but we hope this will change soon.

Stephen Perry. Perry was the young medical student at St. Thomas' Hospital, who, having observed Harold completing a standard cataract operation of the time (ICCE), asked him the following question, which I will now paraphrase: "Do you intend to put a new lens in the eye after removing the old cloudy one?" This single question helped change the course of medical history by giving Harold, who had long been pondering the possibility of developing and implanting an artificial lens, the courage and incentive to mobilize a team and proceed with his landmark operation of November 29, 1949. (Photograph courtesy of Mrs. Perry and Mr. Hugh Williams.)

7

A Simple Question, Mobilization*

"The cure of cataracts was established within perhaps one and one-half hours in Cavendish Square in 1948."

Harold Ridley, Cavendish Square, 1948

Eight years had passed since that fateful day in August of 1940 when the clock began ticking, setting in motion the process leading to the innovation of Harold's "cure of aphakia." Flight Lieutenant Cleaver's wounds were being cared for, and Harold was no doubt studying the effects of the plastic splinters or shrapnel embedded in both eyes of the visually imparied pilot. Harold must have still been pondering how to reach his goal. In retrospect, we now know that he needed something to stimulate him and give him the courage to act.

In 1948, a young medical student asked Harold a very simple question after observing Harold do a standard (for the time) ICCE cataract procedure. According to Harold himself in many of his writings which he handed on to me, that question was all that he needed. He decided then and there to begin active preparations to make and implant the first IOL. He was on the threshold of achieving the long elusive desire to provide a *complete* cure of cataract, providing almost perfect visual rehabilitation. In much simpler terms, and as he preferred to say, he himself was about to "cure aphakia."

---

* Important information and photographs related to Rayner & Keeler, Ltd.'s very important participation in the development of the IOL was kindly provided to me by Mr. Ian Collins, the former Manager and Director of Rayner & Keeler, Ltd. Unfortunately, most of the documentation dealing with Rayner's early history (149 to 1960) has sadly been lost. Two moves of Head Office, where these records were kept, and two severe floods were responsible for this. The surviving records are fairly detailed.

CHAPTER 7

THE PILOT

Harold's careful observation over 8 years of Flight Lieutenant "Mouse" Cleaver's and other pilot's eyes clearly demonstrated that his eyes could tolerate the Plexiglas material that had been embedded in them (the scientific word for such excellent tolerance is "biocompatibility"). Harold could now confirm that this material was suitable and safe for use as an IOL and he, therefore, had no hesitation in selecting it as the lens material of choice for the hoped-for implant operation.

Years later, many naysayers criticized Harold for not completing laboratory studies to confirm the safety of the IOL. They felt that he should performed in-vitro (test tube) analyses or rat or rabbit studies. These accusations were groundless and unfair. In his long observation of Cleaver's eyes, Harold had, in effect, completed a preclinical study of the human eye's tolerance to the Plexiglas material.* It was the best possible study because it involved a *human* rather than an experimental animal.

Harold's study of Cleaver also succeeded in evaluating the now well-known dictum of materials engineering that one should "follow to failure" (ie, follow the material that is being tested for a long period to determine if and when it might fail [ie, degenerate, crack, dissolve, etc]). Harold's follow-up was quite long, 8 years. It is now known that a well-manufactured perspex material is virtually indestructible in the eye.

THE STUDENT

In 1948, a young medical student who is now famous, but soon due to become even more famous (sadly posthumously), became an unknowing "collaborator" by asking Harold, during rounds, if he was planning to put a lens back into a patient's eye from which the cataractous lens had been removed. I will present two versions of this event penned by Harold as follows:

"Ever since Daviel introduced the cataract extraction in 1748, few surgeons had considered the possibility of replacement of the lens.

"Working as his surgeon in 1935, I suggested to my great teacher, A. C. Hudson, and also to my father the possibility of an artificial intraocular lens to restore binocular vision after traumatic cataract but neither was encouraging.

"In 1948 a student at St. Thomas' Hospital saw a cataract operation for the first time and asked if I intended to replace the absent part of the eye.

*"I after that then raised the **courage** (author's underlining) to attempt careful and truly scientific experiments on patients who, after full explanation of the risks, volunteered to advance science and help others. After the War conditions were unfavorable for eye surgery for St. Thomas' Hospital had been repeatedly bombed. Instruments were primitive. Penicillin was the only antibiotic available and there were no anti-inflammatory steroids. However, most fortunately for our research, people during the*

---

*Recall that the usual sequence of testing of a new product is to first do a "preclinical" study in an in-vitro model (see Chapter 6) or in an animal study, followed by a "clinical study" in humans. This is followed in favorable cases by release to the public. The Cleaver study is unusual in that a human was the subject of the preclinical study.

war were accustomed to dangers and a few, for advancement of science were prepared to accept the risks which had been fully explained to them. In those times patients never thought of trying to get compensation money from their much respected hospitals and doctors if anything went wrong."

Harold only learned the name of the student many years later when one of his associates, Mr. Jimmy Phillpot, discovered that the student's name was Stephen Perry. Perry eventually settled with his family in the central English town of Wohlverhampton and served for many years there as a general practitioner. I only learned of his whereabouts a few years ago with the assistance of doctors David Austin, Michael Roper-Hall, and Hugh Williams. During one of Ann and my visits to England, we rang his home telephone number from Mr. Roper-Hall's office, but were sad to learn that he had died a year earlier. However, his widow was indeed aware of his earlier contact with Harold. With the kind assistance of Hugh Williams, she forwarded the photographs seen at the beginning of this chapter.

Some have given Perry almost too much credit, some even asserting that the IOL was his idea—that he should be considered the inventor of the IOL. Harold's statement in the quotations here and in other writings leave little doubt that Perry's input was important in that his simple question helped give Harold the courage he needed to proceed with the very dangerous undertaking that he had been contemplating. Harold already had the idea as early as 1935 or possibly earlier. Note that he had discussed the disadvantages of aphakia and the idea of an artificial lens or lens transplant with his father and his professor.

Sketches made by Harold himself of three eyes that had had cataract surgery (aphakic eyes) made in the 1960s for teaching purposes. These show the problem of post-cataract surgery image magnification caused by thick spectacles or contact lenses, as opposed to an IOL implanted within the physiologic position of the lens in the eye. All three eyes in this drawing are situated so that each looks at an arrow of the same size (top). Recalling that any pair of lenses with a space between them is a Galilean telescope, any magnification would be caused by having the lens of the appliance (contact lens, spectacles, or IOLs) set at a finite distance from the baseline lens in the eye.

With contact lenses the difference between the contact lens and the baseline site is moderate; with spectacles the distance is quite large, since the spectacle is placed relatively far away from the interior of the eye on the patient's nose, whereas the intraocular lens is placed precisely where the lens should be, so there was no distance separating the two lenses. The eyes in all three instances in effect have a negative lens caused as the positive diopter cataractous lens was removed.

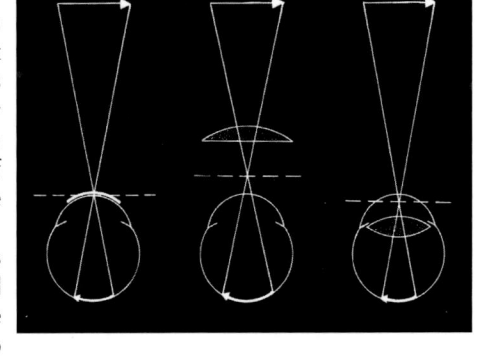

The results of a surgery are bad (anisometropia) if one eye has one amount of magnification and the other eye has another, for example, the high magnification given by an aphakic spectacle in one eye will cause the patient much confusion if the other eye has a different degree or no magnification.

LEFT: Contact lens. The image size of the retina (curved arrow, lower left) is magnified by about 5% because the contact lens does form a mini-Galilean telescope.
MIDDLE: Thick aphakic spectacles placed relatively far in front of the normal site of an IOL. This creates a Galilean telescope of greater power than the contact lens, since the power of any telescope increases with the increase in distance between the two lenses used in the system. The magnification here is up to 25%, more than the contact lens of 5%.
RIGHT: An IOL placed in the correct position in the eye, mimicking the normal lens that we are born with, does not cause any magnification, since the site of the original lens and the site of the new IOL are in exactly the same plane, providing no distance to allow for a Galilean telescope.

CHAPTER 7

I remember well a river walk I had with Harold, when he described to me some of the same events to me but with slightly different emphasis. Note that in the just-cited paragraphs and in this description he emphasized **courage!**

"Many eye surgeons must surely have thought that a new lens for the old would appear one day when science was suitably advanced and I was one of the many who considered but abandoned that possibility before the 1939-43 war. I talked to my father and also my great teacher, A. C. Hudson about a skilled man whose career had been ruined by a small intraocular foreign body that had produced a cataract in one eye. Each of his two eyes could read 6/6 (20/20) but they would not work together. Surely the time would come for someone to attempt the cure of aphakia (the state of the eye after removal of the lens).

"One day a student who had never before been into the eye department saw a cataract extracted by the then fashionable intracapsular method and asked if it was intended to put a new lens in the eye. I replied that this was not usual but I began to think that since even students were then discussing the possibility, the time had surely come for a **courageous** *(author's emphasis) and enterprising surgeon who had achieved all necessary appointments to face the inevitable opposition which would result from a revolutionary operation which offered a new lens for old.*

"What was needed was a young and progressive ophthalmic surgeon with just the right genes, many of them difficult and unpopular, to develop the new cataract operation. When I was age seven, I told my mother that I wanted to be an "inventor." Knowing then that I had the Parker gene, she bought me many books which I could not understand."

Therefore, I believe that Mr. Perry's contributions to the genesis of the IOL were indeed very important. First, unknowingly and most innocently he handed Harold a gentle reminder to proceed forward—of course, not even knowing that Harold had anything such as this on his mind. Second, and most important, his remark reinforced in Harold the necessary courage to proceed with this inherently dangerous project. It was brutally clear to him that implantation of an IOL at that time could possibly have meant the destruction of a patient's eye, not to mention the likelihood of severe ridicule and ostracism by the ophthalmic community, as well as the possibility of serious legal or even criminal consequences.

Harold apparently did not ponder Perry's words for too long; mobilization of his resources and preparations began! As he began locating the necessary collaborators, he stated his basic goal in simplest terms: "To restore the internal optical system of the eye after the cataract extraction." He laid down specific ground rules:

"The optics of aphakic vision had long been known, but the full effects were perhaps not recognized by ophthalmologists. It was considered that the necessity of an external optical aid was an inevitable part of the price to be paid for restoration of visual acuity. Many surgeons, no doubt, had considered the advantages of restoring the internal optical system after cataract extraction but lacked the courage to deliberately insert an intraocular foreign body.

"In the words of Wilfrid Trotter: 'The most powerful antigen known to man is a new idea,' and it was to be expected that an unheralded innovation would arouse criticism in many quarters. Important strategic decisions had to be made.

"Firstly, the work was to be strictly scientific with one aim only: completion of the treatment of cataract.

"There was no thought of financial gain for anyone involved, no grant was requested, and participants carried their own expenses. The material and manufacturing cost of the original implants were supplied at cost price. (All three originators, Ridley, Pike, and Holt agreed to abandon any financial reward and keep the profit purely scientific.)

"Secondly, most careful attention was to be given to details of technique, for without good surgery, the double operation was sure to fail. Thorough evaluation was to be made of every part of the after care with practical assessment of any apparent complication or misfortune. In 1949, surgical instruments were simple, no corticosteroids were available, and the only antibiotic was penicillin.

"Thirdly, the revolutionary rather than evolutionary nature of the project demanded that secrecy be observed until good results of some duration could be shown. Although implants began in 1949, no publication appeared until 1951."

THE OPTICIAN AND THE CHEMIST: THE CURE OF CATARACT

The Fateful One and One-Half Hour Meeting at Cavendish Square

As soon as Harold made the personal decision to proceed with the IOL, he needed to assemble a team to help him design and facilitate the lens. His choice of collaborators was brilliant! He turned first to John Pike, director and senior optical scientist who worked for Rayner & Keeler, Ltd., a leading optical company in England. Ridley and Pike were already well-acquainted, having worked together frequently on other projects. Harold was also well acquainted with Rayner & Keeler, Ltd. The choice of this company turned out to be an absolutely correct one. The meeting at Cavendish Square was about to begin.

Rayner & Keeler, Ltd. was—and remains—a firm that specializes in the manufacture and sales of optical devices.

Cavendish Square, London, was laid out in the 18th century. Harold lived just a few hundred yards north of the buildings seen in these photographs at his town home on 53 Harley Street. This square has assumed great importance in the history of the intraocular lens. It was here that Harold and Mr. Pike of Rayner & Keeler, Ltd. had one of their initial meetings planning of the IOL. This was the conversation that produced the genesis and preliminary design of the first IOL—the meeting where Ridley stated that "the cure of cataracts was established within perhaps one and one-half hours."
TOP: Cavendish Square from an 18th century image, ca. 1765. Note the two beautiful columned buildings just to the right of center.
BOTTOM: The same two buildings in 2002 are seen in the lower photograph of the square.

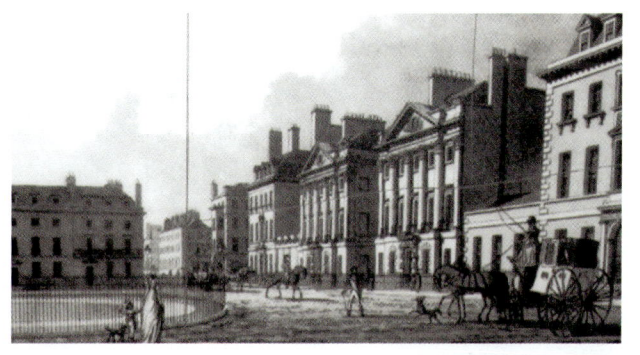

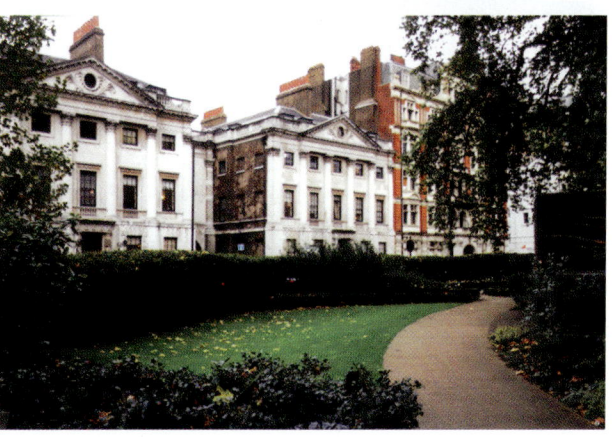

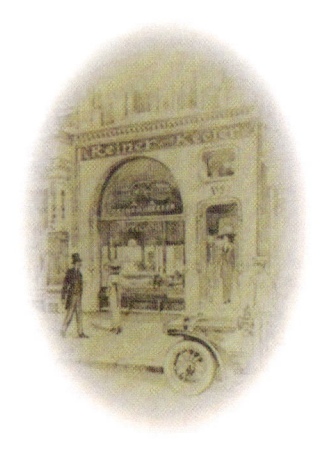

CHAPTER 7

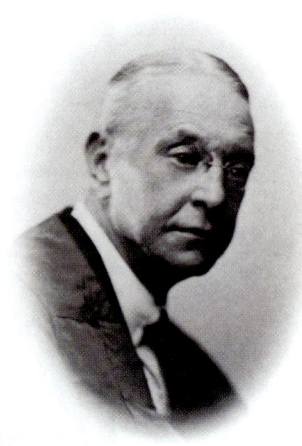

Harold was very fortunate to be able to work with an outstanding optical company, Rayner & Keeler, Ltd. as he proceeded to have a lens manufactured. He had known this company and its brilliant optical scientist, John Pike from previous work they did together.
LEFT: Early photograph of the front of the Rayner & Keeler, Ltd. optical shop in London, early 1900s. It was situated on Bere Street.
RIGHT: The company was co-founded by John Baptiste Reiner, of Austrian decent, in association with Mr. Charles Davis (C. D.) Keeler. They founded and registered their company in 1910. Mr. Reiner died in 1933.

Mr. Jean Baptiste Reiner and Mr. C. D. Keeler founded the company and registered it in 1910. Reiner deemed it prudent to change his company name to Rayner in order to anglicize it. This, he realized, was a good move since his enterprise was located in England. Political and military difficulties for Rayner & Keeler, Ltd., namely the onset of the first World War, existed between England and some of the continental countries and of course the war raged between 1914 and 1918.

Before forming the company, Reiner had completed an apprenticeship as an "art of optician and scientific instrument maker" in 1891 and had gone on to work for E. B. Merowitz, Ltd., a branch of a well-known American optical company.

In 1915, as the first World War raged, Reiner changed the company name change to Rayner & Keeler, Ltd., although he retained his name all of his life. The two founding directors parted company in 1917 when C. D. Keeler resigned and severed all of his interest with company. In 1917, Mr. Henry Morgan was elected to the board of Rayner & Keeler, Ltd. He was an eminent accountant and at one time President of the Society of Incorporated Accountants. He became Chairman of the Board of the company, a post in which he was later succeeded by his brother, Mr. Edward Morgan. Later, a nephew of the latter, Mr. Geoffrey Morgan, became Chairman of Rayner. Mr. Christopher Morgan is now Chairman of Rayner IOLs.

On May 18th, 1918 the Rayner Optical Company took a lease of property at 15 Arundel Mews, Kemp town, Brighton, to be developed as the company's optical workshops. Although only a spectacle prescription glazing factory had been envisaged for this workshop, the new company immediately found itself taken over by the Ministry of Munitions to making optical instruments in support of the war effort. Rayner & Keeler Ltd. still flourishes today in the sales of spectacles and other optical devices; the IOL division manufactures both rigid PMMA IOLs and foldable IOLs.

Mr. Ian Collins was Managing Director of the company as they moved into the 21st century. The Managing Director of the Rayner IOL company today, Mr. Donald Munro, deserves special credit not only for his suburb present management of the company increasing their move into foldable IOLs, but also for leading in the drive to attain knighthood for Harold Ridley in 2001.

Returning to 1948, we will proceed directly to Cavendish Square, a beautiful neighborhood in London. It is just a few hundred yards from Harold's home and offices (rooms) at that time at 53 Harley Street. Harold found a parking place at the Square, and he and Mr. Pike had their initial discussion on the IOL. Harold recounted these times as follows:

"After months of secret thought, I called my friend John Pike, the optical scientist of Rayner's of London with whom I had recently worked on elec-

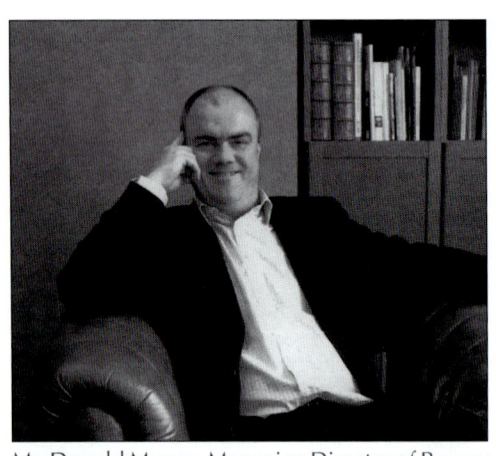

Mr. Donald Munro, Managing Director of Rayner Intraocular Lenses, Ltd. since 1999, having taken over the position from Mr. Ian Collins who had successfully led the company over the several years previous to this. Mr. Munro deserves special credit for playing a critical role in the drive to obtain knighthood for Harold in 2001. In addition to increasing the growth of an already successful IOL company, he also led the company into the era of foldable IOLs.

tronic ophthalmoscopy. I suggested that we meet in my car after completing our routine duties that day.

"So it came about that that two men sitting in a car in Cavendish Square one evening devised all the principles of a new operation."

Ridley wrote:

While seated in the car, I explained the project and invited John Pike to join in a new and exciting venture and he enthusiastically agreed. Within perhaps half an hour, the cure of cataracts was established. We agreed to use an implant made of plastic, chemically sterilized and situated in the posterior chamber—where God had placed the human lens. John Pike was to calculate the necessary optical values required and he would also ask his friend, Dr. John Holt at Imperial Chemical Industries (I.C.I.), to produce some real high quality acrylic."

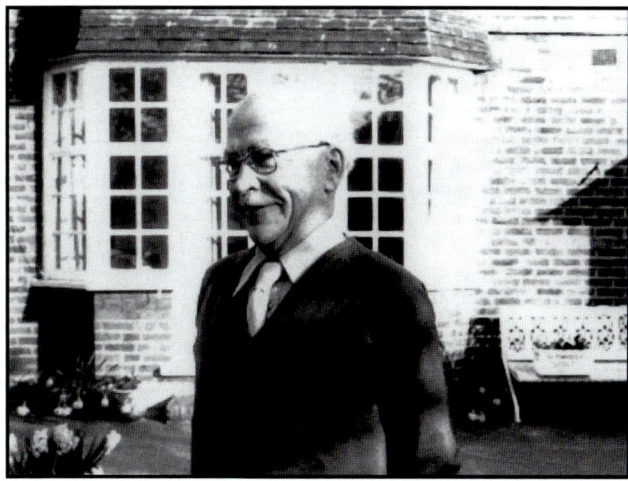

Mr. John Pike at his home.

Pike took the ideas he and Harold had discussed for the IOL back to his company.

His task, working side-by-side with Harold, was to manufacture the artificial lens (Harold often referred to the IOL as a "lenticulus") that would replace the human eye's lens, not only physically but also functionally. Harold knew very well the myriad disadvantages of the aphakic spectacles. He knew that his IOL would eliminate the need for the thick, "pop-bottle-bottom" spectacles that had been used to rehabilitate patients after cataract surgery. The various distortions, aberrations, unwanted magnifications, blurred peripheral vision, and other visual impairments they caused were all too apparent.

As agreed on, Dr. Holt of Imperial Chemical Industries (I.C.I.) produced the needed acrylic (plexiglas Perspex poly(methyl) methacrylate) (Lucite International, Southampton, UK) material necessary for the project.

Perspex was the trade name of the project which was registered in 1934 by I.C.I. as a trademark for their poly(methyl) methacrylate acrylic sheet. In the late 1930s, as a result of Britain's rearmament program, I.C.I.'s total production of Perspex was reserved for the aircraft industry and the material was specifically developed for the use of fighter aircraft. The required properties of transparency, strength, and resistance to heat demanded a high degree of purity and polymerization.

Under Holt's direction, the company synthesized a pure form of the airplane cockpit material that they termed Perspex CQ (clinical quality). This material is the same that is still often used for the manufacture of some IOLs today. This material is a rigid one; even some of the very modern malleable (foldable) IOLs are based on polymer units that are very similar to those of the first IOL.

This is of course the material that Harold had observed in Flight Lieutenant Cleaver's eyes for 8 years. Harold and his team concluded that the acrylic biomaterial was safe and ready to use in human implants.

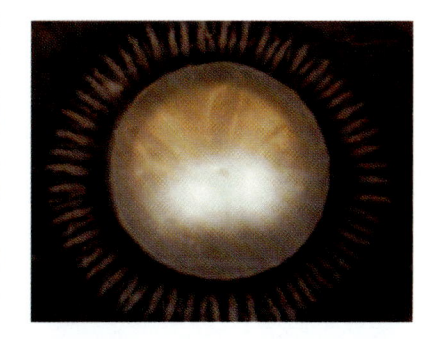

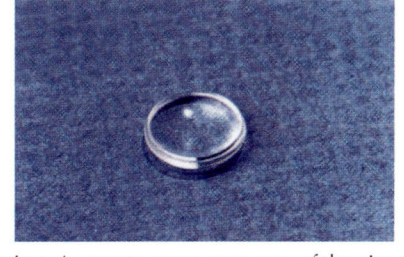

IOL size determination. Accurate measurements of the size of the normal crystalline lens, and even normal lenses that were unchanged in their size were obtained using various techniques.
TOP: This is a photograph from behind of a lens in place in a human eye obtained postmortem, studied by the Miyake-Apple posterior video/photographic technique. The workers at that time did not use this elaborate technique, but simply measured cadaver lenses for sizing. They obtained accurate measurements of the size of the eye and adjacent tissues.
BOTTOM: The Ridley IOL, 1949. This lens was sized as a result of in-vitro examination. Note the groove around the rim of the lens. This lens is one of the first ever made and is in the author's possession.

CHAPTER 7

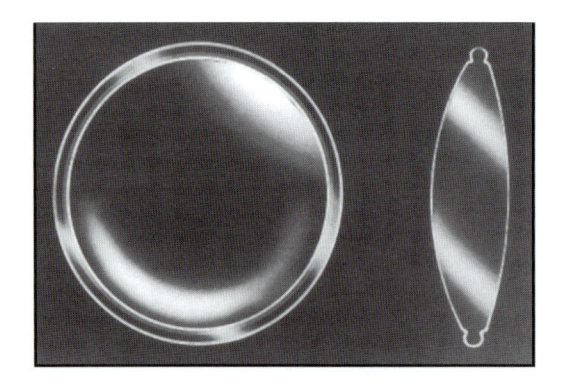

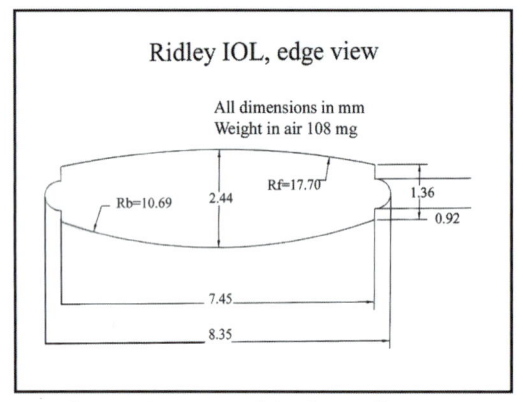

Manufacturer's images of the first Ridley IOL.
TOP: The front and side views can be seen. Note the biconvex shape of the lens and the small ridge that courses around the equator. The latter is designed to help grasp the IOL as it is insterted.
BOTTOM: Rayner's physical specifications and measurements of the various dimensions of the Ridley lens, based on measurements of the human lens.

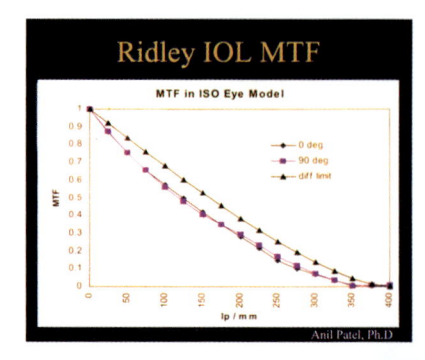

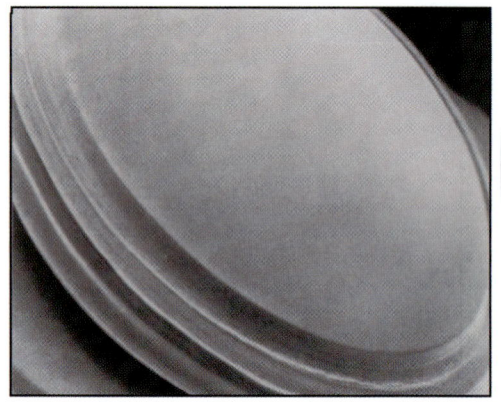

Two means of analysis of the Ridley IOL showing the manufacturing quality available to Rayner and & Keeler, Ltd. at that time. It was excellent and would meet today's standards.
TOP: Dr. Anil Patel, formally of Alcon laboratories, performed an interesting analysis of a Ridley IOL that revealed a manufacturing quality and lens clarity of a 1949 lens that would satisfy today's FDA standards.
BOTTOM: Scanning electron micrograph (SEM) of a Ridley IOL done by the author showing a high power thee-dimensional view of the lens. The Ridley lens was made by compression molding and cetrimide sterilization.

The first lenses were made at Rayner, based on Harold's, Pike's, and other's calculations of size and shape, using the best information available at that time, in particular, research findings from 30 years ago accumulated by the Nobel Prize Laureate Allvar Gullstrand (see Chapter 5). A superb craftsman, Mr. Len Rofe, handmade the lens. He had joined the company in the 1920s. The tradition of excellence in IOL manufacturing that he began was carried on by John Ingram, who continued with this work for many years until his retirement. After Ingram's retirement, he handed his work over to Mr. Mike Ring, who today continues to wear many hats in the company, leading the company in the manufacture of IOLs and other duties.

In addition to John Pike, there were other major contributors to Rayner & Keeler's IOL growth. These included Peter Caudell, John Green, and Ernest Ford. Ernest Ford was important in the advancement of IOLs and was counted as close friend by many surgeons internationally—an important liason between industry and practice.

Pike and the original pioneers who designed the first IOLs were quite correct in utilizing information from their predecessors at Zeiss and from Dr. Allvar Gullstrand, the great Swedish researcher. However, as they applied their calculations and evaluations, there was one factor that they could not have compensated for in advance. They could not fully compensate for the difference in the refractive index (focus power) between the human crystalline lens and the plastic material. They realized that there was a difference, but the only way to get a precise "fit" for the first patients was to try to do theoretical calculations based on their best estimates. The PMMA material has a higher capability to bend light rays. This led to lens power miscalculations in the first 2 cases that Ridley had done, the first being on November 29, 1949. While this was unpleasant, it was not a tragedy, because the patients—both totally blind in each eye with cataracts before the operations—enjoyed markedly improved overall vision and satisfactory central vision after they were discharged. They had thick spectacles in addition to the IOLs to compensate, so this needed to be addressed and changed so that such spectacles would not be necessary.

This flaw was rapidly corrected (see Chapter 8). By the time of the operation on the third patient, the problem no longer existed.

Under John Green, who had joined Rayner in 1962, the small implant department increased in size throughout the 1960s—from a staff of two at the beginning of the decade to six by the end. Although it has been purported that Harold had not anticipated the need for haptics or loops to avoid malpositions, this is not true. Also, Edward Epstein and Harold had designed two variations of his original IOL in an attempt to enhance fixation and thus decrease the incidence of decentration. New techniques were developed for the manufacture and secure fixing of the loops of iris fixation lenses.

Peter Caudell, Instrument Department Manager for Rayner & Keeler, Ltd. who had assisted John Pike from the earliest days of the Ridley lens, recorded that by 1960 Rayner had made 42 different IOL designs that had been used in human eyes. Lens designs with toric optics and Choyce's colored haptic designs were produced during this period. Over 300 ophthalmic surgeons internationally had been supplied with implants.

To meet the continuing rapid increase in demand, the implant department was moved in 1978 to its own building in Wilbury Villas, Hove, East Sussex. The new facility allowed a much needed increase to be made in equipment and personnel. By the end of the decade, Rayner Intraocular, as the company was now called, had increased its staff to 50 people.

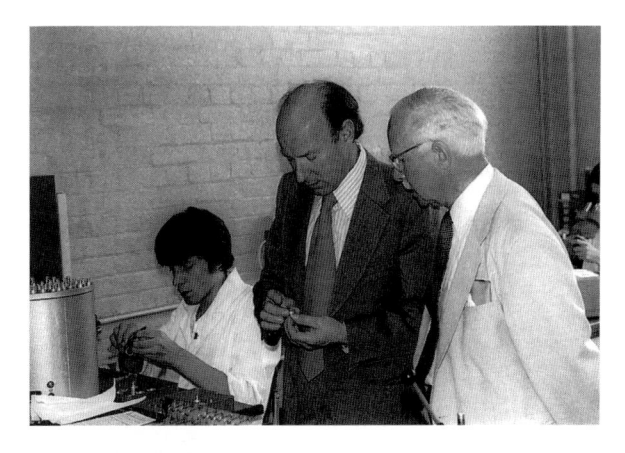

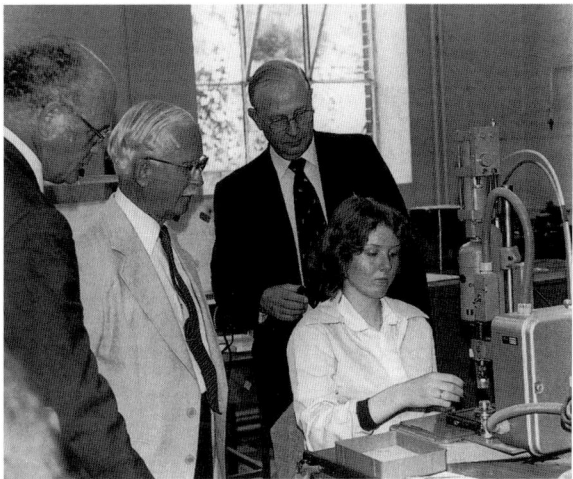

Harold Ridley at a visit to the Rayner & Keeler, Ltd. facility, 1979.
TOP: Mr. Ingham and Harold in conference.
BOTTOM: Three other men were instrumental in the successful establishment of Rayner & Keeler, Ltd. as an important IOL company. These individuals were John Green, Peter Caudell, Instrument Department and Ernest Ford. Two of these three, Ernest Ford (left) and John Green (right) are in consultation with Harold.

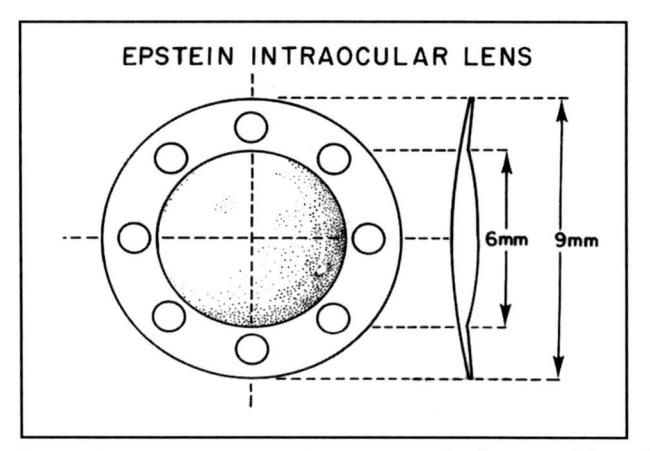

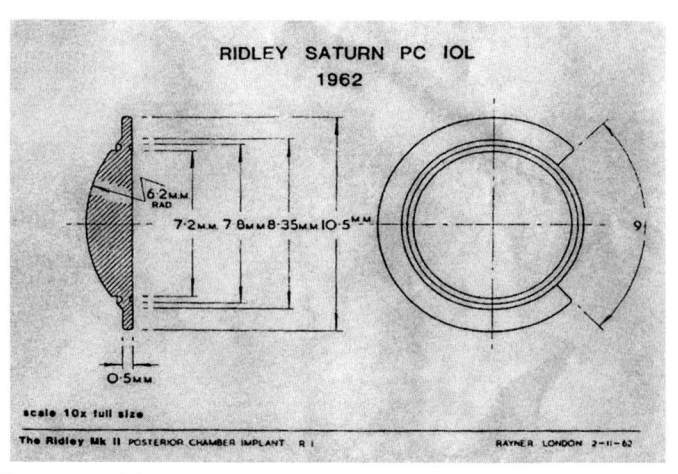

Two early attempts were made to improve the fixation of the Ridley IOL and thus minimize the early problem that existed, namely, decentration (usually an inferiorly directed malposition). The Ridley lens was relatively heavy in air (over 100 mg), as opposed to only a few mg with modern IOLs. Most people therefore regard this as the reason for the decentrations. This was only partly true. However, the most important reason, in my opinion, was surgeons' inability to make a firm lock of the IOL onto the body tissues so there would be no mistake in achieving firm fixation. The two slides shown here illustrate two other means that were attempted—means that were preliminary to the final solution, which occurred definitively by the 1970s with the addition of fixation elements (haptics and loops) attached to the IOL optic.

LEFT: Lens design by Edward Epstein, London. He had holes placed in the periphery of the lens as shown here. The purpose of these holes is to allow fibrous proliferation and fibrous tissue to grow in around and through the holes, in essence, weaving themselves into a right fixation in the lens.

RIGHT: Harold himself tried another approach, essentially making the first attempt at a haptic, by delivering what he termed the Saturn IOL—a lens with a rim around it which more or less mimicked the planet. This was a significant improvement, but was superseded as real haptics comparable to surgeons came into being in the 1970s after the work of Pearce (1975) and Shearing (1977), the pioneers of a return to the posterior chamber with PC-IOLs.

The Surgeon

This was an extremely busy time for Harold, who was working on several projects to which he had applied the insights and information he had gained during World War II. Among other things, he was working on a project to televise eye operations for the first time (Chapter 15). This involved frequent trips to Marconi Wireless, near Cambridge. His nurse, Ms. Doreen Clarke, often recalled the fear she endured on several occasions as they drove at high speeds between the outskirts of London and Cambridge, trying to get everything done.

It has always been amazing to me that Harold could finish two projects simultaneously in October/November 1949: the work at Marconi and the design and manufacture of the first IOL.

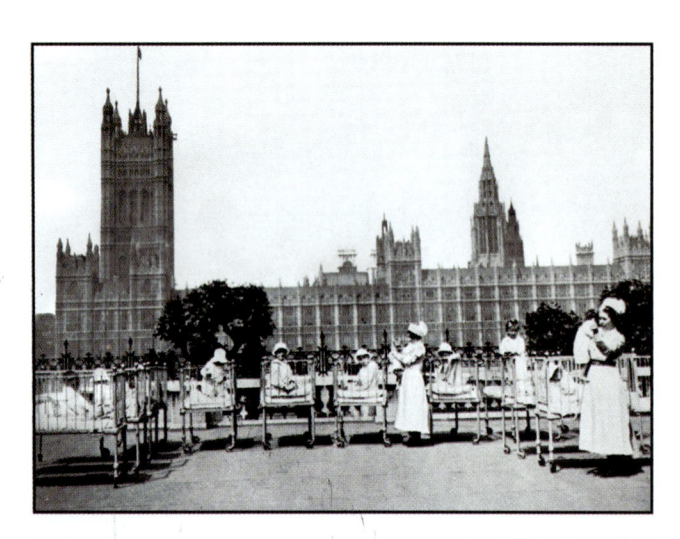

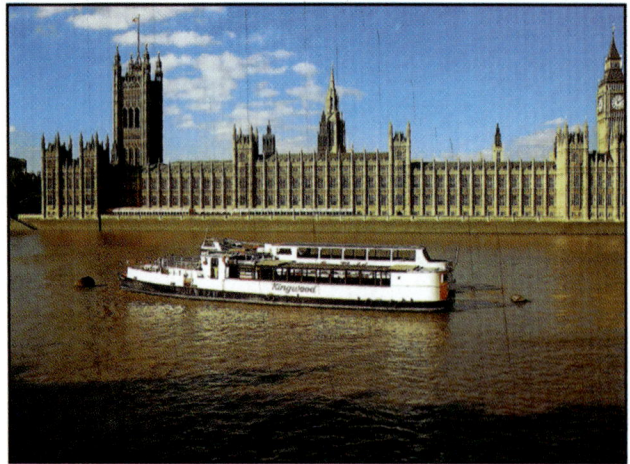

Parliament Building in London.
TOP: Parliament Building just after World War I. Pediatric nurses were able to tend to the children in the sunshine and fresh air.
BOTTOM: Parliament building and Big Ben, ca. 1990s.

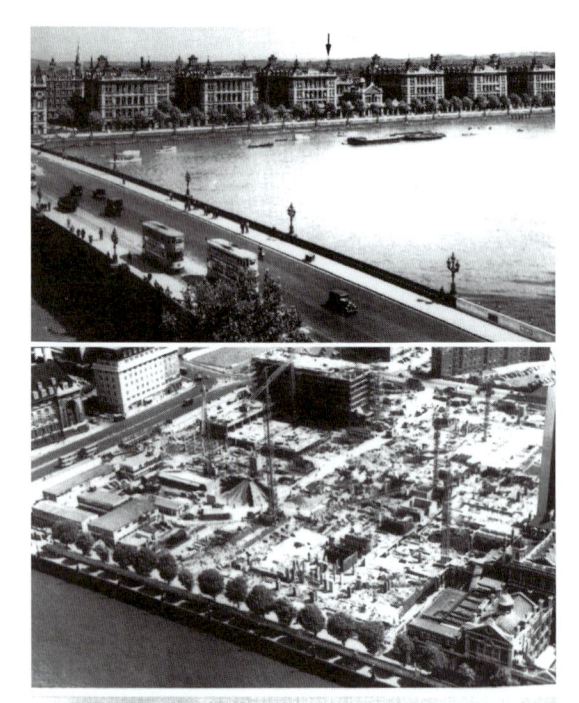

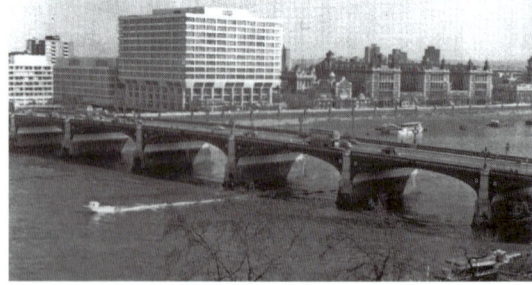

St. Thomas' Hospital.
TOP: St. Thomas' Hospital prior to World War II. Note the stately Italianate design of the structures.
MIDDLE: Extensive damage from German bombing in World War II shows that hospital authorities made the correct decision in proactively moving much of the facility to outlying areas.
BOTTOM: Bombing destroyed the entire group of blocks immediately adjacent to the Westminster Bridge. Today, a new structure is located where the original eye wards once stood.

8

The Operation: November 29, 1949

> *"We must not fail to honor two brave Londoners, (the patient volunteers for the first two operations) who, though well aware of the dangers, risked the loss of an eye so that our future patients might benefit. To them ophthalmology owes a great debt; for all of us involved in the history of intraocular implants they are the true pioneers."*
>
> *Harold Ridley*

Everything was ready.

Harold made plans to perform the world's first IOL implant operation on November 29, 1949 at St. Thomas' Hospital.

There are varying theories as to why he chose St. Thomas' Hospital. Some feel that he was trying to hide his work from others and would have a better chance of doing it there than at Moorfields. Ridley himself offered a more credible reason, pointing out that St. Thomas' Hospital offered a quieter setting where he could do his work without interruption. Also, he had chosen a select staff at St. Thomas', including his operating theater nurse, Ms. Doreen Clarke.

His long-standing emotional attachment to St. Thomas' Hospital based on his training there with "Huddy" and Doyne, not to mention his fond remembrance of Florence Nightingale, whose nursing work was done there, were perhaps other reasons why he decided to do the operation at that facility.

The hospital, a beautiful Italianate structure built in the 1860s, was divided into blocks with central courtyards. The eye wards were located in a block near the Westminster Bridge in a portion of the hospital that had been terribly battered during the Blitz. (Today a large, new, highly functional building is situated at that location, one that is markedly different from the original structures.) The

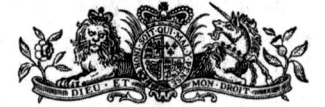

CHAPTER 8

A glance at the November 29, 1949 edition of The London Times shows, in addition to the unusually good weather, articles that clearly indicate that the "clean-up" and rebuilding of the city is continuing. Note especially how St. Paul's Chapel was repaired and renamed the American Chapel in honor of America's participation in the war.

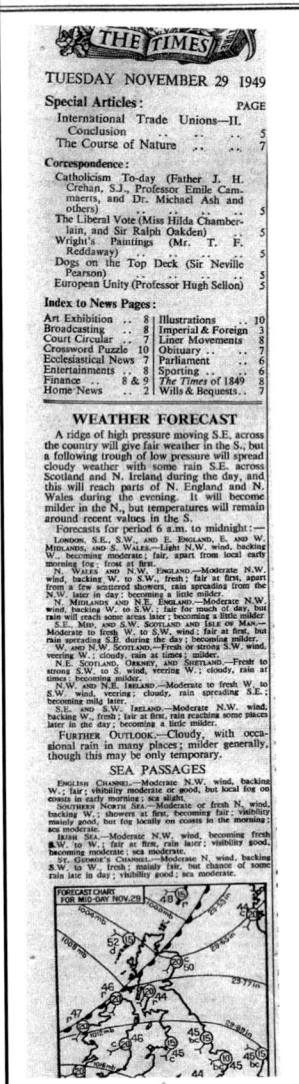

eye wards and the operating theater used for eye operations had been mutilated during the bombing (see page 140). But these parts of the hospital had been repaired to the point where they were once again functional.

Interestingly, the site Ridley chose for the first IOL operation was located just a few hundred feet from where the great artist Claude Monet had lived and worked a half-century earlier (see pages 25 and 26). He had created numerous impressionistic paintings from a third-floor room of the hospital overlooking the Thames River toward Parliament. Monet would no doubt have appreciated the opportunity to have had the good fortune to receive an IOL implant, had such a procedure been available in the early years of the 20th century, rather than going through the difficulties and uncertainties of thick aphakic spectacles that he, as an artist who depended on good vision and accurate color perception, was forced to endure.

The "Brave Londoners"

As mentioned in Chapter 1, the day the operation took place was a quiet London day with unusually good weather for the end of November. Ms. Clarke, who was chosen by Ridley to play a pivotal role in the operation, was a young Florence Nightingale nurse. Operating microscopes did not exist in those days. Someone had to hold a flashlight ("torch") for lighting—a crucial role in the operation. Ms. Clarke, rather than any of the other individuals around the table, many of whom were medical students, was chosen to do this.

THE OPERATION: NOVEMBER 29, 1949

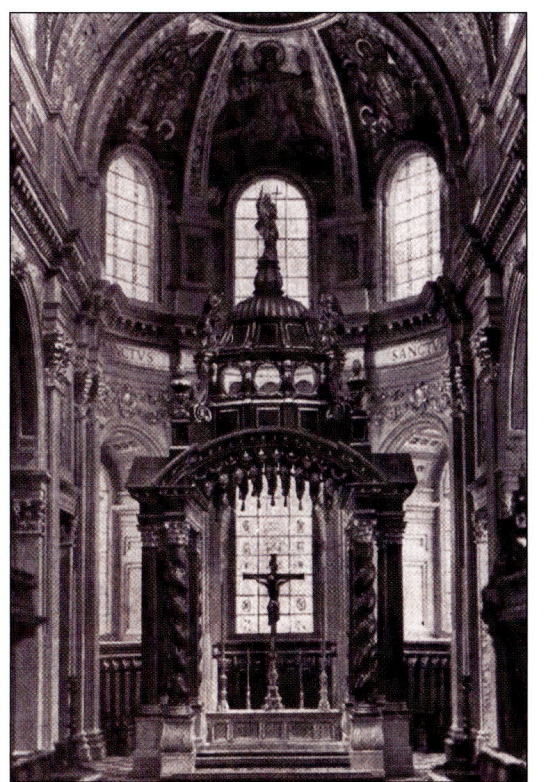

St. Paul's Cathedral. The interior of the American memorial, formerly the Jesus Chapel.

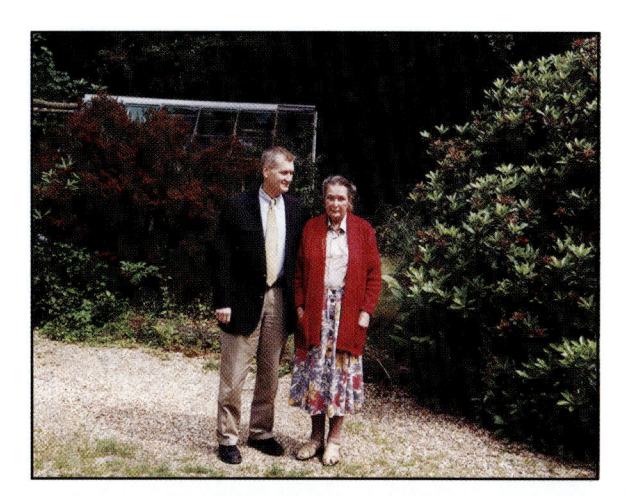

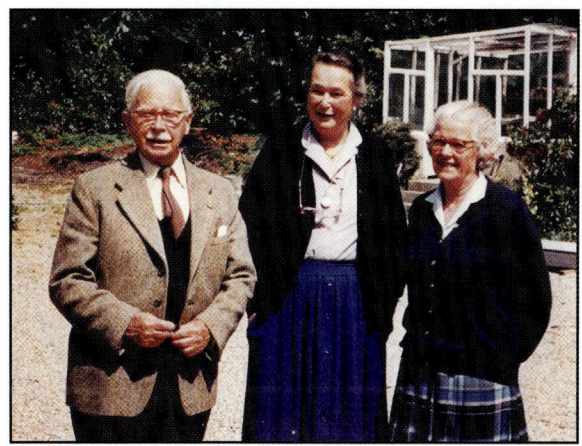

Mrs. Doreen Ogg (nee Clarke) was the nurse for the landmark operation. In addition to her normal duties at surgery, she was designated to hold the light source, essentially a flashlight or "torch," during the procedure.
TOP: The author visits with Mrs. Ogg in Hampshire.
BOTTOM: Harold obviously appreciated Mrs. Ogg's efforts for the rest of his life. He visited her quite frequently. Shown here are Harold, Mrs. Ogg (center), and Mrs. Elisabeth Ridley.

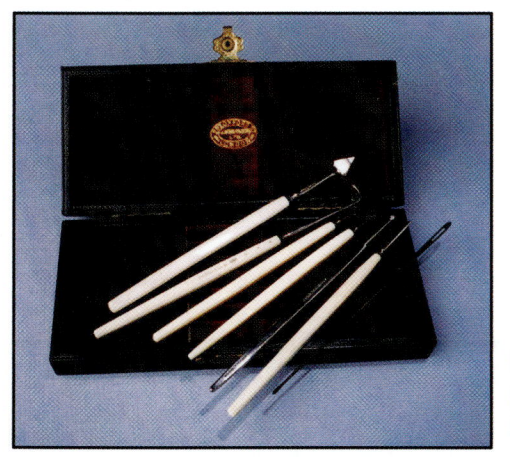

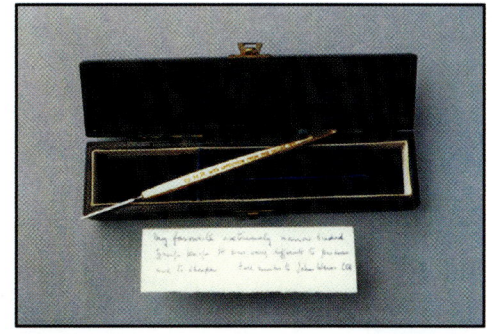

Harold's surgical instruments, which he kept in perfect condition. He used these instruments to place the first IOL in a human eye.

CHAPTER 8

Basic steps for inserting the Ridley IOL (page 81).
TOP LEFT: Step 1-a. Diagnosis. The cataract is clearly visible as a gray opacification behind the dilated pupil.
TOP RIGHT: Step 1-b. Removal of the cataractous lens. The eye has been opened using a special knife termed a Graefe knife. An ECCE is performed by opening the anterior lens capsule using the same knife. This allows access to the inside of the lens. The removal of the lens material is accomplished by applying a gentle pressure.
BOTTOM: Step 2. Implantation of the IOL. The Ridley IOL (upper left) is grasped at its edge by special forceps and inserted into the eye. The goal is to place the IOL through the open anterior capsule into the capsular bag (in-the-bag or capsular fixation). With the instruments available during the early years of lens implantation it was often difficult to consistently get the IOLs into the capsular bag. Actually the lens would often land on the residual front surface of the anterior capsule (on-the-bag fixation). This type is not as secure as "in-the-bag" placement and therefore is partially responsible for some cases of inferior decentration.

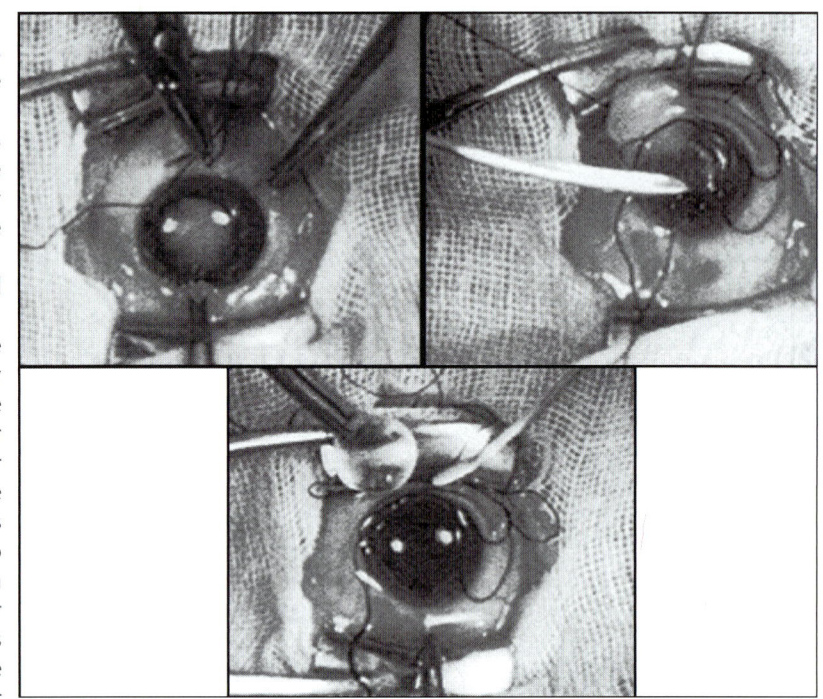

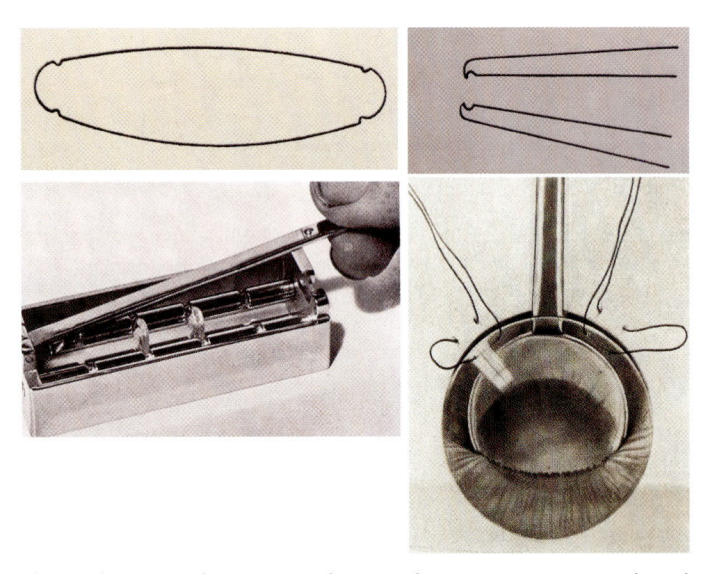

These diagrams demonstrate how early IOLs were grasped and inserted into the eye.
TOP LEFT: A cross-sectional diagram of the IOL showing notches at each equator of the lens. These notches are used for grasping the lens with special forceps used by Harold.
TOP RIGHT: A profile of the lens insertion forceps, showing the slotted tips that firmly grasp the grooved edge of the IOL, resulting in a safe and easy insertion.
BOTTOM LEFT: Harold's early IOLs were displayed in a specialized rack shown here. The top lever holds the lens securely in the grooves and, when opened, indicates the orientation of the lens.
BOTTOM RIGHT: The forceps grasp the lens, and the lens is then inserted into the capsular bag behind the iris.

Harold revealed to me *many times* in writing and in conversations that he considered a few special people, the long forgotten patients who were willing to undergo the operation, as the true heroes in helping bring his innovation to fruition:

"Shortly after the end of World War II, three well-defined groups assembled in London with the intention of completing the cure of cataract only half achieved by Daviel in 1748. The first group, composed of surgeons and nurses, and the second, optical physicists and industrial chemists, were readily found.

"The third group, comprising patients who were willing to collaborate, was more difficult to assemble. For more than a yea, many elderly men and women with strictly monocular cataract were interviewed and invited to risk, from an untried operation, the possible loss of their defective eye in the hope that their personal contribution would widen the parameters of ophthalmology and benefit countless future cataract sufferers. Eventually, two people, one each from two hospitals, volunteered after the object and the dangers of the operation were explained. They displayed not only personal courage, but faith in the venerable institutions and trust in those who worked there. After the first intraocular implants had been fully achieved, other patients were more willing to accept some extra risk to regain their natural sight and be relieved of the disadvantages of cataract glasses."

THE OPERATION: NOVEMBER 29, 1949

The first patient was a 45-year-old nurse named Elizabeth A. She had a total cataract in one eye. The operation, performed in the afternoon, went well with no complications. No photograph or film was made. However, the technique and operative steps were identical to that shown in the illustrations on pages 144 and 159.

Harold had specifically asked Ms. Clarke to write the following in the surgical logbook: "extracapsular ext."(an abbreviation for extracapsular extraction). He told her not to mention the IOL, intending to keep the entire project secret at that time. He had scientific reasons to do this, but, as he explained to me years later, he was also afraid of some sort of professional and perhaps even legal retribution if things had gone wrong. Whether or not this was the right thing to do, it was his decision.

Although the hospital was situated directly across the Thames River from Parliament, no one in the government or elsewhere knew about the procedure. If such an event occurred today, government representatives with myriad television crews would likely be invited and grant funding would probably be requested on the spot!

Regarding the results of the operation, they were fine in terms of the surgical technique and IOL quality. Harold found nothing that would deter him from proceeding forward. The lens itself was fine, but Harold described two "misfortunes" that resulted from the surgeons not being well acquainted with the IOL. There were two things that were difficult to predict in advance, and would be expected to cause complications, and when noted and attended to were easily managed.

I will let Harold describe these in his own words and then let one of the manufactures explain what he felt may have happened during that first landmark implantation.

In Harold's own words:

> "Two surgical misfortunes have to be reported. In Case 1, in which too large a lens was inserted and corneal-scleral sutures were not used, an iris prolapse occurred. By good fortune, however, the eyes settled and is capable of seeing 6/18, though only with the aid of a strong concave spectacle lens.
>
> "Though surgically successful this operation left a high refractive error because the lens proved far too strong, rendering the eye myopic in the high teens. The original optical computations had been based on Gullstrand's figures, though no one could be certain how far from the retina the powerful artificial lens would settle. This first operation was good enough to form the basis to proceed to a second operation. With the skill of Mr. Pike, a second computation was prepared in order to bring the expected postoperative dioptric level to -1 D myopia."

Harold published 4 papers regarding the IOL in rapid succession in 1951-52. These together created a bombshell that introduced a new vocabulary and a major paradigm shift. The pages shown here are from reference #2.
1. Artificial intraocular lenses after cataract extraction. *St. Thomas' Hospital Reports*. 1951;Vol. 7(2nd Series):12-14.
2. Intraocular acrylic lenses. Trans. *OSUK*. 1951;Vol. LXXI:617-621. Also, the 1951 Oxford Ophthalmological Congress.
3. Intraoular acrylic lenses after cataract extraction. *Lancet*. January 19, 1952:118-129.
4. Intraocular acrylic lense—A recent development in the surgery of cataract. *British Journal of Ophthalmology*. March 1952;36:113-122.

The second problem Harold mentioned was really based on the first one. The lens was simply too large and an iris prolapse occurred. In reality, it seems that he had encoun-

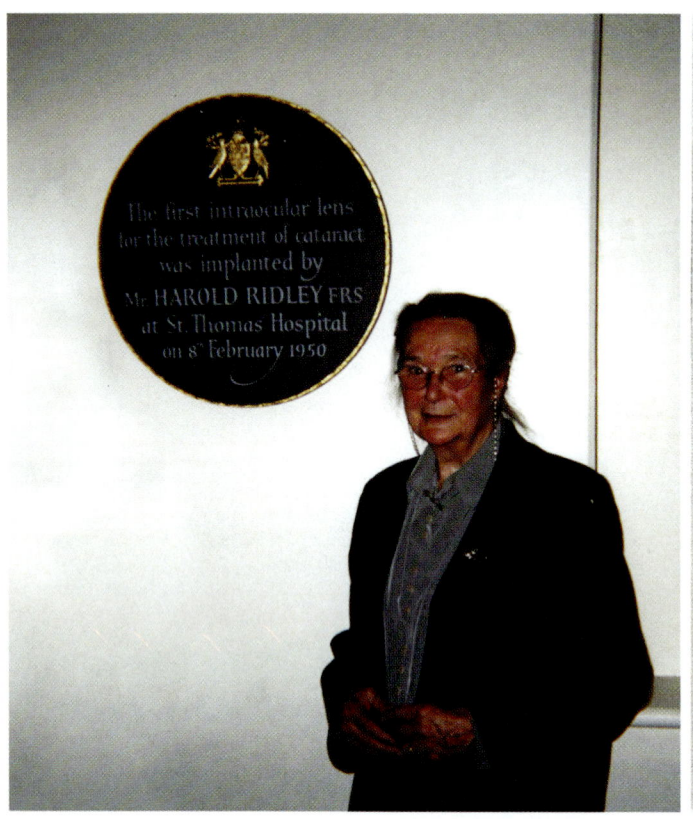

CHAPTER 8

Questions about the exact date of Mr. Ridley's landmark surgery persist. LEFT: Mrs. Doreen Ogg (nee Clarke), the nurse who held the flashlight or "torch" for the landmark operation, strenuously objected to this plaque, which marks the first IOL implant on February 8, 1950. The February date is a logical assumption based on the medical records and the feasibility of doing such an operation as a two-step procedure. RIGHT: A letter from Miss Clarke reiterating her objection to the February date.

Surgical record of Mr. Ridley's original surgery and subsequent follow-up on his IOL implantation technique.

tered only a single "misfortune", namely the lens was too thick front to back (anterior to posterior) that caused both of these problems.

Years later Ian Collins of Rayner & Keeler, Ltd. commented on the results of patient #1, and I believe his findings appear to be correct.

"The first two lenses were mad with raii of 10 mm and 6 mm (biconvex); a lens power in aqueous of +42 D! It is not surprising that these patients ended up highly myopic.

"I have always been puzzled by this 'error'. The curves chosen are identical to those given by Gullstrand for the lens in his No. 2 schematic eye. John Pike, who did the calculations would have known this, and was far too good an optical mathematician to have underestimated the significance of the lens refractive index; for the Gullstrand lens this is 1.416. Was the refractive index of Perspex accurately known in 1949? My feeling is that it wasn't, and that the first calculations were made in the belief that Perspex had a lower refractive index than the 1.49 we now know it has.

"The first lens was implanted by Mr. Ridley at St. Thomas' Hospital on 29 November 1949. Just when he approached Rayners with a request to make this lens is unclear. 1948 and early 1949 have both been quoted but we have no documentary evidence for either.

"The material used was an ICI acrylic known as Transpex 1. In most respects this was identical to the Perspex CQ used today. The only change by ICI that I am aware of was an improvement of the monomer distillation technique. The first two lenses had what Ridley describes as a 'peripheral notch', and not the circumferential grove that was used for lens No. 3 onwards. The specification then remained unchanged throughout the life of the lens and is as shown on the drawing. It was made in one power only—described as was done in those days, as "equivalent to a spectacle correction of +10 D. The power in aqueous was +24 D, the aim being to leave a small amount of postoperative myopia.

"We do no know exactly how many Ridley lenses were made, or how many Ridley himself used. 'About 1000' is probably the best estimate. In this 1960 paper, Ridley refers to his series of 'about 750 operations'. Our records show that the Moorfields continued to order Ridley lenses until 1963, but I do not know if Ridley used these."

Ian Collins, formerly Managing Director, Rayner & Keeler, Ltd.

Of the first 10 cases which were done, four were done at St. Thomas' Hospital and 6 were done at Moorfields. Peter Choyce participated in three early cases (2, 3, and 4) (author's note).

A Lingering Question

One small matter regarding the date of the operation has been discussed and bears mentioning. Ridley always considered the date of his first IOL surgery to be *November 29, 1949*. Indeed, until his death, every publication that mentioned the operation used that date and it became accepted.

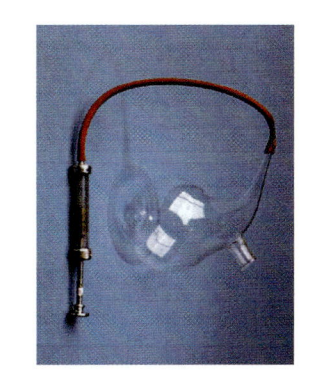

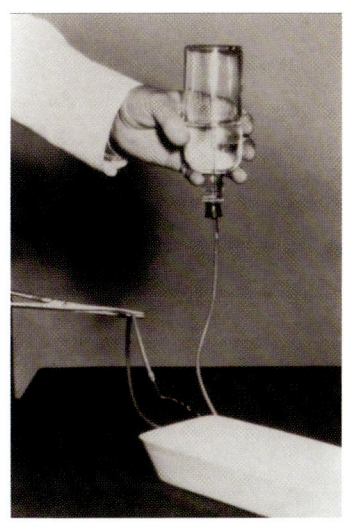

Technological advances in cataract surgery. Bottle and tubing used by Harold for the irrigation-aspiration component of his ECCE.

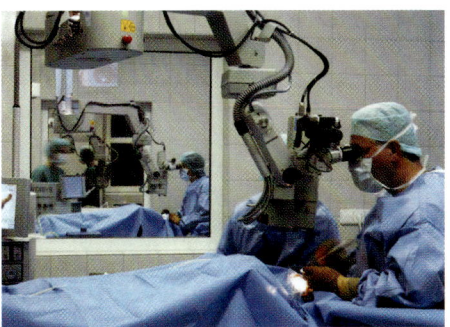

Amazing advances in instrumentation, computer technology and diagnostic/clinical adjuncts have brought Harold's invention into the realm of foldable small incision surgery.

CHAPTER 8

I may have been the first to entertain the possibility of a different date for the actual implantation. In the short biography by Dr. John Sims and myself in 1996, we noted that the implant had been a two-step procedure, the first step being the extracapsular extraction (ie, the removal of the cataractous lens material) on November 29, 1949. The second step, the active insertion of the IOL, was performed after the eye had "quieted down." However, Ridley apparently had lumped this together as one procedure and we left it as such.

In 2001, Dr. David Spalton of St. Thomas' Hospital studied the medical records and noted not only the failure to mention the lens implantation on November 29, 1949, but also the second operation on the same patient on February 8, 1950. This operation was described as a "lenticular graft." Dr. Spalton, therefore, believed this to be the date of the actual implant and a plaque was mounted on the wall at St. Thomas' Hospital to this effect.

I would not have brought this question up, preferring to leave the matter at rest, except for the fact that during one of my two very enjoyable interviews with Ridley's theater nurse, Miss Clarke (now Mrs. Doreen Ogg, having married one of Ridley's former colleagues, Mr. John Ogg), at her retirement home in Hampshire, she strongly insisted that an actual lens was in fact implanted in the patient's eye on the first date—the same day as the extraction. It is difficult to doubt her statement because I found her to be an intelligent, reliable lady with an excellent memory. She gave me detailed information regarding the first IOL operation and events surrounding it.

More than three possibilities exist:

1. A planned primary ECCE and lens implantation
2. A planned primary ECCE and secondary lens implantation, with time for the eye to heal in between the ECCE (November 1949) and lens implantation (February 1950)
3. A primary implantation that later failed and required an IOL exchange, requiring removal of the first IOL and secondary implantation of a new IOL.

The latter would be a very interesting occurence, in that several "firsts" would have occured in Harold's case. This would include: (1) the first implant, (2) the first explant, (3) the first lens removal, and (4) the first lens exchange.

These are the options. I have an opinion that would seem to fit this case, but will not discuss it here.

Whatever the exact truth is, in my opinion, it is not important. It is clear that the operation started on November 29, 1949 and that Ridley wished this to be the official date.

What is important is that on the quiet day of November 29, 1949, a new and daring initiative had begun—a revolutionary advancement that would usher in a golden age of ophthalmology.

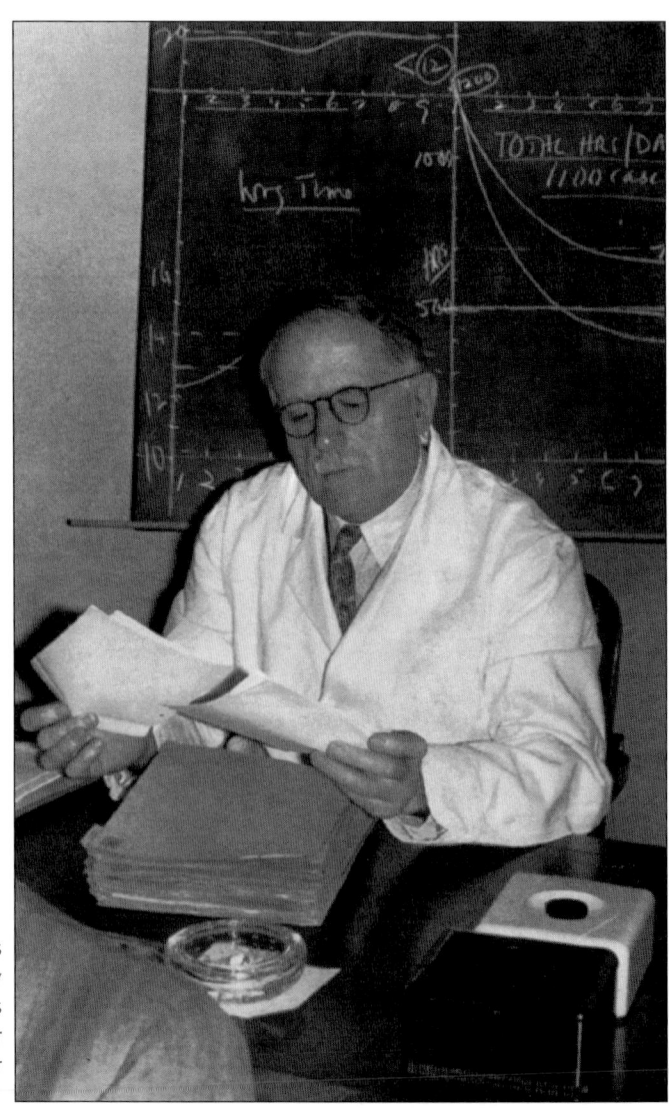

Frederick Ridley. One of Harold's postoperative patients accidentally presented himself to Frederick Ridley for a follow-up examination. After this visit, Harold's operation became public knowledge. Many years prior to this, Frederick Ridley had collaborated with Alexander Fleming in the development of penicillin.

9

Rapid Descent Into a Period of Doldrums

"At the Oxford Congress in 1951, two IOL patients (one whose result was a perfect 20/20 unaided and 20/15 with -0.5 OS) aroused interest and disbelief. There was, however, one powerful opponent, a British ophthalmologist famous for his splendid writings rather than for treatment of patients. He firmly refused repeated requests to look at the patients, so confirming his hostility even at that very early stage. Others showed much interest and a few some measure of support. Without doubt the birth of intraocular implants was greeted with disbelief and often with hostility both in Britain and throughout the world of ophthalmology."

Harold Ridley

A MISTAKE LEADS TO AN EARLY UNVEILING

Harold had planned on keeping his landmark operation under wraps for about two years. This would give him follow-up time before making the surgery public. He wanted to have the time to evaluate his results.

The planned period of preparation was cut short when one of his patients apparently misread a telephone book. Seeking a postoperative visit, the patient mistakenly rang the number of *Frederick* Ridley*—also an ophthalmologist, but no relation to Harold. When he appeared at Frederick Ridley's office, announcing that he was there for his follow-up, the cat, as they say, was forever out of the bag.

---

* Frederick Ridley had already had an illustrious career. He worked with Alexander Fleming in research efforts that lead to the discovery of penicillin. He was an expert in the field of microbiology and bacteriology. He later worked to improve the sterilization of IOLs.

Realizing this, Harold decided it was best to accelerate his plans and tell the world about his invention. He submitted his first publication about the IOL in *The Proceedings of St. Thomas' Hospital* in order to establish priority, and then published two important IOL articles—one in the journal *Lancet* and the other in the publication of the Ophthalmological Society of the United Kingdom.

The articles he wrote and many of his personal papers, which I have read, make it clear that he carefully followed up with his patients and investigated any complications that arose. Some of his critics falsely accused him of not doing this. On the contrary, it is clear from his papers that he documented complications as well as or often better than is typically done even today.

Interestingly, as the news of his IOL operation spread, Harold was actually enjoying better acceptance by surgeons in several foreign countries than in his homeland. In England, only a select few admitted the genius of Ridley's work, including D. Peter Choyce and Edward Epstein. From the very beginning, physicians overseas seemed to be more open to the IOL. Dr. Svyatoslav Fyodorov of the former Soviet Union, a very smart man, heard about the operation and immediately recognized its promise. He promptly made the long trip to England to meet with Harold and see the procedure firsthand. Fyodorov became an absolutely loyal supporter of Harold, and he himself became a prominent pioneer in several fields, including standard cataract surgery and keratorefractive and IOL refractive surgery.

Before we continue with Harold's sojourn at Oxford, I would like to consider the concept of "a prophet is not without honor."

A Prophet in His Own Country

Many great scientists and innovators throughout history have faced rejection. The most severe criticism often seems to come from the innovator's home base, hence the Biblical statement: "A prophet is not without honor, except in his own country, among his own relatives, and in his own house" (Mark 6:4, New King James Version). Harold experienced this to an extreme; he suffered for many years as a result of the intense opposition to his efforts by many of his colleagues in his "own country"—especially in the academic establishment.

I found his plight to be not unlike that of a great but almost unknown German physician, Werner Forssmann (1904-1979), a pioneer in the field of cardiac catheterization. In the late 1920s he was working in a provincial hospital in Eberswald, outside of Berlin, having not been accepted for a position in the great "establishment" hospital in that capital city. He performed a bold and life-threatening experiment on *himself*. At that time it was believed that any insertion of a foreign body into the heart would be fatal. He anesthetized his own elbow, inserted a catheter into his own arm,

Werner Forssmann, Nobel Prize Laureate in Medicine, 1956. LEFT: In 1929 Forssmann, Eberswald, inserted a catheter into his own venous system and heart, proving for the first time that cardiac catheterization could be a safe procedure. RIGHT: Photograph of the original x-ray film that Forssmann had made on himself. The self-inserted catheter passed from a vein in his elbow into his own heart (see arrows).

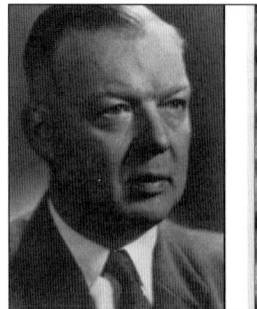

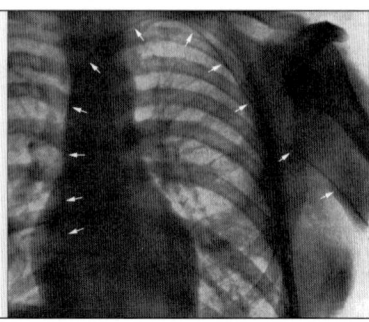

and delivered it through the venous system of his shoulder down into the atrium of his heart. He then ran with the catheter hanging from his arm down two flights of stairs into the basement and obtained an x-ray of his upper body to prove it.

He was immediately fired! Because this work was not done in a "proper" research hospital in a "proper" fashion by a "proper" professor (in this case, the great Professor Sauerbruch of Berlin), Forssmann's accomplishment was ignored, and worse, he was ostracized from the elite and "proper" medical community. They were fully aware of what he did but their jealousies and personal feelings toward him were too intense for them to accept it. The popular press acclaimed his discovery, but the "establishment" scorned him and put him "out to pasture".

Only many years later, after World War II when researchers in New York who were working in this field saw the evidence of his prior work, was he was recognized. They generously and publicly acknowledged his efforts. In 1956 he received a surprise telephone call. He was to share the Nobel Prize for Medicine with Drs. Andre Frederick Couvn and Dickinson W. Richards.

Harold's invention was not life-threatening, but it was certainly career-threatening. Had his early IOL surgery on humans failed he may have been discharged from his hospital and lost his certification to practice. Although medical-legal actions were unusual at that time, he still had an understandable fear that in that event of failure he may have to face a court and jury. Even though the operation was a success, he *still* faced intense rejection, jealousy, and scorn, and was virtually ostracized by some of his peers. For many years he suffered from severe depression because of this. Like Forssmann, he suffered for his gift to humanity.

Though he had many detractors, it speaks volumes about his character that he did not want me to make public the many wrongs he suffered until after he died. Indeed, he was subjected to a long period of much abuse; yet he was unable to mount a defense to answer and quiet his enemies. He did not lack courage; it was simply his nature not to be combative.

A tribute to Harold was organized by the American Intraocular Implant Society in San Francisco in 1979 to celebrate 30 years of the implant. A statement was made by Norman S. Jaffe, MD of Miami Beach, a past president of the Society and himself the director of an important clinical study in Miami that was very helpful in the long run in achieving success with IOLs.

Jaffe recounted the struggle Harold had faced during those early years of implant surgery and expressed envy regarding "the fortitude which Harold possessed while encountering an overwhelming wave of opposition to his innovation, a force that he believed would surely have crushed mere mortals." Dr. Jaffe concluded, "If I had a voice in the process, I would have nominated him for the Nobel Prize in Medicine."

Responding to the ovation given him, Harold remarked wryly, "I cannot help but compare my reception now with that accorded to the innovation of implant surgery 30 years ago."

He described to the audience the opposition that greeted his revolutionary feat, noting that "there was little encouragement offered to him by the profession at that time"—a vast understatement.

> "I was told that intraocular foreign bodies (as his opposition was fond of calling an IOL) would cause glaucoma, sympathetic ophthalmia, and even malignant disease," he recalled. "The only criticism which I seemed to escape was that my object was to make money, since I charged only the standard cataract fee for the more intricate operation."

As I began preparations of this manuscript, several colleagues who had witnessed the injustice Harold suffered requested I "not hold back." They understandably wished that I recount in detail the numerous hindrances and negative encounters that Harold faced throughout his professional life after the implant was born. It was tempting to do so. I am aware of dozens of such episodes—I myself encountered negative opposition from many of my peers in ocular pathology who were loath to accept the new invention and surgical technique. Some felt that I had "sold out" to the new generation of "buccaneers." Peter Choyce in England had had his career very adversely affected by his tenacious support of Harold (see Chapter 10).

However, I have chosen not to dwell on these negative occurrences that were a source of misery, not just to Harold but to others at the time. Harold himself wished for a tempered, nonconfrontational approach—including in this biography. He wrote the following in a letter to me:

"H. R. trusts to David Apple to omit subjects which might be controversial during H. R.'s life-time. Subtle amendments might be made in the obituary after the death. Thank you David."

Harold

I have therefore in this chapter focused on only a few episodes to suffice as examples as to what we encountered. A primary reason for dwelling on this at all is to help answer the question we started with in Chapter 1—why such a long delay, over 25 years, in inventing the cataract-IOL operation. This delay, largely caused by nonmedical reasons, deprived an entire generation of the benefits of this procedure.

From Harold's first presentation at the Oxford Congress onward, the IOL faced huge barriers—just a few of which we will review here.

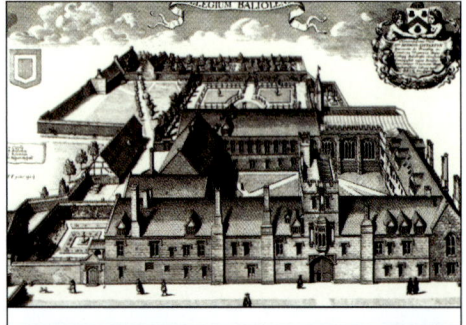

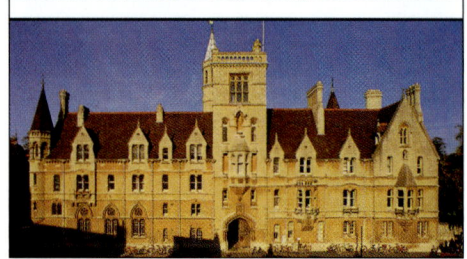

Balliol College, Oxford, traditionally used as a meeting site as well as for housing delegates of the Oxford Ophthalmological Congress.
TOP: Schematic illustration of Balliol College in 1675, by David Loggan.
BOTTOM: Photograph of Balliol College in more recent times.

HAROLD'S FIRST REBUFF

His problems with the British establishment, and especially with Sir Stewart Duke-Elder and Moorfields Eye Hospital, began almost immediately after his work on the implant became public knowledge. In an effort to help the medical community realize the value of the IOL, he decided to make his first major presentation at the Oxford Ophthalmological Congress in July 1951.

The Oxford Congress* was and remains one of the most respected ophthalmological gatherings in the world. I personally have a feeling of great affection for this gathering. In the late 1990s, I had the honor of presenting an honored lecture at that meeting. It was termed the *European Guest Lecture*. The great honor for me is that I am not a European, but I was selected anyway based on my work.

The Congress was founded by Robert Doyne, the father of one of Harold's favorite mentors (Geoffrey Doyne) when he was training in London in the 1930s. The meeting was typically (and still is) held in early July, usually in the facilities of one of the ancient colleges on the university

---

* This discussion and the information therein relates only to the proceeds within the specific Congress, and the events reflect in no way on either the Oxford Ophthalmological Congress or Oxford University.

campus. While the records from the mid-20th century are scanty, some colleagues recall that the 1951 meeting probably was held at Balliol College, one of the oldest on campus with beautiful buildings and courtyards.

Harold had high expectations for this meeting. His first implant had been performed about 18 months earlier and this meeting provided him an opportunity to present some clinical results to a large and well-informed audience. He planned to take two patients to the assembly to present them for examination by the delegates. In addition, he prepared to take a colored cinema of an early operation. This was another innovation he and his colleagues had made at the Marconi Wireless Manufacturing facility near Cambridge in the later months of 1949 (see Chapter 15).

Harold chauffeured these patients and his wife to Oxford from London that day. As was his habit, he cruised along at high speeds. He loved nice cars—one of his favorite non-medical hobbies after fishing (angling).

The two patients had enjoyed virtually perfect results from their surgery, even compared to today's standards. One was 20/20; the other was 20/15 (better than the standard "normal"). Therefore, in his mind, there was absolutely no reason for him not to feel confident and comfortable, with a real expectation that this was to be a landmark day in the history of ophthalmology and eye surgery.

It was indeed a landmark day—but not in the way he expected it to be. Instead, it was the beginning of over 30 years of personal trials and tribulations that led to health problems that plagued him for the rest of his life. Worse, it was the beginning of the above-mentioned unfortunate delay in the implementation of this new procedure—*a delay that deprived an entire generation of patients of the benefits of the IOL.*

The response to Ridley's lecture was disheartening, to say the least. In sharp contrast to his perhaps naive expectations, as morning passed and lunchtime approached, the future of implants was suddenly in jeopardy.

Harold's lecture was well-prepared and presented, and the clinical results were impeccable. Examinations of the patients' eyes or a viewing of a film of the operations that Harold had prepared would have further substantiated the excellent results.

However, not all of the attendees carried out all of the examination that was provided.

Why? To his death, Harold was unable to provide an answer or fully explain the events of that difficult day. However, after years of research, I believe I can now explain what happened—and why the leading ophthalmologist in Britain (perhaps in the world) developed such a hostility toward Harold and his invention.

Sir Stewart Duke-Elder

The established leaders in the field of ophthalmology often sat in or near the front rows of the auditorium at the Oxford Congress. In the 1951 meeting, Sir Stewart Duke-Elder had a prominent place. He often was accompanied by a distinguished guest of high rank, often from another country, and this time was no exception. With him was a distinguished ophthalmologist from the US.

Duke-Elder was undoubtedly one of the most talented and productive ophthalmologists of the time. He was born in a ru-

Harold's major detractor was very powerful.
LEFT: In 1951, Sir Stewart Duke-Elder was the most powerful and influential of the ophthalmologists in the United Kingdom, and, if not the world. He refused to see the two successfully operated patients that Ridley presented in July 1951 in the Oxford lecture. Duke-Elder was termed by some as the "Ophthalmic Aladdin."
RIGHT: Sir Duke-Elder, in academic regalia.

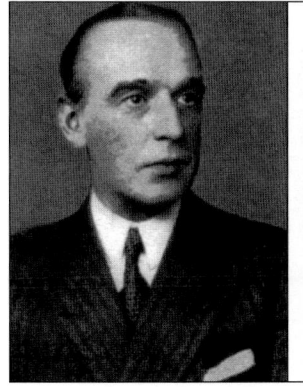

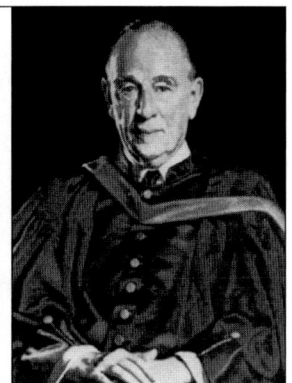

CHAPTER 9

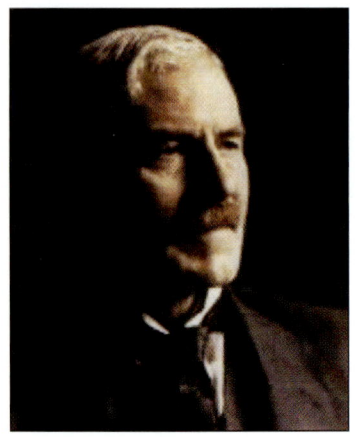

Sir Ramsay MacDonald, Prime Minister of England in the mid-1930s. Duke-Elder became famous and was knighted at a very early age after successfully treating MacDonald's glaucoma.

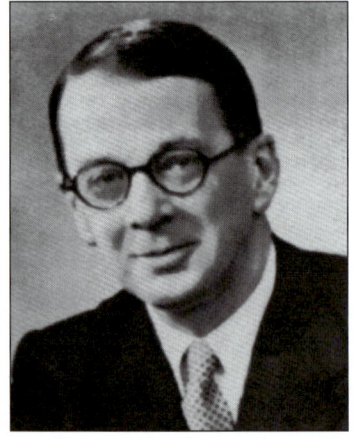

Sir Allen Goldsmith, MD, generally performed all surgical procedures in Duke-Elder's clinical practice.

Norman Ashton was a general pathologist who specialized in pathology of the eye. He worked with Duke-Elder at the Institute of Ophthalmology. He was a friend and colleague of Harold, and nominated him for the Royal Society.

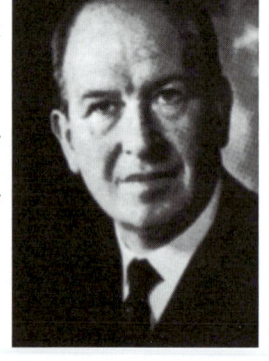

ral area near Dundee, Scotland in 1898. His father was a moderator in the Church of Scotland. An outstanding student at St. Andrew's University, he graduated with the highest honors, his main interests being physics and optics.

Arriving in London to pursue his career in 1923, Duke-Elder took his examinations to become an ophthalmologist. As a junior house officer at St. George's Hospital in London, he gained the attention of some leading ophthalmologists, including Sir John Parsons, a well-respected ophthalmologist and ocular pathologist at that time.

Duke-Elder, like Harold (though older than Harold), was a member of the post-World War I "lost generation." He established an excellent reputation and his academic output flourished during this period, both at home in the British Isles and internationally.

In 1932 he participated in treating the eyes of the then prime minister, Sir Ramsey MacDonald, who had glaucoma that affected both of his eyes. This is a disease characterized by an increased pressure in the eyes. It can progress to blindness if not halted by surgical or medical therapy.

Shortly after the successful treatment of the prime minister, Duke-Elder himself received a knighthood. It was always well known, but not often repeated, that he himself rarely did surgery. In fact, the operations on his patients were performed by Mr. Allen Goldsmith, a superb surgeon. Several sources have told me that he performed virtually all surgical procedures in Duke-Elder's practice. Goldsmith was assumed to have performed the operation on the Prime Minister and he was also knighted.

Duke-Elder did outstanding work at Moorfields Eye Hospital in London and he established a world-famous research institute there, the Institute of Ophthalmology. He worked with the great ocular pathologist Professor Norman Ashton in establishing this productive institution. He was probably best known, and rightly so, as an author, writing many volumes of a didactic nature. Many of the multivolume works of Sir Stewart Duke-Elder were extremely valuable to a whole generation of ophthalmologists (including myself) in the late 20th century. I corresponded once with Duke-Elder and indeed was thrilled and flattered when he requested text and photographs from an article I had written. It was a description of a rare childhood tumor that had originated in the kidneys, but spread to the eye and orbit, a vicious malignancy termed a Wilms' tumor. I of course complied with pleasure and enthusiasm. The requested materials were published in his *System of Ophthalmology*, in the volume covering orbital diseases. Duke-Elder's major source of material was from previous editions that had been published in Germany. They became standard reading for all ophthalmologists-in-training throughout the world. They were noted not only for their factual information, but also for the flowing style of their composition. Much of the work in the preparation of these texts was done by his devoted wife, Phyllis.

At the 1951 Oxford Congress, Harold knew that the illustrious and powerful Duke-Elder would be in the front row listening to his lecture. But he perhaps naively had no reason to suspect that Duke-Elder was soon to classify him as his worst enemy. After all, Duke-Elder had written a sterling letter in support of Harold back in 1935 (see next page) helping him obtain an important position in the London hospital system.

What Harold had not taken into account, again perhaps naively, were a few minor, intervening incidents that must have turned Duke-Elder against him.

One of these incidents dated back to the late 1930s. Ridley was given the duty of arranging and organizing the clinics at Moorfields Eye Hospi-

RAPID DESCENT INTO A PERIOD OF DOLDRUMS

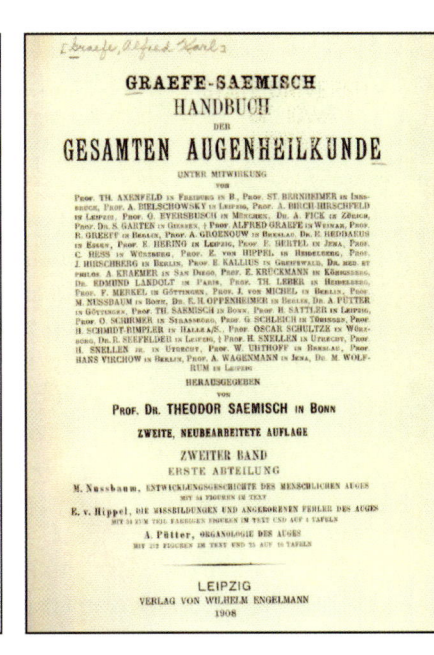

The multivolume works of Sir Stewart Duke-Elder were extremely valuable to an entire generation of ophthalmologists, including the author, in the mid-late 20th century. A major source of material for some volumes was from previous compilations of material published in Germany.

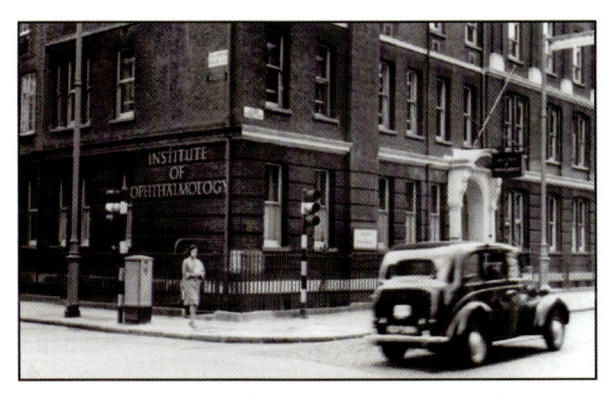

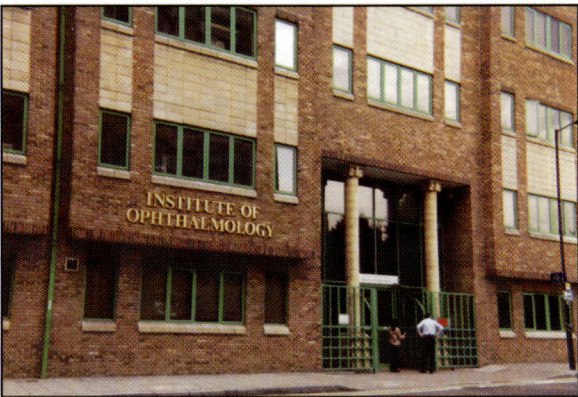

Sir Stewart Duke-Elder had a profound influence on ophthalmology during the middle of the 20th century. The Institute of Ophthalmology was built shortly after World War II, largely due to Duke-Elder's influence.
TOP: Early photograph of the original institute.
BOTTOM: The Institute of Ophthalmology is a modern center for ophthalmologic research and patient care.

Duke-Elder was named a consultant at Moorfields Hospital in 1931. His relationship with the young Ridley appeared to be cordial, as exemplified in his letter of recommendation of 1935 to help Ridley obtain a position at the facility. It was subsequently approved.

157

CHAPTER 9

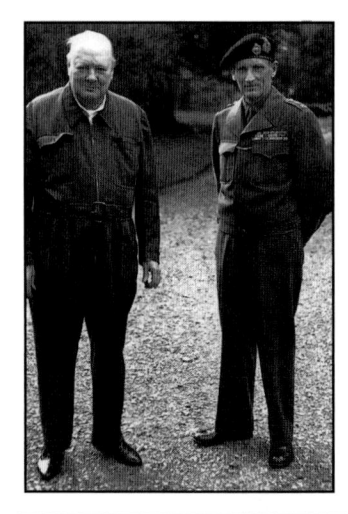

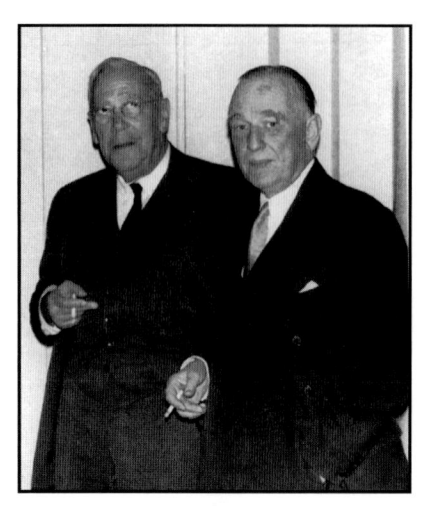

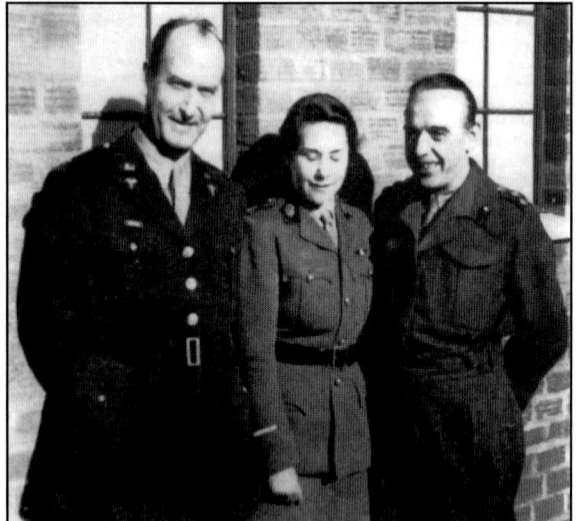

Duke-Elder's circle of colleagues, friends and acquaintances reads like a Who's Who of notable people.
TOP LEFT: Field Marshal Bernard Montgomery (right in this photo) with British Prime Minster Winston Churchill. Montgomery and Duke-Elder were friends. Duke-Elder was a Brigadier General in charge of matters military in ophthalmology, including assignment of duties to ophthalmologists world-wide. He assigned Harold to duty in Ghana in 1943, and the Far East in 1944-1945.
TOP RIGHT: Duke-Elder chats with Alan Woods, Professor and Chairman of Johns Hopkins University.
BOTTOM: Wartime photograph of three of the Allies' leading ophthalmologists. From left: Derrick Vail, Chicago, USA; Susan Vellon, France; Sir Stewart Duke-Elder, UK. Duke-Elder had charge of assigning ophthalmologists to various duties throughout the war.

tal. The rule was that the consultants (staff members), as Harold and Duke-Elder were classified, be present on the days they were assigned to see their patients. Duke-Elder did not believe that rule should apply to him, as a scholar, researcher, and writer. Sometimes, in fact almost always, he would assign a colleague to take his place. Harold had a different opinion—in retrospect as he realized, probably a wrong and certainly politically incorrect one. This precipitated some friction between Harold and Duke-Elder.

While I do not know how this was settled, I do know that Harold lamented later to me that he wished he had used more "political correctness" in solving the problem.

Duke-Elder's unpleasant feelings toward Harold seem to have manifested themselves in the war when he, as the brigadier in charge of all matters military in ophthalmology in the United Kingdom—including duty assignment to ophthalmologists worldwide, sent Ridley to Ghana (see Chapter 13). This was not considered a prime assignment. Many of Harold's colleagues probably would have appreciated the opportunity to avoid the many very dangerous theaters of war; however, Harold would have not flinched at such duties.

After Harold's presentation at the 1951 Oxford Congress, in which he showed his techniques and results, Duke-Elder refused to see either the film or the live patients Harold had brought for examination.

Harold has written several short versions of what happened that day in Oxford. It is important to note that every version that I read among his collected papers, although written at different times and with different emphasis, were thoroughly consistent. There were no exaggerations or changes in the story, or any attempt at embellishment.

"On July 9, 1951 a paper named 'Intraocular Acrylic Lenses' was presented at the Oxford Ophthalmological Congress, which described very simply but clearly the world's earliest successful intraocular implants. The color film of the operation (extracapsular extraction followed by implantation) had, with great difficulty, been made by my team, for no hospital photographer seemed experienced or willing to photograph an eye operation.

"Two of our delighted patients, one of whom could see better than 20/20 unaided, impressed many observers but several well-known ophthalmologists from the USA and the UK showed little interest. A well-known British ophthalmologist repeatedly refused even to look at the implanted lens. An American visitor jumped over a chair and left the hall. It was evident that much courage would be needed to achieve our objective.

"When the presentation of the paper ended there was a little more applause than usual and a few questions. In general there was surprisingly little comment, attributable no doubt to the impact of a new and revolutionary idea. At later meetings some wounding comments were made in many countries. This delayed the cure of aphakia for 25 years so that an entire generation of cataract patients needlessly suffered aphakia.

"In due course further scientific papers giving full details of operations and any complications appeared and in general results were very encouraging, though the need for improved implant fixation was evident. Several surgeons tried a few cases but their results were sometimes not so good as those of the pioneers, so many abandoned implants—leaving their originator once again almost alone in his field and making him vulnerable to a charge of malpractice. Some ophthalmologists abroad were at first almost as discouraged and tried different techniques, lens patterns, and sites. Colleagues in Italy, Netherlands, Russia, etc. made interesting proposals but eventually, the original posterior chamber implantation after extracapsular extraction won through and, I am told something like thirty million patients have benefited from the completion of the cure of cataract."

Harold Ridley

The written records of Harold's presentation revealed several interesting points. There was no question that several people in the audience enjoyed his lecture and were impressed. Some understood the vast implications of the invention. According to Harold himself, he received a substantial ovation, which continued for some time until stopped by the headmaster... but not from everyone.

According to Harold's further notes, Sir Stewart Duke-Elder and his friend from America did not take part in the applause. While no written record was made regarding what was said by the critics, with the exception of John Foster of Leeds' notes that have a very positive tone (see Chapter 6), the response from the front rows was clearly negative. (It was said by Harold that one of the prominent physicians knocked over his chair in his hurry to leave.)

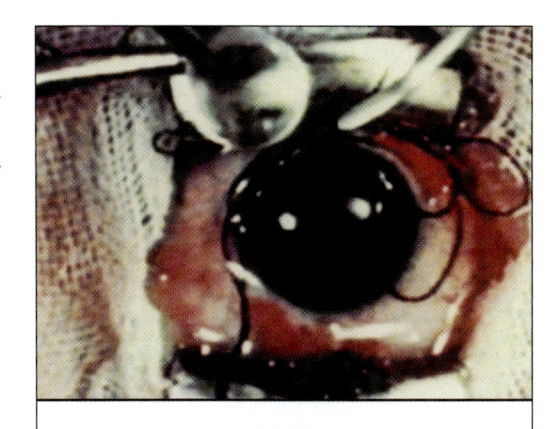

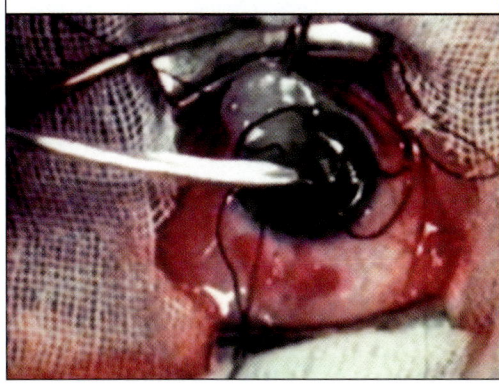

Harold filmed several of his early operations. The colored images shown here were made during a procedure performed at Saint Thomas' Hospital in May of 1951. The general principles he used in this case were those that he used from the beginning.

Since Harold had to present his results earlier than planned, he submitted his first paper to the relatively small transactions of St. Thomas' Hospital. Therefore, his first three IOL-related publications were as follows:

1) Ridley NHL. *Artificial intraocular lenses after cataract extraction.* St. Thomas' Hospital Reports. 1951;Vol. 7 (2nd Series):12-14.
2) Ridley NHL. Intraocular acrylic lenses—A recent development in the surgery of cataract. *British Journal of Ophthalmology.* March 1952;36:113-122. This publication was the "bombshell," the paper that really introduced the world of ophthalmology to a new paradigm, to a new vocabulary, indeed the paper that changed the world.
3) Ridley NHL. Intraocular acrylic lenses after cataract extraction. *Lancet.* January 19, 1952:118-129. This article, published in *Lancet* because of the great prestige, is a summary of the above *British Journal of Ophthalmology* article and the cover is shown here (right, above).

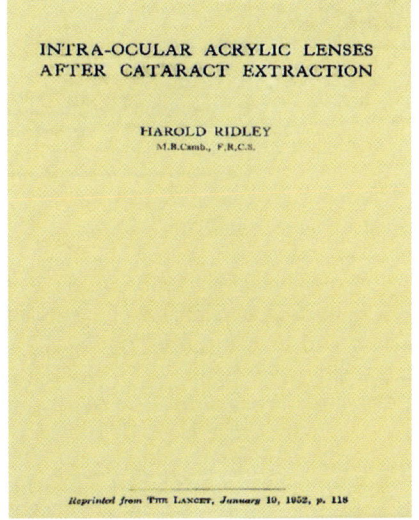

CHAPTER 9

D.E.

During my research of Harold's life, I discovered something that I believe explains Duke-Elder's violent opposition to the development of the IOL and the man who invented it. According to numerous interviews with many of their contemporaries, this opposition was indeed *extreme*, far in excess of a "normal" professional rivalry.

During this same July 9, 1951 presentation to the Oxford Congress, Harold mentioned his experiences with the injured fighter pilots, including "Mouse" Cleaver and likely others, and no doubt he mentioned how the pilots had been a significant factor in the evolution of his invention. He mentioned that the follow-up of these injured patients over time helped prove that the fragments of Plexiglas were well-tolerated and were thus of sufficient biocompatibility (tissue-friendly) to warrant use as an implant, which I believe turned out to be his "preclinical" study (see Chapter 6).

But why would Harold's mention of this episode in the evolution of the IOL have triggered such a negative reaction from Duke-Elder? Some simple detective work I performed not long before the completion of this book, in late 2005, gave me what I am sure is the answer.

I was reviewing the outpatient documentation of the medical examinations performed on the injured eyes of the one pilot that we do have good documentation on, Flight Lieutenant "Mouse" Cleaver from August to October 1940. One examination was performed just 2 months after the injury. When I saw the letters "D.E." on the notes, everything fell into place! "D.E." was Duke-Elder! Shortly after the injury, Cleaver had been transported from South Central England to Moorfields Eye Hospital in London. It was known as the Royal London Ophthalmic Hospital (R.L.O.H.) at that time. He was examined by Duke-Elder, who no doubt further referred him to colleagues within the hospital for further treatment commensurate with his wounds. While at Moorfields, Cleaver was stated to have had 18 operations that were very successful—at least as successful as could be expected from the severity of the injuries. According to our sources, Harold performed many of these operations. I cannot verify this since I have not seen these inpatient or operative records.

Physician's progress note on the patient Flight Lieutenant "Mouse" Cleaver, seen by a physician on September 11, 1940. This was a follow-up examination to assess and treat the eye injuries sustained on August 15. This inset (left) reveals that Cleaver was seen by Duke-Elder (D.E.), having been referred to the Royal London Ophthalmic Hospital (as Moorfields was designated prior to 1956).

As simple as it sounds, I believe what may have gone through Duke-Elder's mind as he listened to Harold's presentation 10 years later in Oxford was: "Why didn't I think of that!"

There he was—the greatest and most influential of all British ophthalmologists, the "ophthalmic Aladdin" as he was sometimes called. He had not seen and made the connection as to what may have been right before his eyes—the idea to invent the IOL. He must have seen what initially all ophthalmologists, including myself, would have seen and no more—an injured pilot. Harold saw exactly the same wounds at another time, but his genius was in connecting this patient's and others' injuries to the idea of the IOL. In effect, what must have gone through Duke-Elders's mind was that Harold had "bested" him by subsequently inventing the intraocular lens! I believe that Duke-Elder knew then and there, in July of 1951, the importance of Harold's invention—a very major discovery that could perhaps challenge his claim as being the doyen of ophthalmology. Duke-Elder was accustomed to being the "general" (he was a brigadier during the war). Events have proven that it tormented him that he had lacked the foresight and genius to have brought it to the world—tormented him and eventually Harold's colleague, Peter Choyce, almost for the remainder of their lives.

After his morning presentation, Harold assembled his passengers and immediately drove back home to London. After that Oxford meeting, Duke-Elder's hostile feelings toward Harold and his invention seemed irrevocable. I have not found any written or oral evidence that shows the contrary.

A Fast Downhill Slope

After that summer's day in Oxford, things began to go rapidly downhill for the new specialty of intraocular lens implantation and Harold's relations with Moorfields Eye Hospital. This has been confirmed in writing and orally by many contemporaries. Duke-Elder had enormous power and an enormous influence there, and it is no secret that apart from Harold himself, relatively few intraocular lenses were implanted at Moorfields for almost 20 years. The hostility apparently filtered down from Duke-Elder through various members of the hospital consultancy staff. Not very many surgeons at Moorfields had many good things to say about the IOL.

Noel Rice, MD held administrative posts at Moorfields for some 25 years (approximately 1970 through 1995). He did not favor implants.
LEFT: Giving a lecture.
RIGHT: Teaching at a "wet lab."

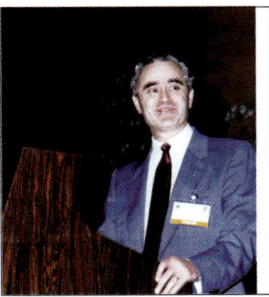

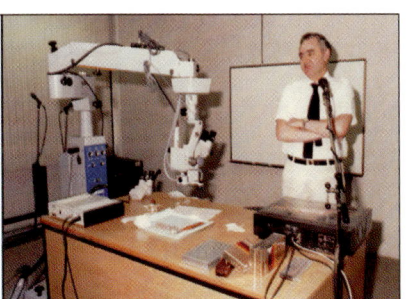

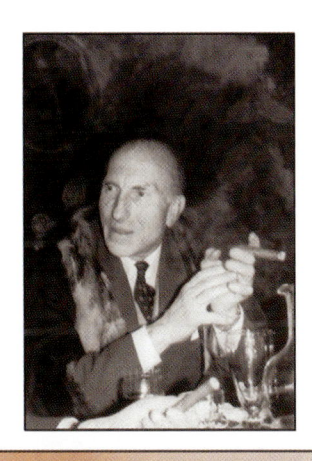

Some "stars" of the 1960s and 70s.
TOP: Dr. Arthur Lim of Singapore was a Fellow at Moorfields Hospital in the 1960s and was well-known with many of the staff. He is shown in this photograph with Dr. Patrick Trevor-Roper, at his left, who also had doubts about implants. He has written a critical letter to the editor questioning them.
BOTTOM: To Arthur Lim's right is my professor from Iowa, Dr. Frederick Blodi of the University of Iowa (left in the photo). I did my eye residency under his tutelage, he is a wonderful man and colleague. He was originally against IOLs but rapidly warmed to their use and eventually had bilateral implants himself. Dr. Lim of Singapore has long been a champion of IOLs for his region in Asia.

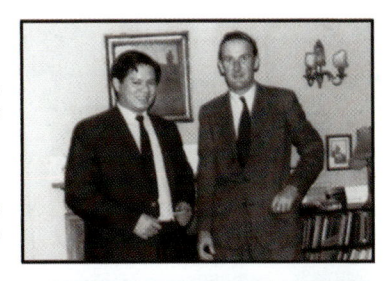

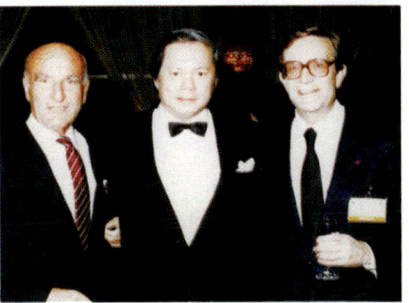

The attitude toward IOL implantation varied within the divisions of Moorfields Hospital and also in regions of the United Kingdom outside of London.
TOP: Dr. Frank Law was a pediatric ophthalmologist at Moorfields who apparently was a supporter of the IOL.
BOTTOM: I was introduced to Professor Michael Roper-Hall of Birmingham by Dr. David Austin. Seen here next to the author, he was a strong advocate for IOL implantation. He worked independently in his lab.

CHAPTER 9

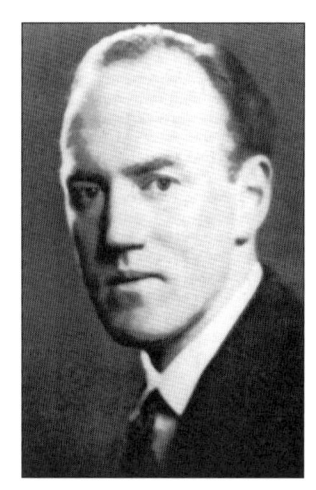

Henry Stallard, MD, an excellent surgeon and author of an important textbook on ophthalmic surgery. He had reservations about intraocular lenses. Incidentally, he was well-known as a world class runner, his accomplishment having been shown in the movie, "Chariots of Fire."

"Despite the magnitude of the surgery that Harold was doing, I cannot recall a single visitor ever attending his operations. Yet with every one, I was witnessing history in the making. I learnt a great deal about lens implantation at this time. It was apparent that this was the way forward, although it was equally apparent that if a surgeon of inadequate skills performed this operation, problems could occur."

Eric Arnott, MD

Even today some blame Harold for the problems in bringing cataract surgery to Moorfields. Some still blame Harold for a perceived lack of scientific methodology in bringing his invention to fruition. We have clearly seen that the often cited complaint that he did not do animal studies is not a viable one. He actually did the important "preclinical" studies by operating on the injured pilot(s) (see Chapter 6).

Because of these intense jealousies and animosities from some members of the establishment, the IOL implant—which was remarkably advanced and successful even in its original version—was rejected by many. The very existence of the IOL was in jeopardy at that time and only survived because of the efforts of several brave individuals who understood Ridley's innovation and kept it alive.

One man who was close to Sir Stewart Duke-Elder, was appointed by him, and worked directly and closely under him in the Institute of Ophthalmology in London was Norman Ashton (see Chapter 17). He managed to remain open-minded. He was an ocular pathologist who recognized the positive attributes of the IOLs and was not afraid to speak out. Ashton was so impressed that he made what might have been a dangerous move at that time. He led a campaign to nominate Harold to membership in the prestigious Royal Society. In contrast to the hostilities toward the implant that swirled around him, Ashton's open-mindedness proved to be the correct course.

"Put Out to Pasture"

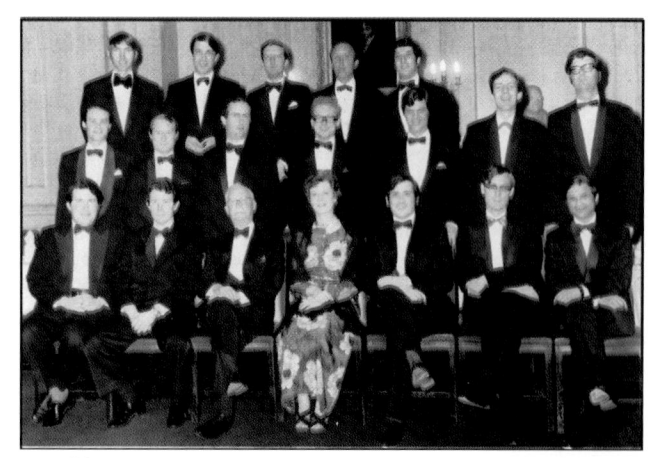

Harold's retirement event in 1971 was purported to be harmonious and amicable. Shortly before his death, however, Ridley reported to the author that it was not. Although the event was officially appropriate, he felt that he was being "sent out to pasture."

Harold's relationship with Moorfields Eye Hospital formally ended in 1971. He was given a good-bye party that publicly appeared amicable. In his private documents he mentioned his despair at that time. He felt that he was put out to pasture. It was therefore not a pleasant departure for him, although he always kept this a secret.

Actually, in retrospect, when Harold discussed this "retirement," he admitted finally that it was a blessing in disguise. He told me, and also our mutual colleague Mr. Eric Arnott about his late years at Keepers Cottage—Eric wrote:

"The Ridleys spent most of their weekends in the tiny thatched cottage by the River Wyle in Stapleford where Harold enjoyed fly-fishing. There we would often reminisce about our lives and careers. He once told me that his children found this constant shift from the Harley Street house in the city to the country quite difficult, as they were always missing out on

parties. Harold was conscious of the debt he owed Elisabeth for bringing up his family and regretted that he had not spent enough time with his children during their development. As so often happens to those who are totally dedicated, the job comes first and the children suffer. Yet despite this, all the Ridley children have made their mark in life."

Indeed they have. Nicholas and David have remained in England and are doing very well and Margaret is married to a Swiss gentleman and lives in Zurich, Switzerland.

The people at Moorfields Eye Hospital today are not in any way associated with the problems of the very early years. Moorfields has established a fine image in regard to its cataract services. However, the record should remain clear. The previously mentioned misunderstandings did occur. Some people at Moorfields hospital were not friendly and helpful to Harold. It is useful to all of us today to be aware that mistakes had been made in order to: 1) help answer the question I stated in Chapter 1, (why did it take so long?), and 2) to help ensure that such problems do not occur again.

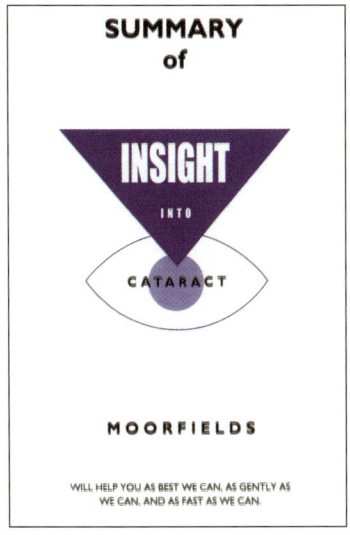

Moorfields Hospital now seeks a new and positive image for its cataract-IOL surgery, as represented by the cover of this promotional brochure.

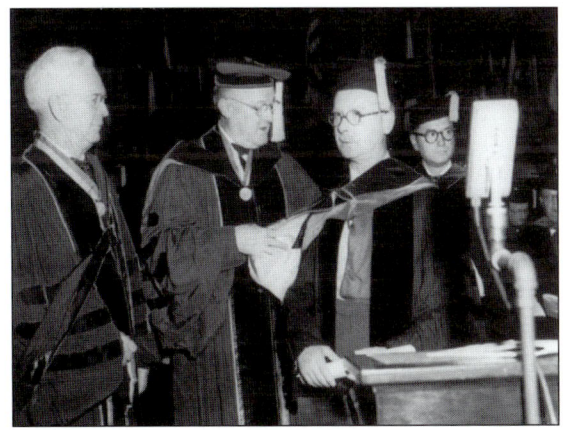

Chicago

There were important positive reactions to Harold's invention in the United States. Harold did the first implant in the United States at a meeting in Chicago in 1952. Dr. Warren Reese of Philadelphia, PA was impressed and became an ardent supporter. Harold gave him some lenses, which he took back to Philadelphia in his private plane and became the first American to implant an IOL. This is detailed in Chapter 10. However, some of the initial reaction was not positive. I will cite two examples.

At another Chicago meeting, Derrick Vail of Chicago, professor and chair at Northwestern University and a close friend of Sir Stewart Duke-Elder, presented a paper at the 57th Session of the American Academy of Ophthalmology and Otolaryngology. Discussing Harold's work, he stated:

> "In spite of Mr. Ridley's remarkably successful run of cases here reported, the operation is one of considerable recklessness. The hazards far exceed the little that is gained in the way of ocular comfort to the patient and the questionable advantage of binocular vision obtained at such an obvious risk.
>
> "Until further work is done and more time has elapsed and more of the risks involved, I do not want such an operation performed on myself nor can I advise it for my patients, willing as they might be to undergo the additional hazards of which they can have no true conception."

Sir Harold Ridley was publicly and ceremoniously honored at a meeting in Chicago, in 1952, but at the same time had been stabbed in the back.

CHAPTER 9

A REJECTION FROM A COLLEAGUE IN OCULAR PATHOLOGY

My first faculty job was at the University of Illinois in Chicago at the Georgiana Dvorak Theobald Laboratory, named after my predecessor in that famous facility. Dr. Theobald was a world-famous ophthalmic pathologist who was quite conservative. She had learned of a complication of an early intraocular lens implant that had been seen in a patient following an injury to the eye. Because of this, she made strong remarks against the use of IOLs—remarks that in retrospect were really related to problems unrelated to the implant and were based on other causes.

She was also unhappy that Harold's innovation was covered in the lay literature, including *Time Magazine*. In those days such things were considered to be a form of advertising—highly unethical. Harold told me that he had nothing to do with that article.

I myself, as an eye pathologist, suffered from ridicule from my peers because of my support of Harold. On one occasion I remember that I classified one of my academic presentations to our Pathology Society originating from material from my Binkhorst Lecture. It was based on research on IOLs, but some of my conservative colleagues in general were not impressed.

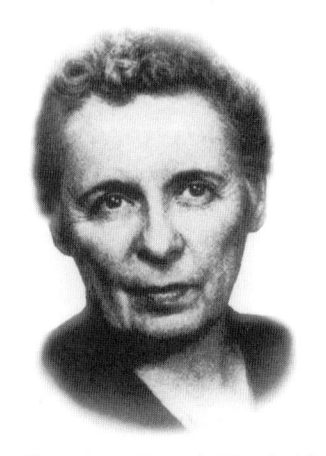

Dr. Georgiana Dvorak Theobald, an ocular pathologist in Chicago, was strongly critical of Harold.

Accounts of restoring vision by cataract extraction and IOL implantation begin to appear in newspapers, exciting the imagination of the general public. This story recounts how the extraction-implantation procedure restored the sight of a 75-year-old priest.

RAPID DESCENT INTO A PERIOD OF DOLDRUMS

Article in *Time Magazine* summarizing Harold's report published in *The Lancet* in 1952. The writer noted that: "US eye specialists are amazed by the news from London. If the plastic lens holds up for five years without trouble, it will be the greatest advance in cataract treatment since the invention of the eye glasses!"

A Different Outcome?

I have often wondered whether the IOL would have been accepted decades earlier, sparing a generation of cataract patients the trouble and distorted vision of the pop-bottle-bottom spectacles. The outcome of the fateful Congress in 1951 may have been different. What if Duke-Elder had not attended that day—or if Harold had been able to have the delegates examine his patients?

We will never know for sure.

What I do know is that as he ended his lecture just before noon and immediately left the auditorium with his wife and patients, he was obviously quite upset. As he drove away, his emotions on the journey home must been far different than those he felt on the drive earlier that morning. It was a terrible, disappointing blow—the intensity of which he could not have expected.

But this was only the beginning.

David Peter Choyce, a very early pioneer in the field of IOLs, who was present on three of the first six operations performed by Harold Ridley in 1949-1950. Choyce is important in the evolution of IOLs from two standpoints. One, his scientific/clinical contributions for over five decades laid the ground work for many future innovations, not only in the field of IOLs but also cornea surgery.
Perhaps, overall his most important contribution was his loyal and very vocal support of Harold Ridley, including over the most difficult period when criticism was often the rule, especially from the establishment. In supporting Harold, he was blocked in his own career advancement.

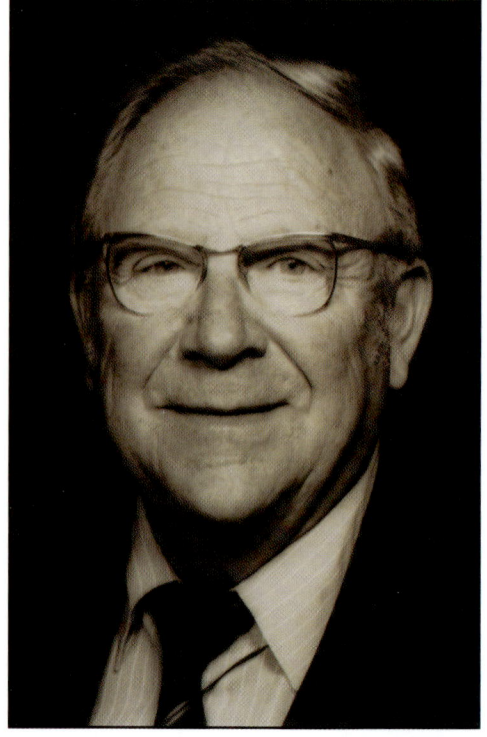

10

A Gradual Ascent to a New Revolution in Surgical Eye Care

"The greatest fear known to man is a new idea. If you have strong reasons to believe in your ideas, have confidence—face the brickbats and go ahead."
   Harold Ridley

"Who would support me before D. Peter Choyce came into the consultant scene? Nearly every surgeon abandoned implants at that time. I was apparently without professional friends, fearful of being charged with malpractice and had very many sleepless hours at night. I wondered if the new cataract operation had been started a generation too soon."
   Harold Ridley

In the early years after 1949 the going was rough. These are just a few of the comments that caused Harold many sleepless nights:
"This operation should never be done."
"The first report was a layman's magazine."
"This operation offends the first principle of eye surgery."
"A foreign body can cause sympathetic ophthalmia and malignant disease."
"The manufacturers should be prosecuted for supplying implants."
"Would you have one of these things put in your son's eye?"
"Dr. Ridley, why don't you GO HOME."
"If any of you ever use an IOL in a hospital that I control, I will most certainly testify against you in legal process."
"The IOL and the phacoemulsification procedure that goes with it represent a time bomb."

CHAPTER 10

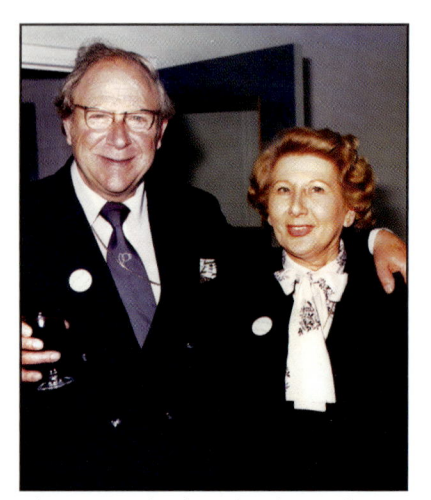

Choyce with his lovely wife Dianna, who was always at his side. She cheered him up even as he was being attacked for espousing Harold and his ideas.

Later in his life, Harold often mentioned to me how depressed he became because of the rejection and scorn that were directed his way. Nevertheless, he knew he was doing the right thing—and his decision was to proceed in spite of the opposition.

Though opposition was fierce, it was not universal. Not every surgeon had abandoned Harold. A handful of courageous, forward-looking professionals stood by him and his IOL idea against the "brickbats" that were thrown at them. These individuals became Harold's loyal friends and are today considered to be some of the true pioneers of IOL surgery. The first and foremost of these allies was D. Peter Choyce.

"Who Would Support Me Before Peter Choyce?"

D. Peter Choyce played a key role in helping Harold make the IOL an accepted, honored reality in ophthalmology. He was important not only for his medical and scientific studies and advances, but perhaps even more importantly, he was a major advocate and mouthpiece for Harold during the dark years of the IOL.

Born on March 1, 1919, D. Peter Choyce was the son of a prominent general surgeon who became director of surgery at the University College Hospital in London. Peter followed his father's example and went into medicine. When World War II came, he was put on reserve status so that he could continue his education. He passed his qualifying examinations in the spring of 1942. He was assigned to duty as a casualty officer at Lewis Ham Hospital in Southeast London, where he treated many victims of the German Blitz. He then became a ship's surgeon on an armed merchant vessel. The ship was damaged during a crossing of the North Atlantic, but managed to sail into the US Navy base in Norfolk, Virginia, for repairs.

While in America, Peter managed to visit some prominent American surgeons. Having taken an early interest in ophthalmology, he made a special trip to New York to visit Dr. Ramon Castroviejo, a prominent eye surgeon who specialized in corneal surgery. This visit helped him come to a decision regarding his medical career, and after the war was over, he returned to London to finish his general surgery work and then begin to study ophthalmology.

Peter secured a fellowship in ophthalmology at Moorfields Eye Hospital in 1949. He had the good fortune to work under Harold and became one of his protégés. This was a major turning point in his career.

His other main teacher at Moorfields was Sir Stewart Duke-Elder, who had for years shown himself to be Harold's active opponent. Unfortunately, as Peter began to believe in Harold's principles and supported him more and more, he soon became a casualty in the longstanding battle between these two leaders. As Peter attempted to progress professionally, Duke-Elder challenged him many times. I will briefly mention three episodes that reflect his feelings about Harold and the IOL.

One episode seemed highly problematic, indeed inappropriate. Peter was simply walking up a flight of stairs in the hospital when Duke-Elder encountered him and asked if he had changed his mind regarding Harold. Peter politely said no, and his relationship with Duke-Elder continued to "tank." Consequently, Duke-Elder treated

Peter in much the same way he treated Harold, attempting to undermine him and block his progress.

When Peter submitted a thesis in an attempt to receive a consultant position at Moorefields, Duke-Elder summarily rejected his application. Later, Peter resubmitted an updated thesis to other examiners and received approval. However, he never was able to practice at Moorfields. Instead, he established a practice several miles east of London at South-End-On-Sea, where he developed a large patient base and worked for 35 years.

Duke-Elder's antagonism toward Peter continued. In the early 1960s, the two physicians attended a meeting in Miami, Florida, of the Section of Ophthalmology of the American Medical Association. Benedetto Strampelli, Joaquin Barraquer, and Peter Choyce had been invited to participate in a symposium on lens implantation. Peter was proud to be associated with such distinguished colleagues and hoped that it meant that at long last his efforts on behalf of Harold and IOL surgeons in general were gaining some recognition. On the whole, what Peter had to say was sympathetically received.

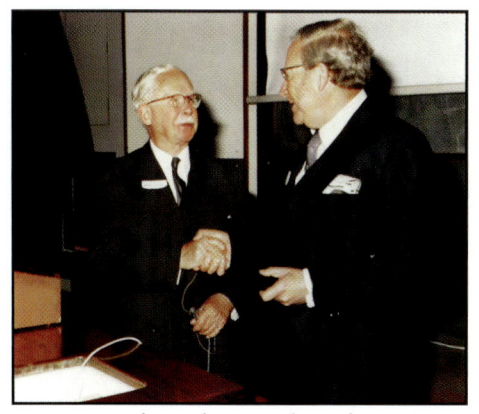

This photograph, taken at an unknown venue, helped cement the concept of their close relationship and Choyce's strong contribution in helping defend Harold and his innovation.

Also on the program was Sir Stewart Duke-Elder, who delivered the very prestigious Proctor Medal Lecture. His thesis was, as always, that the way forward in the solution of ophthalmic problems was by the application of scientific methods. He asserted that the answer did not lie in the application or refinement of surgical skills. Duke-Elder himself rarely, if ever, performed eye surgery.

After his lecture, Duke-Elder invited Peter to have a drink with him in the bar, an invitation that flattered him. After a few scotches (Duke-Elder's favorite drink), Peter said, "I enjoyed your lecture very much, but with great respect, I do think that there are certain areas where the refinement of surgical skills would help not only in the solution of clinical problems, but in the advancement of our scientific understanding of those problems."

Duke-Elder's reply brought Peter back to reality and reminded him that the famous icon of ophthalmology was still terribly opposed to Harold, the IOL, and anyone who considered himself a "Ridley man."

"Frankly, Peter," said Duke-Elder flatly, "I don't give a damn what you think."

Peter continued with his work in support of IOLs, running into obstacle after obstacle. Most of his work was rejected by his contemporaries and it became difficult for him to get things published. Finally, in 1964, he published a work entitled "Intraocular Lenses and Implants." This was basically a compilation of his rejected papers. When I peruse this work today, I am amazed by what Choyce accomplished during those years. For example, he was the first to carefully study measurements of the anterior segment required for implantation of devices into the ocular tissues.

He also did extensive work on anterior chamber lenses. Unfortunately, his strong adherence to this type of lens created some major problems with his peers,

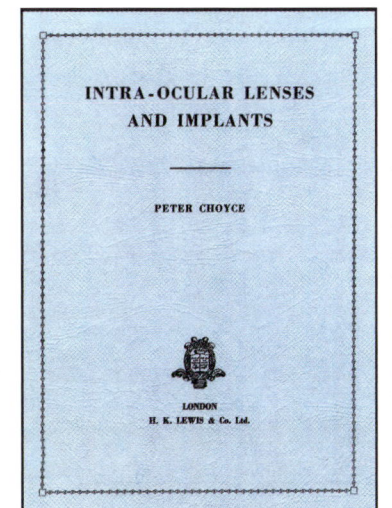

Choyce's support of Harold and his very forward thinking of scientific ideas were, at times, an anathema to the establishment, including the editors of many eye journals. He had been kept out of the important academic institutions such as Moorfields Eye Hospital and, therefore, was forced to establish a private practice east of London at South-End-On-Sea. In some ways, this turned out to be a blessing because it gave him a certain degree of freedom. Frustrated by his inability to publish his material, he wrote and published a thesis, the title of which is seen here. It is a compendium of articles that have been rejected and contain a plethora of new ideas that, today, clearly confirm a vision that very few had. Many innovations and devices he espoused are still used today.

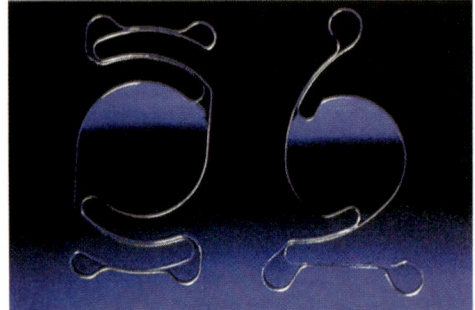

CHAPTER 10

Choyce was an early pioneer of the anterior chamber lens in contrast to Harold's posterior chamber lens and the type that is nearly universal today. He and others proved that anterior chamber lenses, such as the two modern designs seen here, could be safe and effective and used for specific clinical situations. However, as it was learned that the ECCE-posterior chamber IOL, cataract surgery was the procedure of the future; he stuck tenaciously by the AC-IOL, thus retarding his future. It seemed that every complication that occurred with his lens was presented at hospital grand rounds, and everywhere he was subjected to great criticism.

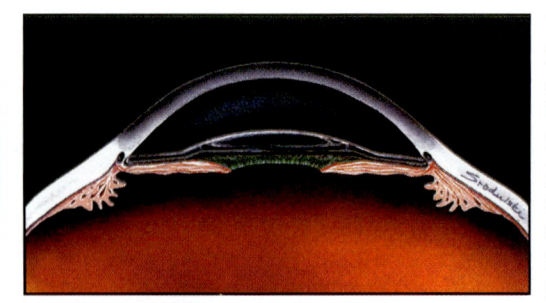

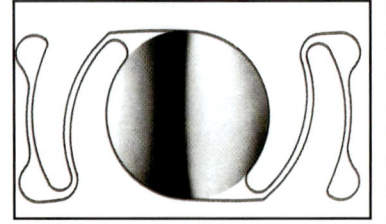

These photographs show the concept of an anterior chamber lens, in which the lens is placed in front of the iris in the anterior chamber, just behind the cornea. A safe outcome is difficult to ensure if the implantation technique is not perfect, and there is less room for error. Note in the lower figure how the lens has four fixation points at each corner, which are inserted into what is called the anterior chamber angle. This is situated immediately adjacent to the aqueous outflow channels of the eye. Disruption of the latter can lead to glaucoma. Choyce would probably feel very vindicated today to note that anterior chamber lenses are still used, including in the very "high tech" phakic IOLs produced by one of the major IOL manufacturers. Still, the posterior chamber lens is the standard.

since these lenses were considered to be highly problematic and indeed did cause significant numbers of complications. His colleagues at Moorfields, of course, noted this, along with their severe criticisms. While Peter probably continued to support his anterior chamber lenses too long, and often with too much gusto, he is now receiving some vindication in the fact that they have made a comeback in use in modern phakic IOLs. Alcon Laboratories, the largest eye care company in the world, has chosen to use an anterior chamber IOL as a preferred phakic IOL and, to date, the results have been excellent.

Peter was responsible for a number of other highly innovative advances related to IOLs, cataracts, refractive surgery, and even orbital surgery. These include being the first to carefully measure the size of pediatric eyes in order to choose the correct IOL for these eyes and then to photographically document a pediatric IOL implantation. He designed a telescopic IOL for use with patients with low vision, and he designed various colored IOLs that could be implanted in patients with damaged irises.

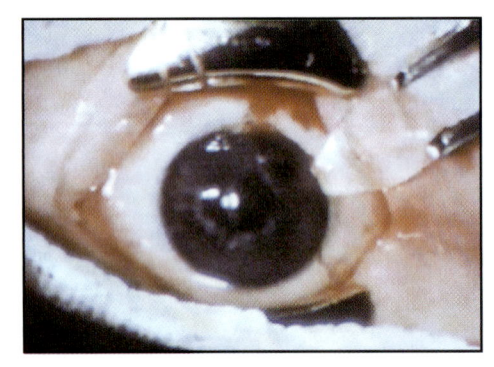

A photograph of Choyce's first pediatric IOL implantation in 1963. His particular lens design at that time was triangular in shape with three fixation points, as is easily visible in this photograph.

Choyce also appeared publicly in many venues, such as during this interview on the BBC in an attempt to authorize implants. During the early years, this was not well accepted by "the establishment" in that it reeked of advertising and commercialism. If it was, it did not turn out to be a highly profitable endeavor, since neither Harold nor Choyce made huge amounts of money.

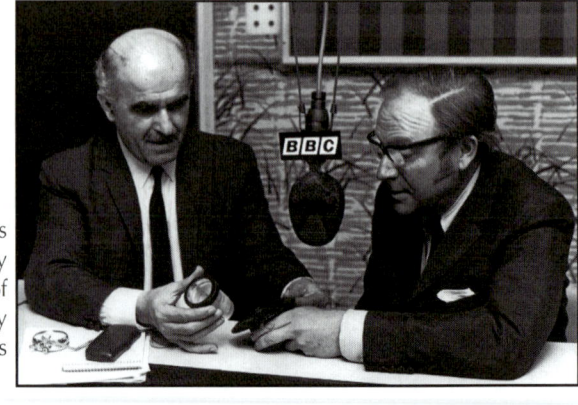

A GRADUAL ASCENT TO A NEW REVOLUTION IN SURGICAL EYE CARE

OTHER SUPPORTERS AND PIONEERS

Edward Epstein also became an advocate of Harold and was one of the first to make any modifications to his lens. Epstein, born in Leeds, England, migrated to South Africa and served in the desert theater of the war against Rommel's army. Following World War II, he continued Ridley's work with IOLs. One of his major achievements was early work on soft, malleable biomaterials, work that was helpful for the development of foldable IOLs. His work was not widely accepted at first, but these of course have become the norm, used in modern small-incision surgery.

Dr. Svyatoslav Fyodorov (Chapter 12) of the then Soviet Union was one of the first to come to study Harold's IOL work. His enthusiasm for the IOL continued unabated throughout the rest of his life, as did his affection for Ridley. His work addressed the fields of both cataract and refractive surgery (see Chapter 12).

The Dutch ophthalmologist Cornelius Binkhorst, now largely underrated and forgotten by many, was another early and important pioneer in lens design. He was among the first, with Harold, to help discern the proper means of fixation of IOLs. Binkhorst was an early advocate of courses designed to teach surgeons about implant techniques. His courses were very popular and were commonly termed "wet labs."

It is noteworthy that Peter Choyce was almost always present at meetings with Harold Ridley. One of Choyce's most important contributions was his role as a "mouth piece," in the positive sense of the word, in that he was able to advocate and defend Harold, who was a modest man unable to slash back and defend sharp criticism. Seated between Choyce on the left and Harold on the right is the great Cornelius Binkhorst.

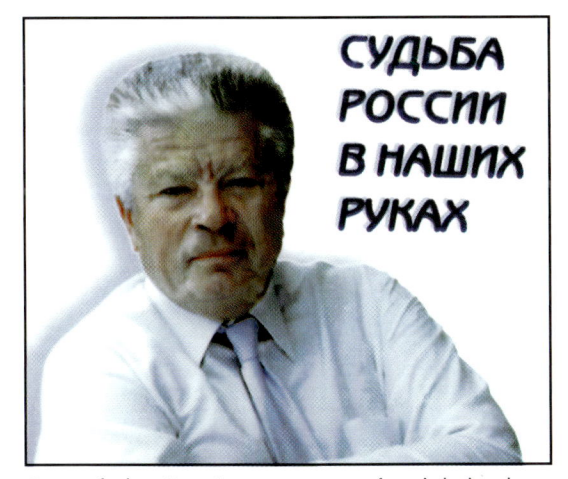

One of the Renaissance men of ophthalmology was Svyatoslav Fyodorov. He lived in Archangel, in the former Soviet Union, at the time of Harold's first implant, and he immediately traveled the long distance to London when he heard about this. He became one of the most forceful and strident supporters of Harold till the end of both of their lives.

His advanced thought and innovations range from radial keratotomy, to classic IOLs, to phakic IOLs, to corneal implants, to cancer treatments, and many more. Perhaps, his position as leader in his country at the time gave him a certain freedom to apply his innovations.

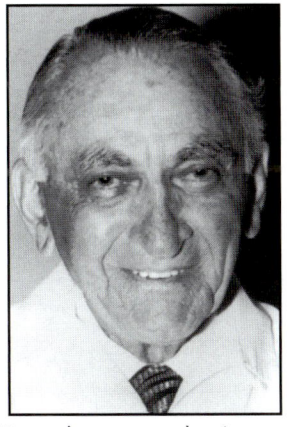

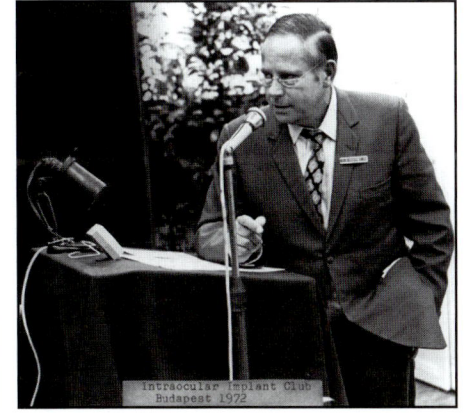

Two other very early pioneers and advocates of Harold Ridley were Edward Epstein of South Africa, left, and Cornelius Binkhorst of the Netherlands, right.

Epstein was in England at the time of the first implant and immediately saw its value. He was one of the first to do various modifications of the IOL. He is still alive, in his 90s, and still presents many important ideas at meetings. Cornelius Binkhorst of Terneuzen, Holland was initially extremely underrated since he advocated a form of iris-supported IOL that turned out to be inferior. However, his greatness and lasting importance emerged when he was the first to reveal some of the theoretic advantages of placing IOLs, as Harold noted, in the site where God wished them to be, in the lens capsular bag. We were able to confirm Binkhorst's ideas in our laboratory in the 1980s. Secondly, Binkhorst was a pioneer in the field of teaching surgery, and many surgeons worldwide made a pilgrimage to his facility to learn the most modern techniques.

CHAPTER 10

Many Americans made the pilgrimage to his home in Terneuzen, Holland to learn the most advanced techniques. The advantage of the wet lab is obvious. Young surgeons-in-training or in transition are able to learn new techniques using artificial eyes before proceeding to operating on living human eyes. I have utilized wet labs in training many young surgeons (page 75) and the Miyake-Apple technique is a wonderful teaching tool (pages 86 to 88).

Philadelphia, Pennsylvania is the location where the IOL was first accepted, widely experimented upon, and given its prominence; a long line of clinicians have espoused Harold's innovation here.

LEFT: The support of Harold began when he did his first implantation in Chicago in 1951. The audience included Dr. Warren Reese of Philadelphia, who immediately became enamored of the technique. Harold gave him five lenses on the spot. Reese returned immediately to Philadelphia and, the next day, became the first American to do an implant, which must have been very successful in that he and his colleagues continue on for many years, making Philadelphia the leader that it was.

RIGHT: Dr. Reese's younger colleague, Turgut Hamdi took up the technique immediately and did many implantations even after Reese had retired. Because of his extremely pleasant personality and his qualities as a surgeon, he was allowed to continue with this daring operation at a very early time in this country—other colleagues could probably not have accomplished it unhindered, but his results left nothing to complain about.

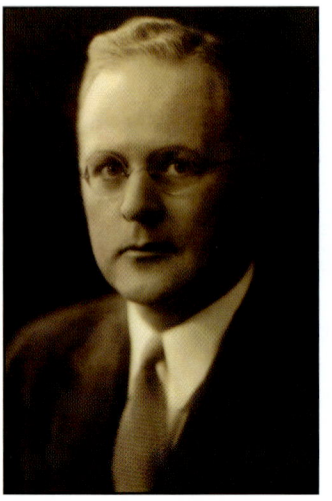

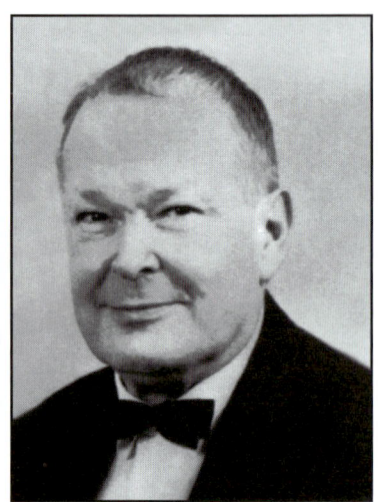

Reese and Hamdi were the first to, to my knowledge, advocate the concept of bi-monofocal technology for IOLs in 1962, and no doubt, they were the most vocal advocates for Harold in the United States at that time. Another surgeon in Philadelphia who is a strong supporter of Harold's, Charles Letocha, kindly supplied the above illustration and many photographs and memorabilia from his collection of Dr. Reese.

THE PHILADELPHIA STORY

Warren Reese, another early IOL advocate—indeed the earliest—was the first American to implant an IOL. He received five or six lenses from Harold in Chicago, as the latter was doing the first implants done on American soil. Reese flew home immediately in his private plane and began doing implants at Wills Eye Hospital in Philadelphia. Reese and particularly his colleague, Turgut Hamdi, became close friends with Harold and advocates of his work. Together, they made Philadelphia one of the most important US cities for intraocular lenses. Hamdi, a much younger man, did many implants over the years at Wills. The conservative "establishment" people were all around but left Hamdi alone. He left them very little to complain about. Miami, Florida, where Norman Jaffe and team later did important studies that helped confirm the efficacy of IOLs, provides an example that shows that an open-minded chairman can change the entire attitude of an institute. The chairman at that time, Dr. Edward Norton, did not inhibit his faculty in the study of IOLs.

We have already noted that Reese and Hamdi were among the first to write about the concept of bifocal or multifocal IOLs, and their ideas have come to fruition with a bang (see Chapters 1 and 11).

A GRADUAL ASCENT TO A NEW REVOLUTION IN SURGICAL EYE CARE

Dr. Charles Letocha of York, Pennsylvania has done a yeoman's service in preserving the heritage and legacy of Harold's invention, beginning with Harold and continuing down to himself and other colleagues, including Dr. David Shusterman. I am grateful personally to Charles for providing both pictorial and moral support.

Munich, 1966

Specialists in all fields of medicine attend the congresses large and small in order to present their latest findings and allow the industry to present new products. This also gives organizers and attendees the opportunity to enjoy nice, relaxing vacations in beautiful venues.

At most congresses of this kind, the vast majority of work presented is excellent science. However, some presentations were based on information that would be profitable to various individuals or companies. Many presenters who discussed findings were not those who did the scientific work themselves, but were hired by companies to disseminate the information. Unfortunately, some of the information presented was not scientifically valid; in other words, it was junk science. Some of the lectures were actually written by professional writers and not the physicians. Some portions of the meetings were devoted to lavish ceremonies, awards, and other events that provided little new clinical input. This still occurs.

A very large meeting took place in 1966: the International Congress of Ophthalmology in Munich, Germany. Although the Germans were the hosts, the most influential person at the 1966 congress was Derrick Vail of Chicago—the president of the International Congress of Ophthalmology. He was a colleague and close supporter of Duke-Elder.

Peter Choyce wanted to make sure that there was a place for IOLs on the program, even just a side room. A rapid exchange of letters between Peter, Derrick Vail, and the German organizers ensued. To make a long story short, the German organizers were very polite, but would not give those wishing to present IOLs a place on the program. They would not even promise that they would be officially recognized.

Peter finally lost his patience and decided, together with several of his colleagues who were already known advocates of implants, to by-

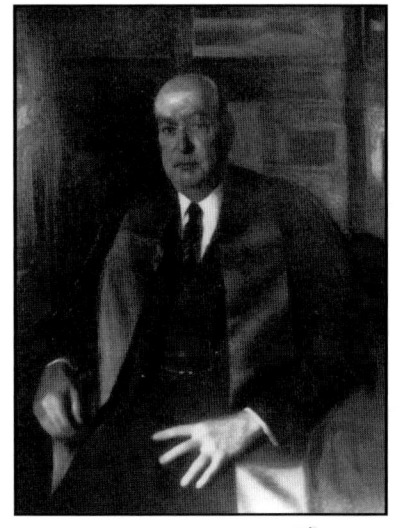

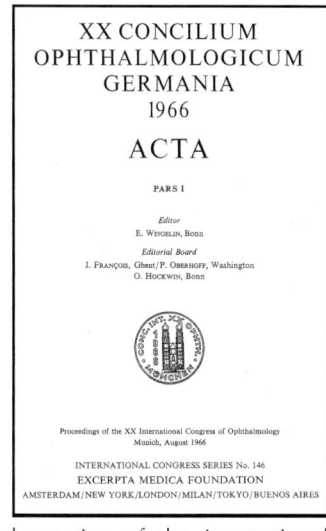

The annual meeting of the International Congress of Ophthalmology in 1966 represented a turning point in the acceptance of Harold and the IOL. This international meeting, held every 4 years in an international location, was scheduled for Munich in 1966. Although ostensibly under the control of the German hosts and local organizers, the president of the organization that year, the guiding light of it, was Dr. Derrick Vail of Chicago.
LEFT: This is a photograph of Derrick Vail in his academic regalia.
RIGHT: This illustration is the title sheet of the proceedings of the Munich meeting

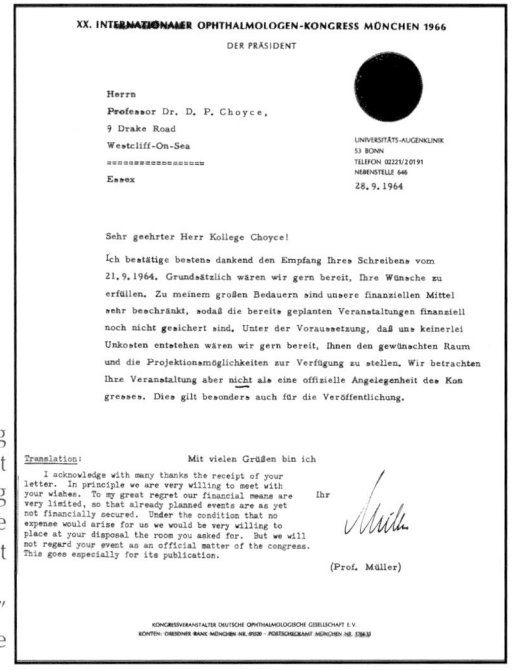

From Mrs. Peter Choyce, I have received a copy of the written interchange among various parties prior to the 1966 Munich meeting. Peter Choyce was somewhat surprised to have received a polite but negative response from the meeting organizers (see the translation of the letter in this photograph at the bottom of the letter). The IOL supporters were given a room for their meeting, but it is clear that they were not given "an official role" in the Congress.
By the time Choyce learned of this, he gave up and decided to do an "end run," and the small group of Harold supporters, lead by Choyce, set up a separate meeting of their own for London.

173

CHAPTER 10

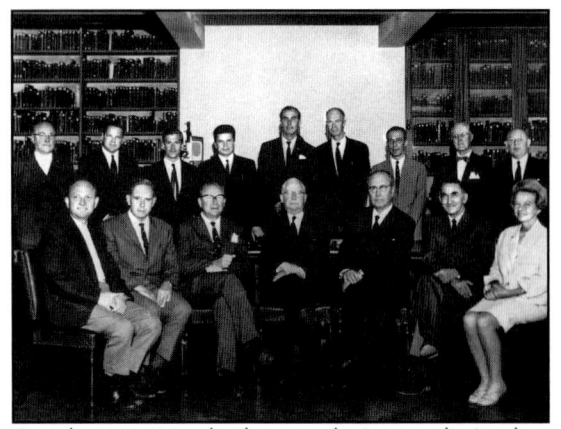

On July 14, 1966, what became the Intraocular Implant Club (IIC) had their first meeting in the Academy of Medicine in London. These pioneers are shown in this photograph. Harold was named the first president. The names of this small pioneering group are as follows: seated from left to right, Jorn Boberg-Ans (Denmark), Cornelius Binkhorst (Holland), Peter Choyce (UK), Harold Ridley (UK), Benedetto Strampelli (Italy), Edward Epstein (South Africa), Mrs. Boberg-Ans (Denmark). Back row: John Pike (UK), Dr. Murto (USA), Michael Roper-Hall (UK), Svyatoslav Fyodorov (USSR), Neil Dallas (USA), C. A. Brown, Dr. Rubenstein, Warren Reese (USA), Leonard Lurie (UK).

pass the main meeting and do an "end run." They formed a society of their own, a club that they named the Intraocular Implant Club (IIC). It was called a club rather than a society because Ridley, its first president, wanted to keep the membership small and focused on medical-clinical discussions on IOLs.

The club's first meeting took place on Bastille Day in 1966, at the Royal Institute of Medicine in London. The venue was just a few hundred feet from Harold's home on Harley Street. He was elected the first president.

PARIS, 1974

By the early 1970s, IOLs had earned somewhat more acceptance, but things were still very tenuous. The IIC had a successful meeting in Budapest in 1972. The next large meeting of the International Congress of Ophthalmology was to occur in Paris in 1974. Duke-Elder's colleague, Vail, was no longer president of the function, but two other anti-Ridley academicians were high-profile in the 1974 meeting: Duke-Elder himself and Jules François of Belgium, the society's president at that time.

As before, the meeting was more or less controlled by the establishment, and Peter again had no luck securing a venue for an IOL meeting or even recognition. He anticipated such problems and decided to try another strategy. On the last day of the meeting, he scheduled a satellite meeting in a building adjacent to the congress center, which was not under their control. He invited all those interested in the future course of implants to attend. This strategy worked magnificently. Not only did the small core group that was already on board attend, but numerous doctors, mainly from America, actually filled the hall! They were not disappointed. Harold Ridley himself was a surprise guest at that meeting.

After this meeting, the IOL, so long in the doldrums, seemed to be on the road to recovery. The club became international and its name was changed to the International Intraocular Implant Club (IIIC).

By the beginning of the 21st century, this group boasted over 300 members, and very informative scientific and social meetings now occur each year.

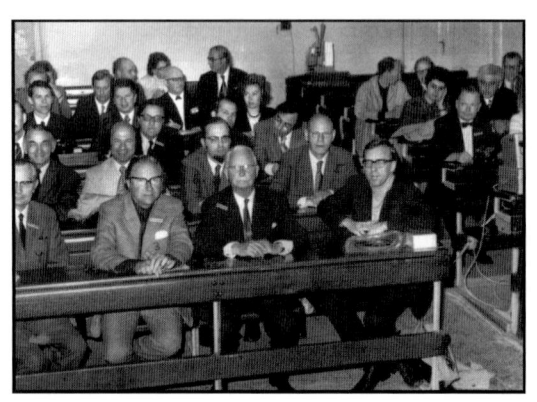

The small gathering in London in 1966 was followed by a meeting with a larger contingent held in Budapest, Hungry in 1972. This is a photograph of the IIC members with Harold and Peter Choyce (left) seated next to Dr. John Worst (right) on the front row. This meeting symbolized a very slow but steady growth of the IIC.

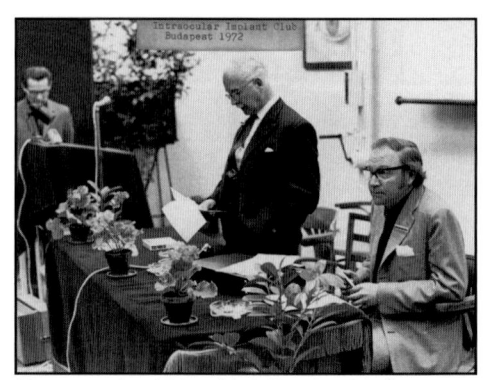

Photograph of Harold delivering his lecture at the 1972 meeting of the IIC in Budapest. Peter Choyce is sitting immediately to his left.

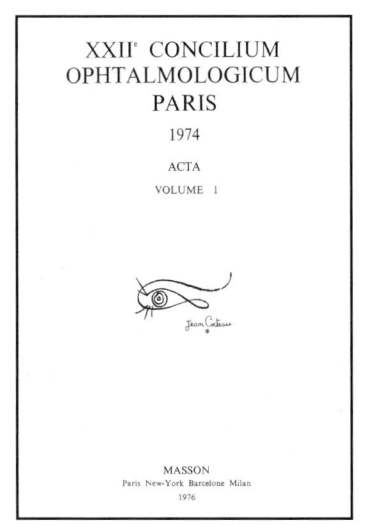

A GRADUAL ASCENT TO A NEW REVOLUTION IN SURGICAL EYE CARE

Another meeting of the International Congress of Ophthalmology was scheduled for Paris in 1974. This is a photograph of the front page of the proceedings of that meeting. This time, the IOL advocates planned something different, namely not to attempt to join in the main meeting but rather to plan a "satellite meeting." The small "satellite meeting" occurred in a building adjacent to the main convention center, starting first with a small number of individuals but joined by many who heard about it and entered the hall with great interest—including, for the first time, a large contingent of Americans. It was a huge success, particularly when Harold Ridley himself entered the packed the room, surprising many. This was not scheduled, but I am sure that Choyce had arranged this. This appeared to be a major turnaround for the society, and it was actually renamed the International Intraocular Implant Club (IIIC) at that time.

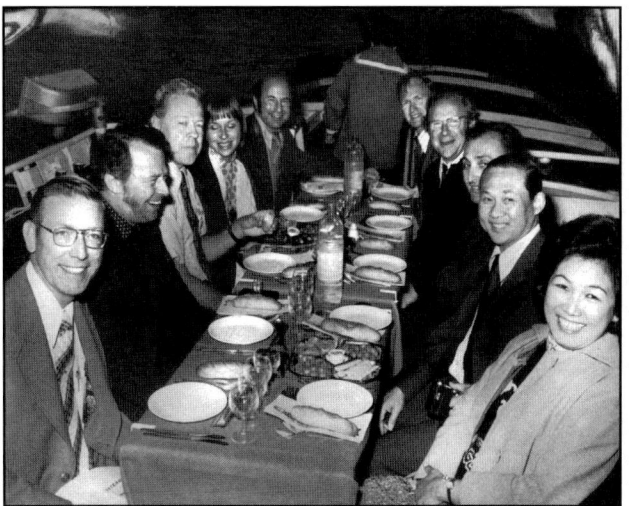

This may be the only photograph that remains from the July 1, 1974 meeting, namely the post-meeting celebration on a small ship (Batteau Mouche) that cruises the Seine River. Here are some of the participants of the meeting at dinner. Peter Choyce is the second to the last person on the far right. The two individuals at the very far right across from each other are Henry Hirschman and Richard Kratz, respectively. The gentleman at the front left is Dr. Robert Drews of Clayton, Missouri, who supplied much of the information regarding this event.

This gathering in Paris represented a new injection of energy leading to further acceptance of the IOL.

"AMERICA'S DOCTOR" PRESCRIBES THE IOL TO THE FDA

In contrast to the very bad start Harold experienced at his first major lecture on the IOL presented at Oxford in 1951, another occurrence almost three decades later had just the opposite effect—a sure disaster turned around into something that can be described as nothing less than a major victory for the IOL, and much more importantly, for humanity.

Most young ophthalmologists-in-training today are provided modern instruments and are free to learn, without interference, modern surgical procedures such as the cataract-IOL operation. Most are too young to remember, and indeed have little interest in looking back at the time when the establishment and some governmental authorities often classified IOL surgeons as "buccaneers" or worse. These were the days when the IOL and its innovators and proponents were under constant attack and the days when the future of the IOL was indeed in jeopardy. I believe it will make all of us more appreciative of what we have and how fortunate we are if we read the short story I am about to tell, a story about the extreme situations that our predecessors were forced to endure.

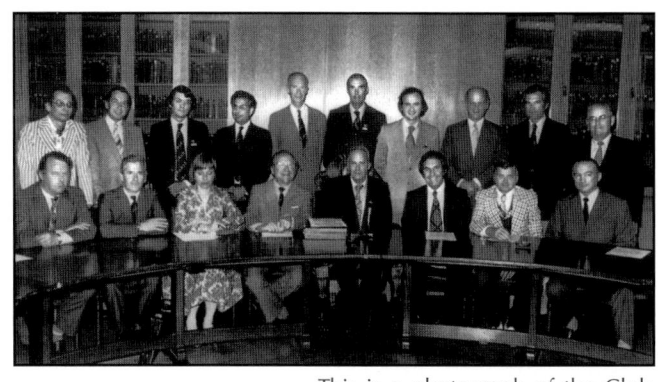

This is a photograph of the Club meeting in 1975 in London. Harold was not present at the time of this photograph.

CHAPTER 10

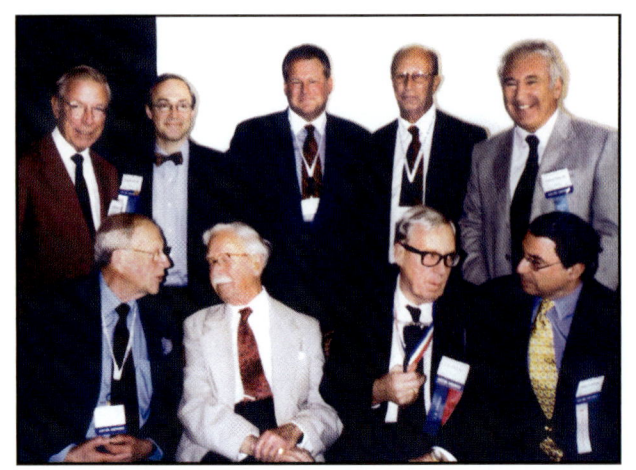

This photograph, courtesy of Jaci Lindstrom of the IIIC, shows one of the last appearances of Harold at a meeting of the IIIC—a group photograph of the presidents and past presidents of the Club. These include, in the front row from left to right, Peter Choyce, Harold, Jan Worst, Steven Obstbaun; and in the back row from left to right, Robert Drews, Doug Koch, Richard Lindstrom, Bo Philipson, and Emanuel Rosen.

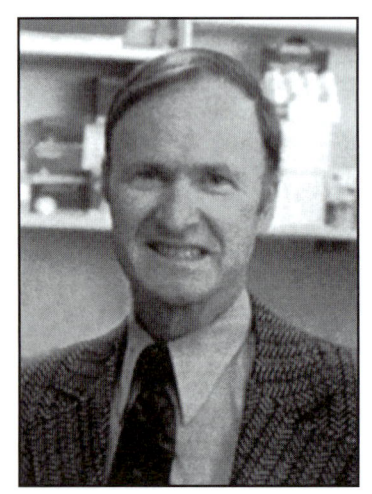

Robert Young had received an implant from Dr. Richard Kratz (above) in 1977 and had an excellent result. Kratz then invited Young to the important meeting in 1977 to testify, and the rest is history. The authorities and bureaucracies found they could not take away something that was "good enough for America's Doctor."

During the early 1970s, complications did indeed occur with implants, most in relation to some companies manufacturing bad designs that were not carefully thought out or well-fabricated. In addition, some surgeons did implantations without careful training and knowledge of how to prevent complications. By 1974, this was coming to a head and several organizations, usually consisting of the same group of people who had been constantly mounting attacks on Mr. Ridley, as well as some public and private organizations, were now weighing in against what was frequently considered to be a dangerous product. Many believed that IOLs were too risky, and the term "time bomb" was often applied to them.

Those against the implant included an organization overseen by Ralph Nader. This group was called Public Citizen, and Dr. Sidney Wolfe, an associate of Nader, actively pursued the IOL. Nader, despite some very useful and life-saving work concerning automobile safety and other consumer-friendly matters, seemed to be overly hostile against the implants. This led to the involvement of the US government, especially the US Food and Drug Administration (FDA). This was supported by many ophthalmologists who were against IOLs. They wanted IOLs out! They saw their practices dwindling as patients began to understand the implications of implants and seek out physicians who implanted them. The FDA declared IOLs a drug, and thus under their jurisdiction. Ophthalmologists were required to report all adverse events involving IOLs to the FDA. These adverse event reports were used in an effort to stop IOLs.

In 1980, Wolfe collected "data" regarding the safety and efficacy of IOLs. Many ophthalmologists before him had distorted or skewed the data. He added up every adverse reaction, even very minor, inconsequential ones that should not have been counted. He took the total number of adverse reactions recorded after a series of IOL implantations and divided it by the number of cases done. He incorrectly concluded that the incidence of problems was over 50%, a ridiculous miscalculation designed to make his case against IOLs. He therefore insisted on a formal hearing by the FDA, no doubt with the intention of removing these lenses from the market.

As the day of that hearing approached, public opinion had been so inflamed that it was clear that IOLs were about to be tarred and feathered and led out the door to oblivion.

A few perceptive ophthalmologists at that time saw this coming and acted. One of these ophthalmologists was one of the finest implant surgeons I have ever known: Dr. Richard Kratz, who at that time practiced in Van Nuys, California.

Kratz, after returning from military service in the Far East in 1948, had continued his training in basic sciences at Moorfields Eye Hospital in London and actually met Harold the year before he did his first implant operation in 1949-50.

Kratz's reputation had grown so much that he frequently treated the rich and famous, including Hollywood stars. One notable and typically successful operation performed by Dr. Kratz was done in 1976 on the fine actor and film star, Robert Young (see photo on the next page). Most of our younger readers may not recall Robert Young. However, those of us who are slightly older recall his television success in *Father Knows Best,* and, important for our present discussion, *Marcus Welby, MD,* where he was seen by millions of people weekly. He was "America's Doctor"!

A GRADUAL ASCENT TO A NEW REVOLUTION IN SURGICAL EYE CARE

Dr. Kratz and his colleagues did some wishful thinking and they hatched a plan involving Mr. Young, who by the time of the important FDA hearing in 1980, had had consistently good vision from his implant surgery. He was 20/20 in both eyes and indeed viewed the operation as an important factor in his ability to continue as an actor. The doctors asked him to testify at the FDA hearing and he agreed to come to Washington to do so.

According to the doctors who attended and were involved, including Dr. Kratz, on the evening before the hearing, Mr. Young did not appear to be entirely fit. This led to intense trepidation that he may not prove to be a good witness the next morning in front of this austere FDA panel, surrounded by a full house of reporters who had heard about Mr. Young's participation. Everyone was therefore on edge.

However, they need not have been. After several surgeons, including Dr. Stephen Obstbaum of New York who showed excellent results obtained on the eyes of a pilot, had presented their cases, Mr. Young took the stand, looked the audience in the eye and simply stated, "Look, I am America's doctor and indeed what is good for America's doctor is good for America." That immediately brought down the house.

However, perhaps his best and most effective commentary occurred in the hallway outside after the meeting was adjourned (which had already been swayed in the direction of IOLs). A huge audience, including the numerous reporters in attendance, gathered outside the room. One reporter asked Mr. Young the following (Dr. Kratz remembers this as if it were yesterday): "Dr. Welby, do you really believe that implants are as useful as you implied?" Mr. Young retorted, "Sir, I am not Dr. Welby. I am only an actor who plays the part of Welby." He then tugged at the man's necktie and continued: "Let me tell you, IOLs saved my career and should be available to all Americans." Apparently, the multitude in this room erupted in applause and the opponents of IOLs were finished at that instant and they knew it. The press corps dispersed to their typewriters and telephones and these stunning events almost immediately were flashed on the afternoon network news shows. Members of Congress who had power over the FDA immediately became caught up in the rapidly unfolding events. Even though the FDA had already made up its mind to ban IOLs, Congress sent a mandate to the FDA to make IOLs available. The FDA and its allies had no choice but to back off and drop their objection to lens implants. The press went away with great things to say about Sir Harold's wonderful invention. The rest is history.

These events in Paris and Washington turned out to be positive. Critics were never again able to orchestrate a concerted organized attack. Marcus Welby was truly "America's Doctor"—a doctor who made a difference.

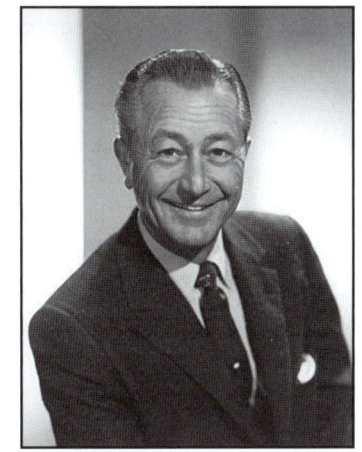

At the 1980 meeting, the anti-IOL forces had a goal of removing IOLs from the market. The presentation of a series of successfully operated and happy patients was not enough to convince the authorities regarding the safety and efficacy of the IOL. It took strong words from actor Robert Young (seen here) famous for *Father Knows Best* and especially at that time, *Marcus Welby, MD*, "America's Doctor."

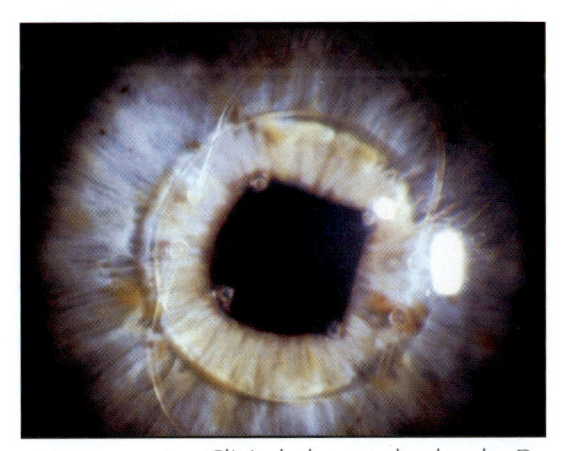

Clinical photograph taken by Dr. Steven Ostbaum of the eye of an airline pilot. Dr. Ostbaum had operated on a cataract for this pilot in the late 1970s. This is an example of a lens that is affixed to the iris.
The result was presented to the packed-house meeting in 1980, where the IOL was being attacked.

Unstoppable Forward Movement

It is unfortunate that, beginning with Sit Stewart Duke-Elder and Derrick Vail, several prominent surgeons in the 1950s and 1960s, many representing the academic establishment in Europe and the United States, treated Harold and his lens with disdain.

CHAPTER 10

While it was certainly reasonable for those in the ophthalmology establishment to approach the IOL procedure with caution and conservatism, their reactions created an unhappy situation, not only in human terms because of the discourteous and unpleasant actions often directed toward Harold, but also because energy for productive research was often siphoned away. New development was often limited by the prejudice expressed against it.

When discussing these issues Harold always brings up the name of his friend Peter. He recalled:

"Peter Choyce courageously became a fervent supporter of IOLs, in spite of having received a personal warning from Duke-Elder against cooperating with me."

The forward momentum of the IOL that followed the meeting at the 1974 International Congress of Ophthalmology, along with Robert Young's testimony before the FDA, was backed by mounting scientific evidence.

Pioneering work was conducted by Dr. Jose Barraquer in Spain, Robert Drews in Missouri, and Norman Jaffe and his team in Miami, Florida. The latter team did an important clinical study that was clearly positive for the specialty. By the mid-1980s, our work in Salt Lake City, Utah had been publicized. Our team, the Apple Korps, had elucidated the many complications of IOL surgery and found ways to avoid them. Our correlative studies in the laboratory on the new techniques, such as hydrodissection, capsulorrhexis, PCO prevention, decentration prevention, biocompatibility issues, and phacoemulsification, were also introduced.

All these findings were tied to Kelman's phacoemulsification techniques, helping establish the modern field of small incision surgery with intraocular lenses. Suddenly, a bright, new world for IOLs had come into being. A few bumps in the road were still ahead, but Harold's innovation had finally climbed from the abyss to the forefront and was not to be stopped.

Dr. Robert Drews of St. Louis, Missouri was a prominent American cataract IOL surgeon who was a witness to the events of the 1974 International Congress of Ophthalmology (ICO) in Paris. He is seen in the group picture on the River Seine on page 175. He always seemed to exude a feeling of optimism, as seen in a comment he penned:

"Five thousand years, 250 years, 40 years ago; what will the future hold? I think the time is coming when information processing will advance to the state that we can begin to make inroads in providing pseudo-visual input for the blind. But no matter what brilliant achievements are made in the future, Ridley's place in history remains secure. Ridley has stated that he looks forward to meeting Daviel in heaven. I think that Daviel will be flanked by millions and millions of people who have had their cataractous lenses replaced with the ultra-clear vision of lens implants!"

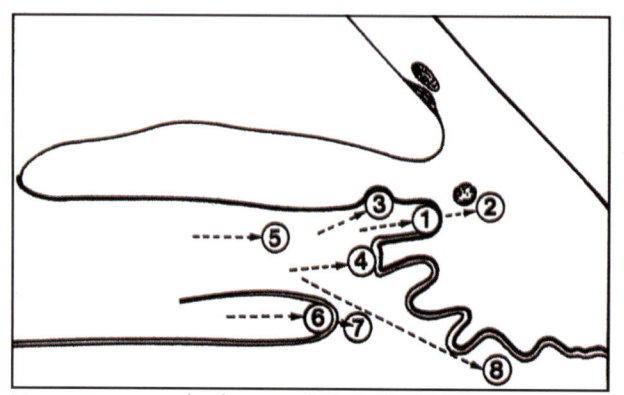

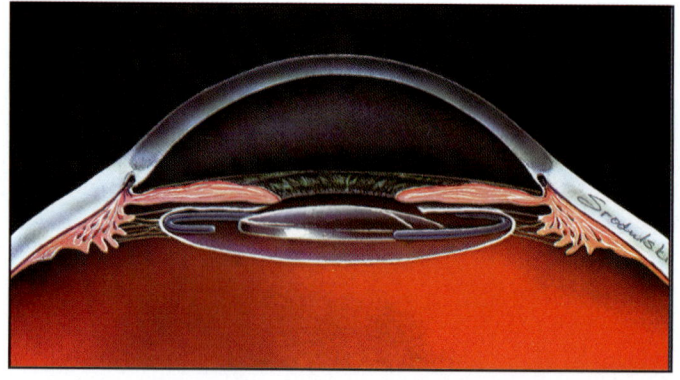

Most surgeons today have settled on the posterior chamber IOL as their lens of choice. This was a lens originally recommended by Ridley.

Malposition can be caused by problems with the IOL design (ie, too heavy) or may relate to problems in the surgeon's surgical technique. Whenever implant surgery is done, the haptics or loops must be targeted and placed in a specific location, in general known as the lens capsular bag.

LEFT: This diagram shows the multiple sites where lens haptics could land if careful and accurate surgery is not accomplished. The ideal place for the lens haptic is site #6 nicely, snuggly sequestered within the lens capsular bag. The numbers 1, 2, and 3 connote fixation of the other main type of IOL, the anterior chamber lens.

RIGHT: Schematic illustration showing ideal placement of a 3-piece posterior chamber IOL perfectly and symmetrically implanted within the lens capsular bag. (Kris Szyolski completed this drawing.)

11

The Good, the Bad, and the Ugly: Evolution of IOLs, Ups and Downs

"If you were trained sometime between the 1950s and the 1970s, you have witnessed and participated in nearly the entire development of modern cataract surgery, as we know it. Where we go from here is unknown, but certainly all we do today will be history tomorrow. As Prospero said in The Tempest, t*he past is but a prologue."*

Norman Medow, MD, New York

"My lens is an adaptation of the original Ridley IOL. All implanters are the children of Mr. Ridley."

Steven Shearing, MD, Las Vegas

The initial meeting between Harold and me in 1985 (Chapter 4, pages 58 and 59) was made possible because of some scientific/analytic research on IOLs I had performed. This work was done in my laboratory between 1981 (IOL #1) and 1984. It was highly technical, especially for that time.

In 1984, Dr. Randall Olson and I prepared a National Institute of Health (Federal) grant application in order to help us fund further research on IOLs. I do not believe that some of the referees understood the implications of Harold's work. Their anti-IOL stance not only reflected the already simmering aversion to Harold and his invention that many had—mostly from the academic establishment. They were also not enthusiastic about the application of pathology to this type of project. Some of the referees even at that late date (1984) felt that IOLs would not last. Even after the convincing testimony of "America's Doctor," Marcus Welby (Robert Young), in 1980, they were still skeptical (Chapter 10). This episode was one of many examples when I was criticized for devoting my pathology talents to the realm of the "buccaneers."

CHAPTER 11

We survived the negative answer from the Federal Government but were pleased that our work was useful in eventually helping surgeons avoid IOL-related complications.

In this chapter, I will briefly outline a few examples of IOL-related complications that we have studied. I realize this is highly technical, complicated, and perhaps uninteresting for some readers, but I hope it provides a brief overview of some examples regarding the types of complications and diseases that needed and still need to be addressed. These studies were also useful over the years in helping perfect the cataract-IOL operation.

Some complications did develop with Harold's early IOL implants. In retrospect, these complications were unusual, but his critics often magnified their intensity and exaggerated their clinical significance.

The success of any prosthetic device implanted in the body, including the IOL, depends primarily on three factors: (1) the design of the device, (2) the quality of the material used to fabricate the device, and (3) the quality of surgery during the insertion process of the device. Problems relating to all three of these factors appeared at various stages in the evolution of the IOL.

Early on, one of the main reasons for the complications arising from Harold's IOL implants had nothing to do with the IOL quality but involved the lack of skill of some of the surgeons who performed the procedures.

Harold listened to the criticisms and worked to improve the procedure and the lenses. At one point, he even changed his lens type from the original circular (disc) posterior chamber IOL to a tripod anterior chamber lens. This turned out to be less satisfactory than the original design. The ophthalmology world made many attempts over the coming decades to change or improve the IOL. However, several problematic designs were introduced that caused additional complications—the BAD and the UGLY. Finally, some of these actually did advance the design in a positive way—the GOOD.

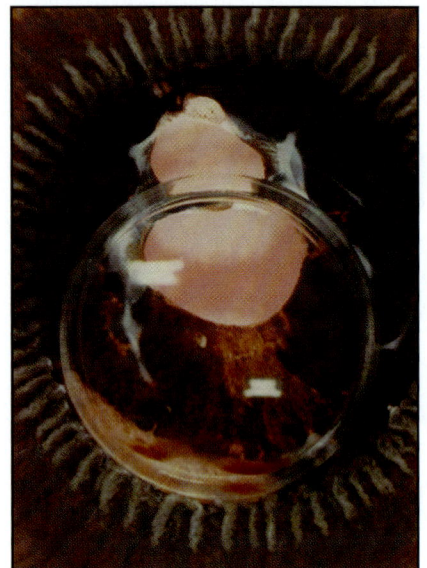

Inferior (downward) malpositioned or decentered Ridley IOL. This is a view from behind, using the Miyake-Apple posterior video/photographic technique, which permits us to locate the position of the IOL as if the observer were standing at the back of the eye looking forward through the pupil (the white space just beyond the lens in this photograph).

Many of the important landmarks of the eye can be seen. The multiple elevations that circle for 360 degrees around the lens are termed the ciliary processes. They are connected with the periphery of the normal lens and its outer capsule and hold it in place. In addition, the cells (epithelia) of the ciliary processes secrete a watery or aqueous fluid termed the aqueous humor. This fluid passes through the eye at a normal predetermined rate. If the exit of this fluid is blocked in any way, the pressure in the eye may increase, causing the very common condition of glaucoma (increased intraocular pressure).

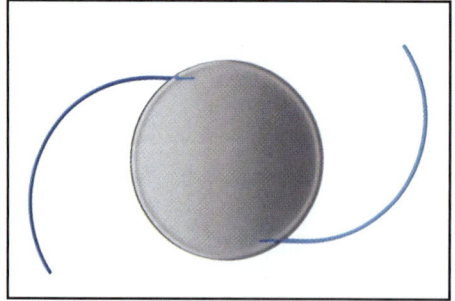

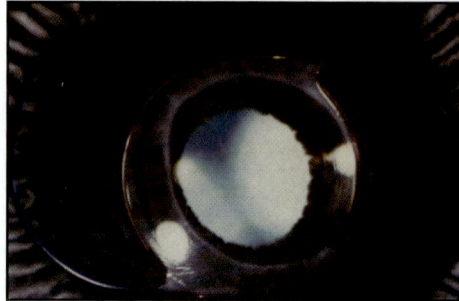

After many years of experimentation with many IOL designs, engineers and researchers concluded that the two basic profiles seen in this figure were the best in terms of fixation and IOL stability within the eye. Note in each case that two haptics or loops were added to the optic. This provided the lens with a stable site on which to fixate.
LEFT: A so-called 3-piece IOL (see page 180), in which the optic is made from one material and the 2 haptics are derived from a secondary type of material.
RIGHT: One-piece IOL design in which the entire lens consists of a single piece of PMMA. In essence, the lenses are cut much as is done with a cookie cutter when preparing cookies in the kitchen.

Recall that as my relationship with Harold matured, my goal was to focus my efforts on two broad categories and functions: firstly, to support him as a friend and as one who was highly deserving of recognition and honors for what he had done, and secondly, to continue the scientific studies on IOLs—which indeed continued up to the time of his death and continue even today.

Table 11-1
EVOLUTION OF THE IOL

I. 1949-1954
Original Ridley posterior chamber, PMMA IOL manufactured by Rayner & Keeler, Ltd.

II. 1952-1962
Early anterior chamber IOLs

III. 1953-1973
Iris-supported IOL. These include iridocapsular IOLs implanted after ECCE

IV. 1963-1992
Transition toward modern anterior chamber IOLs

V. 1977-1992
Transition to and maturation of rigid PMMA posterior chamber IOLs

VI. 1992-2000
Mature PMMA rigid IOLs

Standard capsular IOLs designed specifically for in-the-bag implantation
    Anterior chamber IOLs
    Kelman (flexibility)
    Choyce (footplates)
    Clemente (no-hole three-point fixation)

VII. 1990s-present
Foldable small incision IOLs
Specialized IOLs, eg, accommodative, phakic, toric, telescopic, and others (see Preface).

Following is a list and brief discussion of a few complications of cataract-IOL surgery that I have researched and helped present or treat by informing surgeons regarding the nature of and cause of these and other complications:

1. Lens malpositions (decentration)
2. Material problems (haptic/loop degenerations, optic operations
3. Secondary cataracts (posterior capsule opacification [PCO])
4. Infections (endophthalmitis, uveitis, toxic lens syndrome, toxic anterior segment syndrome [TASS])

CHAPTER 11

IOL Design: Haptics and Loops: Solving the Problem of Decentration

The primary complication that arose with Harold's original posterior chamber lenses was termed "inferior decentration" or the migration of the implanted lens downward in the eye, out of the desired location. Small to moderate shifts were inconsequential. Even the large shifts did not happen as often as was purported at the time, and it rarely caused major visual loss.

Peter Choyce noted the following:

"Actually, he was also not perturbed if a patient's implant dislocated into the posterior segment of the eye, as the material was inert and little damage would be done to the eye. On one occasion, I was assisting him with an operation on a paratrooper. It was important that this patient retain his binocular vision (the vision of the two eyes being used together) so that he could keep his job in the army. Harold had already implanted two lenses on previous operations, both of which were now lying in the patient's vitreous cavity, having been previously dislocated. Harold was now inserting yet another implant. I said to him: 'He will now almost be able to play poker-dice, with his three implants.' Harold was not impressed."

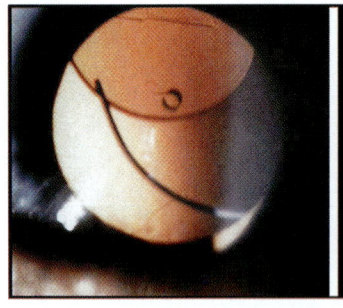

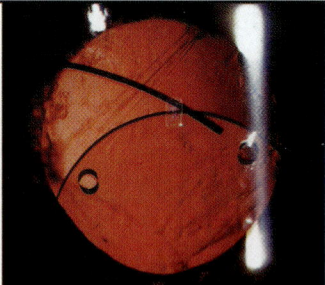

It was thought that the plastic lens was simply too heavy and, therefore, would sink down into the eye. This was true in part, but other factors came into play. The weight factor was actually somewhat negated by the fact that when the IOL is placed in fluid, it became more buoyant. The actual weight of Ridley's IOL was approximately 100 mg. However, within the aqueous solution of the eye, it is effectively decreased to just a few milligrams.

Having observed hundreds of explant specimens and cadaver eyes, it is my strong belief that the main problem was the fact that Harold did not have the advantage of the wonderful anterior capsulotomy technique that we have today, termed the continuous circular curvilinear capsulorhexis (CCC). By having a smooth, intact opening in the front capsule of the lens just large enough to allow insertion of the lenses within the capsular bag, unwanted tears in the surrounding capsule were avoided, and the lens had more support to prevent it from sinking in the eye. When the changes in the surgical technology which occurred in the 1980s, the incidence of this problem radically decreased.

We know today that in general, the best design of any IOL, regardless of whether it is made of two materials or a single material, involves a central optical component designed for vision or as a platform for other specialized functions, such as multifocality, plus two fixation elements on either side of the optic. These are called "haptics" (or "loops") when they are fabricated from suturelike material. In England, John Pearce (1975) was a pioneer in the use of one-piece haptic-IOLs, and in the United States, Steven Shearing (1977) was a pioneer in the use of "loop" PC-IOLs.

In a conversation with Dr. Steven Shearing, one of the first to design a flexible looped posterior chapter IOL, Harold noted, "I'm convinced that the posterior chamber is the right place for the human lens as nature has decided before us and

When the surgeon fails to place the haptics in the proper location, all sorts of lens movement and decentrations may occur. The two decentrations seen here have whimsical names, although of course to the patient, he or she would prefer avoidance of the name and achievement of a good result.
LEFT: Upward lens decentration, termed a sunrise syndrome, based on the final location of the haptics.
RIGHT: This form of decentration is termed a sunset syndrome, reminiscent of the evening sun going down. Both of these forms were caused by the surgeon failing to properly implant the lens haptics in the desired location.

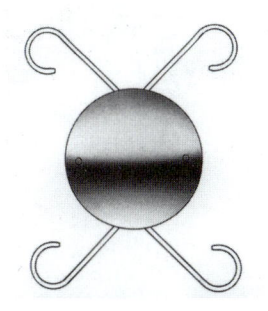

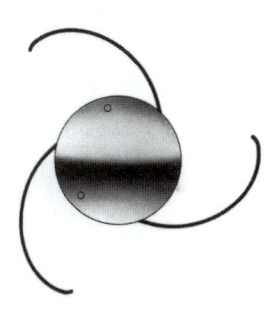

THE GOOD, THE BAD, AND THE UGLY: EVOLUTION OF IOLS, UPS AND DOWNS

For many, many years, lens designers and surgeons, in an effort to improve fixation and essentially make the lens "hold still" within the eye, placed all sorts of types, designs, and numbers of haptics on lenses. This was a laudable goal, but in fact the multiple extra "wires" within the eye could rarely be controlled and these would often scrape against tissues and cause all sorts of problems.
LEFT: Four haptics are present.
RIGHT: Three haptics are present, reminiscent of an airplane propeller.

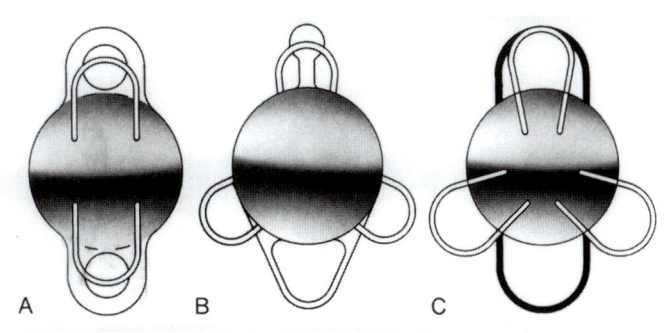

The 3 lenses labeled A, B, and C in this figure represent attempts to tightly fixate the IOL to the surrounding iris tissue in order to avoid lens movement and decentrations.
A, B, C: The multiple extensions and loops could cause damage by scraping (chafing) against adjacent tissues, these turned out to be unsuitable.

God indeed before that. I am particularly impressed with the design of Shearing's IOL."

Shearing was likewise complimentary:

> "My lens is an adaptation of the original Ridley IOL. All lens implanters are the children of Dr. Ridley. I am glad he is pleased with my contribution. There is no doubt that had the technology been available at the time Dr. Ridley was active, he would have come up with a similar design."

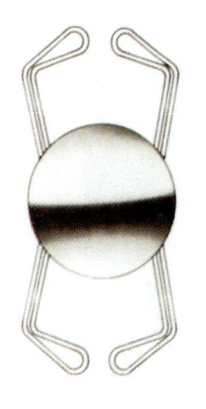

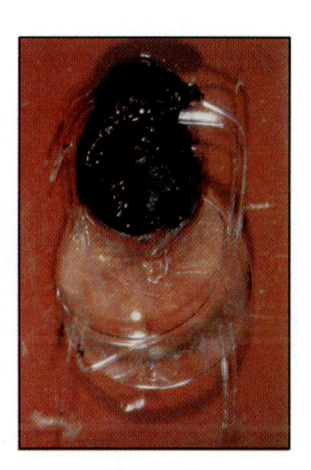

Before this was discovered, numerous designs were attempted to lock the lens in place to prevent decentration. Many IOLs were developed. Many were developed by company engineers collaborating with surgeons. Some surgeons attached multiple haptics and loops to the lens optic in a number of configurations. As we studied these configurations, my colleagues and I often joked that some of the earlier designs would have made better IUDs than IOLs.

The problem with such complicated designs is that they can erode into tissue and break into blood vessels, causing serious problems. When trying to remove these lenses, the eye tissues can be damaged, often causing disastrous results, including the loss of the eye.

A turning point was reached when researchers and surgeons finally realized that such complicated devices were dangerous and could not be tolerated by the eye. A return to simplicity—almost approaching that of Ridley's original lens design using only single haptic or loops with the optic—enabled IOLs to survive.

Even with the right haptic design, however, decentration can occur if the haptics are not inserted correctly into the eye. In order for the lens to remain in the right position, both haptics should be inserted in a symmetrical fashion. When this is not done

This figure exemplifies what happens when extra or extraneous loops on a lens lead to too much contact with the adjacent delicate tissues of the eye.
LEFT: Sketch of a particular lens type showing four pairs of loops.
RIGHT: This is a photograph of the same lens illustrated in the left diagram showing a disaster, namely incarceration of iris tissue and blood within the mulitple loops, necessitating removal of the IOL.

CHAPTER 11

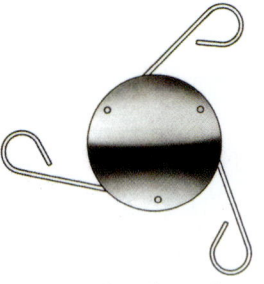

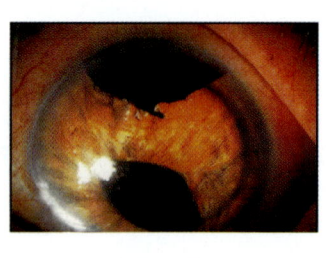

An example of a 3-loop IOL that caused extensive damage requiring removal because of excessive tissue contact.
LEFT: Sketch of the IOL.
RIGHT: An eye following removal of the type of IOL seen on the left, showing the extensive damage that occurred not only as the tissue was contacted by the IOL, but also during the very difficult surgical removal process. Notice the large irregular gaps in the iris that were created as the surgeon carried out the difficult removal procedure.

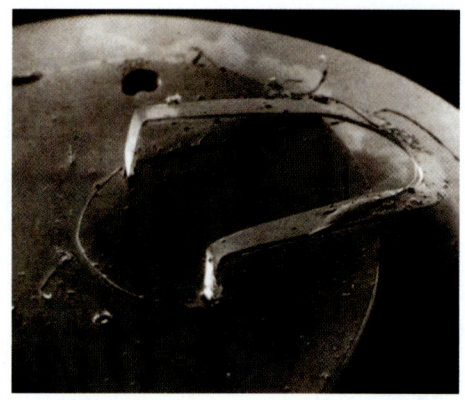

In addition to problems with the number of haptics (or loops) in excessive numbers, the material chosen for haptics may be inappropriate. This scanning electron micrograph demonstrates an example. The lens designer had a strong wish to ensure that the lens remain tightly fixed in position and therefore used a metallic material to clamp the lens in place. This also did not work because the very sharp and rough edges of the metal were not "tissue friendly" in the eye.

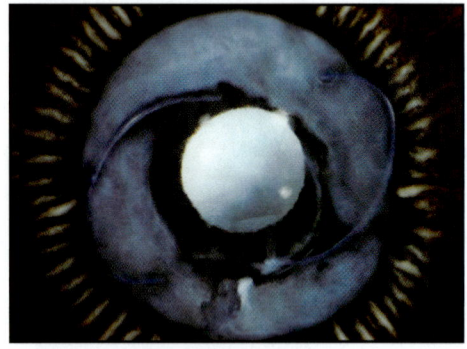

This is a photograph from behind (Miyake-Apple posterior video/photographic technique) showing two problems that had occurred in surgery. First, note the large donut-shaped mass of white material surrounding the center of the IOL. This represents poorly removed cataractous material and would have the potential to become a secondary cataract (see pages 188 and 189). Also, the haptic material of this lens (stained blue in this photograph) would occasionally undergo an alteration or form of biodegradation so that it was not stable in the eye. Lenses of this type have been removed from the market.

(and in the early years it was difficult to do), the lens can move or rotate in one direction or the other.

By the mid-1980s, we finally learned the importance of securing both haptics symmetrically into the evacuated capsular bag. This was a major breakthrough. (The early to mid-1980s, by the way, was a pivotal period for IOLs. The information and experience gained during those years have brought us to where we are today.)

Another malpositioning problem with the IOL surgical technique was the heavy-handedness of some surgeons when inserting the lens. This could cause breakage of the zonules that normally hold the lens in place. The zonules are normally intact all around the lens. However, when broken, there is no reliable chance for the permanent, secure fixation of the lens.

In the 1980s, several breakthroughs were achieved to markedly reduce this potential problem. One important innovation was the introduction of a lubricating material called Healon, manufactured by Pharmacia, Corp (Uppsula, Sweden), which could be used to coat the IOL or used within the eye as a lubricating material. This made possible much safer and smoother surgery with less damage to tissues.

When surgeons learned how to make the above-mentioned CCC (page 180), the smooth-edge cut into the capsule for insertion of the lens, there was another decrease in the rate of complications. In other words, when surgeons found a means to reduce the number of tears in the capsule, there was a marked increase in the probability of proper centration. The CCC was first publicized by Drs. Thomas Neuhann in Munich and Howard Gimbel in Calgary, Alberta, Canada, and according to some, Dr. Calvin Ferrco of North Dakota.

THE GOOD, THE BAD, AND THE UGLY: EVOLUTION OF IOLS, UPS AND DOWNS

MATERIAL PROBLEMS

The problem of the biocompatibility of the implant material was a major one for several decades after Harold's first implant. As it turns out, Flight Lieutenant Cleaver's experience with Harold's choice of material—the PMMA that was used in the cockpits of the World War II airplanes—actually did very well for the IOL's *optic component*. It was the choice of the *haptic material* that often caused problems. Some haptic materials broke down or dissolved over long periods. Nylon, for example, was used for a while and would usually break down.

Problems could, of course, occur with the optic biomaterial itself, including breakdown or destruction due to fracture or cracking. In other instances, certain types of materials could opacify. Another difficulty was related to polishing. When bad manufacturing techniques were used and the edges of the lens were not smoothed out but remained sharp, with sandpaperlike surfaces, the edges of the optic could erode and cut into the adjacent tissues of the iris. Fortunately, these problems have largely been dealt with and now rarely cause complications.

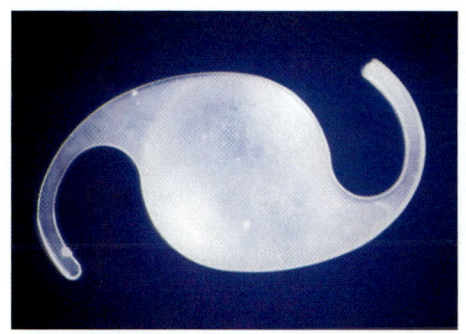

Regarding biocompatibility, in addition to having problems with various subunits of the lens (haptics or loops), the entire lens has been known to undergo a degeneration as seen here. This entire lens is opaque, perhaps because it was fabricated from faulty material. Researchers are carefully working to be sure that this type of problem does not recur.

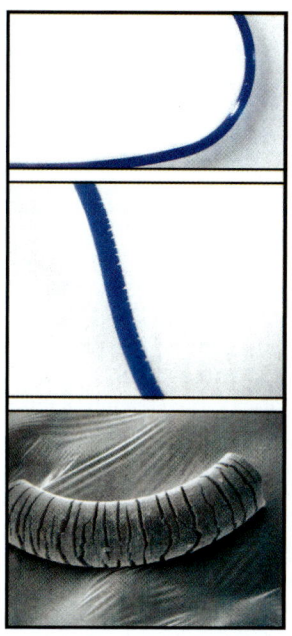

These photographs illustrate the concept of alterations of the loop.
MIDDLE: The blue loop material as photographed with a normal microscope shows numerous parallel clefts, which represent a breakdown and hence loss of strength and stability of this material.
BOTTOM: This high-power photograph is a scanning electron micrograph that shows in detail the surface alterations that occur. This, therefore, represents a biomaterials problem directly affecting the haptic of the IOL.

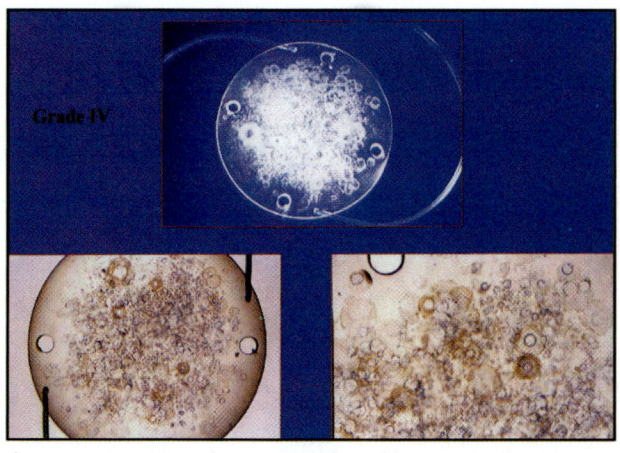

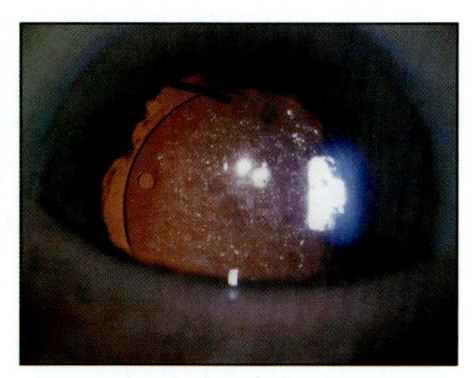

These opaque IOLs show examples of lens optic degeneration (as opposed to the haptic changes seen in a previous photograph). These all represent a disease called "snowflake degeneration," in which poorly manufactured PMMA optics begin to spontaneously crack after 1 to 2 years in the eye.
TOP LEFT: Photograph of an IOL after removal. BOTTOM LEFT: Two higher power photographs. RIGHT: Clinical photograph.

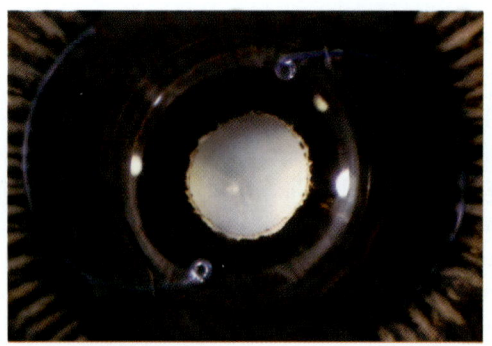

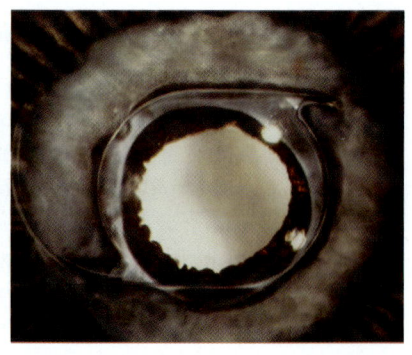

CHAPTER 11

Secondary cataract is a condition in which residual elements of the original cataract returning or regrowing following removal of the cataractous material and implantation of the IOL, causing a secondary opacity. In the past this has been a very common complication (over 50% of cases). It is now better controlled, down to 5% to 10%.

LEFT: The best means to avoid a secondary cataract is to do a very thorough removal of the lens during the primary operation, as was done in the case shown here, as viewed from behind with the Miyake-Apple technique.

RIGHT: The cleanup of this eye was not as thorough, and extensive cortical material (the donut-shaped gray mass) remains in place and is poised to grow over the visual axis to cause the problem that we term secondary cataract.

SECONDARY CATARACTS
(POSTERIOR CAPSULAR OPACIFICATION)

Two surgery-related problems triggered criticism for decades after Harold's initial implant.

The discussion of decentration and posterior capsular opacification (PCO) below brings up an important point regarding the quality of Harold's surgery and his honesty in reporting any problems. His naysayers said he did not report them, an accusation that was categorically *not true!* He discussed these complications from his *very first case,* as noted here: "The two most persistent major complications of my procedure were IOL decentration and posterior capsule opacification."

Harold himself noted these complications of extracapsular cataract extraction with IOL implantation in his earliest patients. Harold recorded these complications in his initial reports. In his first 1951 publications, he described lens decentration, remarking, "Apparently, the most difficult problem was to retain the lens position." Shortly thereafter, he wrote of the difficulty of "devising a method of inserting (the lens) in the eye and retaining it in position." These comments, of course, related to the fundamental issue of lens fixation that is paramount to proper IOL centration and avoidance of decentration, which have been topics of numerous research projects for the past half century.

He also immediately recognized the problem of PCO. In the initial 1951 report, he noted "thickening of the posterior lens capsule is a possible complication not easy to treat." In one report, he designated it as "the principle complication." One of his early cases, which "required division of the posterior capsule from behind," probably represents the first reported mention of the need for secondary posterior capsulotomy after IOL implantation. He recognized that "complete removal of cortical and capsular remnants has sometimes called for considerable perseverance and prolonged irrigation," a recognition of what still remains important is sometimes overlooked in modern procedures—the need for adequate hydrodissection-enhanced cortical clean-up.

It has taken almost half a century, but we are optimistic about achieving control of these two complications. Researchers are beginning to verify this in experimental and clinical studies, and we are seeing very positive results in our laboratory studies of human eyes obtained postmortem with posterior chamber IOLs. Control of decentration and PCO is becoming more necessary now that IOL implantation is emerging as a refractive procedure and mandates almost perfect optical rehabilitation—as opposed to the former goals of simply removing opaque lens material and achieving safe but often less than optimal visual rehabilitation.

Harold's reporting and thoughtful management of these conditions refutes the allegations of naysayers who state the contrary.

A secondary cataract can occur when the surgeon fails to remove all of the cataract tissue during the initial procedure. When this happens, the cataract may actually grow again as the cells proliferate and block the visual axis. About 20 years ago, the incidence of PCO was 50% and was the second most costly surgical procedure that the United States Medicare system had to pay. The number-one cost was the primary cataract operation itself!

We often hear about *laser surgery* for cataracts, but in reality, the only time laser surgery is used for cataracts is when the laser is used to drill a hole in the secondary cataract. A relatively simple maneuver is now used to dramatically lower the risk of this complication. It is called "hydrodissection." The surgeon literally sprays fluid under a very low pressure into the evacuated capsule after the cataract is removed in order to wash out any remaining cells in the capsule that could proliferate to cause a secondary cataract.

The key figures in the development of this procedure include Dr. Kenneth Faust of Leesville, Florida, who coined the term "hydrodissection;" Dr. Howard Fine, who coined the term "cortical cleaving hydrodissection" and popularized this as an important clinical procedure; and researchers in my laboratory who gave it the name "subcapsular hydrodissection." Dr. Ehud Assia of Tel Aviv is another key individual who did research with us in this field. He called the procedure a "subcapsular hydrodissection."

Early surgeons used a knife to cut an opening in the capsule to allow passage of light. Today, the treatment for secondary cataracts is to use a laser to drill a hole into

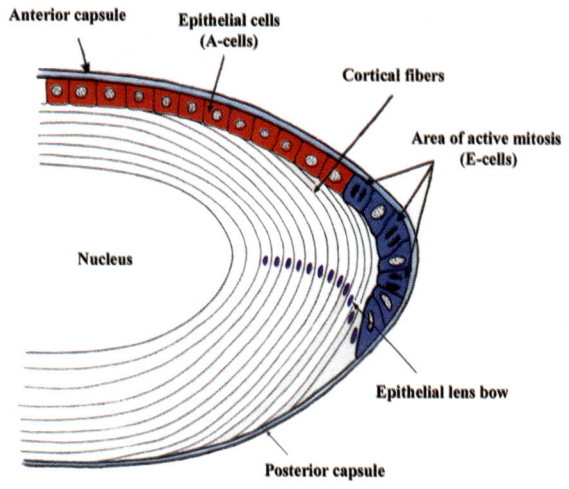

It is tempting to consider the lens as simply amorphous hyaline acellular structure (just like a camera lens), but in reality a biological lens has structure and is made up of cells. The cells are the elements that can proliferate and cause the primary cataract. These same cells, if not completely removed from the eye, can recur again, causing a secondary cataract and leading to the need for a Nd:YAG laser posterior capsulotomy. In this diagram, the cells that are blue in color (labeled E-cells) are the culprits.

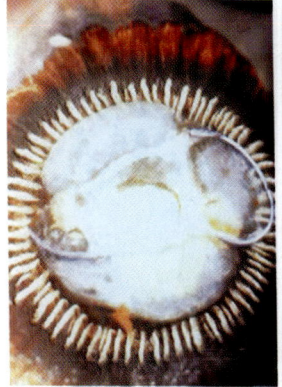

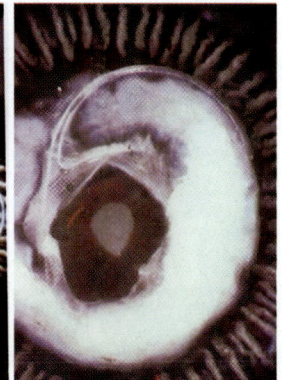

Two examples of secondary cataract as viewed from behind with the Miyake-Apple technique. Both eyes had extensive retained or regrown cataractous material as evidenced by the masses of white material seen overlying the region of the optical component of the IOL.
LEFT: This is an eye that has not been treated for the secondary cataract, so the visual axis is totally clouded by the ingrowth of secondary cells, which causes the central white mass.
RIGHT: The main treatment of this condition is with a laser, a procedure termed the Nd:YAG laser posterior capsulotomy. Notice in this figure how the geometric four-sided cut has been made into the back of the IOL so that the hazy material is absent in that region and the pupil in front of it is visible.
It used to be stated in many regions that the most common cause of blindness was cataract and the second most common cause was treated cataract, namely, the common secondary cataract that often occurred. This is now rapidly changing, and the incidence of secondary cataract is decreasing.

CHAPTER 11

the defective lens. As noted above, this complication used to occur in up to 50% of IOL implant cases. Thanks to many breakthroughs, including hydrodissection, the incidence of secondary cataract development during the past 10 years has been cut down to less than 10% on the average!

Charles Kelman's invention of the technique of phacoemulsification—literally using the technique of a dentist's drill to help dissolve and evacuate the cataractous lens material—must also be mentioned here. The fluid passage through the eye during phacoemulsification is an excellent additive to the already complicated hydrodissection. Phacoemulsification has played a major role in producing the wonderful results that we see today. A well-performed phacoemulsification helps remove lens epithelial cells.

INFECTIONS (ENDOPHTHALMITIS)

Another surgery-related problem that sometimes caused complications after IOL implants was endophthalmitis (infection of the eye). This could happen because of poor sterilization practices or badly manufactured products and often led to loss of the eye. This still occurs occasionally, but in general is under control. An intraocular inflammation or infection of the uvea is called a uveitis.

Over the years, there has always been a danger of infection in the eye when any surgical procedure was done. In several chapters, we have noted that the couching procedure was commonly marred by inflammation and infection, usually caused by a dirty, infected couching needle. This also occurs, although much rarer, after standard cataract surgery as we know it today.

LEFT: Photograph of an eye with postimplant endophthalmitis (total infection of the interior of the eye after the cataract surgery), requiring enucleation, with no hope of restoring the eye. It is filled with pus.

RIGHT: Another case of endophthalmitis viewed at the microscopic level showing the various substructures of the eye. The dark material in the center represents pus, namely acute inflammatory cells and bacterial organisms.

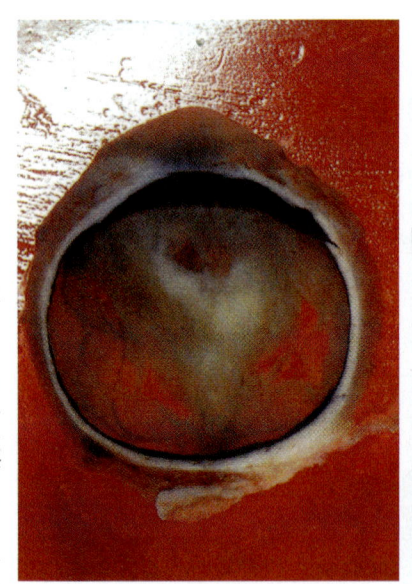

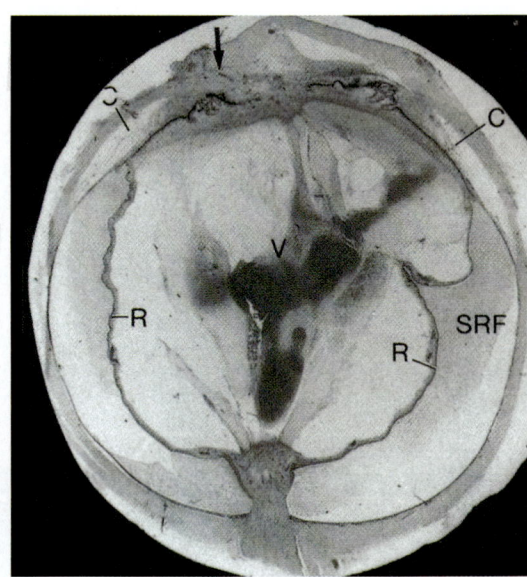

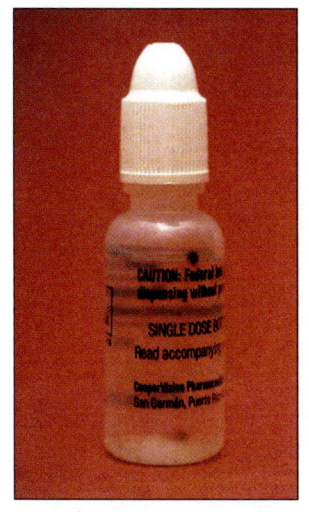

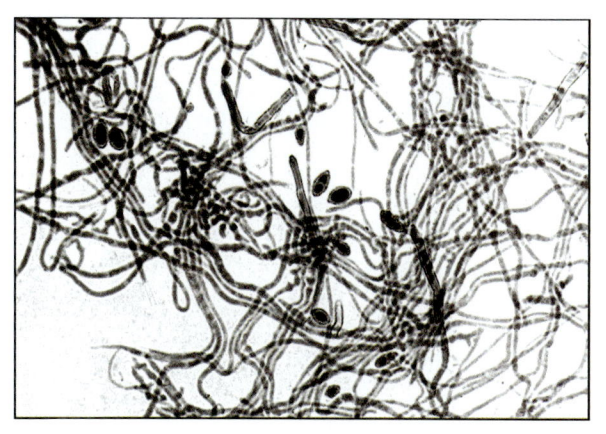

THE GOOD, THE BAD, AND THE UGLY: EVOLUTION OF IOLS, UPS AND DOWNS

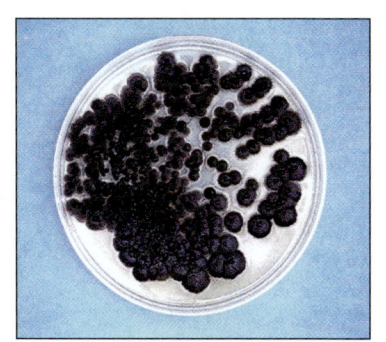

Over the years various pharmacologic agents, ointments, drops, and IOLs themselves would rarely cause reactions, sometimes due to faulty manufacture, sometimes due to misuse in the operating room. The case shown here is an example of that, showing an example of a fungus endophthalmitis that developed after use of specific eye drops.

In the 1980s we saw several cases of anterior segment inflammation, both infectious and non-infectious. It was termed toxic lens syndrome by many surgeons, although this was something of a misnomer because it was not usually caused by the "lens" itself. Presently, the name toxic anterior segment syndrome (TASS) is used. In general, infections caused by faulty eye medications are now fewer and fewer, and avoidable if properly manufactured, as well as adhering to techniques in the operating room. Occasional outbreaks do occur that are genreally manageable if diagnosed properly.

LEFT: Photograph of a bottle irrigating solution. An operating room nurse noticed the dark spot on the interior wall of the bottle. Contamination was suspected.

MIDDLE: Sabourand's agar plate from the bottle of irrigating solution reveals dark growths that are recognized as fungus.

RIGHT: Multiple colonies of fungus, namely *ulocladium sp.*

EVOLUTIONARY EXCELLENCE

These examples are just a few of the types of complications that implant surgeons used to encounter at a high rate. Things are much improved today. The evolution of IOL materials, design, and implantation procedures—and particularly the innovations of the 1980s—have made possible the wonders of the highly specialized ophthalmic surgery that is practiced far and wide today. Those wonders include the foldable IOL—a lens made of malleable rather than rigid materials similar to PMMA that can be folded like a taco and, after the cataractous lens substance is removed by phacoemulsification, introduced into the eye through a small incision. In Chapter 1, we introduced the component of multifocal and bifocal IOLs, and in Chapter 12 we will briefly discuss the use of IOLs for correction of refractive errors such as myopia (near sightedness) or presbyopia.

Hopefully, the BAD and the UGLY have been left to the past, and we can now look forward to the GOOD; who knows where else the future may take us?

On a tomb in the Church of Santa Maria Maggiore in Florence was found an inscription which read: "Here lies Salvino degli Armati, Inventor of Spectacles. May God pardon him his sins."
Nuova Enciclopedia Italianoa, Sixth Edition.

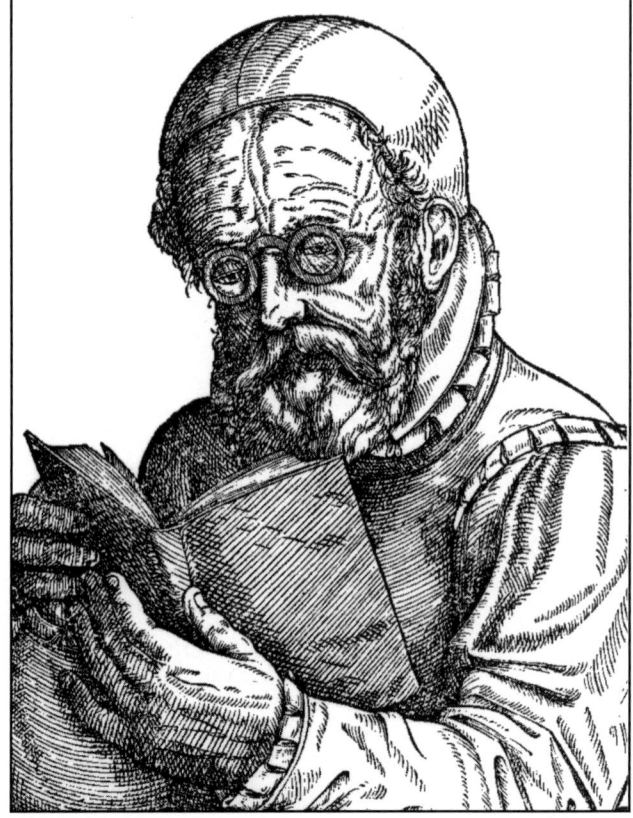

Spectacles have been in existence for centuries; an example of an early bespectacled scholar is seen in this photograph. Aphakic spectacles for use after cataract surgery have been available since the 17th century.

There has been a never-ending quest for individuals to have the opportunity to "get rid of their glasses," no matter what the origin of the need, in order to achieve cosmesis, comfort, and other desirable results.

12

Let's Get Rid of Our Glasses

> *"According to the* Nuova Enciclopedia Italiana *(sixth edition), the following quotation is written on a tomb in the church of Santa Maria Maggiore in Florence, Italy: Here lies Salvino degli Armati, Inventor of Spectacles. May God pardon him his sins."*

> *"The story of Harold Ridley and intraocular lenses is the foundation of refractive surgery. Modern refractive surgery has helped millions of people reduce their dependence on glasses and contact lenses."*
>
> Steven Schallhorn, MD, 2006; Captain, US Navy

Modern cataract surgery is not only a means of removing and replacing an opaque lens, it is now essentially a refractive procedure. With appropriate lens power calculations, sometimes combined with a corneal molding via incisions or suture alterations, a patient's refractive error can be eliminated.

People have worn spectacles for centuries; many for just as long have wished that they did not have to. It is a natural instinct to want to get rid of glasses. Most people feel that they might not look good in glasses and do not like the inconvenience and expense of having to wear and care for them.

Since at least the 17th century, thick postcataract aphakic spectacles were the main and often the only means of achieving visual rehabilitation after removal of the opaque, cataractous lens. Since this time, these glasses were undesirable because of the unwanted optical effects and aberrations that invariably occurred. As we have noted previously, looking through these thick spectacles is like looking through the bottom of a cola bottle, with many distortions. Worse, in the under-

CHAPTER 12

privileged world the use of aphakic spectacles was often disastrous. When a patient's glasses were lost or broken, more often than not, they could not be replaced. Without glasses, the vision of these patients was often worse than before the operation.

There are individuals who have refractive errors such as nearsightedness whose vision may improve to normal with standard spectacles or contact lenses. However, they would simply like to "get rid of the spectacles" and be able to have the same high-quality vision without the need of these devices. The subspecialty of refractive surgery is simply defined as a type of surgery designed primarily to correct such errors as nearsightedness, farsightedness, and astigmatism—as opposed to surgery to remove an opacity such as the lens and thus cure blindness. The former has emerged and become very popular during the past two decades.

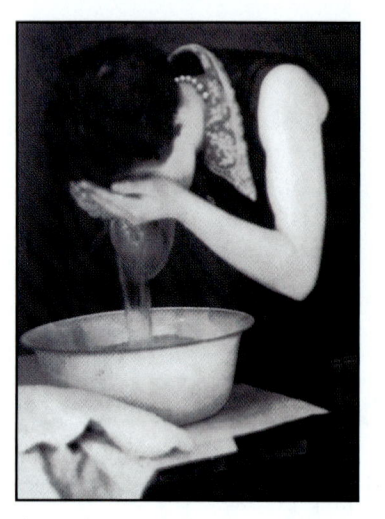

In the late 19th and early 20th centuries (and probably still today), books have been written describing unique methods for curing imperfect sight, especially myopia (nearsightedness), without spectacles. Unfortunately, time and experience have shown that many of these methods were of absolutely no use. Spectacles and later contact lenses remained the only practical means of curing the main refractive errors, astigmatism, and presbyopia (the farsightedness of aging).

Two definitions are important in differentiating standard cataract-IOL surgery and refractive surgery.

Cataract-IOL surgery is performed to improve vision in patients with visual disability or indeed to cure blindness in the partially blind patient. As has been emphasized in several previous chapters (see Chapters 5 and 6), it is a visual rehabilitation.

Refractive surgery is a vision correction surgery and is not performed on a patient with frank visual disability or blindness, but rather generally performed on a patients who are correctible to a good or excellent visual acuity (20/20 or 6/6) when wearing a device or appliance such as glasses or contact lenses. The usual goal is to enable the patient to function without any device.

Patients who require refractive surgery are not merely people who desire a cosmetic procedure or who might be categorized as "vain." Even if this was the case, this is in no way an objectionable reason. Rather, refractive surgery is justifiable for many firm, obvious medical reasons (eg, the inability to tolerate contact lenses or important occupational reason). A very obvious example is the need for a pilot to have continuous perfect vision to carry out the duties of this occupation. Comments in this chapter by Steven Schallhorn, Captain, US Navy (see following) and a recent article in *The New York Times* by David S. Cloud refer specifically to the issue of aviator's vision. In the June 20, 2006 edition of *The New York Times,* Cloud writes:

> *"Nearly a third of every 1,000-member Naval Academy class now undergoes the procedure, part of a booming trend among military personnel with poor vision. Unlike in the civilian world, where eye surgery is still largely done for convenience or vanity, the procedure's popularity in the armed forces is transforming career choices and daily life in subtle but far-reaching ways.*

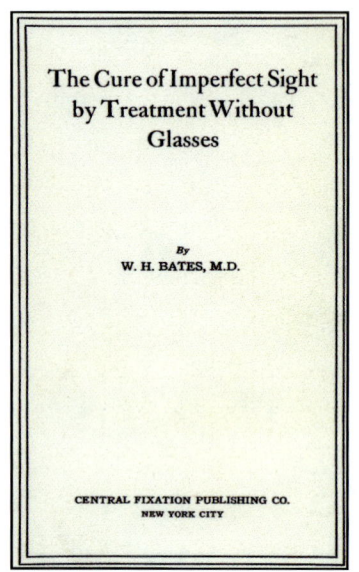

For many years, health care deliverers have attempted to correct errors of refraction, especially nearsightedness or myopia, by various nonmedical means, for example as seen here with eye washing. In general, these have often been within the realm of the charlatan or quack and have not been successful.

Today, better means are available to truly say that we are on the trail of attacking and hopefully minimizing the need for visual appliances such as glasses and contact lenses.

> **Table 12-1**
>
> ## TYPES OF REFRACTIVE SURGERY
>
> I. Corneal refractive surgery
>   A. Incisional, corneal surgery (either with a surgical knife or a machine)
>   1. Radial keratotomy
>   2. Keratomileusis
>
>   B. Laser corneal surgery
>   1. Photorefractive keratectomy (PRK) (laser only, no surgical flap)
>   2. Laser-assisted keratomileusis (LASIK) (combined laser and surgical flap)
>
> II. IOL refractive surgery
>   A. Refractive lens exchange
>   B. Phakic IOLs
>   C. Multifocal IOLs
>   D. Toric IOLs for astigmatism

"Again fighter pilots can now remain in the cockpit longer, reducing annual recruiting needs. And recruits whose bad vision once would have a disqualified them from the Special Forces are now eligible, making the competition for these coveted slots even tougher."

In recent years, there has been a race among proponents of the various types of refractive surgery to establish the supremacy of their particular techniques. Major categories of refractive surgery are listed in Table 12-1.

A detailed discussion of refractive surgery techniques is beyond the scope of this book. My main goal is to demonstrate the close relationship between cataract-IOL and refractive surgery, both in evolution and with regard to techniques and goals of the surgical procedures. This relationship is not well known to the general public and indeed is not even well known to some eye care professionals.

The paradigm has changed today. Cataract surgery is always a simultaneous refractive surgery. With the cataract operation, it is no longer enough to remove the opaque lens and insert an IOL that gives the patient an approximate correction. The goal is to achieve a correction of all parameters. Techniques are now used to bypass the cornea and simply insert an IOL over the normal lens of a patient with a high refractive error and thus utilize the IOL itself to correct the error (phakic IOLs). The technique of refractive lens exchange has been determined to be safe and is now popular. This is a technique in which the crystalline lens is removed and an IOL is inserted with the correct final necessary power recalculated. In other words, the goal is to perfect vision (emmetropia) by recalculating the power of the IOL necessary to achieve perfect or almost perfect vision in a given patient.

We live in a new world, and it is useful that physicians and patients alike understand the relationship between basic cataract-IOL surgery and refractive surgery. I have asked Dr. Stephen Schallhorn, Captain, US Navy, one of the world's most prominent cataract and corneal surgeons, to send me his comments regarding the evolutionary process from pure cataract-IOL surgery to refractive surgery to a combination of both. Schallhorn has a very important task in treating pilots who of course require excellent vision. His comments reflect very clearly in a few paragraphs what has happened, namely the transitional process between early cataract surgery and what will be required today and in the future from ophthalmologists.

His comments are as follows:

"We take for granted advances that have occurred in medicine. This is no more apparent than that of the modern cataract procedure. While the surgery may only take 15 minutes to perform, this belies the complexity of the procedure and the effort that has gone into its development over the years. Advances have made this procedure one of the most successful in the history of medicine. What was once the leading cause of blindness in the world can now be cured with a single surgical procedure. Millions have benefited.

"Cataracts are a natural result of the human aging process in which the lens inside our eye becomes cloudy and opaque. Simply removing the cataract is only half of the solution to restoring vision. Without replacing the cataract with a lens inside the eye, either special contact lenses or thick coke-bottle glasses are needed to regain vision. The vision through these glasses is usually inadequate due to optical aberrations and visual distortion. Here we come to the pioneer work of Harold Ridley as described by another pillar in the ophthalmic field of intraocular lens implantation, Dr. David Apple.

"The story of the intraocular lens really starts with Mr. Ridley's observation of a fighter pilot named 'Mouse' Cleaver. 'Mouse' was flying a Hurricane fighter in the 1940 Battle of Britain when he came under enemy fire. Shards of his canopy were embedded into his eyes. The Plexiglas did not seem to cause inflammation in the eye, as almost every other foreign substance would. Ridley had the foresight to realize that this material could be crafted as a lens and placed in the eye after cataract removal. He then worked with industry to produce and implant lenses. It sounds simple, but it certainly wasn't as David appropriately describes in this book. Mr. Ridley was vilified for many years by colleagues. Thank goodness he persevered.

"This is an amazing story and especially personal to me as a fighter pilot and ophthalmologist. The innovation of IOLs has its roots in aviation. Reducing dependence on cumbersome and visually-disabling glasses, the story here of Mr. Ridley and IOLs is the foundation of refractive surgery. Modern refractive surgery has helped millions of people reduce their dependence on glasses and contact lenses. I developed refractive surgery programs to do the same for aviators. Over 1,000 Navy and Marine aviators have been successfully treated and returned to flying and over 500 students have entered flight training after refractive surgery who otherwise would not have qualified. We have come full circle since Mr. Ridley's pioneer work in the 1940s. A fighter pilot helped start a new field and now we are helping aviators.

"Everyone who has or will undergo a cataract procedure owes a debt of gratitude to the innovation, perseverance, and determination of a true hero to humanity, Mr. Harold Ridley."

Corneal Refractive Surgery

The first type of surgery to come into common usage was the incisional form (see Table 12-1). This method is not new. In fact, it was attempted over a century ago, at

LET'S GET RID OF OUR GLASSES

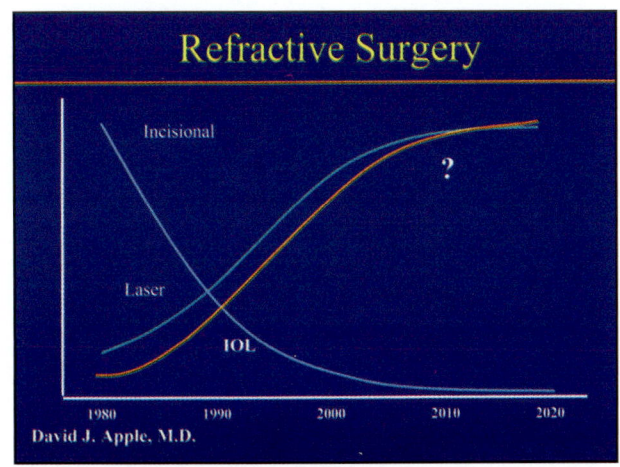

Medical/surgical means of correcting errors of refraction (myopia, hyperopia, presbyopia, astigmatism) have long been dreamed of but results have improved only during the 20th century. There are basically two forms of refractive corrections that are invoked now, namely incisional correction and correction using IOLs. At present, it seems that there is a contest regarding which form will be most accepted first by clinicians. At the moment, there seems to be a swing in pendulum back toward IOLs with refractive capabilities (eg, multifocal IOLs [see Chapter 1]).

TOP (left): A graph correlating the relative incidence of the 2 techniques as seen in the American market.

BOTTOM (left): One of the first examples of an incisional keratopathy, actually a radiokeratotomy performed experimentally in rabbits, work of Professor L. J. Lans, Leiden, 1896. This obviously provided stimulus for Sato and Fyodorov to perform their great work in the fields of radiokeratotomy.

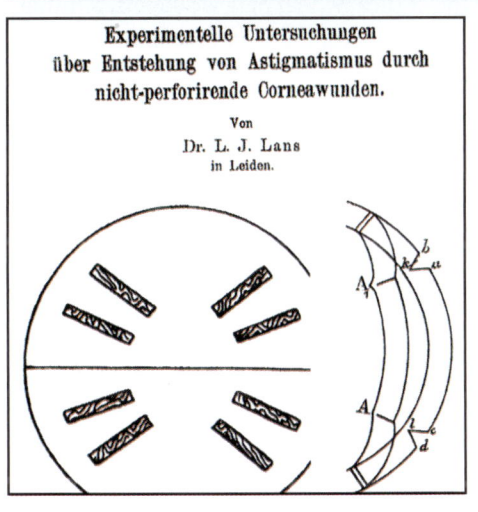

least on an experimental basis. A Dutch physician, Leendert Jan Lans was doing corneal operations on experimental animals. A perusal of the photographs from his early article in the German literature shows that he was actually doing what we now call radial keratotomy (ie, placing radial incisions or slits into the cornea. In doing so, he made the cornea flatter, thus providing a correction for myopia (nearsightedness). Radial keratotomy became a common and popular clinical procedure, implemented in early years by Sato in Japan and not long thereafter by Svyatoslav Fyodorov in the Soviet Union.

Fyodorov's work was very instrumental in truly "getting the ball rolling" in the field of refractive surgery. He was an innovative surgeon who, in addition to popular-

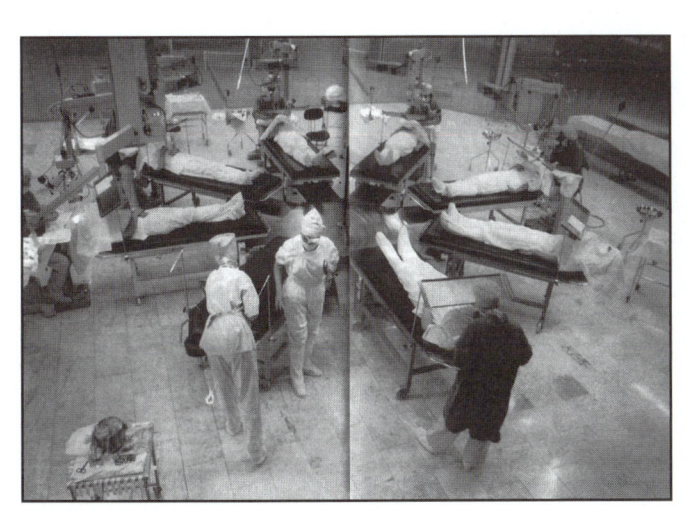

The most famous conception of Fyodorov is the large assembly line that he set up in his Moscow facility to increase the efficiency of radiokeratotomy performance that was done by several surgeons in one sitting. A surgeon manned each station (bed) and gave his or her designated incision as the patient was slowly turned around on the stations, so that at the end of the operation, the complete radiokeratotomy done in rabbits over 100 years ago was completed.

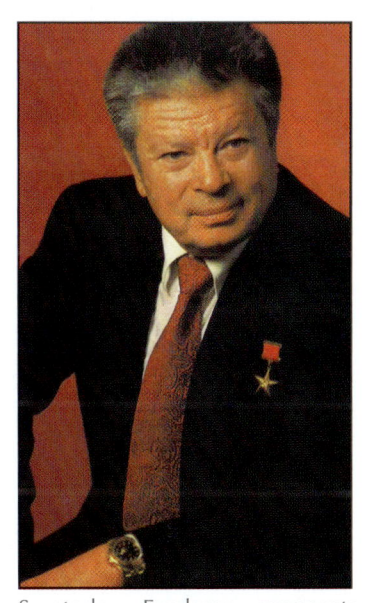

Svyatoslav Fyodorov represents one of the great figures in anterior segment surgery, both refractive and IOL surgery. He is best known as one of the founders of incisional refractive surgery, most specifically radiokeratotomy. Also, he was one of the very first in 1951 to recognize the validity and greatness of Ridley's work as he invented the IOL, including the application of Ridley's IOLs for various types of refractive surgery.

Fyodorov remained a loyal supporter of Ridley throughout his life.

izing the radial keratotomy technique, developed the well-known surgical suite (operating room or operating theater) in which the operating tables were placed in a circle and the patients were moved around so that each surgeon would be able to place a slit in the patient's cornea at the appropriate angle. It functioned like a "Detroit assembly line" and by the time the patient was finished, multiple radial incisions were complete. Fyodorov worked virtually as a capitalist in his large communist nation for many years, and he established several clinics across the entire span of his country.

Another type of incisional refractive surgery is keratomileusis, which is performing a surgical incision into the cornea. It is designed to flatten the cornea and change the refractive error. Dr. Jose Barraquer in Bogotá, Colombia pioneered this. This procedure is basically the forerunner of the modern LASIK technique that is very popular today.

Laser refractive surgery is a popular technique, but there are two possible disadvantages. First, there is a surgical entrance into the cornea, which may weaken it, although this has not been a broad problem. Second, the technique is irreversible. The incisional and laser techniques are far beyond the scope of this book, although I want to again emphasize that the optical principles used with these and also with IOL refractive surgery are those developed not only by the early pioneers in centuries gone by, but also by surgeons and rescuers working first in the field of cataract-IOL surgery.

Intraocular Lens Refractive Surgery

The possibility of using IOLs as a means of refractive surgery became a reality the day that Harold invented the IOL. His revolutionary procedure opened the door to numerous advancements (see Preface), including the broad field of refractive vision-enhancing devices that may at first glance seem unrelated but are not; devices that are used universally today.

Among the first surgeons to clinically apply the technique of IOL refractive surgery were Peter Choyce in England, Dr. B. Strampelli in Italy, and Dr. Barraquer in Colombia. Among other things, Choyce authored a monograph in 1964 that offered schematic illustrations of the various types of IOLs that could be manufactured to correct the major refractive errors. These were done beginning in the 1950s, using the anterior chamber IOL designs that were available at that time. In general, progress in this area was slow because some of these lenses failed due to improper design and surgical techniques. It is a well-known story that Dr. Barraquer had implanted numerous phakic AC IOLs into patients solely for vision corrective refractive surgery without removal of the patient's lens. A huge number had

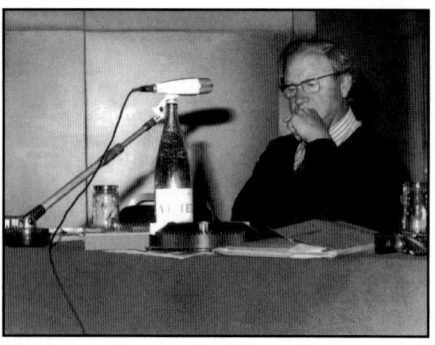

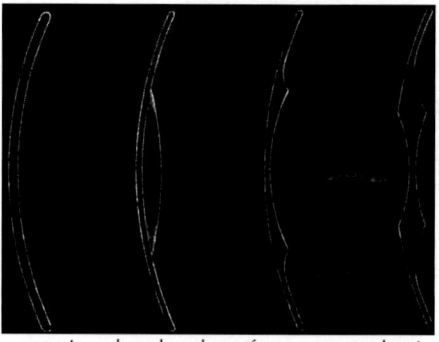

Choyce and several of his colleagues, utilizing anterior chamber lens formats as a basis, designed several lenses for treatment of most types of refractive errors.
LEFT: Choyce pondering the topic of refractive surgery.
RIGHT: A drawing by Choyce showing several types of anterior chamber IOLs (each individually designed for treatment of the various refractive areas, ranging from ametropia [no problems] to advanced myopia [near sightedness]).

to be removed because of complications. These were sent to Dr. Robert Drews in St. Louis, MO who reported these in the literature. This put a halt on the technique on the IOL refractive surgery and indeed almost fatally injured the reputation of IOLs in general. The reason these lenses failed was not because of Dr. Barraquer's technique (he was then the best) and was not a slur against IOLs in general. The failure in his cases occurred because he only had access to some of the poorly designed lenses that had been manufactured.

Nevertheless, the groundwork was established.

Peter Choyce also played an important role in the broad field of refractive surgery that was very important no matter what the technique. To my knowledge, he was the first to take systematic and scientific measurements of the various anterior structures into which corneal incisions had to be made or IOLs had to be implanted, regardless of whether they are phakic or aphakic. In the early years, one of the main reasons for IOL failure, and still today in rare cases, was improper sizing of the lens so that the haptics did not become situated in the correct position. This violated one of the major laws of biomedical engineering and organ transplantation, namely the requirement that the device be correctly fixated (see Chapter 11). Only recently have more precise measurements been made with modern techniques such as ultrasound biomicroscopy.

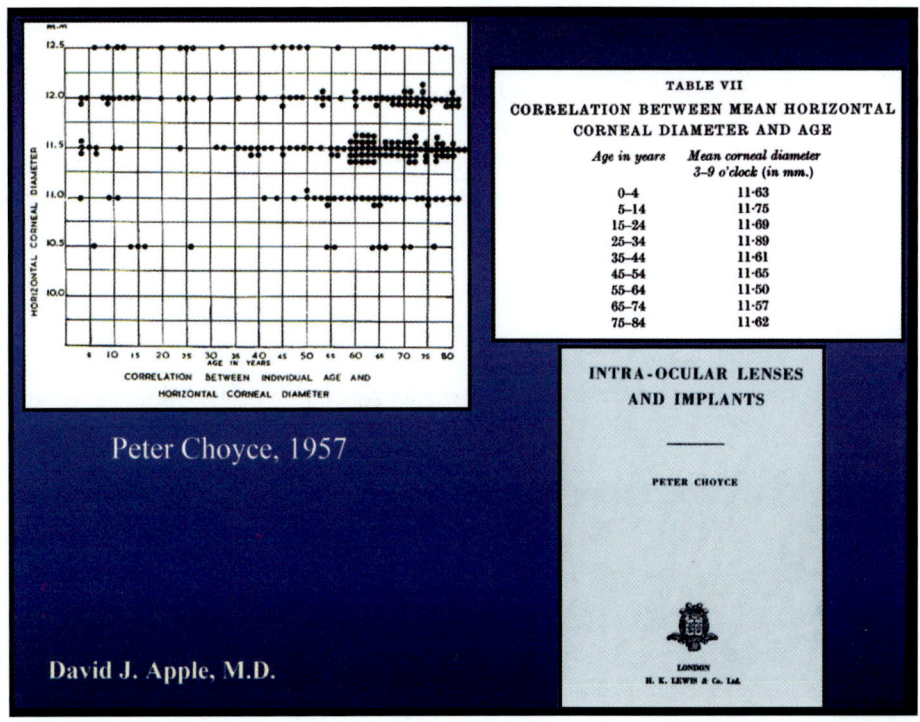

One of Choyce's greatest contributions was his success in performing measurements of the eye tissues that were relevant for various types of implantation. There were no serious attempts at measuring the various tissue sizes in the eye prior to his work, so it was difficult to get a good "fit" of the IOL in a given eye. Therefore, it is no wonder that decentrations were often seen at an unacceptable level. These illustrations are from his 1957 textbook, a book consisting of multiple articles that were turned down for publications in the "establishment" literature, and which he therefore published himself. Many of these were masterpieces.

Choyce, based on teachings from Ridley in collaboration with others, did work on corneal devices, including the device called a keratoprosthesis as seen here. This might be considered an attempt to form a "bionic cornea."
TOP: High-power photograph of a keratoprosthesis.
BOTTOM: The main function of the keratoprosthesis is to remove opaque, useless corneal tissue (upper left), implant the keratoprosthesis, and achieve a result as seen on the upper right where the visual axis is clear.

Choyce also bridged the basic areas of corneal and IOL refractive surgery by doing early work in the field of corneal modification and corneal implants. He and his British colleague, Dr. Michael Roper-Hall, did work in terms of changing the shape of the cornea, doing implants in the cornea, not only for refractive purposes but also to treat diseases. A major example of the latter is an early form of what some today call an "artificial or bionic" cornea, the keratoprosthesis.

SVYATOSLAV FYODOROV

Moving ahead to the 1980s, we come again to Svyatoslav Fyodorov, who played an immense role in virtually all aspects of cataract and refractive surgery. His was an amazing record. He played a prime role in the development of basic IOL surgery. In 1950, as soon as he had heard of Harold's original implantations, he immediately traveled the long distance from his home in the northern reaches of the Soviet Union to London to become familiar with the technique.

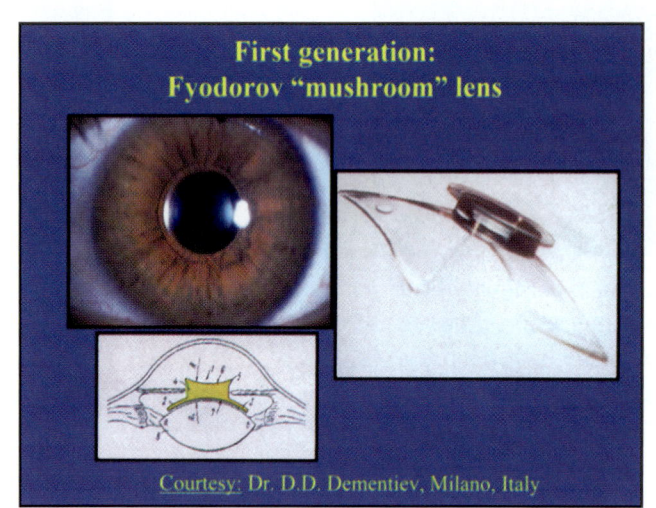

Until the day of his death, Fyodorov was a devoted friend and adamant supporter of Harold—none was more loyal and Fyodorov participated in the major events honoring Harold, until shortly before his death. He was truly a faithful follower and his close attention to details learned from the Ridley School in London helped him achieve fine results in the far northern reaches of the former Soviet Union and eventually Moscow. He played a huge role in incisional refractive surgery, as just mentioned with radial keratotomy. He was a major player in the development of phakic IOLs.

In addition to Choyce's primary work with refractive IOLs, Fyodorov also worked in this field, his first design being what was termed the "mushroom" lens as seen here in the clinical photograph and in sketches. It was a "phakic lens" designed to be placed on the crystalline lens and intended to change the patient's refraction so that glasses could indeed be discarded. In essence, it was a cosmetic procedure.

I personally had the opportunity to meet him many times at various functions just prior to his untimely death in 2000. He died in a helicopter crash. He had been involved in the rough-and-tumble world of Soviet politics and was a presidential candidate at one time.

PHAKIC INTRAOCULAR LENSES

Fyodorov had the vision to recognize a very important aspect of Harold's invention, namely, that the IOL was not only important in and of itself, but that it was also important in leading surgeons and researchers to explore the new techniques of microsurgery as applied to the eye. Having designed IOLs for normal cataract surgery (aphakic IOLs), IOLs implanted in patients in which the crystalline lens had been removed, Fyodorov was one of the first to design and popularize a type of refractive IOL, the phakic IOL. An aphakic IOL is designed to be implanted for the purposes of correcting refractive errors without removing the patient's own lens. The eye remains phakic (with a lens) and the surgeon then calculates the power

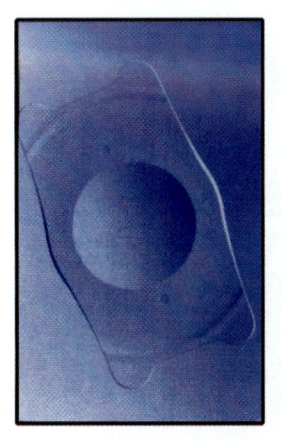

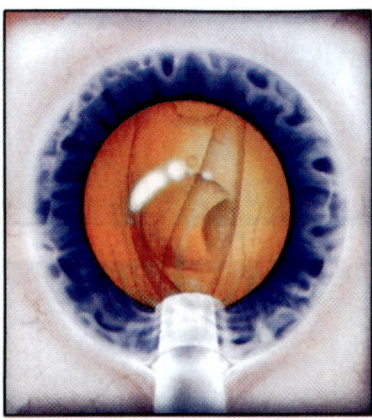

LET'S GET RID OF OUR GLASSES

The lens sketch shown here shows a phakic IOL, a foldable-style lens that can be introduced in the eye after folding through a small incision. It then opens up on the patient's lens and can be effective in changing the patient's refraction.

necessary for the additional IOL, which is then fitted in the eye in tandem with the patient's own normal lens.

In the early years of its use, during a period when this would have been considered malpractice in the United States and some other countries, Fyodorov had the freedom in his country to implant IOLs in patients who were basically normal except for the refractive error. The IOL would be placed adjacent to the patient's own lens for the sole purpose of changing refractive or focusing power of the eye. The required thickness of the IOL could be calculated by performing preoperative measurements and determining the degree of nearsightedness or farsightedness. The principles for this type of work were of course based on the early work by Harold, Choyce, and others in London.

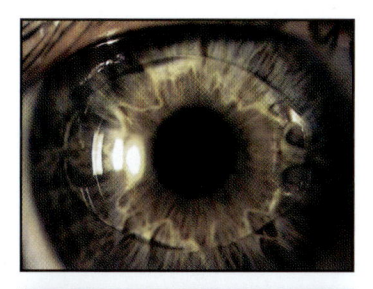

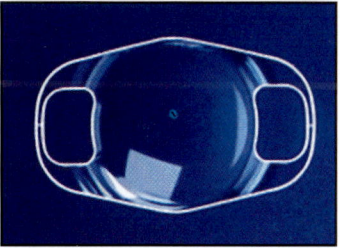

Many phakic IOL designs have been marketed. One of the most popular is called the intraocular contact lens (ICL). It is manufactured by Staar Surgical Corporation, which received approval from the United States Food and Drug Administration in 2006. The lens seems to work very well in most cases, but a few cases of secondary cataract have been shown to form, perhaps caused by the IOL touching the patient's lens.

The Verisyse IOL, manufactured by Advanced Medical Optics (AMO), is another example of a phakic IOL design that is placed in the eye. It is attached to the iris adjacent to the clear, crystalline lens. Alcon Corporation markets an anterior chamber phakic IOL—something that would make Peter Choyce, who campaigned for this IOL type for many years, very happy.

A recent innovation had been the introduction of a variation of the former iris claw lens, termed now the Varices lens (an IOL that actually can be attached to the front of the iris at 2 sites, as seen here and thus provide a refractive change while the patient's own lens is still in place).
TOP: Clinical photograph.
BOTTOM: Artist drawing.

BIFOCAL AND MULTIFOCAL INTRAOCULAR LENSES

Bifocal and multifocal IOLs have been a dream for many years. We saw in Chapter 1 that Hamdi and Reese were the first to suggest such an IOL. The first bifocal IOL that was manufactured by IOLab Corporation and the implant was a design by John Pierce in England.

Multifocal lenses have been tried extensively throughout the 1980s and 1990s and have had their ups and downs. Successful multifocal IOLs would be highly desirable

CHAPTER 12

The laser-related refractive procedures are beyond the scope of this text. LASIK has become immensely popular over the years, although intraocular lens refractive surgery seems to be having a resurgence.

Some refractive surgeons now also deal with cosmetic issues (eg, pearls placed on the sclera [upper right] and others). Much of this draws a fine line between pure medical treatment and cosmetic treatment, but whatever the market bears will be provided.

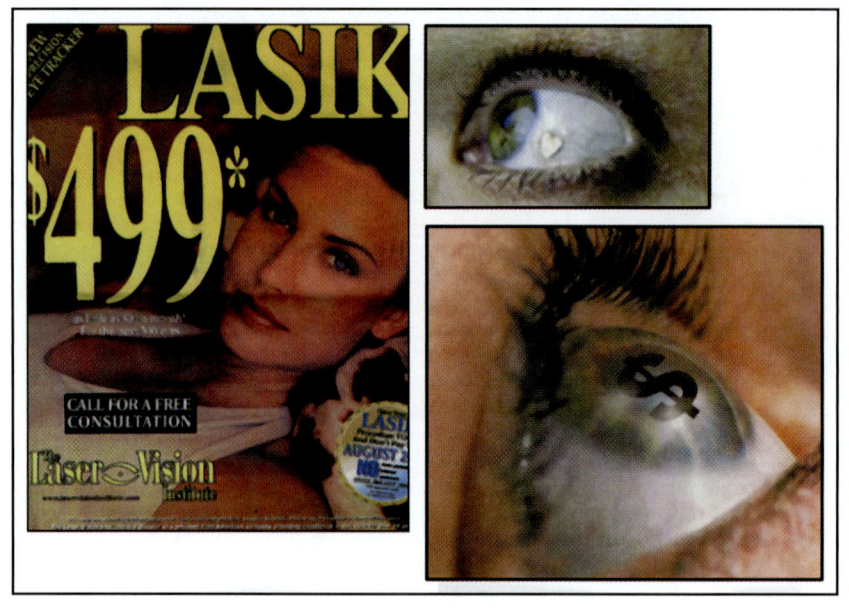

because they would permit focus through all ranges from very near to very far, impossible with regular IOLs. The concentric rings of a multifocal lens are cut into the front surface of the IOL optic (see Chapter 1), thus allowing for vision at both near and far. They are therefore ideal in that they can function as IOLs to not only replace cataractous lenses that have been removed but also to precisely correct refractive errors.

The Start of Something Big

Harold's invention of the IOL not only vastly extended the horizon of possibilities available to patients with vision problems (see Preface) but also helped launched a new medical-industrial complex.

The IOL began to be sold as a profitable product, and when surgical techniques such as laser therapy and numerous new pharmacologic entities came into existence, eye care became a huge business. It has almost come to the point that some types of refractive surgery are in reality a cosmetic surgery. Indeed, some clinics are arranged in a way that ophthalmology offices and surgical suites are placed in or adjacent to the practices of cosmetic plastic surgeons.

Surely, Harold would have been surprised but very pleased at the changes that have been brought about by his invention over 50 years ago. Knowing him well, the only comment he would have would be the possibility that extensive manpower would be taken away from the primary goal of curing blindness, in lieu of surgeons doing cosmetic surgery. I do not believe this has happened, but we should guard against that for the future.

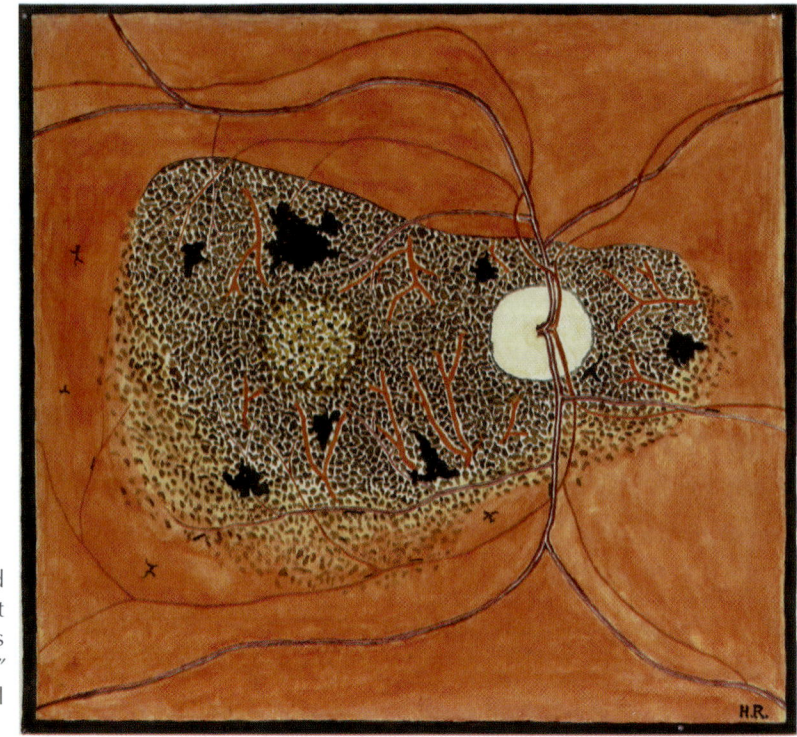

A color fundus drawing (a drawing made by Harold himself) showing the important changes that can occur in the retina and macular region. This rendition is termed by many the *"Ridley fundus."* It has become a classic and is used in virtually all articles and texts that deal with onchocerciasis.

13

Innovations in Addition to the Intraocular Lens

"I hope you will not forget to mention the Ridley Foundation. Some people think we might have done more entertaining, but alcoholic parties as opposed to small gatherings of friends do not greatly appeal to us. Please mention too the active work we undertook in tropical countries almost every year, for no one else did this sort of thing at that time."

Harold Ridley

TROPICAL OPHTHALMOLOGY: ONCHOCERCIASIS (RIVER BLINDNESS) AND CATARACT-IOL SURGERY IN THE DEVELOPING WORLD

Although Harold's invention of the IOL provided a procedure that finally made cataract surgery successful and complete, he showed foresight, creativity, and innovation in several other areas related to the science of the eye.

Table 13-1 lists, in no particular order, several subspecialties of ophthalmology that probably represent a large cross-section, possibly 70% to 90% of the clinical specialty. Note that Harold did work in most of these areas throughout the years, even while he was busy first inventing and then defending his cataract-IOL procedure.

Harold was particularly proud of his efforts in the field of tropical ophthalmology, namely diagnosis and treatment of eye diseases in many underprivileged areas of the world. For example, large surgery centers are being set up in many

CHAPTER 13

Table 13-1
SUBSPECIALTIES OF CLINICAL OPHTHALMOLOGY

1. Cataract-IOL surgery (Chapters 1 through 12)
2. Corneal and refractive surgery
   a. Corneal incisional refractive surgery, eg, radial keratotomy, keratomileusis (Chapter 12)
   b. Corneal laser refractive surgery, eg, LASIK
   c. Specialized IOLs designed for refractive surgery (Chapter 12)
3. Retinal optic nerve diseases including nutritional amblyopia and age-related macular degeneration (Chapter 14)
4. Eye plastic surgery (cosmetic and aesthetic), including artificial irides to alter iris appearance and/or color (Chapter 7)
5. Diagnostic and teaching techniques, including television in ophthalmology, telediagnosis (Chapter 15)
6. Glaucoma, including optic nerve (disc) analysis (Chapter 15)
7. Non-invasive diagnosis of the retina and optic nerve (Chapter 15)
8. Neuro-ophthalmology, including optic nerve diseases (Chapter 15)
9. Ocular oncology (Tumors)   (Chapter 15)
10. Pediatric ophthalmology, including pediatric IOLs (Chapter 15)
11. Tropical ophthalmology, including nutritional and infectious diseases (Chapters 13 and 14)

Harold had an intense interest in tropical ophthalmology (ie, treatment of patients in the underprivileged world). This was based in part on the fact that his mother was raised in India, that there was much contact of English people with the various countries of the Empire, including many poor countries, and he traveled extensively in the various countries that we today would term the underprivileged world.

LEFT: Title page of Harold's classic article on ocular onchocerciasis, published as a supplement to the *British Journal of Ophthalmology* in 1945. Being inducted into the army in 1943 as a major, he was sent by Brigadier Sir Stewart Duke-Elder, in charge of all things related to ophthalmology and the military, to Ghana in Africa. This was not a battle area and it was not considered a desirable assignment. However, as was typical with his intellect, he made the best of this assignment and indeed made several important discoveries in addition to river blindness, vitamin A deficiency, leprosy, and others while serving in this and other regions of the developing world.

RIGHT TOP: Title page of another article on tropical diseases by Harold.

RIGHT BOTTOM: Still another article dealing with toxoplasmosis. His work on onchocerciasis is his best known work with the exception, of course, of the IOL.

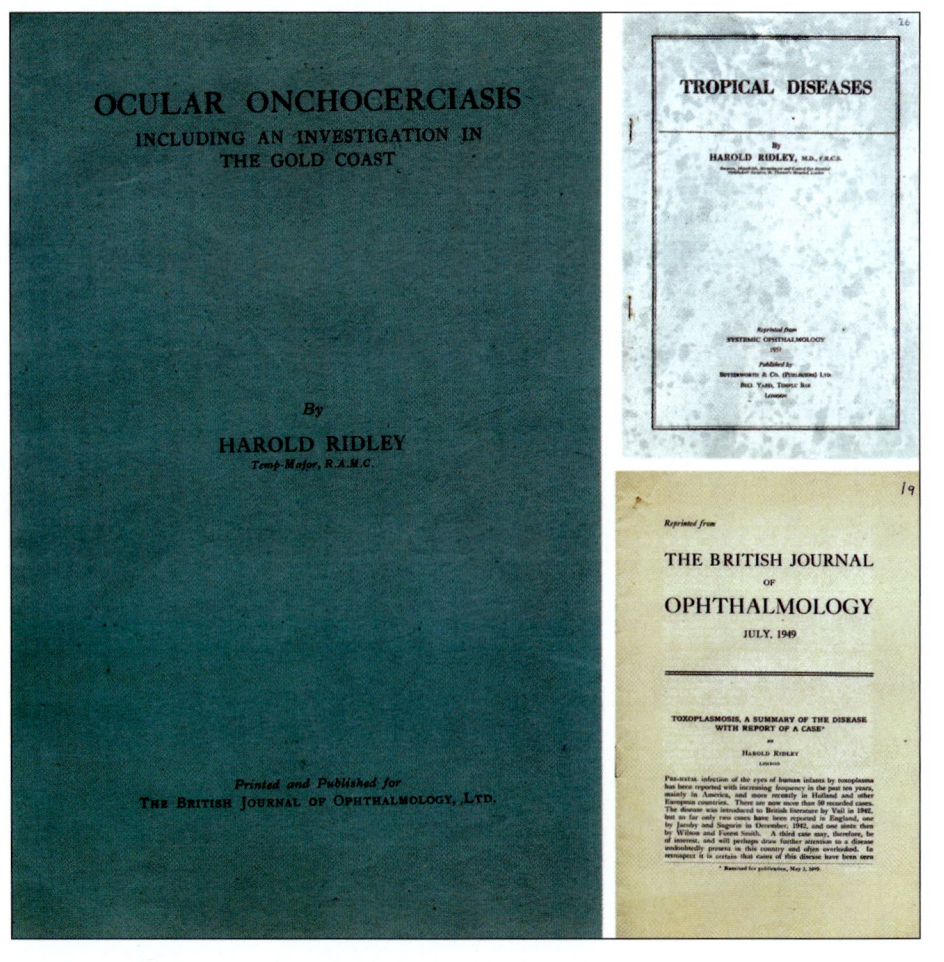

countries, usually sponsored by governmental or nongovernmental organizations or private philanthropy.

Many physicians and surgeons throughout the world are now providing eye care and setting up treatment centers for underprivileged patients in the undeveloped world. However, few people know that Harold and his colleagues were among the first to recognize the need for such activities and, indeed, were active in these fields well over half a century ago. The problem of world blindness is massive, almost incomprehensible. Early on, I learned that:

One blind person = a tragedy.

Ten blind persons = a disaster.

One million blind persons = a statistic.

Harold's work in the field of tropical ophthalmology has been almost unknown or forgotten, and certainly, it is rarely cited in reports or lectures given by workers in this field. As was so often the case, his modesty, self-effacement, and inability to market himself have in part been responsible for this. I personally was unsure of his interest in tropical ophthalmology until I began a careful reading of his personal papers. These papers clearly reveal the intensity of his activity as well as his sincerity. Note in the opening quote his comment regarding "alcoholic parties." He disliked the waste that he claimed to have often seen when various charities, bureaucracies, etc came to various countries and attempted to help with the cataract problem. Also, as noted in his quote, he was frustrated because he was not remembered as a pioneer worker in this field.

In his letters, I found a correspondence from a very well-known and important worker in the field, John Wilson, a blind gentleman who was a true leader in all areas of tropical ophthalmology, Director of the Royal Commonwealth Society for the Blind, and an early worker with the WHO's Global Program for the Prevention of Blindness. A read through the paragraphs of this letter confirms, from an impeccable source, Harold's activities and successful achievements in multiple endeavors: onchocerciasis (river blindness), the establishment of cataract-IOL facilities, and important activities in treatment of vitamin A deficiency, for which he has received virtually no acknowledgment.

Dear Mr. Ridley,

Your voice on the radio and on the telephone brought back so many memories of those days, now some 50 years ago, when you, Duke-Elder and Frank Law helped us to establish the medical activities of the Royal Commonwealth Society for the Blind. Over the intervening years that organization has become the leading nongovernmental agency in developing, with the World Health Organization, the Global Program for the Prevention of Blindness.

Even earlier, you identified onchocerciasis in Northern Ghana at the start of what, over the years, has become an impressively successful control project. WHO's Annual Report, published this February, said that over the 25 year control period, 34 million people have been protected from onchocerciasis in West Africa, and more than 400,000 cases of blindness have been prevented. They add that 11 million children, born since 1974 in the control area, are not at risk of onchocerciasis. Economically, 25 million hectares of land, previously unoccupied for fear of the disease, has now

CHAPTER 13

been brought into fertile production, which they say is enough to feed 17 million people annually.

Jean and I were recently in India where we were told that last year, 3 million cataract operations were performed in the Indian subcontinent, some 60% of them using IOL technology. I think you knew Dr. Venkataswamy in Madurai; last year his group of hospitals performed 135,000 cataract operations, some 80% of them with lens implants. His unit, which now manufactures the lenses, has developed an international market, reducing the unit cost to about $20. Here again, your outstanding initiative in developing lens implant technology was the foundation for all that development.

I remember also when you went, on behalf of the Society, to Central Africa and in what was then Northern Rhodesia, identified vitamin A deficiency as the main reason for the very high prevalence of child blindness in the Luapula area. Previously, it had been thought that it was the result of the malpractices of tribal medicine men. Now of course, xerophthalmia is one of the priorities of the Global Program, though there is still much to do in controlling that disease, which is linked to so many cultural practices.

I remember that you also advised on the surgical treatment of eye complications associated with leprosy in India. With the use of multi-drug therapy, that obscene disease has been impressively reduced in recent years, but still, there are many cases of leprosy related to blindness.

Since I retired as Director of the Royal Commonwealth Society for the Blind in 1983, I have been working with the United Nations on their program for the prevention of other causes of disability. We have established the 'IMPACT Program' with foundations in many countries, and though many tasks remain, good progress is being made with the control of some orthopedic conditions, hearing impairment, and what is now probably the largest category of disability mental impairment. However, the Prevention of Blindness Program, which you did so much to initiate, remains the most successful model.

You kindly invited Jean and me to visit you sometime in Stapleford. My daughter, with her family, lives in Devon, and we will probably be visiting her in July. If I may, I will telephone to you nearer that date if it is possible for us to visit Salisbury for an hour or so in the course of our journey to the West Country.

Meanwhile, with every good wish and the greatest admiration for the incomparable contribution you have made to ophthalmology.

Yours sincerely,

John Wilson

There is one reference in this letter that reveals an important and very unfortunate fact—the reference to Duke-Elder. Both Harold and Duke-Elder must have shared similar and sometimes identical goals in improving eye care. It is unfortunate that they veered off course and developed their terrible animosity later on as Harold moved forward with his IOLs (Chapter 9).

One of the most satisfying successes of my work at the biodevice center in Charleston consisted of a series of efforts to contribute in helping improve cataract/IOL surgery in order that a correct technology transfer be made to the various underprivileged populations. Harold Ridley himself was a true pioneer in this field, and I learned a considerable amount about this from him. Further discussion of cataract surgery follows a brief summary of his highly respected work in the field of onchocerciasis.

SHIPPED OUT

Having served through the time of the phony war, during the invasion of France and the Battle of Britain, Harold was finally inducted into the British Royal Army in May of 1941, entering at the rank of temporary major.

Sir Stewart Duke-Elder was in charge of ophthalmology-related activities in the British services and was responsible for the assignments of surgeons. It is clear that Harold was not afraid to dodge bullets if necessary. He was raised in an environment very much influenced by military matters. Indeed, there were very few years of the 20th century when one war or another was not ravaging the many unfortunate populations of the world. Harold had hoped to be sent to a combat area where he could utilize his surgical experience. Instead, he was surprised to learn that he had been billeted to West Africa—far away from the action. This was a stunning disappointment. He suspected (probably correctly) that Duke-Elder wanted to "farm him out" away from the areas of greatest importance in the war. No active combat was taking place in West Africa at all.

Harold arrived in Ghana, West Africa, shortly after his marriage to Elisabeth Weatherhill on May 10, 1941. He was appointed part-time sanitation officer and headquartered at the capital city of Accra. Rather than dwell on this problem or sink into disappointment and boredom, he honorably began his duties.

He immediately established excellent relations with the inhabitants of the region. They helped him move his personal items and paraphernalia to his field hospital. His most important possessions were his boxes of medical equipment. His slit lamp (biomicroscope) was powered by a primitive electrical supply that was barely sufficient to provide the illumination required.

ATTACKING RIVER BLINDNESS

Many other men in Harold's circumstances would have kicked back and enjoyed doing little or nothing; that was not his style. He quickly turned his attention to a detailed study of onchocerciasis, a disease transmitted by a certain type of fly. Also called "river blindness," onchocerciasis is recognized as the fourth most common cause of blindness on the earth.

The river banks in the regions where this condition occurs teem with the black flies whose multiple bites distribute microscopic parasitic worms into victims. The worms' offspring swarm through the tissues of the afflicted individual's body, especially the skin and eyes.

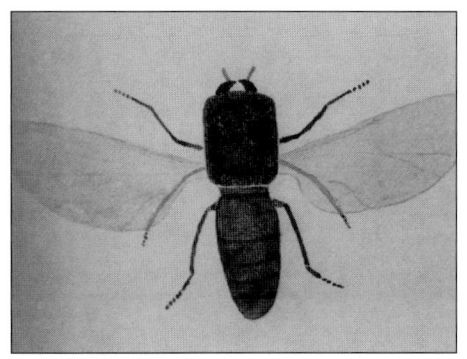

An illustration of the fly that transmits river blindness.

CHAPTER 13

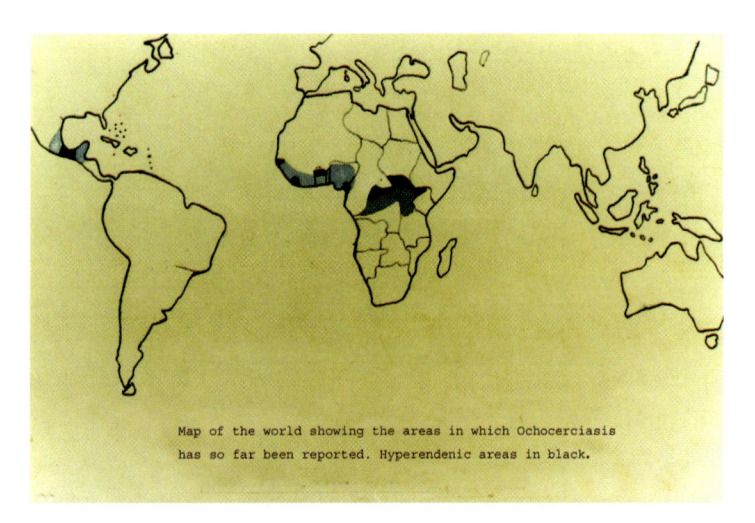

Map of the world showing the areas in which Ochocerciasis has so far been reported. Hyperendemic areas in black.

Field maps used by Harold himself during his sojourn in Ghana to indicate where concentrations of river blindness had been reported.
TOP: A world map showing both sides of endemic areas in blue and black.
BOTTOM: A map of Ghana and the African Gold Coast showing an area of increased incidence of river blindness.

According to the International Lion's Club, river blindness has an enormous economic impact around the world, preventing people from working, harvesting crops, receiving an education, and caring for children. In Harold's time, the disease was endemic in Central America, Central Africa, and Western Africa—especially on the Gold Coast of Africa, precisely where he was assigned for military duty.

Until his time, with the exception of work done by a Belgian researcher, there had been very little systematic study into this condition, and he seized upon the opportunity. His previous interests had run mostly in the direction of surgical diseases of the eyes. This new interest, which involved medical therapy rather than surgery, was therefore a significant, if temporary, change of course for him.

In Accra, Harold met a British General, Brigadier G. M. Findlay, AMS (Army Military Service) with whom he pursued investigations on onchocerciasis. Ridley, General Findlay, and a Captain John Holden journeyed to Funsi, 90 minutes north of Accra, to study the disease.

Using his slit-lamp, powered only by a 12-volt battery, they worked for 2 weeks. The conditions on site were primitive. Most of the work, not only the actual clinical examinations, diagnoses, documentations, treatments, pathologic analyses, and even fundus (retinal) paintings were done by Harold himself. They discovered that 90% of the region's patients had onchocerciasis, and 10% of these were blind.

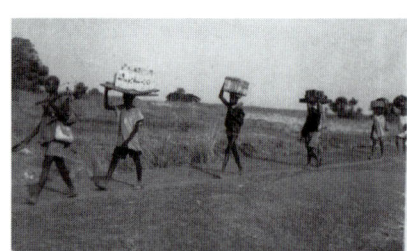

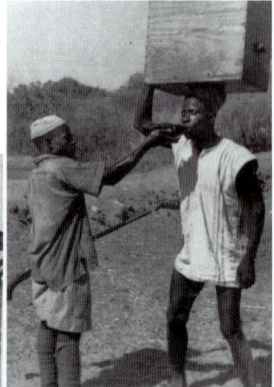

Photographs of Harold's entourage bringing equipment and supplies to his encampment where he set up a field clinic.
TOP: Photograph of the movement of boxes in the usual fashion for this region.
BOTTOM: A group photograph of Harold's team, who he found to be very helpful as he pursued his clinical treatments and research.

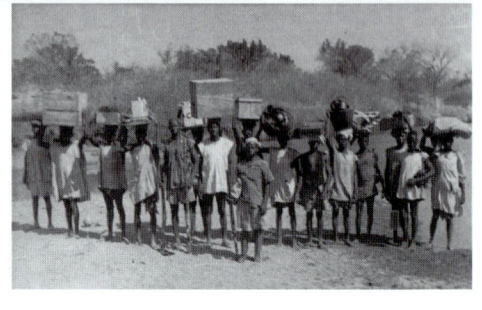

Harold was able to obtain tissue samples from affected patients, and he presented these to a colleague who was able to make photomicrographs that showed the organisms. As Harold confirmed, the disease also affected the inside and back of the eye, the retina, and optic nerve.

Life in the African bush was interesting, to say the least. In his notes, Harold wrote:

> *"After marching for some four hours, we had to spend the night in the bush and chose for our camp the middle of the Great North Road, which was firm ground, clear of vegetation and, apart from lions and other wild animals, safe from traffic. We lit fires and everyone kept in close contact. We had taken the precaution of ordering whisky by parcel "post" and saw it arrive on the heads of porters who carried also flaming torches made from dry elephant grass to light the way and discourage lions. After the long march and ample whiskey, we slept well."*

After he returned from the bush, Ridley made a sketch of the posterior pole (retina) of a typical eye with this condition, showing the intense pigmentation that occurred surrounding the optic nerve and macular region. This is now called the "Ridley fundus" by workers in the field.

He wrote a classic monograph entitled *Ocular Onchocerciasis*. It was published in 1945 in a supplement of the *British Journal of Ophthalmology* and became a landmark. In it, Ridley described the condition, illustrated important clinical and pathologic features, and changed the way many think of this disease.

The groundbreaking article he wrote stimulated further research throughout the years, which is now leading to an increase in our ability to treat the disease. For example, the pharmaceutical giant Merck developed a new treatment direction for the condition—a drug named Mectizan—and in 1987 announced its decision to donate Mectizan in whatever amounts needed to prevent onchocerciasis for as long as necessary. The Jimmy Carter Center, in collaboration with the International Lion's Clubs, have supported a 2004 initiative to underwrite and facilitate 50 million treatments.

As it turned out, Harold did more for humanity during his tour of duty in Africa than he could ever have done as a war surgeon. The attention he called to river blindness and the light he shed on it constitutes one of his most important contributions to mankind. By turning a disappointing assignment into an opportunity, Ridley worked under primitive conditions to fight a terrible disease.

His success in this conflict—one that was far different than he thought he would be fighting during the war—brought a sense of pride to him that was equal to, if not even greater than, that which he derived from his later invention of the IOL. Although his modesty and inability to "sell" himself politically resulted in his failure to receive the credit he deserved for his landmark work, he knew what he had done. And that was enough.

While in Africa, Harold did not confine himself to his work with river blindness. He also investigated the condition termed xerophthalmia—a corneal condition that afflicted people throughout the underprivileged world, especially children. He was one of the first to discover that a simple, small dose of vitamin A could have a massive effect on xerophthalmia. This discovery was another that

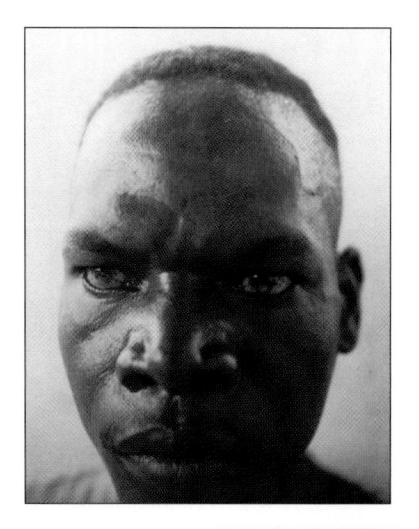

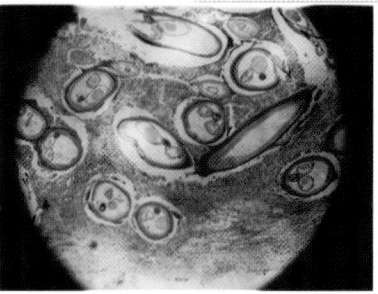

Photographs showing primary clinical and pathologic features of the disease.
TOP: A common facial appearance showing lumps about the nose due to infiltration of clumps of the organism and surrounding fibrosis.
BOTTOM: A photomicrograph obtained showing the microscopic appearance of the organisms that cause river blindness. Notice the central clusters of organisms that are enmeshed in fibrous tissue, which creates the then scars seen on the skin, as well as in the eye.

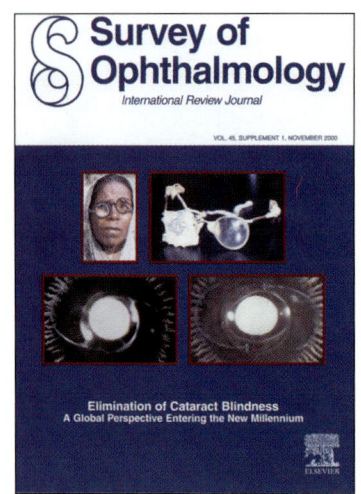

CHAPTER 13

gave him great satisfaction throughout his life. Today, vitamin A is being used with immense success by WHO and other groups to fend off this disease.

Harold also treated ocular leprosy, a disease commonly regarded as incurable. In several of our river walks, he spoke of his attempts to do surgery for leprosy, performing what he felt may have been the first successful corneal graft on a leper. He did not record his data.

These early efforts in tropical ophthalmology during the war led to his early involvement with John Wilson and his Royal Commonwealth Society for the Blind, a major consortium of government and nongovernment organizations dedicated to fighting blindness, especially in the developing world.

One other disease that commonly affects individuals in the developing world and remains one of the top two or three blinding diseases today is trachoma. Harold did not do original work in this field—at least he never mentioned it to me, nor have I been able to find anything about it in the documentation he left behind. This appears to be the only major disease categorized as "tropical ophthalmology" in which he did not do independent research or clinical trials.

Later, Ridley recalled his war-time service:

> *"I am quite proud of my war record, which must have made some colleagues jealous for though I joined the Army late, I had been able to do a lot of useful work and much more than friends in uniform. When in the Army, I luckily met onchocerciasis and malnutrition. I even got Army engineers to make, out of a crashed Spitfire, a trephine for keratoplasty corneal transplantation (author's note) and myself made apparatus for treating retinal detachment, which proved successful. I also got plastic materials from the Dental Department from which I fashioned acceptable and greatly appreciated artificial eyes. After the war, I was appointed the Civilian Consultant in Ophthalmology to the Ministry of Defense (Army), and most unusually, held this post until my formal retirement in 1971."*

APPLYING LABORATORY TECHNOLOGY TO CATARACT-IOL SURGERY IN THE DEVELOPING WORLD

My first foray in the field of developing world ophthalmology was in the 1970s during my ophthalmology residency at the University of Iowa. I spent several weeks in

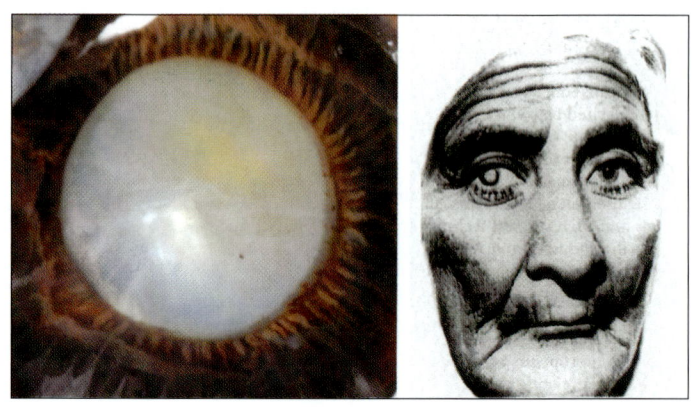

Another prime interest as would be expected for Ridley and also myself is the issue of cataract surgery in the developing world. For many years, there was strong resistance to using Harold's IOL in underprivileged areas because of multiple reasons, including the typical naysayer mentality, as well as financial and logistical obstacles in obtaining the necessary lenses and supplies for implantation. In 1999 I began working with the World Health Organization on this problem, and my interest in this culminated in the publication of a review article in the *Survey of Ophthalmology* as noted here. This represented one of the first attempts at focusing an institution (at that time, the Storm Eye Institute) on problems of blindness in the developing world.

Cataracts in many of the poorer countries are often quite advanced because the patients are unable to seek or obtain treatment. One often sees a triad in older patients, namely white hair, white skin, and a white lens. People simply expect to have this condition and in the past have not had incentive to seek out treatment.
LEFT: A photograph from behind, Miyake-Apple posterior view, showing an extremely dense cataract, that was obviously situated in this eye for many years until the patient's death.
RIGHT: Photograph of the triad of white hair, white wrinkled skin, and a white lens.

INNOVATIONS IN ADDITION TO THE INTRAOCULAR LENS

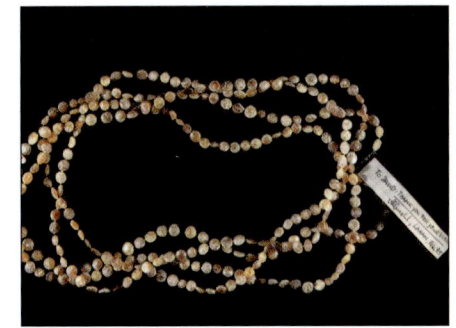

The problem of cataract is so severe in many developing countries in which the incidence and prevalence is enormous. Cataract is by far the most common cause of blindness. Sixty percent of all blindness is indeed caused by this disease.

In order to demonstrate this in a very undeniable fashion, some surgeons in Nepal prepared a necklace for me that was made entirely of removed cataractous lenses from a myriad of patients. This provides an excellent object lesson as to the very high incidence of cataract and also emphasizes the need for better availability of treatment.

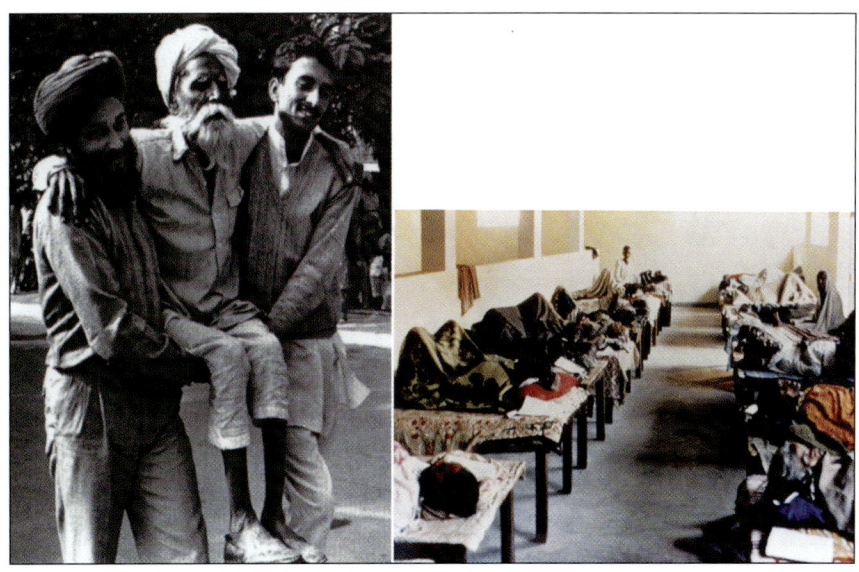

Until recently, many patients were treated in eye camps with only minimal quality gadgetry available for surgery, but this is now improving.

LEFT: It is a severe financial burden to have so many people develop cataracts and be unable to take care of themselves, be unable to work, and need such assistance to try to obtain help for their cataract.

RIGHT: A ward in India showing a myriad of patients with cataract during their recovering phase after surgery.

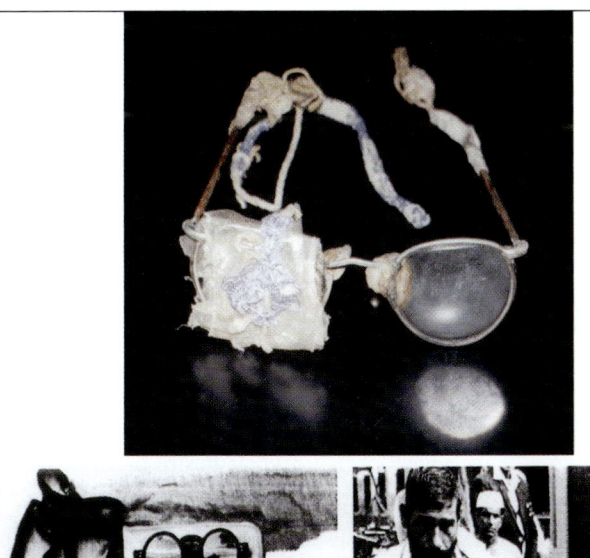

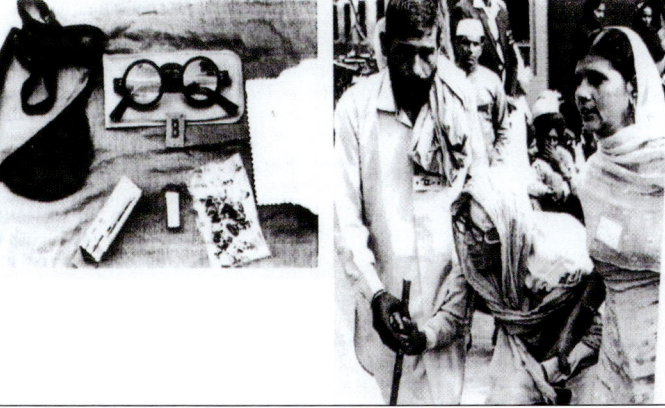

In the past, the most common visual rehabilitation after cataract surgery was the use of the thick aphakic spectacles that we have mentioned several times in this text. These provide a marginal improvement in vision at best, and if complications ensue, the final vision after surgery can indeed be less than the vision from the preoperative cataract.

One major problem in a developing world situation is the fact that patients often damage, break, or even lose their spectacles and have no opportunity to replace them. These patients end up more blind than when they began their ordeal.

LEFT: A kit used to provide aphakic spectacles after surgery to patients in a developing world situation.

RIGHT: Postoperative appearance of a patient leaving the operating suite with the typical aphakic spectacles. Her new vision is probably nowhere close to perfect and she will be fortunate if she is able to retain her spectacles and continue with any improved vision at all.

CHAPTER 13

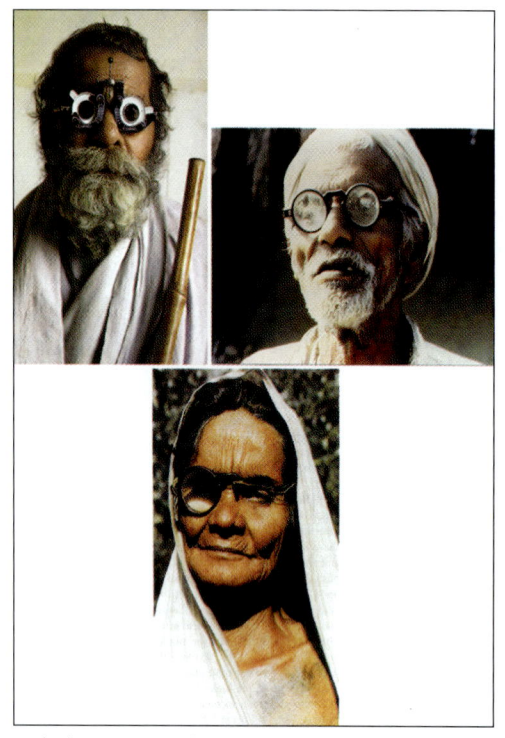

Aphakic spectacles in a developing world situation.
UPPER LEFT: This desperate man was able to obtain an ophthalmologist's trial frame to use for his aphakic spectacles, which had been lost.
UPPER RIGHT: Another patient with aphakic spectacles.
BOTTOM: A lady with broken spectacles; only the right eye has the normal magnified vision that is required for sight.

the back country of Nigeria under the auspices of a charitable organization called Project Focus. My adventure got off to a terrible start. I had hardly arrived at the main Nigeria Airport in Lagos when I was assaulted by several young men. During the assault, I received a severe corneal abrasion in one eye, which later necessitated that I perform all of my surgery there using only my good eye. I had to wear a patch on the other eye for the entire time. To make matters worse, these young gentlemen absconded with three full bags of ophthalmic instruments and medicine as well as personal items. I am sure that some of the medicine and eye drops helped set up many medical "practices" with "medicine men." I am sure that there were many, many dilated pupils in the eyes of villagers throughout the surrounding areas over the next several weeks thereafter. The robbers were an exception; as soon as I made my way to the eye facility over 100 miles from that airport, all by myself, I began working with an absolutely wonderful staff and duly performed my quota of cataract operations, of course without implants. I learned for the first time the marked disadvantages of "pre-Harold Ridley" cataract surgery with no IOL. In particular, I saw the many catastrophes that occurred when patients left the hospital and often lost or broke their glasses, their thick aphakic spectacles, that in effect were their lifeline to sight. They had no hope of obtaining new ones. Because of this, they were often condemned to a worse vision than they had before their surgery.

After I returned home, I had a clear sense as to what was needed to improve the chances of underprivileged people getting proper cataract care. At that time, I had hardly even heard of IOLs. As has been noted earlier, almost all of our professors were against them. However, after I had time to think about it, it was clear that the IOL would be what was needed. Of course, very importantly, they needed a successfully implanted IOL at that time. In the 1970s, this was not at all forthcoming. Even into the 1980s, many surgeons and much of the bureaucracy, which often controlled the overseas "establishment" working in the field of tropical ophthalmology, were not advocates of IOLs.

I was very fortunate to have had a wonderful young Indian eye surgeon who worked with me as a research fellow (a member of the Apple Korps) very early in my career, ca. 1969. Her name was Dr. G. Natchair, the wife of Dr. G. Nam and the sister of the legendary Dr. Venkataswamy, Madurai, India. It was fortunate that I had gotten to know them then. After my experience in Nigeria I had a great desire to work in the field of tropical medicine, and I jumped at the opportunity to work with this team at their home base in Maduri, India. My team developed a working relationship with Dr. Venkataswamy's team on two levels. First, we advised them on IOL designs and styles that would best fit their needs, and we arranged for what are called wet-lab teaching sessions (practice operations on fresh cadaver eyes). Several doctors, residents, and other surgeons in training came to Charleston and had the opportunity to use our Miyake-Apple technique (described in detail in Chapter 5). Second, we developed a working relationship with their hospital and with the SEVA foundation, located in the San Francisco Bay area. We assisted them in creating and building their own IOL manufacturing facility in Maduri, and they have succeeded in manufacturing beautiful state-of-the-art one-piece posterior lenses since the mid 1980s.

BRINGING LIGHT TO THE UNDERPRIVILEGED WORLD: INTRODUCING THE MODERN CATARACT-IOL OPERATION

In 2000, after having worked in the field of tropical ophthalmology off and on for about 25 years, with greater intensity for the previous 5 years—about 5 years after I met Harold—my team, the "Apple Korps," wrote a monograph on the issues and problems of cataract surgery in the underprivileged world. This was written 50 years after the first IOL implant. This appeared in the *Survey of Ophthalmology,* volume 45, supplement 1, November 2000. The goal of transitioning from the thick spectacles of the past to the permanent IOL placement was foremost in our minds as we prepared this manuscript.

Even into the early 1990s, it was frustrating to note that the problems that prevented the delivery of modern cataract IOL surgery to the developing world still existed. As usual, many individuals in the field of ophthalmology continued to be strongly against IOLs. Many of the naysayers were in the academic establishments, including the American Academy of Ophthalmology and the American Ophthalmologic Society. As late as 1990, it was sometimes a chore to get manuscripts or presentations on IOLs accepted. Some of the highest authorities at the National Eye Institute of the National Institutes of Health—the United States government's medical arm—were strongly against IOLs. This, therefore, delayed their study on use both for the industrialized world and especially for the developing world.

These problems were exacerbated by some glitches; some were serious. One was what I consider to be an unpardonable act: some companies sent IOLs to the developing world, but the lenses they sent had been rejected by the FDA or otherwise declared defective. In some cases, they did this for a tax write-off. In other cases, they actually sold these lenses. This sort of thing did little to encourage IOL initiatives in underprivileged populations.

I was pleased to be part of a meeting held at the World Health Organization (WHO) in Geneva, Switzerland, on December 3, 1990. The meeting was entitled "The Use of Intraocular Lenses in Cataract Surgery in the Developing Countries." Based on my research in this field, I was invited to attend by Dr. Bjorn Tylefors, the Director at that

In 1990, the World Health Organization Committee on Prevention of Blindness sponsored a meeting in Geneva regarding the topic of IOLs in the developing world. Until that time, IOLs were generally not deemed proper for use in underprivileged countries for the various reasons cited above (ie, various prejudices, costs, logistics, etc.). I consider this meeting to have been a major turning point, and the interchange there in effect "got the ball rolling" in increasing the desire for dissemination of implants in the developing world. Colleagues with whom I have worked and are in this photograph included Dr. Peter Choyce, Dr. David Yorston, and Dr. Bjorn Tylefors.

Shortly after the Geneva meeting, Dr. Tylefors, Program Director of the Prevent Blindness Division of the World Health Organization, Geneva, visited my department in Charleston where we pondered various means to help improve the world's ability to bring IOLs into the developing world. Also at this meeting we discussed the use of so-called "wet lab," which are basically practice surgeries for doctors-in-training using experimental animal eyes or human eyes obtained postmortem. Following this meeting, dozens of individuals came to my laboratory in Charleston and began the process of learning the modern techniques of cataract IOL surgery.

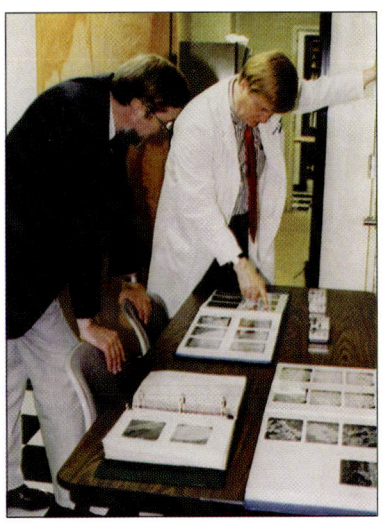

CHAPTER 13

Photographs of our IOL center laboratory in the mid-1990s, showing a visit of surgeons from overseas locations. The surgeon performing the operation using the Miyake-Apple technique, in which she can visualize the progress of her surgery on a television monitor, is Dr. G. Natchair, who was one of the very first research fellows that I had working for me when I began my career at the University of Illinois in Chicago back in 1970. She now has matured to the codirectorship of one of the most important clinics in Madurai, India: the Arvand Facility. They have also advanced to the point where they make IOLs that are of good quality and are sold under the name Aurolab. Dr. Natchair's husband stands directly to my left in this photograph.

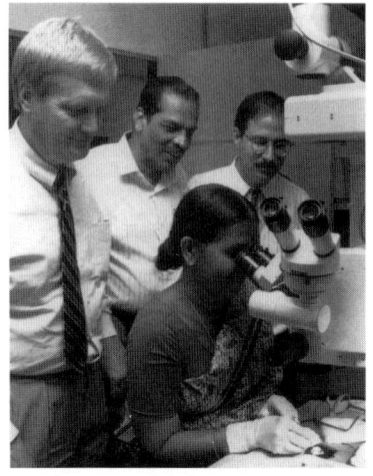

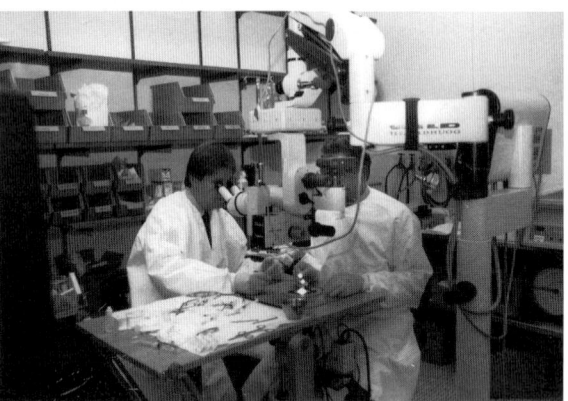

In the 1970s and especially in the 1980s, a whole cluster of poorly made anterior chamber lenses was released on the market. These were very damaging, caused many problems, and were often sold to developing world countries as a tax deduction in order to gain some financial relief from failed products. The numerous lenses seen on the front of this brochure clearly indicate that there are so many designs that one cannot be sure which one might be better than the other.

Also, lenses of this type, made by many companies that were often of questionable quality, gave the whole group of anterior chamber lenses an inappropriately bad name. Therefore, when there turned out to be a proper use for such lenses, they were often refused.

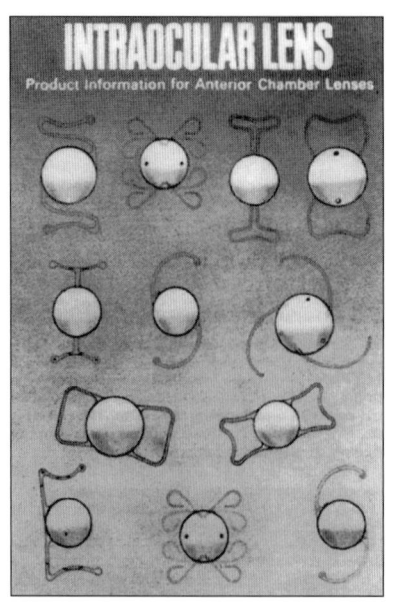

time of the Prevention of Blindness Division of the WHO. Dr. Peter Choyce, of course a loyal colleague of Harold during the tough years, was also invited. The meeting was a turning point.

Numerous capable professionals formally agreed to begin initiatives to provide IOL surgery to the developing countries. Dr. Bjorn Tylefors, as the leader of this group, deserves our gratitude. Despite opposition, including from high-ranking individuals from several countries including the United States, Dr. Tylefors, not an eye surgeon himself, clearly recognized the value of IOLs and was, therefore, a strong supporter to finally get the ball rolling.

I personally invited Dr. Tylefors to my laboratory and facility in Charleston, where we later discussed the implementation of the initiative. Meetings of this type were instrumental in providing information as to the correct type of lens to be used in these situations. Prior to this, there was practically no real differentiation among many interested parties between good and bad designs. I believe I provided significant help in that sense.

My own efforts to help bring IOL surgery to the developing world continued through the decade of the 1990s but were cut short by my illnesses. One of my proudest legacies was the implementation of teaching centers for young surgeons serving underprivileged populations. In these teaching centers, called wet labs, in which we utilized the Miyake-Apple posterior video/photographic technique, surgeons were taught new techniques, shown new IOLs, and were able to see their own mistakes on the video. This proved to be a powerful teaching tool.

Ridley's experience in the underdeveloped world instilled in him a deeply felt need to help underprivileged populations. Almost immediately after he invented the IOL in 1949, he realized the enormous impact this innovation could have in the underprivileged world. There, the triad of white hair, wrinkled skin, and white eye (from cataract) was considered to be a natural phenomenon that could not be avoided; blindness was a common condition of age. In the rare occasions that cataracts were removed, it was either through the process of couching or using the unsatisfactory combination of ICCE and then replacing the natural lens with the poor substitute of thick spectacles that distorted vision.

The problem of cataracts in the developing world is a massive one. In my opinion—an opinion that is shared by most although not proven statistically—cataracts are associated with ultraviolet radiation, basically sunshine, as well as other environmental and genetic factors. This is the reason why they are much more common in geographical zones with extensive sunshine, where many of the developing nations are located.

Ridley realized that if his invention could be applied to the poorer areas of the world, wonderful results could be achieved. Unfortunately, an immediate application was not to be. Skepticism, envy, and early complications from IOL surgery had hindered the acceptance of IOLs even in the most advanced nations. In developing countries, the problems were augmented by bureaucratic tangles, and financial and logistical problems that would have to be added to the pile.

Progress in the fight to bring modern IOL surgery to struggling nations was consequently slow.

*Ridley Establishes a Foundation**

Long after his war service, Ridley set up a foundation for two main purposes. One was to help needy people, such as nurses and their families who found themselves in dire financial situations. The other was to promote ophthalmologic services to underprivileged countries.

He registered the charity in March, 1967. It was, he said,

"financed by all the money which I had inherited from both parents, amounting to about £21,000. My father likewise had earned all his own money. I financed the foundation by seven annual installments to reduce tax, and at the end of the time, inflation was just beginning which made the later installments rather a burden because my hospital salary ended when I became due for my pension in 1971.

"I had established a scheme," he continued, "largely with cooperation from the Royal Empire (later Commonwealth) Society for the Blind, which was set up largely from my monograph on Ocular Onchocerciasis (river blindness), whereby visits were made to certain countries in the Empire which were in need because local ophthalmic services were inadequate..."

To set this work in motion, Ridley, his wife, and a nurse from St. Thomas' Hospital traveled to various needy countries, demonstrating surgical techniques and afterward helping assist local surgeons perform the operations. The "pastoral" visits, as he called them, had many wonderful results, such as reducing blindness in children in the Luapula Valley by 90%. Today, medical missions to third-world countries are common. This was not the case when Ridley was doing them. Later in life, Ridley referred to the "active work we undertook in tropical countries almost every year," and pointed

---

* An update on the Ridley Foundation submitted by Harold's son Nicholas can be found in the appendix of this book.

CHAPTER 13

out that "no one else did this sort of thing at that time." Ridley's foundation was a no-nonsense organization, dedicated solely to humanitarian and charitable causes.

Since the turn of the millennium, Harold's (and other's) goal to deliver IOLs to the third world is finally beginning to be realized. There is still much to be done. I know my old friend and mentor would have been delighted to note the progress to date, but work is far from finished. In some countries, the waiting list for cataract surgery continues to grow at a rate of 14,000 new cases a day—5 million new cases each year. As of the year 2000, there were an estimated 50 million blind people in the world, about half of these suffering from unoperated cataracts, 90% of these in developing countries.

As John Wilson wrote to Harold in the letter included earlier in this chapter, "Your outstanding initiative in developing lens implant technology was the foundation for all that development." It is up to us to continue such initiatives as we continue forward in the 21st century.

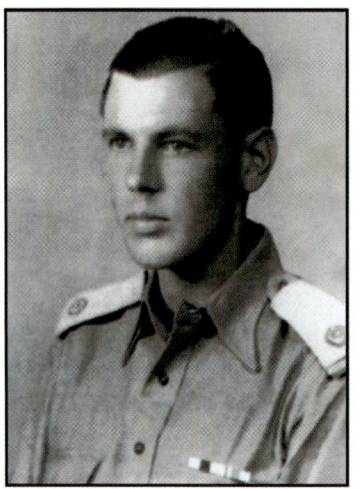

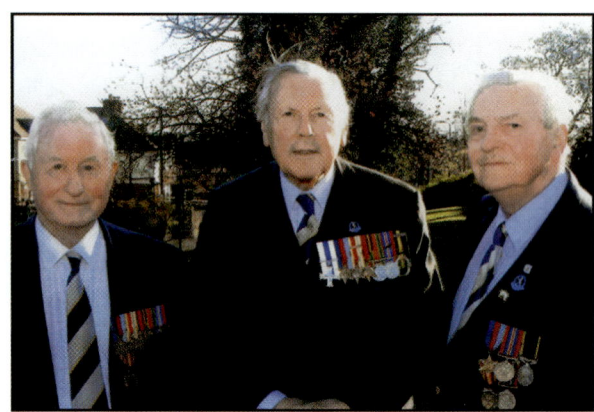

Mr. John Winstanley, a genuine war hero and practice partner with Harold Ridley at St. Thomas' Hospital for decades. Like most other surgeons at St. Thomas' and Moorfields during the early years of the IOL, he did not implant IOLs. He was a good friend of Harold and was not against the IOL, but simply did not want to make the transition to it at a relatively late age.
LEFT: Photograph of John at the time of his entrance into the military as a private at the age of 18. He was immediately transferred to the Japanese theater of war and his incredible success led to rapid promotion.
RIGHT: John (center) at a recent meeting with friends from the war era.

I had known the Winstanleys earlier, but in the year 2005, I had the opportunity to visit them at their home near Oxford, reminisce about Harold, and obtain important information for this book.
LEFT: The Winstanleys enjoying the casual lifestyle.
RIGHT: Photograph of myself with John during that visit.

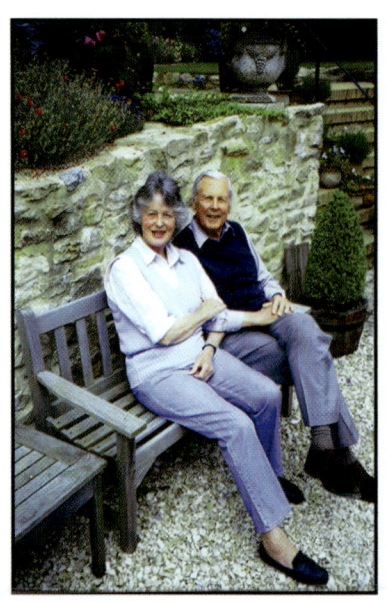

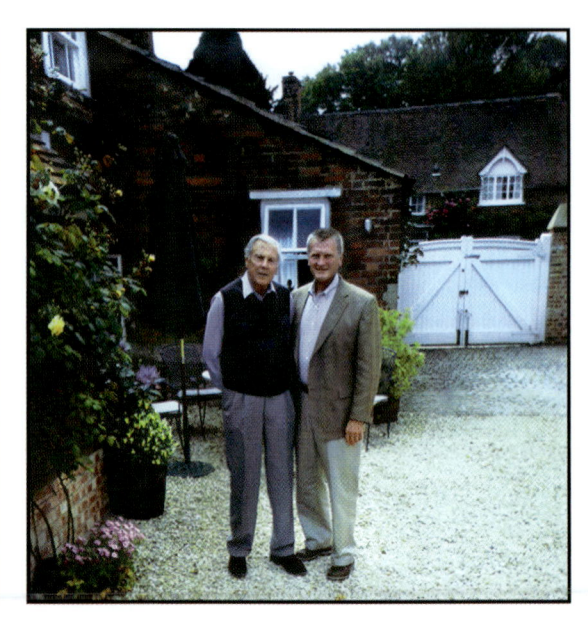

14

Released Prisoners of War in Thailand and Burma

> THE BRITISH JOURNAL OF OPHTHALMOLOGY
> DECEMBER, 1945
>
> COMMUNICATIONS
>
> OCULAR MANIFESTATIONS OF MALNUTRITION IN RELEASED PRISONERS OF WAR FROM THAILAND
>
> BY HAROLD RIDLEY, Major, R.A.M.C.
>
> OPPORTUNITY has presented itself for the examination of the eyes of some 500 released allied prisoners of War and internees from Thailand who considered that there sight had deteriorated during captivity. Among these no less than 100 cases of amblyopia have been seen in 17 days, and many of those whose corrected vision is normal have subclinical vascular lesions of the eyes. The majority of these men are to be repatriated immediately and many will shortly be attending the ophthalmic clinics of the United Kingdom. In Rangoon it has been possible to examine large numbers who have as yet had no opportunity to improve, and the findings are a guide to the prominent features of syndrome which may be less evident by the time the men reach home.
>
> The barbarity with which these men were treated caused the death of thousands from malnutrition and intercurrent disease. For the purpose of this report it is sufficient to record that the food was inadequate in quantity, especially in view of the heavy labour which had to be performed and that it was lacking in variety, being especially deficient in protein, fats and vitamins. Red Cross parcels were hardly ever distributed and drugs for the treatment of severe

Harold was transferred to the pacific theater of war in 1944, having finished his duties in Ghana as described in Chapter 13. He was immediately saddened by the appearance of literally thousands of malnourished, emaciated former prisoners. However, he was astute enough, as usual, to take an opportunity to study the eye findings of these patients, many of whom had severe visual loss. From these studies came a very important paper that was very prescient in perhaps helping lead scientists to new developments in the fields of macular degeneration and optic nerve.

NUTRITIONAL AMBLYOPIA: INVOLVEMENT OF THE OPTIC NERVE AND MACULA

"Failure of the choriocapillaris to nourish the outer retinal layers at the macula may be significant."

Harold Ridley, 1945

For many years after World War II, Mr. John Winstanley was a consultant ophthalmologist with Harold at St. Thomas' Hospital. He was an authentic war hero in the Burma theater of war. He was very helpful to me in two interviews regarding the status of the war that Harold entered on the other side of the world from Southern England, where Harold had his earlier encounter with the carnage of war during the Battle of Britain.

After serving for 18 months in Ghana, having completed his studies on river blindness, he received a transfer. He went first to India.

> *"In Calcutta,"* he explained, *"we basically had nothing to do with no assignments. Finally, I was transferred to Rangoon, Burma, where life began again. I treated over 200 released Allied prisoners of war in Rangoon and Singapore who suffered from nutritional amblyopia while Japanese prisoners of war."*

A major catastrophe of the Burma military campaign, as well the conflicts in Thailand and elsewhere in the Pacific theater of war, was the capture and enslavement of thousands of Allied soldiers who were forced to labor on such projects as the Burma Road. Similar to the Bataan death marches in the Philippines, the soldiers were grossly undernourished and many died of starvation and disease.

CHAPTER 14

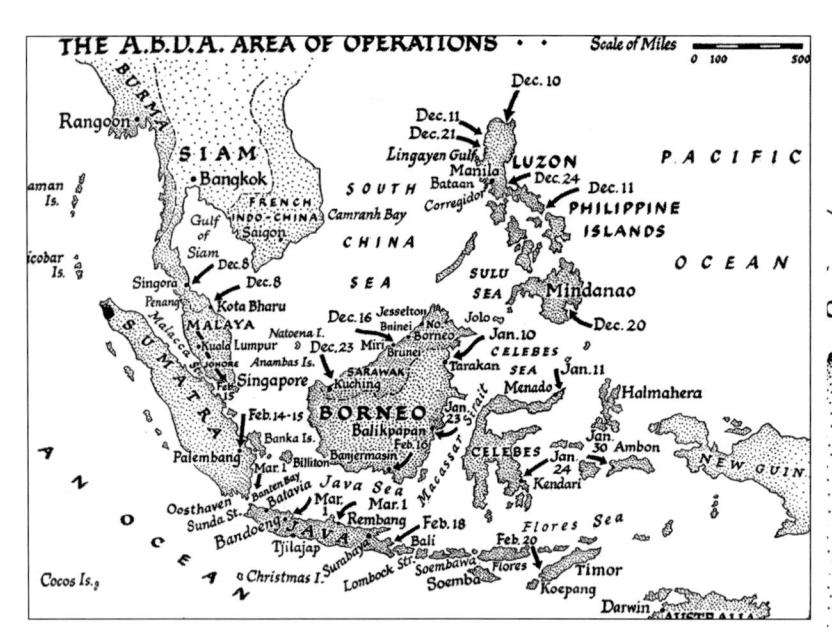

Burma-Thailand theater of war.
There was severe loss of life as well as unbelievable mistreatment of soldiers and prisoners with marked malnutrition. This occurred especially when prisoners were forced by the Japanese to do slave labor on the "Burma Road." After fierce fighting, the British and other Allied Forces were able to clear the Japanese forces from the region.

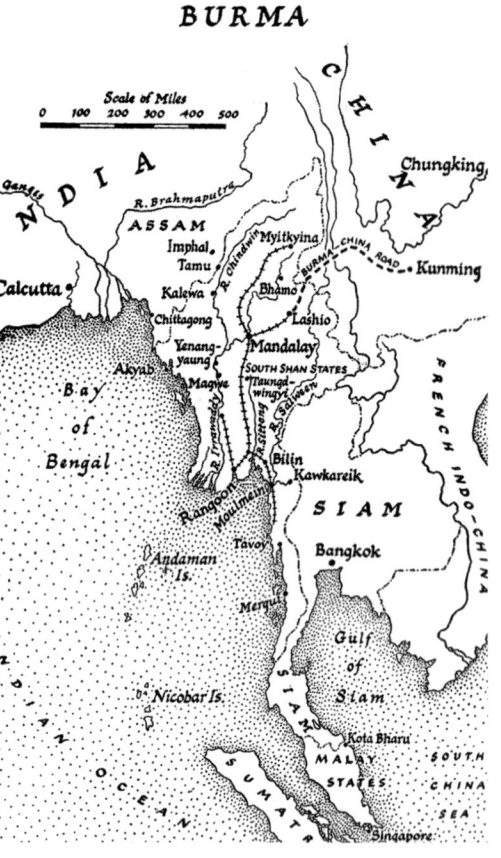

Harold noted:

> "Many of the prisoners had worked on the Burma Railway. Starved and ill-treated, they had developed sudden central scotoma, sometimes relieved by good diet if available. Some made a partial recovery within six weeks of release. However, the advanced cases, though given a vitamin-rich diet were irreversible."

Harold's examinations of the recently released prisoners of war revealed two basic patterns as viewed by examination of the eye with the ophthalmoscope. Both conditions caused nutritional amblyopia, which by definition means loss of vision (amblyopia) due to malnourishment.

The first and main manifestation of the condition was classic optic atrophy—a disease that had been long suspected even without good visual confirmation. Only since the invention of the ophthalmoscope in the mid-19th century by Helmholtz and Babbage (see Chapter 5) could it be viewed clinically. It is seen most commonly in populations in underprivileged regions or during atypical situations such as war when the incidence of malnutrition increases.

The second manifestation of the condition Harold observed was somewhat similar to what is seen today as age-related macular degeneration (ARMD). In this disease the primary site of one's central 20/20 (6/6) vision, the macula, is situated just lateral or temporal (toward the ear) from the optic nerve, and is affected in various ways.

Although people do not at first think of ARMD as a form of diet-related amblyopia, Harold made a few observations in his paper that I consider prescient. He noted:

> "It is uncertain whether disturbance in a visual pathway originates in the retina or optic nerve. Failure of the choriocapillaris to nourish the outer retinal layers at the macula may be significant."

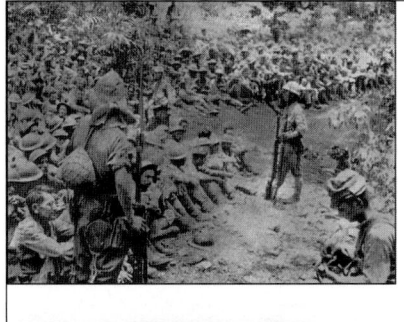

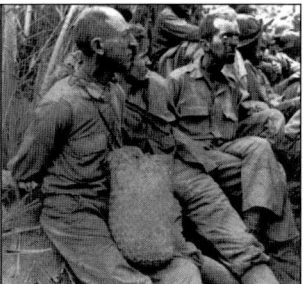

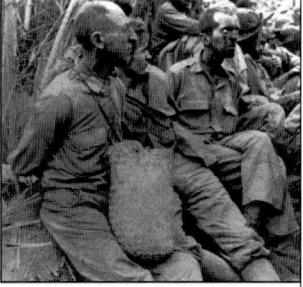

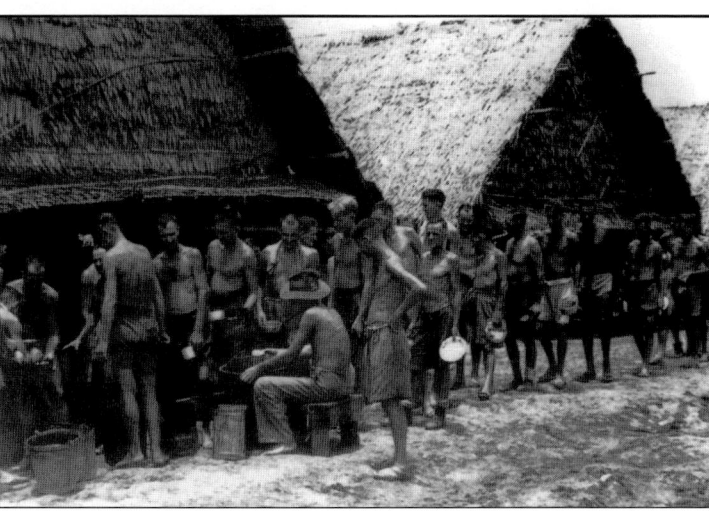

TOP LEFT and RIGHT: Still under the thumbs of Japanese guards.
BOTTOM: Other clusters of prisoners.

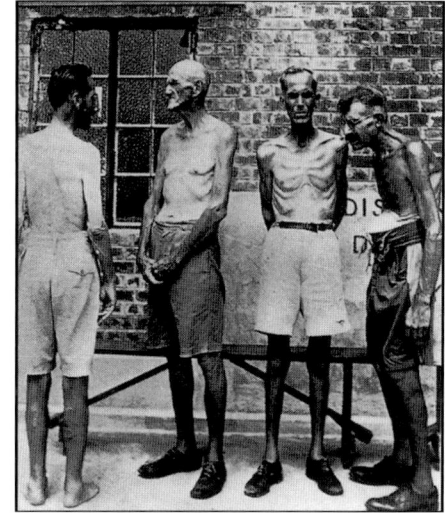

We now know that vascular problems, at the level of the choriocapillaris, the small capillary sized vessels that supply the retina and its associated pigmented layer, are at least partly the cause of ARMD. It is possible that the malnutrition suffered by these servicemen had affected their maculas in a fashion analogous to what occurs with ARMD.

Regardless of the details regarding the etiology of these conditions, the therapy initiated on the returning prisoners by Harold and his colleagues anticipated some of the principles of therapy that we use today, almost 65 years later, for ARMD. He spoke of using "multivitamin therapy" for his patients, many of whom experienced an improvement. This was a logical treatment; he was undoubtedly not the first to consider this. However, his linkage of the process to choriocapillaris involvement associated with the choice of therapy revealed advanced thinking for that time.

The use of this type of therapy was logical since the problems were obviously nutrition-based. Ridley noted in his paper that the virtual epidemic of starvation that occurred in this large theater of war was the first that made possible a study of a large population of individuals with this disease—a total of over 500 within his region, 200 of whom he examined personally.

In some ways, his multivitamin therapy can be seen as a forerunner to one of today's practices of treating eye conditions with varying forms of multivitamins and other pharmacologic agents. People have used herbal, pharmaceutical, and other nutritional concoctions for centuries to treat all kinds of aliments, including those of the eye. In his classic work in the 16th century, Georg Bartisch (see Chapter 5) wrote about using medicinal agents for almost all of the eye diseases that he was aware of, including cataract, glaucoma, and others. We know now that most of these were useless

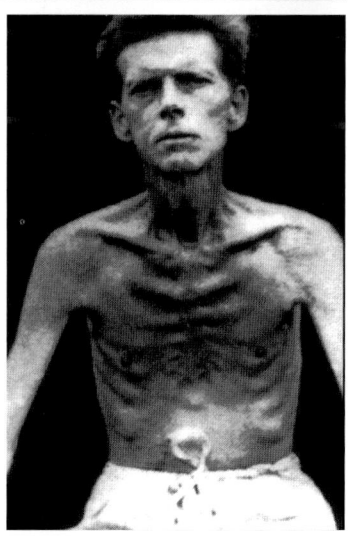

TOP and BOTTOM: The physical appearance seen in these two photographs are typical of the general physical emaciation of each released prisoner.

CHAPTER 14

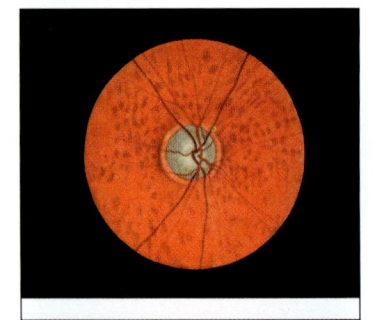

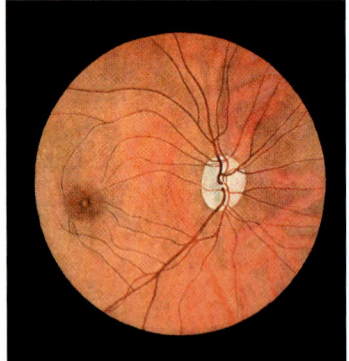

Early fundus drawings, 19th century, showing examples of nutritional amblyopia with optic nerve atrophy.

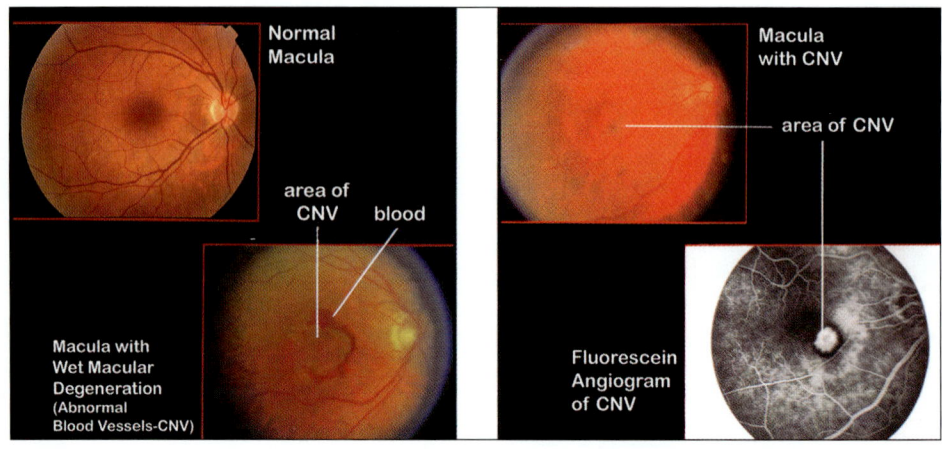

Clinical fundus photographs showing age-related macular degeneration (ARMD).
LEFT: Normal macula.
RIGHT: A patient with ARMD with abnormal blood vessels that are bleeding.

remedies, bordering on quackery, but this doesn't mean that all such remedies were ineffective. Even today, certain nutritional products claim to hold the key to curing a wide spectrum of diseases and conditions. We know some of these are valid, at least within limits, yet others have proven to be false if not dangerous claims.

Not surprisingly, this sort of thing has made some people skeptical about attempts to cure diseases with various concoctions in the absence of scientific analysis and testing. This was not possible in 1945 when Ridley and his team were provided with hundreds of "test cases" as they worked to restore sight to released prisoners of war. They did not have the opportunity to scientifically "think it over" and wait for results of long-term clinical studies. They needed to act quickly if sight was to be restored to these service men.

Multivitamins are today in common use for macular disease. Their final role is still unknown. However, other forms of ancillary therapy and treatments are now being studied in a concerted attempt to cut back or eraddicate this condition. Direct laser therapy to the damaged macular region is a mainstay of therapy, but is only helpful in selected cases. Another experimental treatment modality is the implantation of a telescopic IOL (see Chapter 16, page 242). This futuristic idea was actually first conceived by our colleague, Peter Choyce.

Ridley's work on nutritional amblyopia with the released prisoners of war in Burma, like his work on river blindness in Ghana, once again proved his thoughtful determination to apply whatever was available locally wherever he was, in whatever way he could to provide a clinically useful innovation.

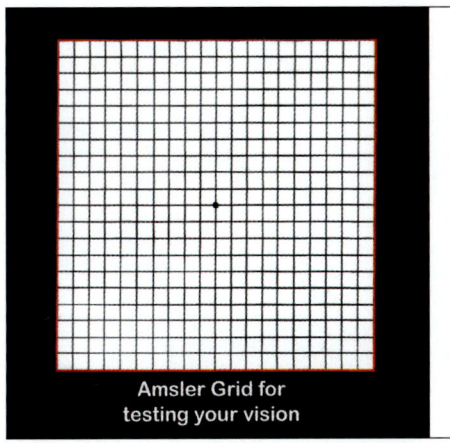

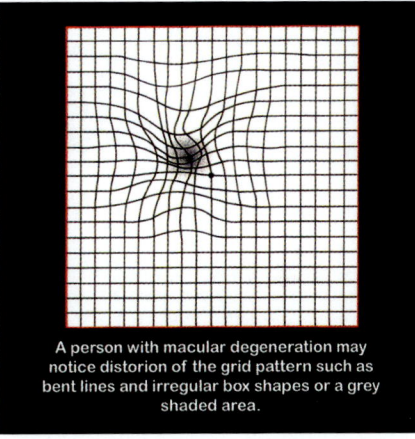

RELEASED PRISONERS OF WAR IN THAILAND AND BURMA

A person with macular degeneration may notice distorion of the grid pattern such as bent lines and irregular box shapes or a grey shaded area.

Amsler Grid for testing your vision

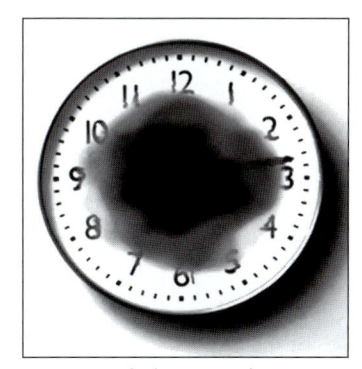

Disease of the macular region may cause a central scotoma (loss of vision).

The Amsler Grid, a special test for central retinal (macular) function.
LEFT: Normal appearance.
RIGHT: A person with macular degeneration may notice distortion of the grid pattern, such as bent lines, irregular box shapes, or a gray shaded area.

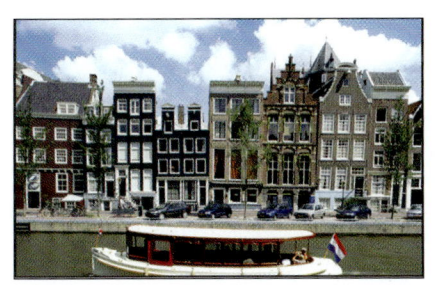

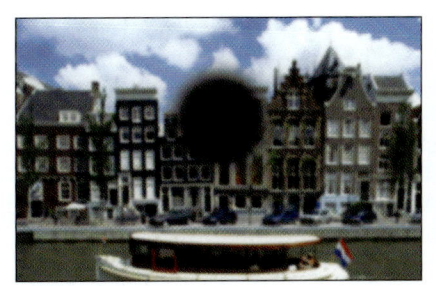

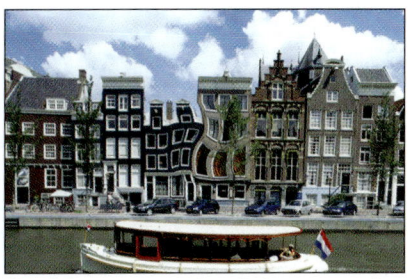

A view of the canals. LEFT: Normal vision. CENTER: Central scotoma (visual loss caused by degeneration of underlying macula). RIGHT: Visual distortions caused by deposition of fluid in the macular region.

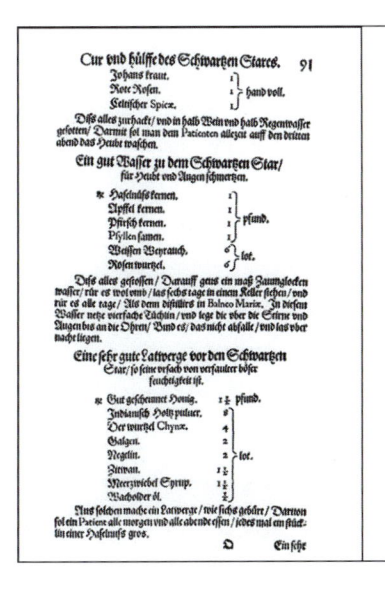

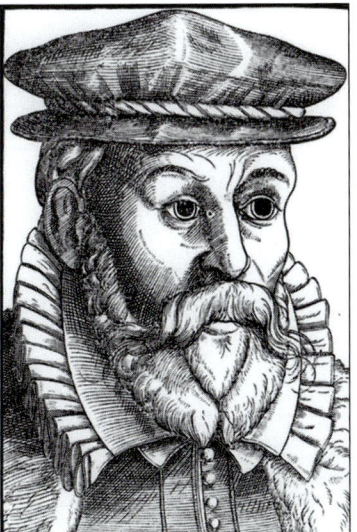

Medicinal remedies for eye diseases have been available for centuries, as is evidenced by the image in Georg Bartisch's 16th century textbook on ophthalmology.
LEFT: An ophthalmic recipe.
RIGHT: Acute glaucoma with bilateral dilated pupils. Ophthalmologists concocted various medicinal recipes to treat this.

225

CHAPTER 14

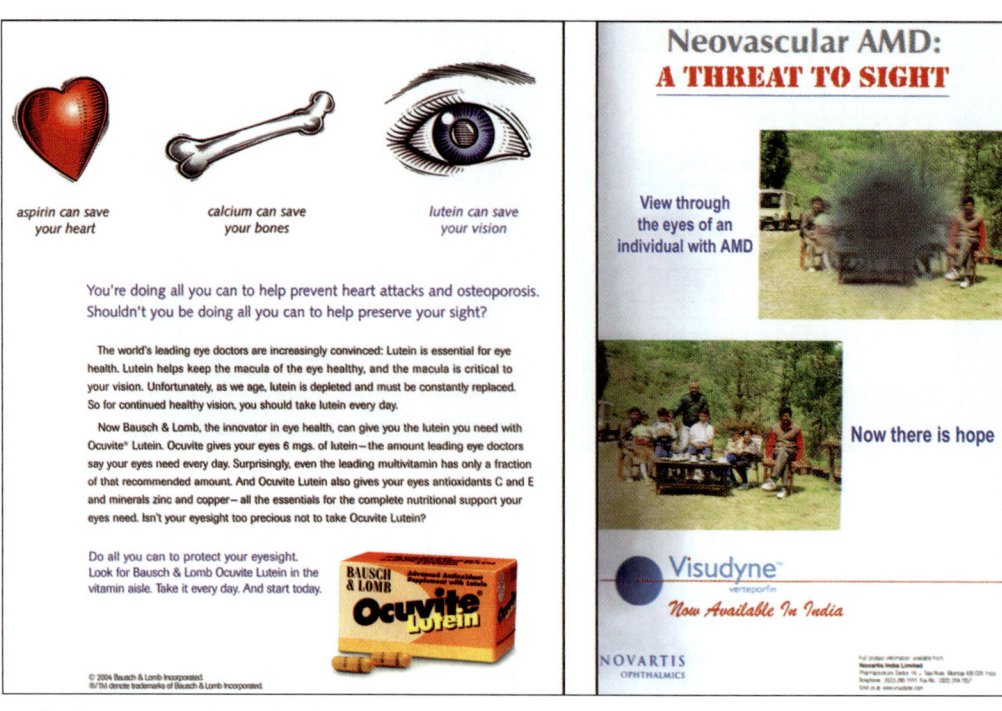

Medical treatment of macular diseases. Just as Harold treated amblyopia of released prisoners who he suspected may have choriocapillaris problems, physicians today are also treating ARMD patients with multivitamins and other medical therapies.
LEFT: Ocuvite (Bausch & Lomb), a multivitamin with zinc.
RIGHT: Visudyne (Novartis). It is activated by light, forming reactive oxygen radicals that destroy neovascular endothelium (new abnormal blood vessels) in the choriocapillaris under the macula. These abnormal vessels are the cause of ARMD, just as Harold has postulated that these same vessels may be significant in the causation of some of the amblyopias he saw in the prisoners of war.

Harold always had an interest in retinal-optic nerve diseases even though those were not his specialties. These reports on retinal topics were from his early years.
LEFT: 1935.
RIGHT: 1937.

SIMPLE DETACHMENT OF THE RETINA   101

Reprinted from
THE BRITISH JOURNAL OF OPHTHALMOLOGY,
February, 1935.

SOME PRACTICAL POINTS IN THE TREATMENT OF SIMPLE DETACHMENT OF THE RETINA

BY

HAROLD RIDLEY

SENIOR RESIDENT OFFICER, MOORFIELDS EYE HOSPITAL

OF late, with improvements in technique, operations for detachment of the retina have become much more frequent. Though at the moment diathermy operations are in almost universal favour, there is considerable variation in method and application, and a few notes based on first-hand experience, either as operator or assistant, of a large number of cases recently dealt with at Moorfields may be of interest.

The problem, like any other in surgery, consists of two parts— diagnosis and treatment. From the surgical aspect a simple retinal detachment should be regarded as a secondary lesion following a retinal tear, and on this latter our attention must be concentrated. Diagnosis consists of localization of the hole.

Localization of the hole may be simple or very difficult. In many cases a very shrewd idea can be obtained even without the use of the ophthalmoscope. A patient seen wearing a high myopic correction is most likely to have a large tear in the upper half of the retina some distance from the periphery; an emmetrope or hypermetrope a disinsertion in the lower temporal quadrant. The patient's history, if reliable, is of great importance; for instance, flashes of light in the lower nasal field followed by a shadow beginning in the same situation is almost pathognomonic of a hole in the upper temporal quadrant. Unfortunately, a shadow beginning in the upper half of the field is not such a reliable guide to the situation of the hole, for subretinal fluid leaking through a hole above tends to sink under the action of gravity

---

Reprinted from

THE BRITISH JOURNAL
OF
OPHTHALMOLOGY
FEBRUARY, 1936

CYSTIC RETINAL DETACHMENTS

BY

HAROLD RIDLEY

LONDON

IT is only in comparatively recent years, since detachment of the retina became other than a hopeless condition, that its varieties have been studied. The vast majority of simple detachments are characterised by the presence of a hole which is in all probability the *fons et origo mali*. In myopes the hole is most commonly horseshoe-shaped and in the upper temporal quadrant, and in emmetropes and hypermetropes a disinsertion in the lower temporal quadrant of the retina. There is, however, a much rarer type in which no hole is present and is, in fact, a cystic detachment which is not widely recognised and has only previously been reported in single cases by British writers.

Comment was made by the writer on this subject in the *Brit. Jl. of Ophthal.* of February, 1935, but a description of the condition may be repeated.

The cysts reported hereafter occurred in persons of middle-age. The history given was that an opacity was suddenly noticed in some part of the nasal field and that this did not later increase as is usual in detachments. It seems also that the sensation of movement experienced with a billowy detachment does not occur. Central vision was unimpaired though a scotoma corresponding to the detached area was found. In two patients the condition was bilateral. All the cysts were temporal and extended to the periphery of the retina, three being in the upper quadrant and five in the

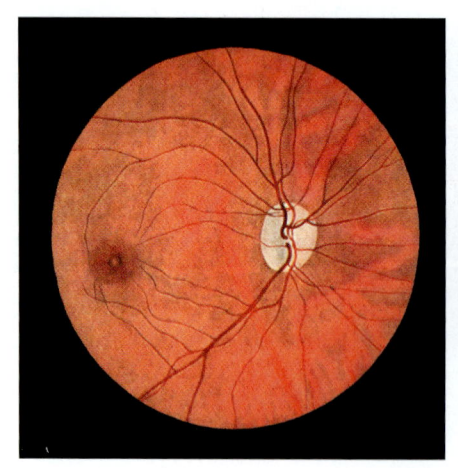

The advance to fundus photography.
TOP LEFT: In the year just after the invention of the ophthalmoscope, most retinal images were preserved by artists' drawings.
TOP RIGHT: As the technology advanced, photographic images of the fundus became a reality.
BOTTOM: The early fundus camera, like this one circa 1910, were bulky, cumbersome, and complicated to use.

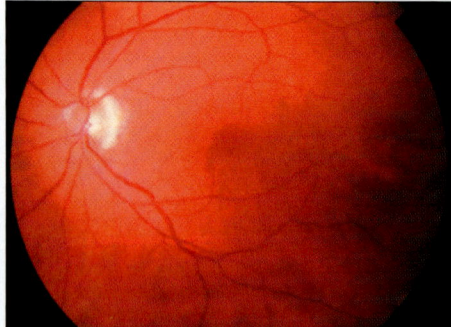

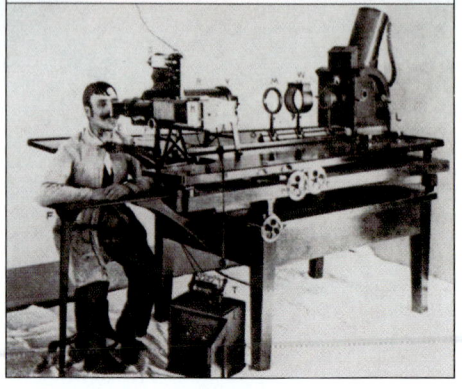

15

Technical Applications from World War II

"Harold Ridley invented the concept of the laser scanning ophthalmoscope (LSO) in the 1940s and 1950s. All he had to do was wait for the invention of the laser! His work finally came to fruition in 1979 through 1983 thanks to the efforts of Dr. Martin Mainster and colleagues."

David Apple, MD

Harold had what one calls the "golden touch." By that I mean he worked successfully on the topic at hand, taking advantage of the situations that came his way. His many successes included excursions into nonsurgical areas of ophthalmology—something few are aware of. One of his successes involved an innovation in the field of noninvasive diagnosis of the optic nerve and retina—far, far away from intraocular lens surgery. He published several papers related to the optic nerve and retina. After the end of World War II he was able to apply new technology developed during those years to enhance diagnosis and treatment of retinal and optic nerve diseases. These applications have become increasingly important today since there are now many options available for the treatment of diseases affecting the retina and optic nerve, especially ARMD (see Chapter 14).

While working in close concert with his colleagues who were doing brilliant work in the technical department at St. Thomas' Hospital, he developed a number of electronic devices that were of particular use in the eye sciences—too many to describe in this chapter. We will discuss only two of them here; both were significant advancements that led to innovations and inventions that are still very useful today and have had a marked impact on diagnosis, education, and patient care.

Harold was working on these innovations in the field of electronics during precisely the same period of time when he was making final preparations for the implantation of the IOL. It is amazing that he was able to keep up with the de-

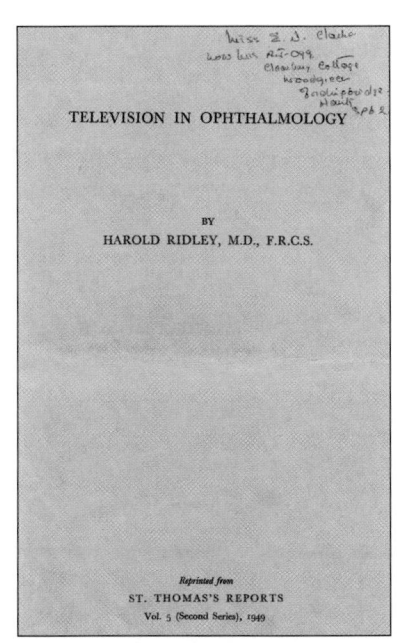

Harold was one of the first to apply TV technology to ophthalmology.

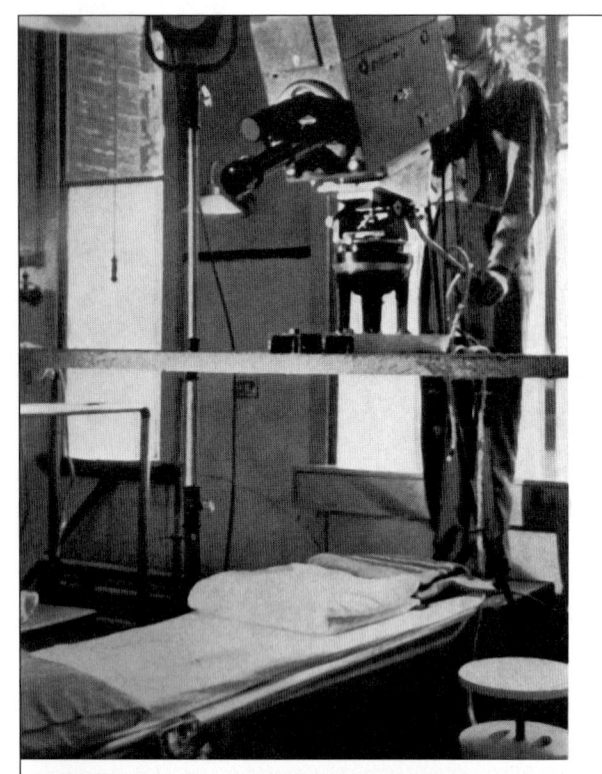

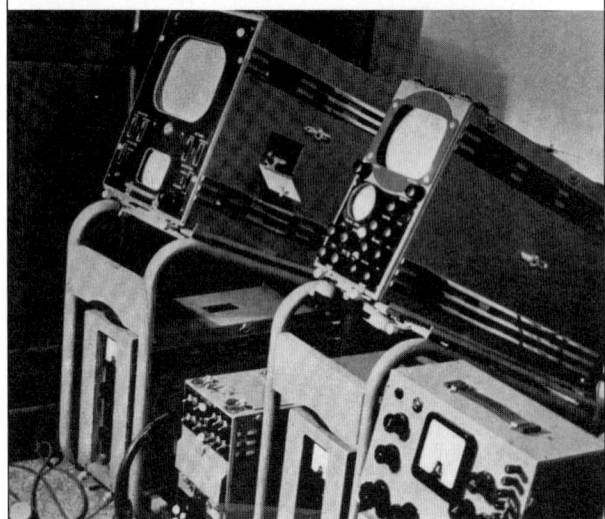

Harold and his team applied television technology to the eye.
TOP: Ridley and colleagues succeeded in televising eye operations in black and white as well as in color.
BOTTOM: Early 5-inch television monitors were used to view the first television images of the fundus (retina and optic nerve).

mands of multiple projects. But we are fortunate that he did; they turned out to be highly beneficial not only to the field of ophthalmology, but to medicine as a whole.

Televising Eye Operations

Throughout 1949 Harold traveled—actually speeded, over 100 miles per hour—back and forth from London to the small city of Chelmsford, just outside Cambridge, where the Marconi Wireless Telegraph Co. had offices, technical facilities, and manufacturing facilities. Working with colleagues both there and at St. Thomas', he was working on experiments with televising ophthalmic operations, not only in black and white, but also in color.

Dr. John Sims and I wrote about this stage of his career. We included the following statements from Harold:

"Cooperating again with Marconi's Wireless Telegraph Company and Pye Electronics' Company, and with additional help from John Pike of the Rayner's Company, as well as colleagues from St. Thomas' Hospital, including several brilliant workers in the field of electronics (Mr. Peter Styles and Dr. P. Bauwens of St. Thomas' Hospital), fundus pictures were produced. The first pictures were obtained by indirect ophthalmoscopy, transferred onto an electric apparatus and later by the 'Flying Spot' Ophthalmoscope.

"Fundus pictures good enough to have been televised to other cities were produced. However, with the apparatus then available, more detailed examination of the inner eye was not achieved. We hoped to try selected wavelengths, etc., but had neither time nor money to spare. My great teacher, A. C. Hudson (Huddy) did not support my attempts to produce electronic retinoscopy, or later, intraocular lens implants, for that matter, but we did remain the best of friends.

"Monochrome fundus pictures were produced and shown at the Oxford Congress in 1950, along with full color televised operations conducted earlier at St. Thomas' Hospital."

Two colleagues from St. Thomas' Hospital assisted Harold in these efforts—Ms. Doreen Clarke (now Mrs. Ogg), his loyal nurse assistant on the November 29, 1949 operation (see Chapter 1), and Mr. Jimmy S. Phillpot. These two volunteered to be "patients" for the television experiments, and the images of their eyes have ensured them a small place in ophthalmic history.

It was possible to televise operations on the external eyes in both black and white and color. However, with the early technology, it was only possible to film operations inside the eyes in black and white. After his successes in filming surgery of eyes viewed

TECHNICAL APPLICATIONS FROM WORLD WAR II

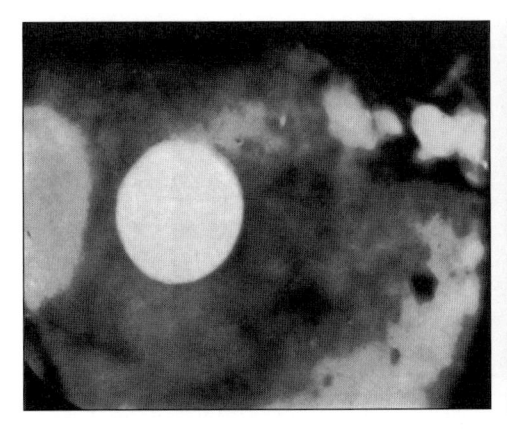

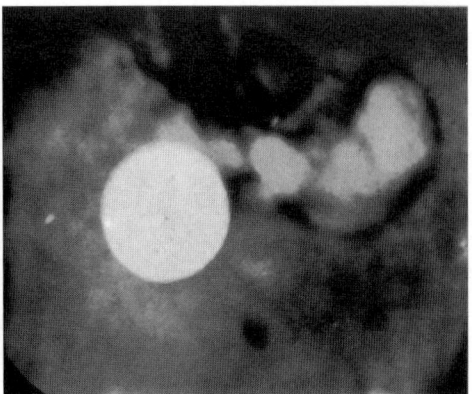

LEFT: Photograph taken from the monitor showing optic disc, macula, and pigmentation from past choroiditis televised by indirect ophthalmoscopy. The bright circle is reflected light.
RIGHT: Another image of televised indirect ophthalmoscopy image showing a choroidal scar with pigmentation.

on the outside, he worked on being able to televise operations deep within eye. He called this "intraocular television."

In order to have a proper perspective of the cutting-edge nature of Ridley's work with television, it must be remembered that although television had been around for decades, experimentation with the viable technology at that time was still quite new. In fact, I can remember as a child seeing television for the first time in 1950 at the home of more affluent neighbors who could afford the relatively expensive devices, peering with wonder into a very small screen with a very fuzzy picture.

It is not clear exactly who televised the first eye operations. Although Harold did not claim this honor for himself, there is no doubt that he was at least an early pioneer in this field.

It was Harold's full intent to develop a system of telediagnosis. This would allow, for example, a doctor in Salisbury to send a televised image of a patient's problematic eye condition to an expert in London and get a diagnosis back immediately. He was quite precise with this idea. This technique is now used routinely with the excellent advantage and result that he predicted.

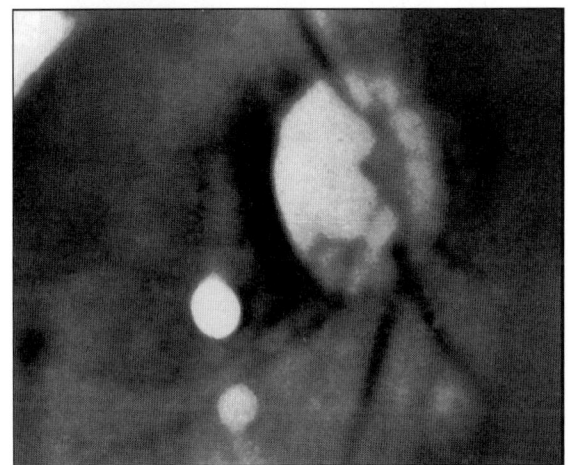

Photograph taken from the television monitor showing a normal retina. This picture is a photograph of one of Harold's assistants' eyes, and is blurry due to the difficulty of pulling the image off the small screen. However, the salient structures are still easily identified. This is one of the first televised views of the interior of an eye ever made.

NONINVASIVE DIAGNOSIS OF THE RETINA AND OPTIC NERVE

Another important result of Ridley's foray into electronics was his contribution to the field of noninvasive diagnosis of the retina and optic nerve. I have prepared the following list to outline the evolution of the pathways of innovations that have enhanced our ability to perform noninvasive (without a biopsy or surgery) diagnosis of diseases of the posterior pole (retina and optic nerve, ocular fundus, or fundus oculi). Harold's contriutions were to numbers 6 and 7, namely standard TV analysis and LSO (SLO).

Optic Nerve and Retina Evaluation
1. Prior to 1851: No practical techniques were available. The optic nerve and surrounding retina had remained "terra incognita" for millennia. Proper clinical examination could not be carried out.

CHAPTER 15

> **RECENT METHODS OF FUNDUS EXAMINATION INCLUDING ELECTRONIC OPHTHALMOSCOPY**
>
> HAROLD RIDLEY (London)
>
> THE origins of modern ophthalmology may fairly be said to date from Helmholtz's discovery of ophthalmoscopy in 1851. He employed very crude apparatus, viewing the fundus through a battery of clear glass plates set at an angle so that light from an outside source could be reflected into the eye. A concave lens was incorporated so permitting a clear image of the fundus if either or both eyes were myopic (Fig. 190).
>
> FIG. 190. 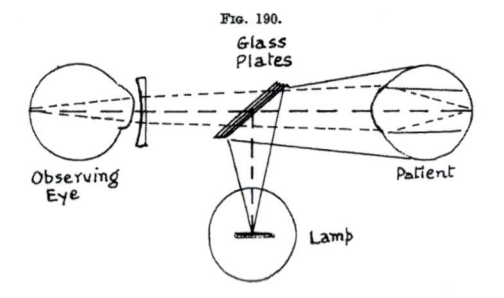
>
> Helmholtz evidently did not know of the invention four years earlier by our own Charles Babbage who used a glass mirror with a clear hole in the middle like our well-remembered non-luminous instruments (Fig. 191). Had our ophthalmologists followed up this invention, the origin of ophthalmoscopy would have been British.

As Harold's work on television and ophthalmology evolved, he eventually developed the technology that led to the invention of the laser scanning ophthalmoscope (LSO). He had the idea, he just had to wait for the invention of the laser!

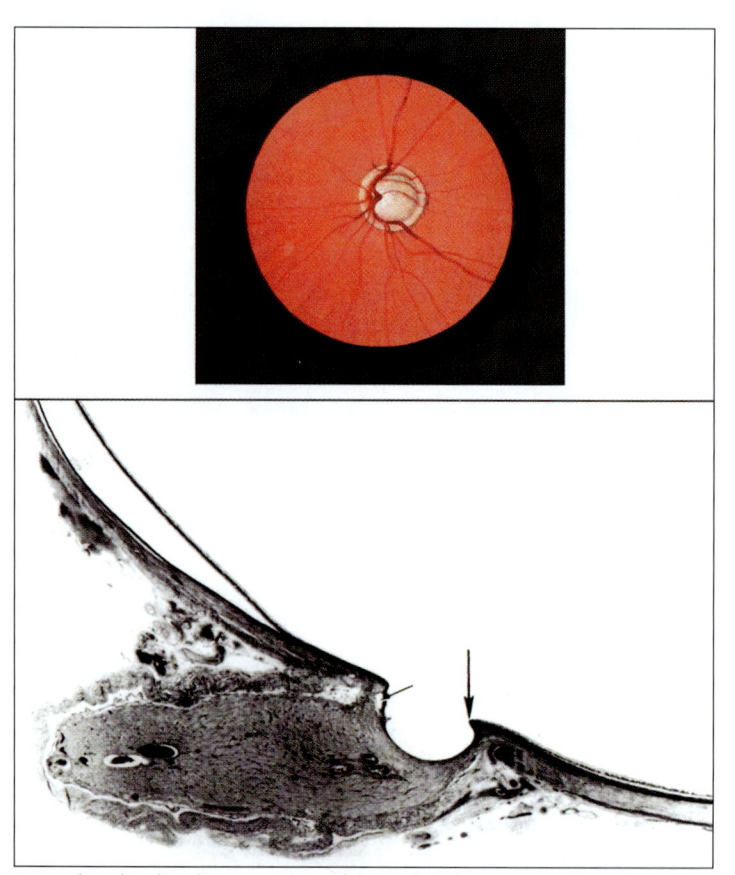

Immediately after the invention of the ophthalmoscope, the only means of documenting optic nerve pathology was via the artist's brush.
TOP: An excellent artist's rendering of a large glaucomatous excavation of the optic nerve head, classic for this condition.
BOTTOM: Pathology cross-section of the retina-optic nerve from my collection, showing the typical glaucomatous evacuation (demarcated by arrows) that forms as the intraocular pressure pushes back against the damaged nerve, resulting in damage to both the nerve head and retinal nerve fibers.

2. 1851: Hermann von Helmoltz's discovery of the ophthalmoscope (almost simultaneously described by Charles Babbage in England) enabled the first views into the eye, including the posterior pole.
3. Mid-19th century: Histopathological (microscopic) analysis of autopsy eyes and research material provided for the first time a view of the substructure of the eye tissues. Normal histology (classic light microscopy) was supplemented in the mid-20th century by electron microscopy.
4. Latter part of 19th century and early 20th century: The initial technique for viewing and analyzing the optic nerve and retina after clinical examination with von Helmoltz's ophthalmoscope was with painted images made by extremely brilliant and talented artists.
5. Early 20th century: Techniques for optic nerve and retinal photography were developed, which at first were cumbersome, but provided real images as opposed to earlier drawings.

TECHNICAL APPLICATIONS FROM WORLD WAR II

6. 1940s onward: The application of television technology to the retina, optic nerve, and surrounding tissues was studied by Ridley and his colleagues at St. Thomas' Hospital (Peter Styles, and others at Marconi Wireless Telegraph Corp. and Pye Corp.). Ridley and his team succeeded in televising eye operations in both black and white and in color and in examining the fundus tissues with television technology.

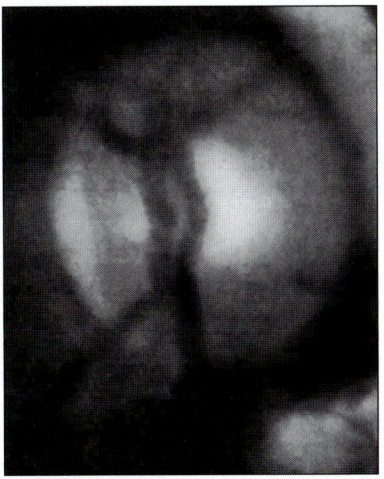

Photograph via the TV monitor of the eye of one of Harold's assistants showing the optic disc as seen by indirect ophthalmoscopy.

7. 1980s and 1990s: Ridley published his team's original work on what evolved into a paper that provided a classic description of his "flying spot" ophthalmoscope. This work then evolved into the laser scanning ophthalmoscope (LSO), (also termed a scanning laser polimeter or SLO). This is now a well-accepted means of noninvasive examination of the back of the eye. All Harold and his team had to do was wait a few decades for the invention of the laser.

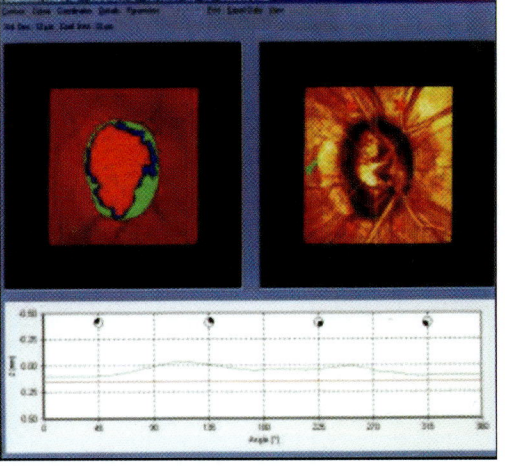

Electric evaluation of the optic nerve head. The area of the cup appears red.
TOP: The optic nerve head on this eye shows a normal cup.
BOTTOM: The margin of the optic disc is narrow by a large cup, as enclosed by the large red area.

Nerve fiber layer analysis in both the optic nerve and retina was further improved by the introduction of computerized optical coherence tomography (OCT).

The latter two tests—LSO or SLO and OCT—now provide the examiner with the ability to in essence generate histological cuts of the tissue, providing the same advantages that microscopy would, but without any need for invasion into the tissues.

The list shows that Harold made two important contributions to these diagnostic modalities, namely, the use of television for the diagnosis and recording of surgery, and not long thereafter, the development of the laser scanning ophthalmoscope (LSO). Together with today's high-quality OCT, this technology makes the diagnosis of certain forms of eye diseases much more practical and available.

Harold's contributions in this area have been verified by experts, including Dr. Martin Mainster, who helped develop the mature procedure of laser scanning ophthalmoscopy from 1979 to 1983. Mainster, now one of the world's experts in this field, and his colleagues did their work without knowledge of the early British efforts in the field. Another expert in this field is Dr. Barry Masters, formerly of the Uniformed Armed Services Medical School in Washington, DC. In a review article, Masters confirmed how Harold's work laid the groundwork for this device once laser technology became available.

As his work in electronics evolved, Harold prepared to present it at the meeting of the International Congress of Ophthalmology (ICO) in 1950. However, he was deprived of an official position in the organization by his colleague, Sir Stewart Duke-Elder.

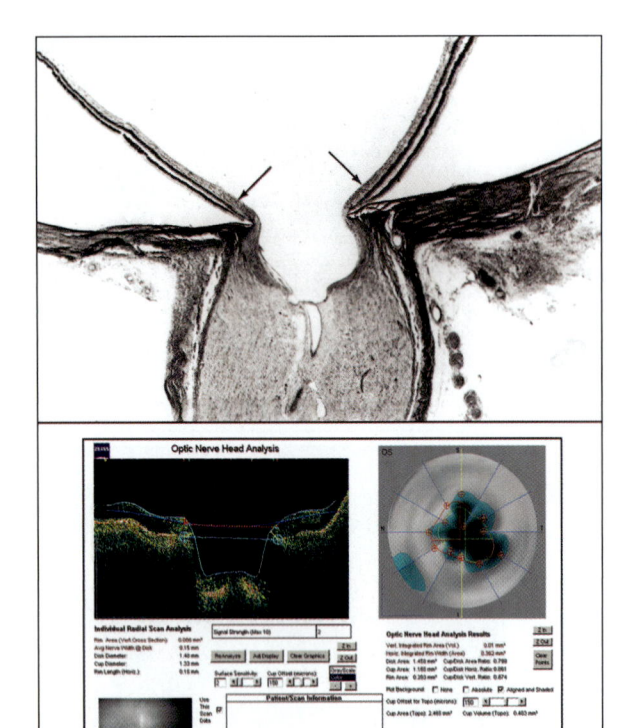

CHAPTER 15

This slight represented yet another in a series of problems the he had with the master. However, Harold said that he overcame what he considered a problem by going ahead and proceeding with his presentations at St. Thomas'. In his words:

"I overcame this without problems (or so it seems), by putting on the dramatic televised operations at St. Thomas' Hospital, and also electronic ophthalmoscopy. These demonstrations were wonders to many participants, some of whom (from Norway, for instance) had never seen TV in any form. After the Congress, Duke-Elder refereed my demonstrations, but as a sign of things to come, never offered congratulations,

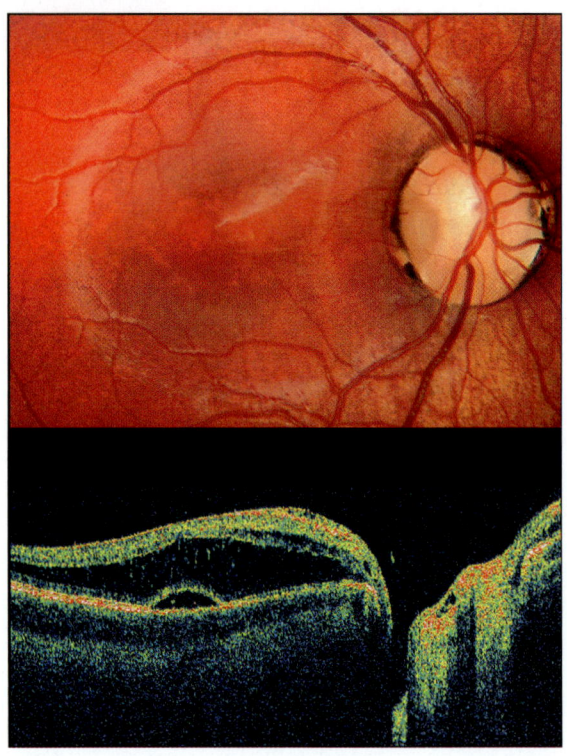

Histologic versus digital diagnosis of an optic nerve in glaucoma.
TOP: The very deep cup is easily recognizable in this cross section (demarcated by arrows).
BOTTOM: The image at left is almost identical to that seen in the histological section above.

Digital analysis of the optic cup, optic pit. An optic pit is a colobomatous (congenital) condition often accompanied by an associated swelling of the macula (macular edema).
TOP: Clinical photograph of a temporal optic pit. There is a large accumulation to the left of the nerve in the retina.
BOTTOM: This is a digital image of the same retina and optic nerve as above. This shows an excellent view of the colobomatous excavation of the nerve (right). Notice that the retina (left) has cystic cavities that contain edema fluid.

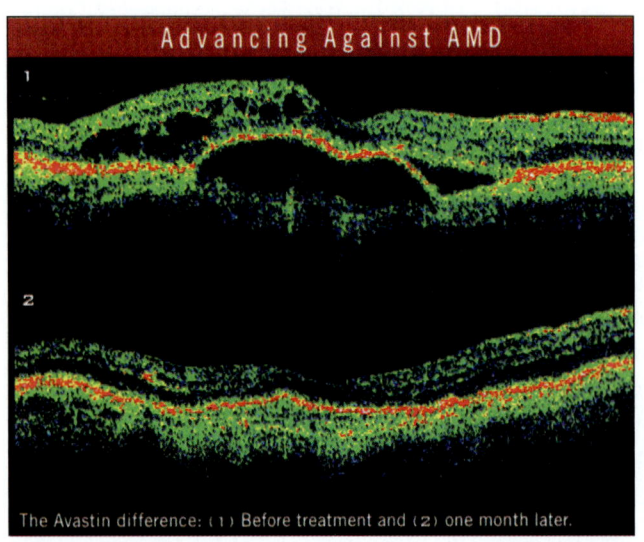

Digital image showing a successful treatment of ARMD using Avastin (Genentech, Inc., San Francisco, CA).
TOP: A photograph before treatment, with multiple sites of deposition of fluid within cysts in the retina.
BOTTOM: One month after treatment these lesions have disappeared, indicating a successful treatment.

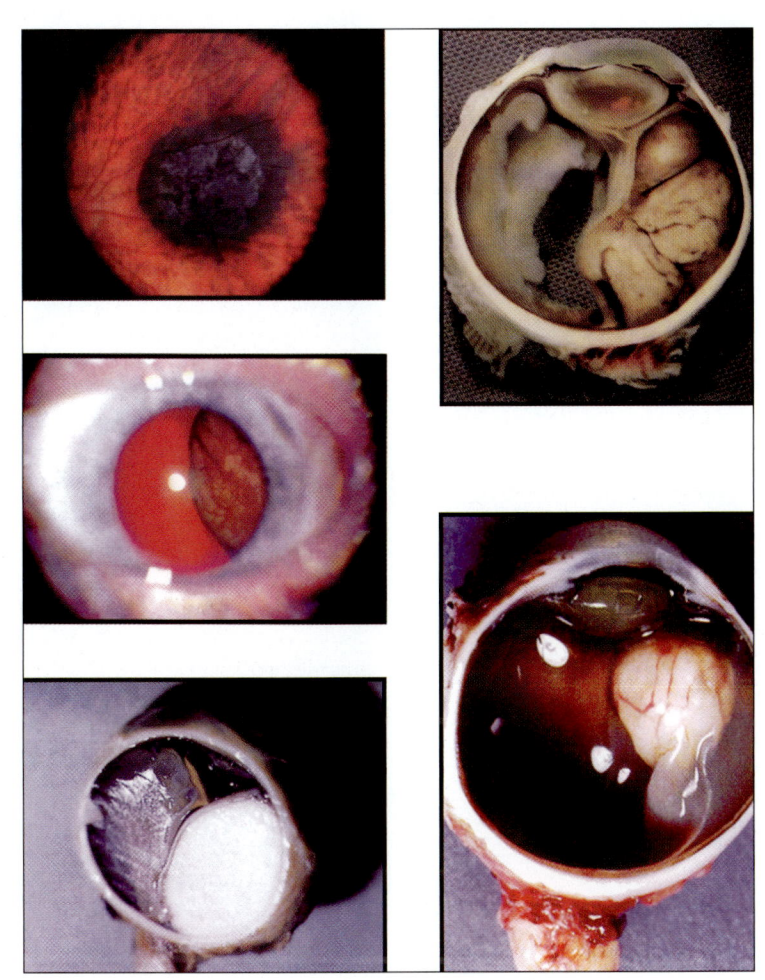

TECHNICAL APPLICATIONS FROM WORLD WAR II

Malignant cancers sometimes arise in the eye. This is a series of five cases from my collection to illustrate these tumors. They are malignant melanomas that arise from the pigmented tissues of the eye, the uvea. This consists of the iris, ciliary body, and choroid. The picture on the upper left, is a clinical photograph. The four others are eyes that have been opened to exhibit the tumor mass.

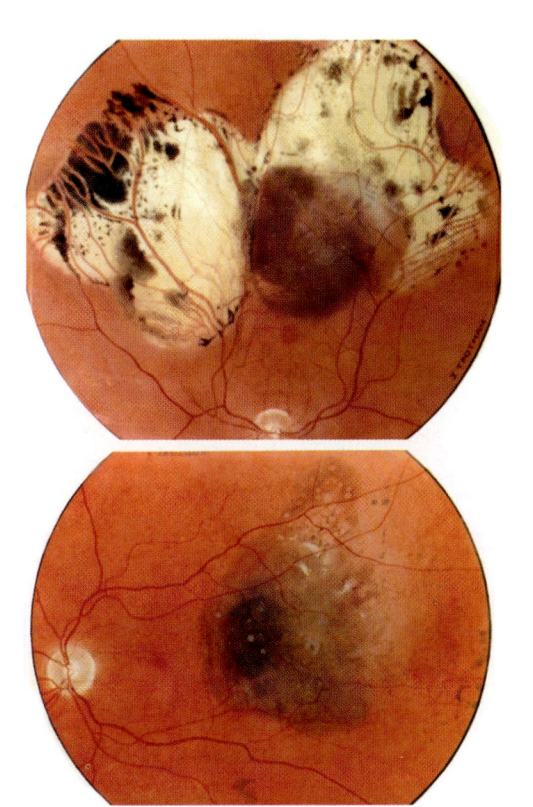

Radiation treatment of melanotic (pigmented) neoplasm).
TOP: A large, treated tumor mass.
BOTTOM: Post-treatment. This not only destroys (hopefully) the cancer, but also destroys some of the surrounding retina. This is evidenced by the scarring and dark pigment accumulations around the tumor. At least the patient still retains his or her eye, as surgical remaval was avoided.

nor even mentioned the name of the producer. I thought that he was just jealous and just carried on with my hospital work and with my research."

Harold also did a brief clinical study on intraocular tumors—an attempt to destroy or eradicate them without having to remove the patient's eye. He was not the first to experiment in this area, but again it reveals his initiative to work with whatever was at hand. There are three possible techniques to do a localized treatment: surgical excision, destruction of the tumor by light (photocoagulation), and radiation. He presented some successful cases at a meeting in Budapest.

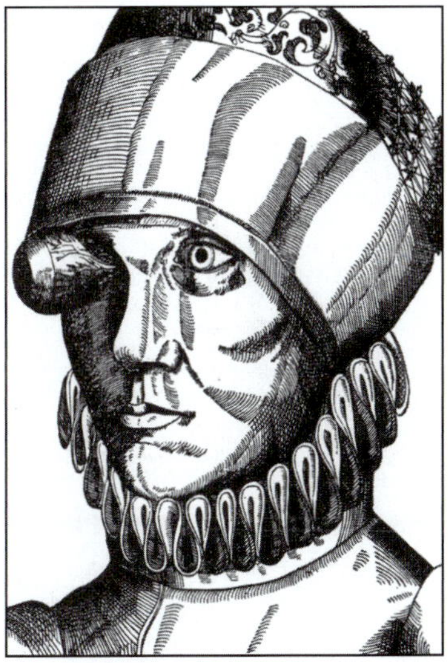

Eye cancers have existed since the beginning of the human race. This is a picture of one illustrated in Georg Bartisch's 16th century textbook. Prior to the modern era, most tumors simply grew (as seen here) and the patient would invariably die. Eye tumors in adults are almost invariably malignant melanomas. In children the tumors grow from the retina (retinoblastomas).

235

CHAPTER 15

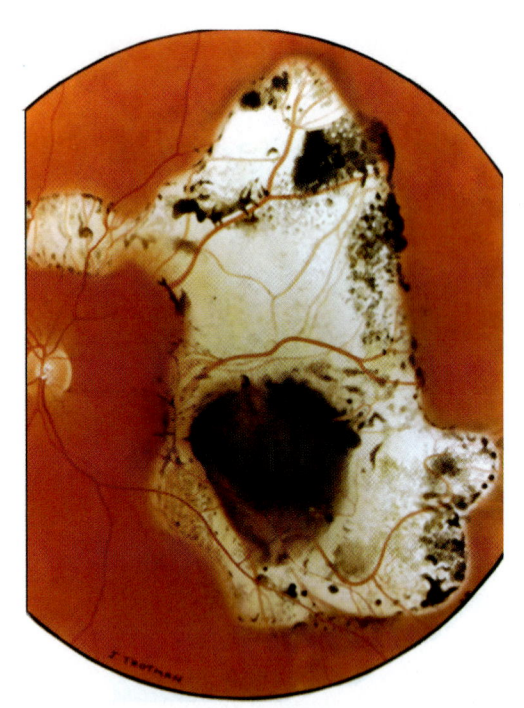

Harold's research efforts on intraocular tumors were cut short because it was difficult to concentrate on other projects, since he was busy improving and defending IOLs. This occupied the lion's share of his time and energies for the rest of his life.

Treatment of a very large tumor. Compare the size of the mass at the area of treatment on and around it with the apparent size of the optic nerve (left). With the various techniques of local therapy, one hopes to destroy the tumor cells without having to remove the patient's eye.

16

Biomedical Engineering and Artificial Organ Transplantation

"The field of bioengineering can be traced back to a British doctor, Harold Ridley, who treated wounded pilots in World War II. His observation led to the plastic lenses used in cataract patients today.

"Ridley, an ophthalmologist and surgeon, noticed the eyes didn't react with inflammation to the plastic even when embedded deep into the interior of the eye. Normally, the body reacts to reject any foreign material.

"After the war, Ridley began experimenting with the Plexiglas and eventually used it to fashion an artificial lens to replace the clouded-over lenses in people with cataracts. **It took decades, but the medical community eventually accepted Ridley's lenses as a standard treatment for cataracts**" *[emphasis added].*

Buddy Ratner, PhD, Director of the University of Washington's Engineered Biomaterials Center, Seattle, Washington, 2004

Modern medical implants, for example artificial hearts or kidneys, are no longer particularly novel concepts. We are now benefiting from the advances of technology that occurred through the 20th century. However in Harold's time, much of this technology was still just science fiction. Even the most cutting-edge thinkers in 1949 considered the idea of putting foreign material such as plastic, silicone, nylon, Teflon, etc *into* the body to take the place of vital organs such as the heart or eye to be heresy.

---

* In this book I have listed many of the numerous synonyms of this material. These include poly(methyl) methacrylate (PMMA), acrylic, Plexiglas, Transpex, Perspex, Perspex CQ (clinical quality), the latter being a special modification of material used in cockpit canopies to make it suitable for implantation in the eye.

CHAPTER 16

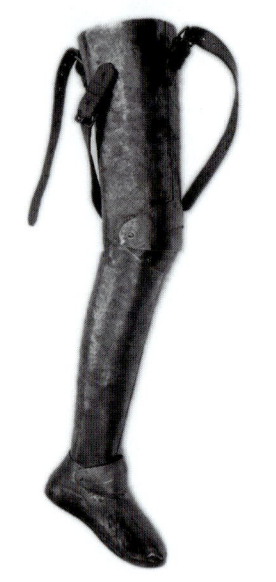

Early prosthetic leg, medieval Germany.

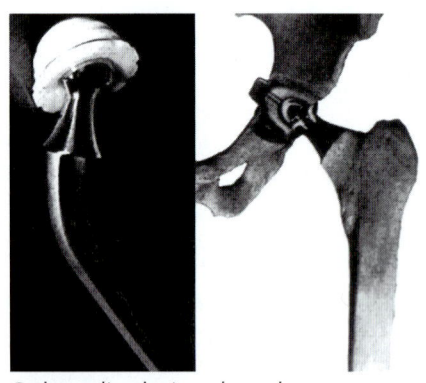

Orthopedic devices have been a part of therapeutic medicine for a long time.
LEFT: A more recent ball and socket hardware design for hip replacement.
RIGHT: Early hip replacement hardware circa the early 20th century.

Harold's implantation of a plastic intraocular lens on November 29, 1949, was more than heretical. To my knowledge, it was the first foray anyone in any specialty had made into the science of implanting prosthetic devices in the delicate, vital internal tissues of the body. The eye is certainly a delicate organ, and surgeons were clearly afraid to disturb its interior by inserting something foreign into it. But, having studied the reactions (or lack of them) in pilot's eyes, including Cleaver's eyes for many years and conjuring up the necessary courage after his encounter with the student, Stephen Perry, in 1948 (see the front page of Chapter 7, page 128), Harold did operation number one on November 29, 1949, and it worked!

Devices designed for many purposes had been in existence for years, but to my knowledge most if not all of these were prostheses designed to provide structural support or to provide a splint to serve a function, for example, various dental prostheses. I am not aware of any report prior to 1949 of an actual implant of a replacement device into the heart, lungs, kidney, brain, eye, or other vital organ of the body. Most surgeons were afraid to or were unable to touch the very vulnerable and delicate tissues of the body that were critical and indispensable.

In other words, I believe that Harold did something revolutionary that day in 1949 that was far above simply beginning the era of inserting plastic into the eye. It was a move into unknown territory. Just as the ancients could not see into the eye and therefore gave it mystical properties (Chapter 2), implantation of foreign devices into vital body organs did not occur until Harold's first IOL operation.

Harold broke ground to become a pioneer in the special field we now call *biomedical engineering,* with special application in this case to transplants (transplantology) and artificial devices.

In the specific field of ophthalmology, Harold's first IOL operation opened a whole new realm of possibilities (see Preface). The changes his innovation set in motion have led to a wide spectrum of phenomenal advances both in device design and surgical techniques—from very simple things—to what is essentially intraocular plastic surgery—to complex electronic devices.

Much more complicated uses for Ridley's original advancements have already been studied. Jim Deacon, one of my former fellows in the "Apple Korps," was an early investigator in the field of injectable IOLs. This involves injecting a polymer that is liquid or close to liquid state at the time of injection into the eye. The material then "hardens" just enough to form an effective intraocular lens within the eye. Such a device would have many uses, the most obvious being that it could function as an accommodative lens. One can design the lens so that it hardens just enough to be able to change its thickness; the lens thickens or thins by adjusting itself appropri-

An IOL used for cosmesis.
TOP LEFT: Placement of an early Choyce artificial iris IOL designed to improve cosmetic appearance or to repair a damaged iris.
BOTTOM LEFT: Close-up of patient after implantation of a Choyce model artificial iris (right eye).
RIGHT: Modern one-piece, all polymethylmethacrylate (PMMA) artificial iris IOL; the central optics of course are clear and the surrounding iris portion and haptics are made of colored PMMA.

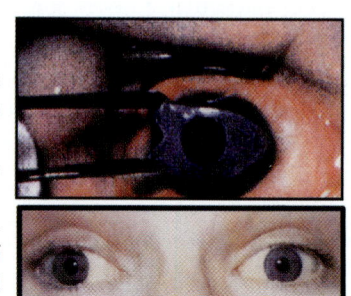

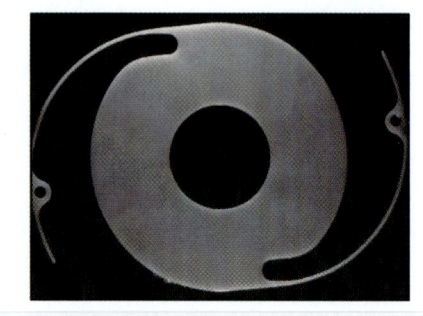

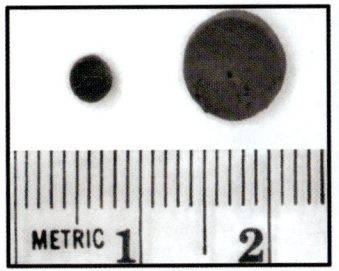

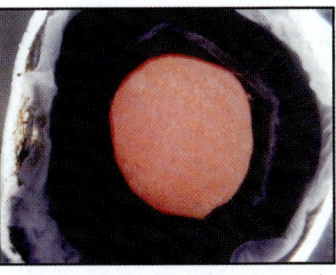

BIOMEDICAL ENGINEERING AND ARTIFICIAL ORGAN TRANSPLANTATION

The theory of an expandable IOL. This is a portion of a toy made from hydrogel material. It is designed to expand when immersed in water. We performed an experiment by making a crude "disc" IOL. We made a slice of the leg of a toy soldier and placed it in water.
LEFT: The experiment confirmed that the "lens" expanded after being immersed under water.
RIGHT: We placed a disc in a rabbit eye and confirmed that it might potentially serve as an IOL.

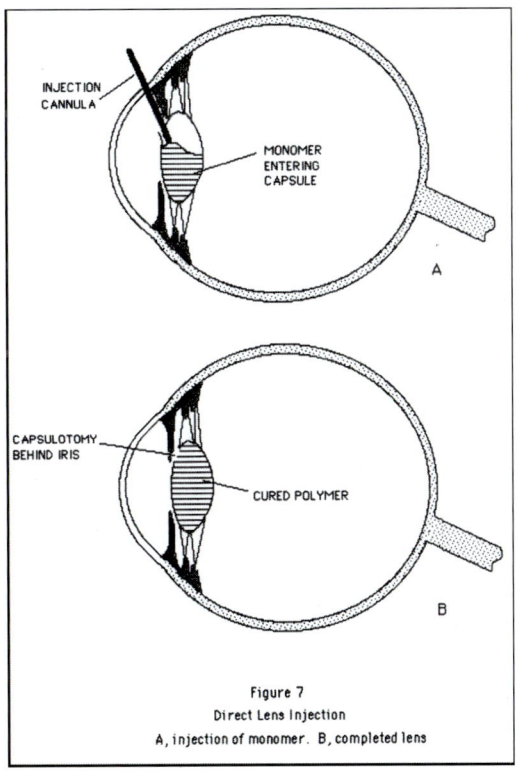

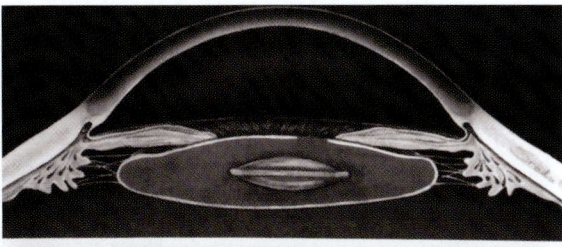

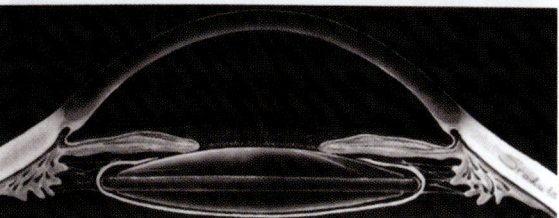

Schematic illustration showing the concept of an expandable IOL. (Courtesy of Stephen Siepser, Michael Blumenthal, Ehud Assia, Guy Kleinmann, and David Apple.)
TOP: The disc-shaped IOL is implanted in the dry state.
BOTTOM: After a few minutes in aqueous, the disc expanded to become a full-size lens.

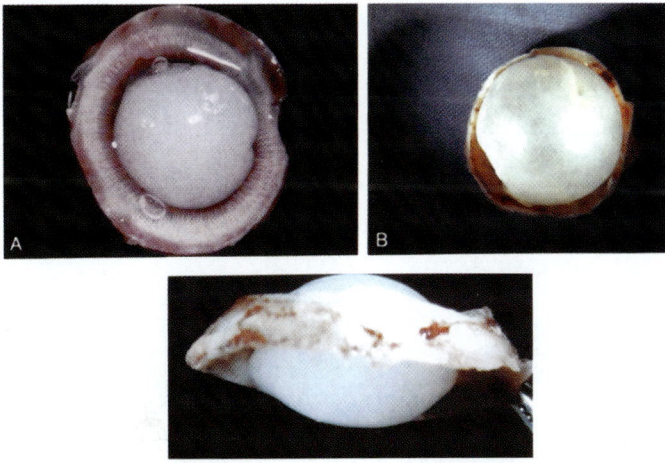

Diagram showing one proposed technique of direct lens injection (the injectable lens). This was designed by Jim Deacon, MS, a former fellow in my laboratory.
TOP: Injection cannula entering capsule and dispensing monomer into the capsule.
BOTTOM: Surgery is complete. The fully formed injectable lens fills the capsular bag.

The injectable IOL. These are three examples of experimentally injected polymer materials (not optically clear, but white for this experiment). Note how they have all formed into physiologically shaped lenses in the capsular bags of the animals.

CHAPTER 16

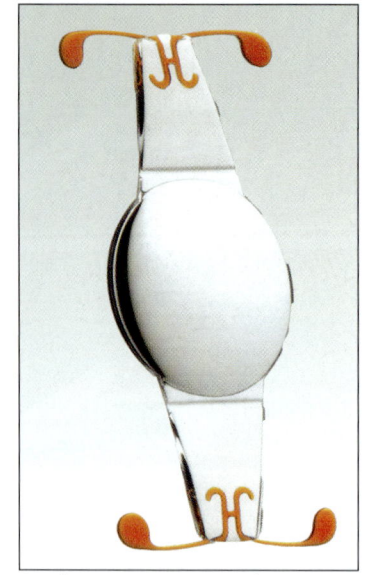

Single optic accommodative IOL. The lens is designed so that the optic moves forward and backward as the ciliary muscle expands and contracts. This appropriately changes the refractive power of the eye for near and far vision.

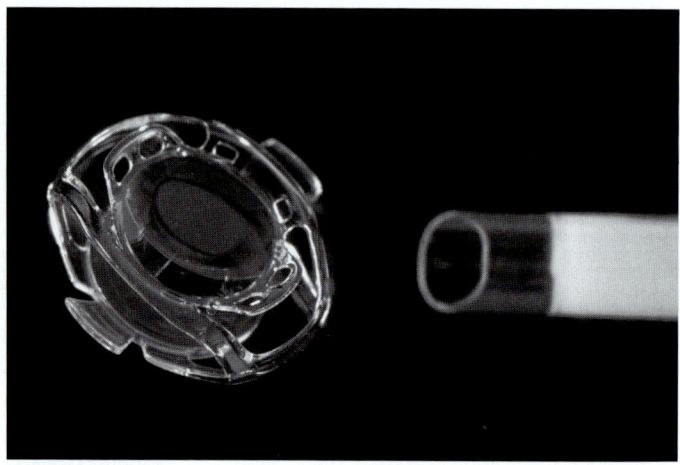

Dual optic accommodative IOL. There are two optics that are designed to appropriately change positions to provide accommodation.

ately according to the wishes of the individual's brain to allow both near and distant vision. This is possible because the lens can change its thickness upon impulses from the brain. We have done enough experiments in this field to verify that this is a viable possibility for the future.

Another example is the technologically more complex telescopic intraocular lens, also pioneered in its original form by Peter Choyce (see Chapter 10). It can be useful in any patients who might be assisted by a low vision aid. With a lens such as this, the simple optic of the IOL is replaced by a miniature Galilean telescopic device that uses the lens optic as a platform. The most common disease requiring a low vision aid is age-related macular degeneration (ARMD), but there are other such diseases where the power of an intraocular telescopic lens might be useful.

Finally, there have been numerous attempts to produce a "bionic eye." For example, the development of an artificial retina consisting of devices implanted inside the eye that utilize microchips to create vision is a move in this direction. The successful creation of implants of that nature would be a true miracle for those patients with complete or near total blindness—for example, those suffering with advanced retinitis pigmentosa.

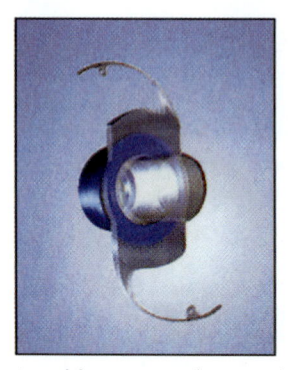

An old concept of Peter Choyce's is being revived, namely the telescopic IOL. A major use for this design is to help patients with low vision. This is a manufacturer's diagram showing the general shape of the telescope framework and the fixation haptics.

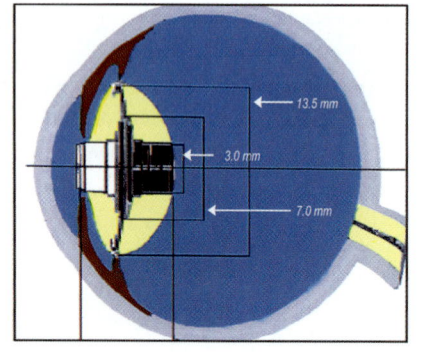

The field of bioengineered medical devices is expanding and has become a driving economic force throughout the industrialized world. The medical device industry is a 70 billion dollar business and still growing. Great strides in many specialties such as cardiology and orthopedics are being made, with breakthroughs being achieved regularly, thanks in part to digital electronics and new materials. In ophthalmology, the field of refractive surgery and the applications of what Harold would have termed "electronics" is rapidly growing. What is going on is truly miraculous.

I have done a search of the literature on this topic and conclude that Harold has clearly been a true pioneer in the field.

I am not alone in this assertion. Dr. Buddy Ratner, professor and chair of the Department of Bioengineering at the University of Washington School of Medicine in Seattle is one of many who have been aware of the literature. Dr. Ratner has publicly declared that Harold was indeed one of the pioneers, if not *the* pioneer who provided the focus and drive to successfully introduce prosthetic devices into all organ systems of the body.

To summarize, I believe it is important to document not only Harold's heretofore largely unknown or forgotten cataract operation, but also to note that he helped pioneer the general use and worldwide dissemination of permanent implantable intraocular prosthetics or biodevices—in short, artificial "tissues or organs" designed to remain permanently in a delicate tissue/organ of the body.

This is taken for granted today, but was a "bombshell" then in the 1940s and early 1950s. The strife that ensued was, in a limited way, similar to what is occurring today on a national/international level with respect to stem cell and cloning research. His invention helped propel not only ophthalmology, but indeed general medicine into a new era. It helped generate a new subspecialty that we now term biomedical engineering, which has grown rapidly over the past two decades.

Harold himself was probably not aware of the more universal significance of his invention, but we believe history will show that the introduction of these broad conceptual ideas and innovations were as important as the basic visual rehabilitative benefits of the IOL itself.

In other words, in the long run I believe that this may be Harold's most important contribution to the world—even transcending the wonderful benefits of the intraocular lens itself.

Harold's aptitude for electronics was passed on to his youngest son, David, who is the proprietor of a company that provides devices offering various forms of assistance to handicapped people. His innovations have been very clever and it has been obvious to me that, like his father, his motivation is not just money, but a true interest in the welfare of his patients.

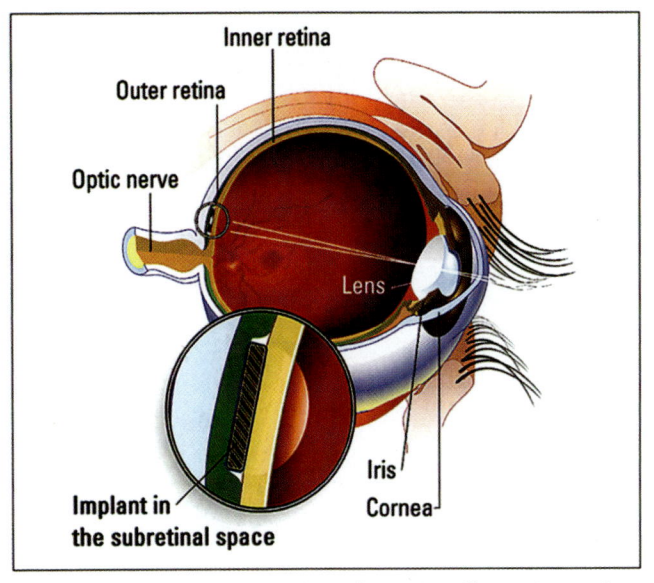

A schematic illustration of a proposed "artificial eye" using microchip technology. With this proposed model, the implant is placed in the subretinal space.

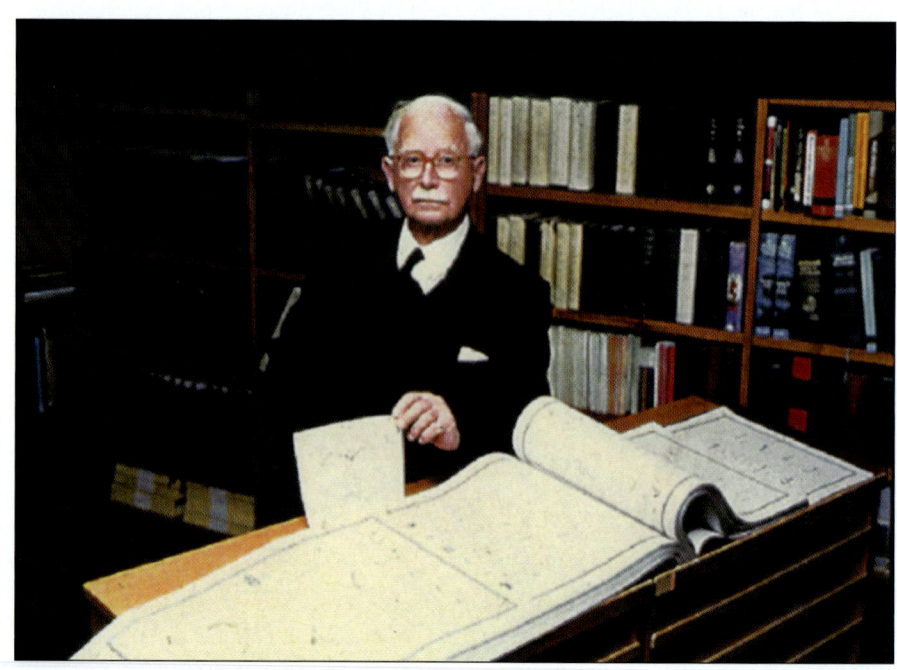

In 1979, Harold was honored in San Francisco by the American Academy of Ophthalmology and Otolaryngology with a handsome, leather-bound volume entitled *A Salute to Dr. Harold Ridley*. The volume had been signed by some 4,000 appreciative American ophthalmologists.

17

Honors, Many Received "Long After I Should Have Been Gone"

"On behalf of the leadership and membership of the American Society of Cataract and Refractive Surgery (ASCRS), we would like to invite you to be our honored guests at the upcoming Symposium on Cataract, IOL and Refractive Surgery to be held in Seattle, Washington on April 9-14, 1999. You will be honored as one of the outstanding ophthalmologists of this century, and equally important, this will be an opportunity to celebrate and honor you for the 50th anniversary of your invention of the IOL. The entire world of ophthalmology will look forward to this opportunity to present you this well deserved honor on this 50th year celebration."

ASCRS Program Committee, 1999

After decades of abuse and professional ostracism, Harold Ridley finally received recognition and honors for inventing the IOL. But they came, as he said, "long after I should have left this world."

Sadly, he was right. From an actuarial standpoint, the expected lifespan of a male born in England or Wales in 1906 was only 48 years, and that did not include the influence of war, which would have decreased it even further. If he had died at age 48 as the actuarial tables had predicted, he would have died without receiving a single honor for his remarkable, world-changing work. In fact, if he had died at age 72, a full 24 years older than the average lifespan, he likewise would have died without an honor to his name.

My own experience was quite different. I began receiving honors just a few years after I began my work in the field of IOLs. I was in my mid-40s; I began working with IOLs at the "right time." The major awards included the Jan Kiewiet de Jonge Award, the Binkhorst Lecture and Award, and soon thereafter, the ASCRS Innovation Medal (now known as the Kelman Medal).

CHAPTER 17

I received these awards rapidly, one following the other, because of timing; I was at the right place at the right time. The true innovator, Harold, (and indeed several other pioneers) lived through most of his life experiencing so much negative feedback and receiving few or no honors or recognitions. The honors to Harold did come, finally, and in this chapter we will focus on a small sampling of these.

A Book Signed by Grateful Surgeons

In 1979, recognition came from a group that meant a lot to Harold, namely, the surgeons who were the ones who really tried and evaluated his invention. Thanks to the efforts of Dr. Ken Hoffer and his colleagues at the IOL Implant Society (today the American Society of Cataract and Refractive Surgery [ASCRS]), Harold received a very meaningful recognition at the 1979 American Academy of Ophthalmology and Otolaryngology meeting in San Francisco, CA. He was presented with a large, leather-bound volume entitled, *A Salute to Dr. Harold Ridley*. Four thousand or so American ophthalmologists had signed the book—ophthalmologists who, by that time, were beginning to recognize what he had done for their specialty.

"Around 1974 some American surgeons became keenly interested in the cure of aphakia, mainly employing the Dutch method, though the majority verdict was still against any form of implant. However by 1979 in San Francisco it was evident that implants were at last beginning to be an accepted part of ophthalmic surgery and I was awarded a prize book containing signatures of 4,000 colleagues worldwide. However the precise method was still in doubt though gradually extracapsular extraction with posterior chamber lenticulus—my original procedure—was chosen and is now almost universally employed. I told the audience by your tribute today, you have saved my career from anticlimax."

Harold Ridley

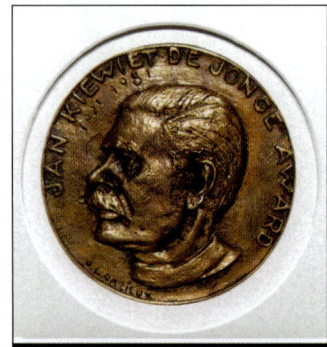

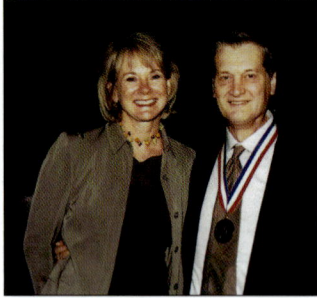

I received honors soon after entering the field of cataract-IOL research, in the beginning of my collaboration with Harold
TOP: The Jan Kiewiet de Jonge Medal, presented by the European Society of Cataract and Refractive Surgery.
BOTTOM: With my wife Ann after I received the ASCRS Innovators' Medal (now known as the Kelman Medal).

Election to the Royal Society

The first major award Ridley received from a scholarly institution was undoubtedly the one of which he was most proud. In 1986, just before his 80th birthday, he was inducted into the Royal Society, one of the—if not the—most erudite scientific societies in the country, perhaps the world. The society has deep historical roots dating back to the time of Sir Isaac Newton and was founded in the 17th century.

A prospective member has to be nominated for induction into the Royal Society. The identity of the two gentlemen who nominated Harold provides an interesting insight regarding the various feelings that still existed toward the IOL, both positive and negative. Neither of the nominators was an ophthalmologist! One of the two nominators was Norman Ashton, a general pathologist who turned his attention to ocular pathology and worked with Duke-

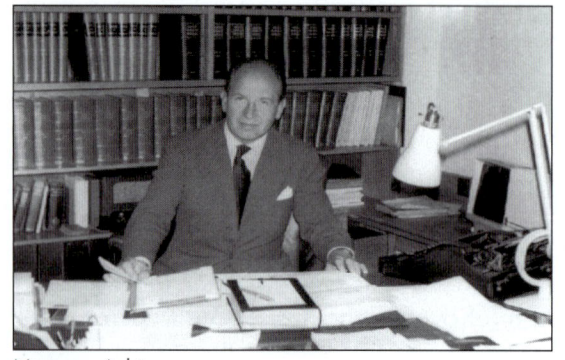

Norman Ashton.

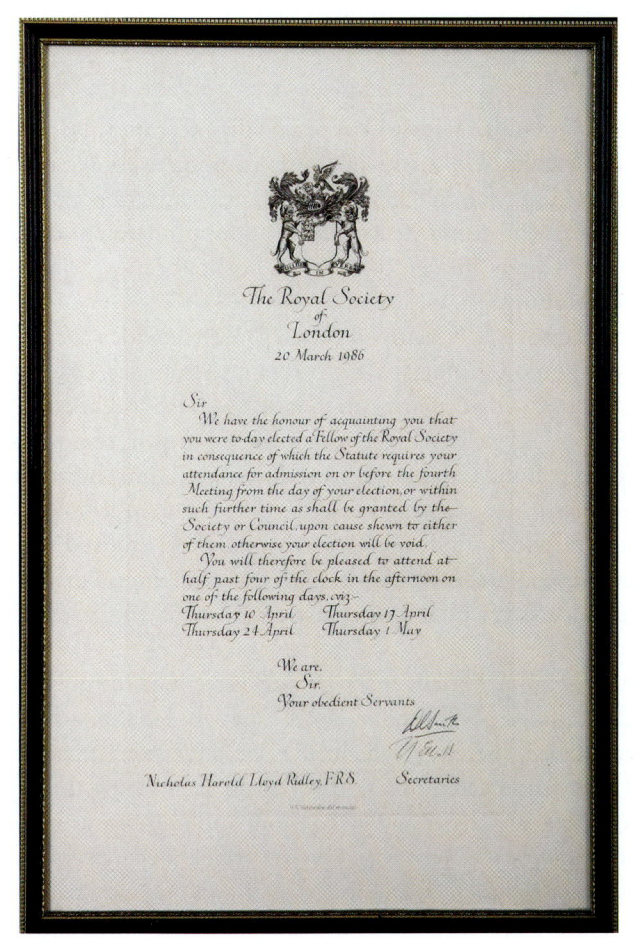

HONORS, MANY RECEIVED "LONG AFTER I SHOULD HAVE BEEN GONE"

Harold was inducted into the Royal Society of London on March 20, 1986.

Elder at the Institute of Ophthalmology in London. Since he was not a surgeon, he certainly had no ax to grind regarding the implant. He viewed it from his perspective as a noninterested observer; he clearly saw the value of the IOL. He did not carry the baggage of jealousies or other issues that were for so long a problem among many of Harold's colleagues. The second nomination was forwarded by an expert in the field of butterflies and moths, Mr. E. B. Ford, FRS, Oxford. He knew about Harold's work and could appreciate its importance, although the specialty was far removed from his realm of knowledge.

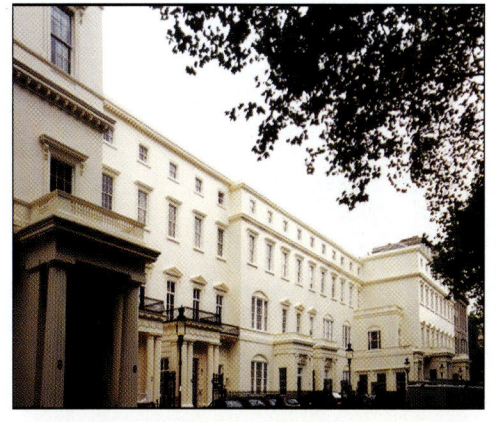

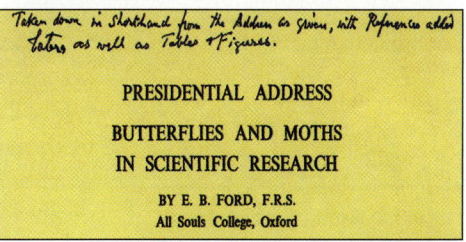

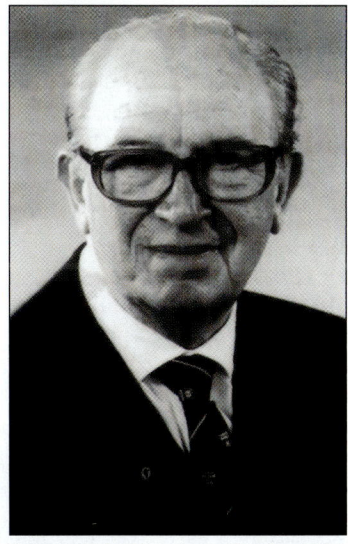

One of the honors of which he was most proud was his induction into the Royal Society in 1986.
TOP: The Royal Society headquarters in London.
MIDDLE: A protion of a publication by Mr. E. B. Ford, FRS, an expert in the study of butterflies and moths, nominated Mr. Ridley for membership in the Royal Society. Note that he had no real connection to ophthalmology or eye surgery, but truly respected Harold's work.
BOTTOM: Norman Ashton, the great pathologist at the Institute of Ophthalmology.

247

CHAPTER 17

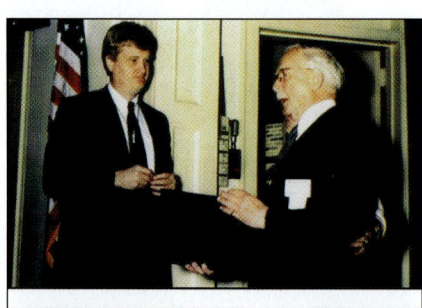

AN HONORARY DOCTOR'S DEGREE

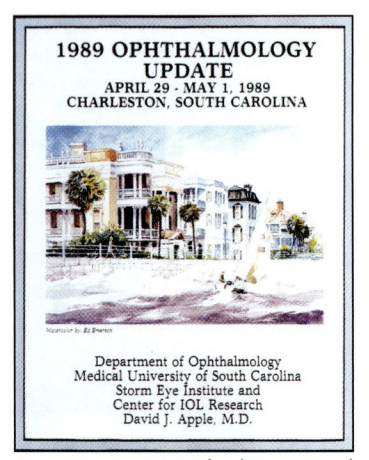

Announcement of the annual meeting of our opthalmology department at the Medical University of South Carolina in conjunction with conferring an honorary doctorate degree on Harold in April and May 1989.

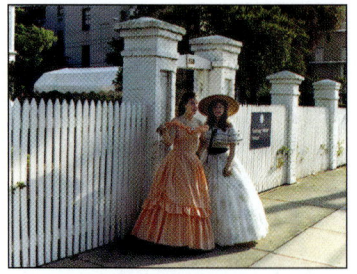

The Ridleys enjoyed the *Gone with the Wind* atmosphere of an American southern city.

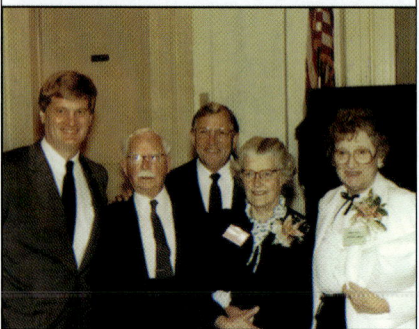

One of the accomplishments of which I am personally most proud is my work in promoting a drive at the Medical University of South Carolina to confer an honorary doctorate degree on Harold in May 1989. This was 40 years after the first implant.

My research on the IOL had confirmed without a doubt the potential safety and efficacy of the implant, and I was amazed that he had not yet been so honored at any academic institution of learning.

At the time I was Professor and Chairman of the Ophthalmology Department at the Medical University of South Carolina, having just moved from Salt Lake a few years earlier to help rebuild a floundering department, to raise funds for and help build a new facility (see pages 69 and 73), as well as further the work of our IOL research center.

I presented my idea to honor Harold to the university administration. It was not received with enthusiasm. Apparently, honoring a foreign surgeon whose work was still difficult for the public to understand because few had enjoyed the benefits of the surgery was not deemed a compelling initiative at that time. Further, Harold was not a donor to the university, which is often a prerequisite in the granting of such degrees—today's reality.

I all but gave up, but not quite. I finally made my way directly to the president of the university, former South Carolina governor, Dr. James Edwards. He showed great vision in quickly approving my idea. I, therefore, scheduled a special session. It had to be held outside of the normal graduation ceremony normally held each spring. I am not sure why it was not held at the regular ceremony; perhaps our application was too late. We, therefore, chose to confer the degree on Harold at our annual departmental meeting. It was an academic meeting devoted to teaching residents and updating participants in practice. Our residents would present the results of their research. At that time, these meetings were major events that helped rebuild the scholarship of the department.

The Ridleys were invited to Charleston. Upon arrival, they were immediately attracted to the city's British heritage and also to the southern, *Gone With the Wind*-type charm that was not difficult to find there. Not only did this visit further cement my relationship with Harold and his wife, but my mother also had a chance to get to know them. They immediately established a close friendship, one that lasted throughout the rest of their lives and enriched both of their visits to Charleston. The Ridleys even encouraged my mother to come to Salisbury to spend her remaining years near them.

Dr. Edwards and I presented the diploma, a Doctor of Humane Letters, to Harold on April 29, 1989. Prior to that moment, I had rarely, if ever, seen such a smile on Harold's face. It was the face and smile I have shown in the Preface. Several prominent surgeons traveled to Charleston to witness this event, the first such honor presented to Harold from a university. This, combined with his induction into the Royal Society a few years earlier, led to marked improvement in the general well being of the Ridleys, who for so long had been virtual outcasts.

Harold received an honorary doctorate degree from the Medical University of South Carolina.
TOP: He received his diploma from the author and also President James Edwards.
BOTTOM: Left to right: the author, Harold, Medical University of South Carolina President and former Governor Dr. James Edwards, Mrs. Ridley, and the author's mother Margaret Apple are all smiles after the presentation.

Among his remarks at the Ceremony were the following, which summarize the phases of his professional life from A-Z:

> "When, in 1951, implant surgery was announced, it aroused great criticism, much of it hostile. Some said, 'this operation should never be done,' and others stated that 'it offended the first principles of ophthalmic surgery, and foretold glaucoma, sympathetic ophthalmia, and even malignant disease.'

> "Not everyone seemed to understand that the new operation was designed to cure aphakia and was not simply to make cataract glasses unnecessary. Fortunately, there were a few physicians, both in Europe and America, who had insight and they were encouraged by results that provided success within reach. Some of these early cases remained successful for more than 30 years, but others developed complications, most often dislocation, which served to stimulate research into the causation and treatment.

> "Now, after 40 years, a fifth generation of implants has been developed, mainly in the United States, but finality in implant design and placement have still not been achieved. However, extracapsular extraction and a much improved fixation that could not safely be provided by technology of the 1950s, is increasingly favored. Surely it is right to copy nature as closely as possible.

> "Those who have the benefit of successful implants may well be the most delighted and grateful people we see. Their surgical and visual problems have been overcome, and it remains only to congratulate each one and say 'farewell.'

CELEBRATING THE INTRAOCULAR LENS' 50TH ANNIVERSARY AT THE ROYAL ALBERT SCIENCE MUSEUM

An event that brought Harold to a new and improved relationship with his colleagues in his own country was scheduled for November 29, 1999, precisely the 50th anniversary of the implant. Rayner & Keeler, Ltd, the manufacturers of Harold's original IOL, organized the meeting.

The event was scheduled to be held, quite appropriately, among the exhibits of World War II aircraft in the Royal Albert Science Museum. Donald Munro, Rayner & Keeler's managing director, asked me if I would chair the session because of my close acquaintance with Harold. I agreed with great pleasure and excitement, but shortly thereafter became ill and had to have heavy treatment with surgery, chemotherapy, and radiation. This kept me from going to the meeting myself. However, I asked my wife, Ann, to attend. Ann took her daughter, Jacqueline, and I was told by several sources, that the comments Ann delivered on my behalf were very well received. I am sure they were better than I probably could have done myself.

This gala event gave Harold the opportunity to be surrounded by many colleagues, including those who had accepted him early on and even some of his early critics who had changed their feelings. Some of these colleagues had come from great distances, in particular, Svyatoslav Fyodorov, from what is now the former Soviet Union.

The Queen Mother, the mother of Queen Elizabeth II, was invited. At the age of 100 she had had a pair of IOLs successfully implanted by one of Harold's protégés, Dr. John Pearce. However, just prior to the event, she became ill and could not attend. She died not long afterwards.

Ridley saw several of his colleagues for the last time at this meeting.

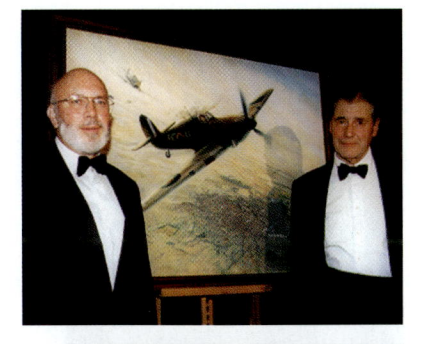

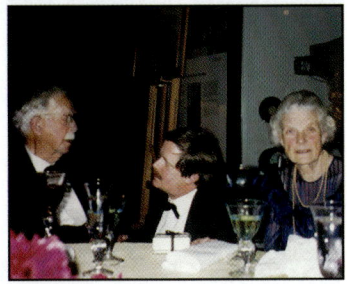

At the Science Museum in London, November 1999, the 50th year of the invention of the IOL.
TOP: Dr Eric Arnott (right), next to an image of Flight Lieutenant "Mouse" Cleaver's Hurricane being shot down. Recall that Eric later implanted an IOL in one of Cleaver's eyes 40 years after the operation.
BOTTOM: Harold's younger son David (center) flanked by Harold and Elisabeth.

CHAPTER 17

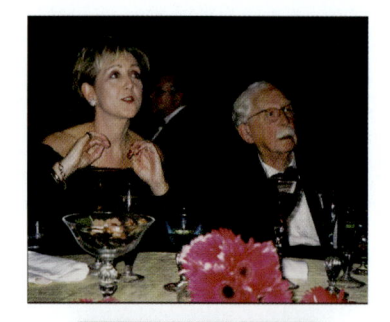

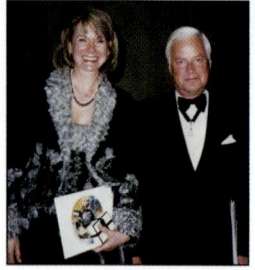

At the Science Museum, 1999.
TOP: Lauretta Ridley (left), the wife of Nicholas (Harold's older son), with Harold.
BOTTOM: My wife Ann with Nicholas Ridley, Harold's older son.

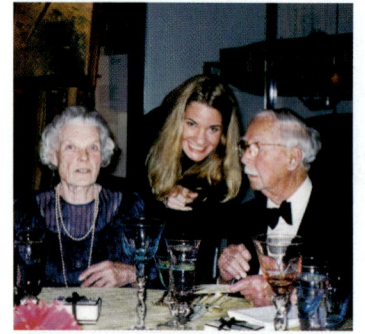

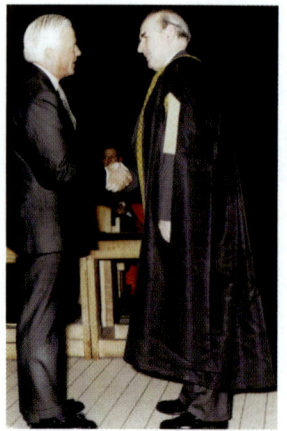

Harold received an honorary degree for the University of London. His son Nicholas (left) received the honor for him.

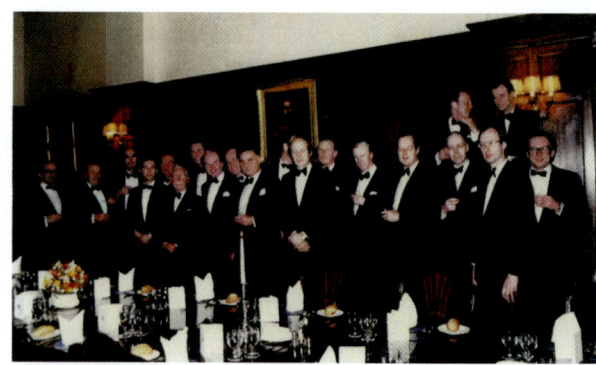

Colleagues in London at St. Thomas' Hospital celebrate Harold's 80th birthday in 1986.

ASCRS honors

Harold Ridley, MD, FRCS, FRS

and 50 years of intraocular lens implantation

April 10, 1999

ASCRS Symposium on
Cataract, IOL and Refractive Surgery

Elisabeth and Harold with our daughter Jacqueline (center).

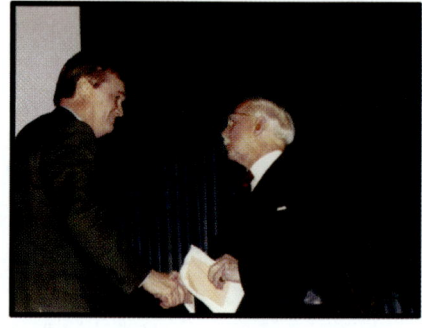

Ophthalmology Hall of Fame.
LEFT: Documentation of the award to Harold on the 50th anniversary of the IOL.
RIGHT: I participated in the Hall of Fame ceremony. Myself (left) with Harold.

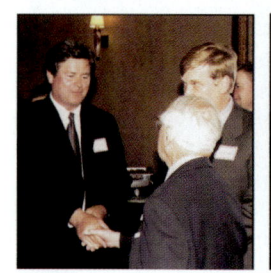

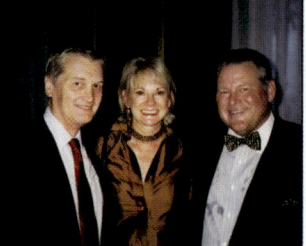

ASCRS in Seattle, 1999. The Ophthalmology Hall of Fame. A pre-meeting gathering of Harold's close friends.
LEFT: Dr. Jim Davison of Marshalltown, Iowa greets Harold.
RIGHT: Ann and myself with Dr. Richard Lindstrom of Minneapolis, Minnesota.

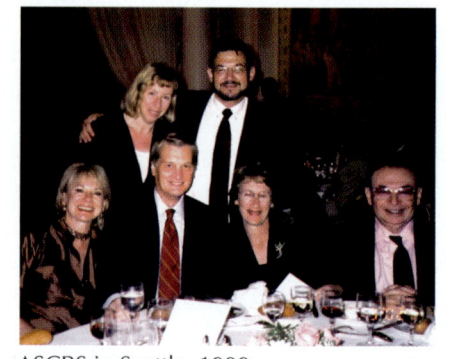

ASCRS in Seattle, 1999.
Left to right, seated: Ann and Dr. David Apple, Vicky and Dr. Howard Fine.
Standing: Ayala and Dr. Ehud Assia.

Election to Ophthalmology Hall of Fame

In 1999, Harold was inducted into the Ophthalmology Hall of Fame at the annual meeting of the American Society of Cataract and Refractive Surgery in Seattle, WA. This surprised no one and I was honored to be able to help present the award to him at the meeting. At the dinner held after the formal meeting sponsored by Rayner & Keeler, Ltd., he had another opportunity to again meet and renew friendships with several of his colleagues.

For me, something special happened at the event.

Dr. Lorenz E. Zimmerman, the guru of ocular pathology and one of my mentors under whom I worked in the early 1970s as a Research Fellow at the Armed Forces Institute of Pathology at Walter Reed Hospital in Washington, D.C., was also honored at that meeting. "Zim," as we called him, must have at first been skeptical about the IOL and even questioned my involvement with them. However, as the IOL was slowly being accepted almost everywhere, this skepticism changed. My former pathology professor and I had a pleasant reunion at that meeting.

We had to fly in a small plane to a special function. Sitting diagonally from Harold on that flight, it was almost eerie to observe him next to the PMMA (Plexiglas) window of the plane. In a sense, that is where it all began.

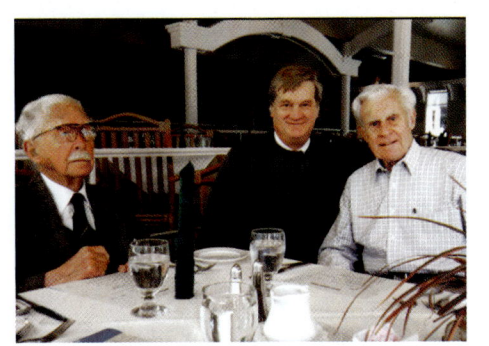

Seattle, 1999. This was a wonderful opportunity to have a reunion with not only Harold (left), but also my former mentor in ocular pathology at the Armed Forces Institute of Pathology at the Walter Reed Hospital, Dr. Lorenz E. Zimmerman (right).

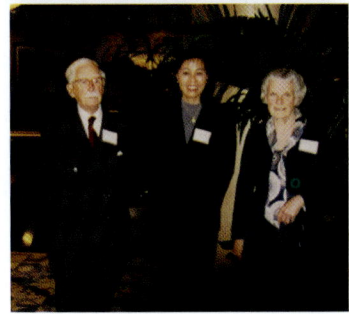

ASCRS in Seattle, 1999.
TOP: Dr. Kensaku Miyake with the Ridleys.
BOTTOM: The Ridleys with Dr. Qun Peng, one of my special Apple Korps team members.

A Long and Illustrious List

The awards mentioned here are only the tip of the iceberg. He received several other distinguished awards later in his life, including the Gullstrand Medal and the Gonin Medal, which is awarded every 4 years. The European Intraocular Implant Lens Council established a special Ridley lecture in his honor.

Recognitions flooded in from all over the world as the IOL was finally accepted. In one, a full-page tribute announced: "Mr. Ridley's Vision Gave Us Ours." Such accolades became common, a far cry from the often vicious criticism of the past.

While the honors and recognitions were very much appreciated by Harold, they were not the source of his greatest career satisfaction. That was reserved for the actual benefits his invention brought to so many millions of people throughout the world. In his own words, "My reward is the success of my very lucky advance of science and the knowledge that so many millions have been helped to minimize the effects of old age."

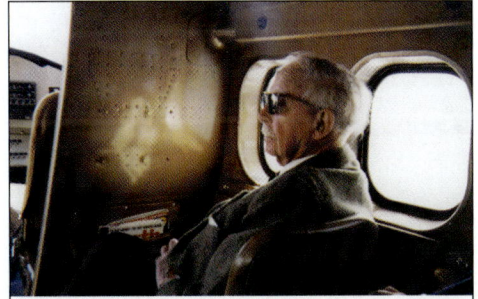

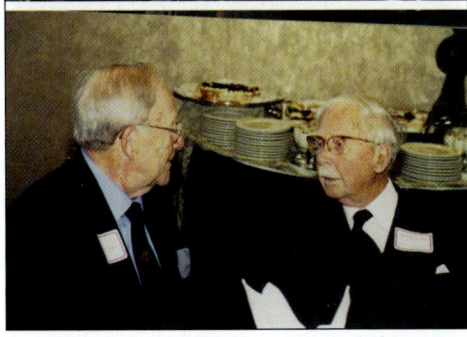

To attend one of the functions of the 1999 ASCRS meetings, we had to take a short flight.
TOP: It was an eerie feeling flying next to Harold adjacent to a Plexiglas (PMMA) window—it seemed that the cycle was complete.
BOTTOM: Harold talks with his oldest and closest colleague, Peter Choyce, MD. This was one of their final meetings.

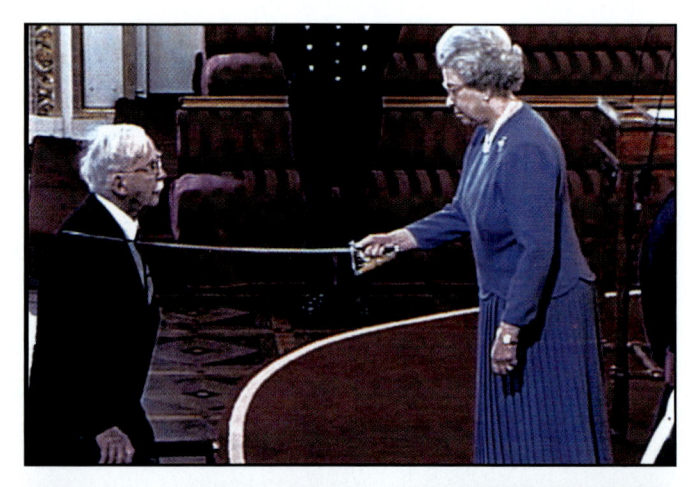

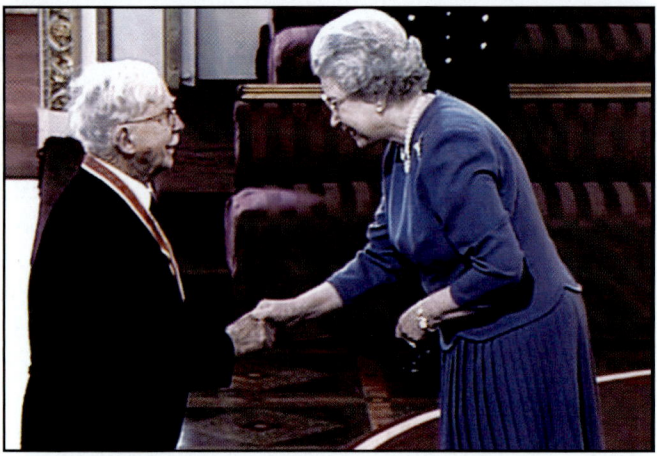

Sir Harold Ridley.
TOP: Sir Harold Ridley kneels as he receives knighthood from Queen Elizabeth II of England on February 9, 2000.
BOTTOM: Sir Harold Ridley receives a smile and congratulatory handshake from Queen Elizabeth II.

18

Knighthood and the End

"Throughout the centuries there were men who took first steps down new roads armed with nothing but their own vision. Their goals differed, but they all had this in common: that the step was first, the road new, the vision unborrowed and the response they received—hatred. The great creators—the thinkers, the artists, the scientists, the inventors—stood alone against the men of their time. Every great new thought was opposed. Every great new invention was denounced. The first motor was considered foolish. The airplane was considered impossible. The power loom was considered vicious. Anesthesia was considered sinful. But the men of unborrowed vision went ahead. They fought, they suffered and they paid. But they won."

The Fountainhead, Ayn Rand, 1944

"WHAT WAS A MIRACLE YESTERDAY REMAINS A MIRACLE TODAY AND FOREVER"

Referring to the implant that had just been installed into her eye, a patient made the following statement to her surgeon, Dr. Bob Drews, St. Louis, MO; "What was a miracle yesterday remains a miracle today and forever." Personally, every time I see or speak with a happy patient with an IOL in his or her eye(s), I think back to a statement that Harold loved the most and quoted everywhere—a statement made by one of his very first patients as he sat up from the operating table (of course with no spectacles) after his surgery, "Gentlemen, I can see all of you quite clearly."

CHAPTER 18

Letter from the author to British Prime Minister Margaret Thatcher urging her to reconsider the decision to bestow knighthood on Mr. Ridley. I received no response.

This is routine today, but can you imagine Harold's reaction as he heard that for the first time? Because of his efforts, that type of statement has been made untold millions of times. I do suppose it does become almost routine to some patients today who demand perfection and more—for example, the executive who needs to be back in the office after lunch—or better yet—who would like to be on the golf course just a few hours after surgery. It has become routine to both doctors and patients.

Several years ago many people, myself included, began to recognize that Harold deserved a high honor. Being British, a knighthood would be the obvious goal. Most of us interested in this issue never considered the possibility of a Nobel Prize, although the sheer number of people who have benefited from his successful "Gift to the World" as we discussed in Chapter 1 would seem to make him a prime candidate. However, the Nobel Prize Committee generally rewards scientists for basic research (eg, work at the molecular level). We therefore went for the ultimate honor that we deemed was due him and that he would treasure, knighthood.

Letters from colleagues near and far were written to the British authorities regarding this. They carried return addresses ranging from Shreveport, LA, to the vast plains of the Soviet Union. I myself started writing in 1985. Colleagues in the United Kingdom and on the European continent tried to accelerate the process. Key people at Rayner & Keeler, Ltd, the business organization that knew and appreciated him most, including Christopher Morgan (one of the company's early directors) and today's director, Donald Munro, were very helpful at different levels of the process.

Our goal remained elusive. All attempts were either ignored or turned down. It seemed clear that there were individuals with connections to the authorities that had the ability to block or at least slow down this process. Harold was getting very old, however, and since knighthood cannot be granted posthumously, timing had become acute.

Finally, on November 3, 1999, I received a response to a letter I had written to Prime Minister Tony Blair. The response was written on behalf of his wife, Ms. Cherie Booth, QC, and mailed to me by Ms. Louise Brown. Apparently, my letter had been forwarded to the right people.

Response to a letter I wrote on behalf of Harold to British Prime Minister Tony Blair. It was passed on via his wife Cherie Booth QC. He was knighted 3 months later.

Success at Last

Not long after the November 3rd correspondence, I received a telephone call from Donald Munro, the current Managing Director (from 2000 to the present) of Rayner, Ltd., with magnificent news. He himself had long been a champion of Harold Ridley and had campaigned long and hard for him to be knighted. He had written a letter to an authority in the government's Office of Science and Technology, asking for his support in helping move along our goal of Harold's being knighted. The government authority explained that when he had received Munro's letter, he had simultaneously heard some very good news about Harold, though he was not at liberty to state it publicly.

The authority's words were few but clear:

> *Mr. Munro: I was already aware of his possible consideration when you wrote, due to my position on the Science and Technology Honors Committee. That position also prevents me from using my influence as you requested. However, (between us) a high honor has been, nevertheless, bestowed, and I am sure that you will be as delighted for Ridley as I am.*

He couldn't say it directly or publicly, but those were the magic words.

When the news came officially, it stated that Harold was to be knighted by Queen Elizabeth II in Buckingham Palace on February 9, 2000, less than 4 months after my having received the response from #10 Downing Street.

Once it was announced that he was to be knighted, numerous messages of congratulations poured in. He asked his son, Nicholas, to send a letter on his behalf to all his friends and colleagues in lieu of a personal letter or Christmas card. In that letter, he noted that he, among other things, had reached the age of 93½ but remained able to conduct a peaceful life at home with Elisabeth at his side.

Nicholas wrote the following in his behalf:

> *Most importantly, my father considers himself privileged to have been able to pioneer the cure of aphakia and to have been able to advance medical science. He feels that he has been more than adequately awarded by old age, during which time he has seen that intraocular lens implants are now everyday surgery. Equally importantly, my father is acutely aware that the success of intraocular lens surgery is a tribute to the ophthalmic profession as a whole and he is extremely proud that it was pioneered in England.*

I wanted very much to go to the ceremony, but the admission was for the family of the awardees. I nevertheless enjoyed the ceremony in absentia having later received a complete video of the proceedings.

Peter Choyce tells a wonderful story regarding the 60 to 90 seconds that Queen Elizabeth II and Harold were together on the podium during the ceremony. A perusal of the video confirmed to me that the queen was indeed conversing freely with Harold. After the ceremony, everyone was dying to know what she said. Harold's answer with a smile, "I couldn't hear a damn thing!"

In spite of that, he was now a Knight of England: *Sir Harold Ridley*. He had finally driven past the naysayers. I was glad to be one of the several who helped him, and he had finally received what he deserved.

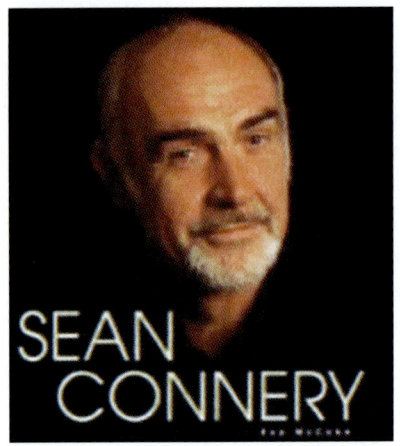

CHAPTER 18

Actor Sean Connery was knighted the same day and honored in the same ceremony as Sir Harold Ridley.

The complaint is often heard that some of the individuals receiving knighthood may not have the qualifications that those in academia think they should have. It must be remembered, however, that knighthood is apparently for honoring people with different agendas and occupations. I was pleased to note as I read the list of those who were knighted that day, the actor Sean Connery was honored in the same ceremony. We always, of course, loved him as James Bond, but I enjoyed many of his other appearances. I was particularly fond of his role as General Urquart in the great historical film, *"A Bridge Too Far."*

Harold was also given a medal. He was certainly gratified by the ceremony and the honors, but was also weary from the ceremony and all the attention he had received. Not long afterward, on my last visit to his home, I asked to see the medal. I had to smile when he revealed that he had put it aside and couldn't find it. At any rate, it has been found and is in safe hands now with his oldest son, Nicholas.

Confronting Old Age

Old age is the down side of not dying young. When Harold knelt before the queen to be knighted, he was 93 years old and partially deaf. My wife, Ann, and I felt that his deafness was the main obstacle to communication in his later years. He had been the recipient of the sight-saving IOL surgery he himself had invented. He actually loved to tell anyone who was within hearing distance about that. He was very proud to have been the recipient of his own invention.

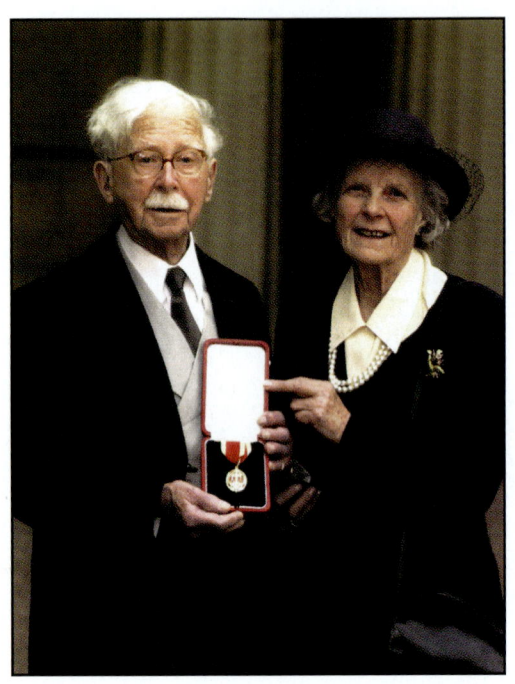

Sir Harold and Mrs. Ridley show the medal received at the knighthood ceremony.

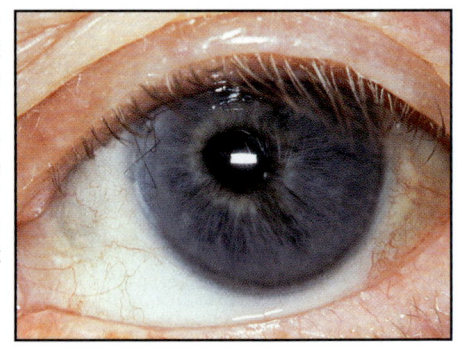

Sir Harold Ridley was very proud to be the recipient of his own invention—the intraocular lens (IOL). This is a close-up of Sir Harold's operated eye done in the early 1990s at St. Thomas' Hospital. This photgraph was taken by Dr. Jan Worst of the Netherlands.

"In spite of the good which has resulted and having fulfilled God's orders," Harold said, *"I am now in a state of depression, thinking mainly of the many small mistakes I have made in life. If I had my time over again, I should probably make much the same mistakes, but not in the end have so much good fortune.*

"I doubt if I could go through the stresses again but I thank God for giving me a job which was really worth doing. I must confess that I feel rewarded when colleagues now at last say, 'Ridley was right!'"

Almost a decade earlier, Harold wrote a letter to his brother, Allder. The letter reveals that even then, in his 80s, Harold was dealing with depression and questions regarding the course his life had taken. He wrote:

"Last Friday I was presented with the Galen Gold Medal in Therapeutics by the Worshipful Society of Apothecaries of London… I explained that I felt like the prodigal son returning after many years in disgrace and being given the fatted calf. Truly, the profession treated me most unkindly and for 20 years I could not get over to colleagues the importance of my operation (due largely to Duke-Elder who did not like anything done except through his institute).

"So many of us become depressed when the peak of life has passed and all of us must fight off senile depression. I have been exceedingly lucky to be able to continue professional activities until the age of 83, but my turn has now come, too. God gave me a job to do which was really worth while and which, it seems, no other man in England and perhaps in the world was willing to take on because it inevitably meant telling all one's colleagues that they did not know how to cure, as opposed to treat, cataract. I had to be prepared for problems which certainly arrived, but strangely I am myself one of the beneficiaries of my own operation.

"In spite of my errors, I can feel that my life has been worth living and will remain a milestone in surgery, and one which millions require treatment for every year. Nevertheless, like you, I get quite severe depression at times. The higher the peak one has climbed, the greater the distance to fall, and I find that I have more enemies than the handful I knew of. What an interesting, if worrying, era we were born into and in spite of two world wars I think we were truly lucky for we have seen great changes in the world."

About that same time he was showing a group his first televised film and telling about the beginnings of the IOL, he wrote, "All my peers and teachers and almost without exception my contemporary colleagues have passed away, and I am now a living fossil."

In letters to me during his last years, Sir Harold made several telling comments. One letter contained a statement that made me sad for his aged condition, but at the same time made me smile, knowing that he had not lost his dry sense of humor. "I am suffering now from lack of judgment and am really unfit for work," he wrote, "Elisabeth wants me to give up driving, except of course to get her to the hairdresser."

CHAPTER 18

THE END OF A LONG AND FRUITFUL JOURNEY

In May of 2001, I attended the annual meeting of the American Ophthalmology Society. I delivered a lecture in a morning session and then returned to my hotel room that afternoon. Not long after I had become settled in the room to relax I received a phone call from my assistant in Charleston. She informed me that Harold had been hospitalized in Salisbury because of a severe cerebrovascular hemorrhage. The prognosis was poor. I am not ashamed to say that, all alone in my room, I broke into profuse tears that lasted for a long time.

The lecture I had just given had addressed the topic of complications of some of the most modern IOLs. Scattered throughout the lecture were several mentions of Harold, including some citations regarding how one or more of his early observations directly applied to modern cataract IOL operations. At the very end, I closed with a few remarks and some illustrations intended to share with the audience my feelings of gratitude for what he had done. Harold passed away two days later.

The organization that hosted my lecture, the American Ophthalmology Society, has been around for over 100 years and requires members to write a thesis and be selected and elected by the membership. In the past, many of its members were not very supportive of Harold; of these, the most prominent was Dr. Derrick Vail.

THE FAREWELL

Ann and I went to England to attend the small funeral service at the 1100-year-old St. Mary's Church in Swinstead, East Anglia. The church was located near the estate where Harold's eldest son, Nicholas, and his lovely wife, Lauretta, live. This was an opportunity to meet those who were close and loyal to Harold, including his three children, several surgeon colleagues and their families, and the people of Rayner, Ltd, who had never failed to support him, even in the darkest days. Donald Munro, Rayner's managing director, who did much to support the efforts for knighthood, was among them.

True to form, Harold had requested that his eyes be removed and submitted to a laboratory for future use in either teaching or research. I do not think this was emotionally palatable for his family members, however, and therefore was not done.

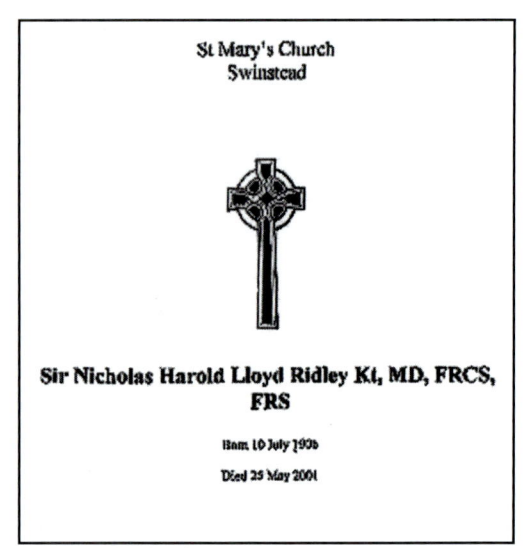

Sir Harold's death announcement.

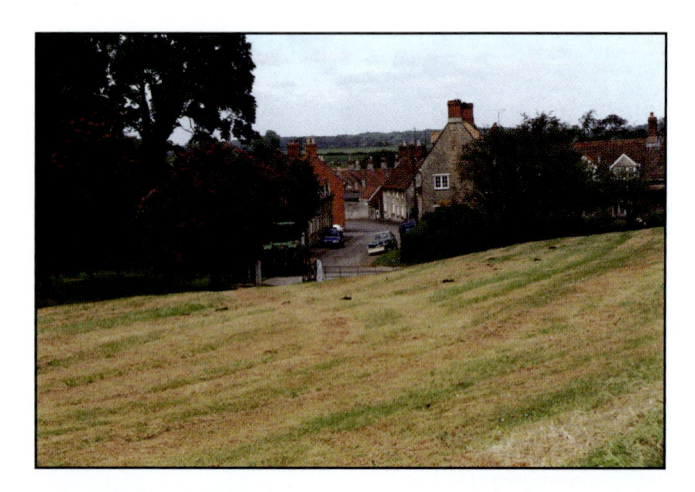

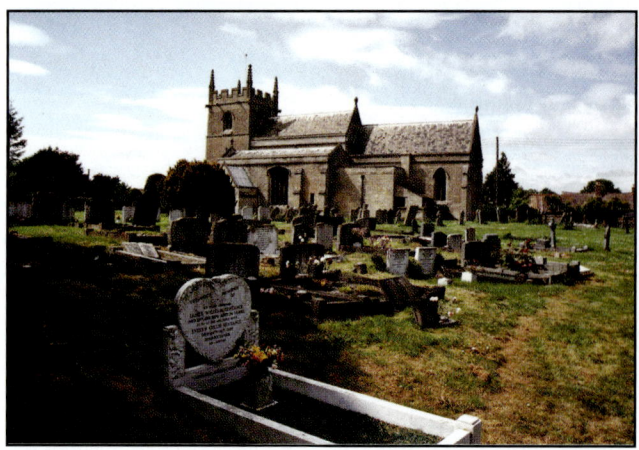

TOP: View of the village of Swinstead, East Anglia, from St. Mary's Church.
BOTTOM: The 1100-year-old St. Mary's Church.

KNIGHTHOOD AND THE END

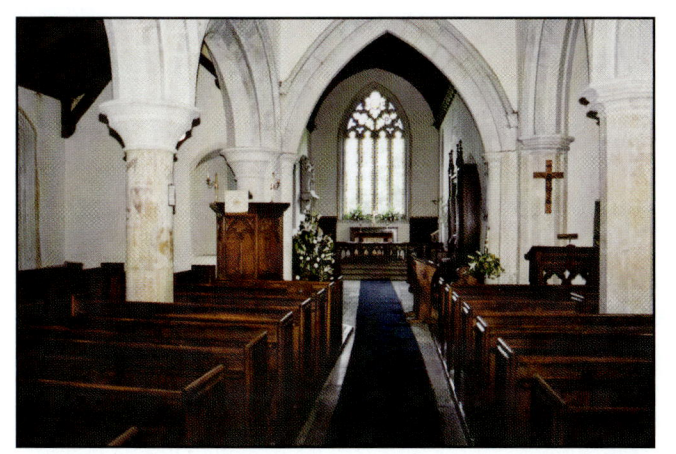

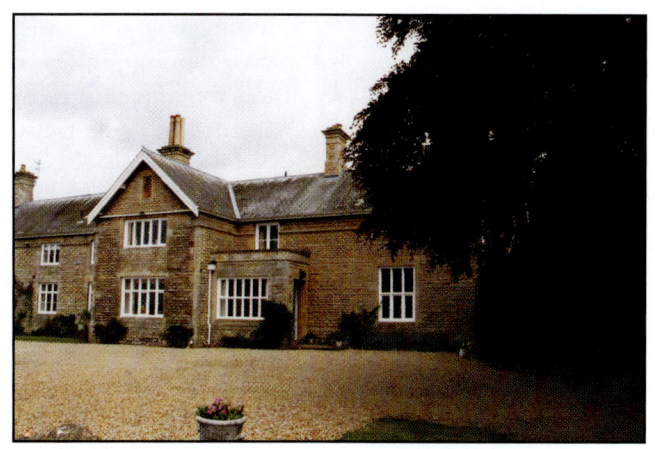

LEFT: Interior of St. Mary's Church, where the funeral of Sir Harold Ridley was held.
RIGHT: St. Mary's Church is located on the estate of Sir Harold's oldest son, Nicholas. Pictured is the main house on the estate.

As Ann and I drove away from the services and the subsequent reception at Nicholas's home thereafter, we drove past a sign posting the region of the birthplace of Sir Isaac Newton at Woolsthorpe-by-Colsterworth, just a few miles away. We detoured to see the modest structure. Newton's work on optics had been very helpful to Harold as he prepared for the implant.

It was a sad time, but we were comforted knowing that Ridley had lived a long life of 94 years and had realized that millions of people worldwide, including himself, had benefited from the operation and implants that he first made a reality.

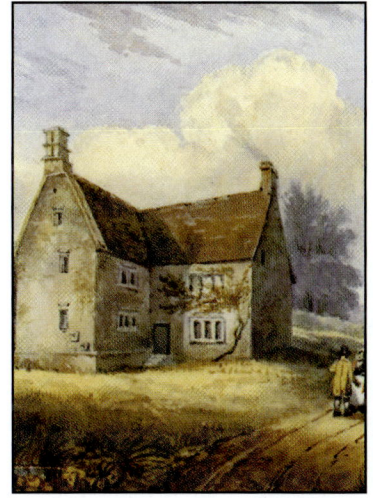

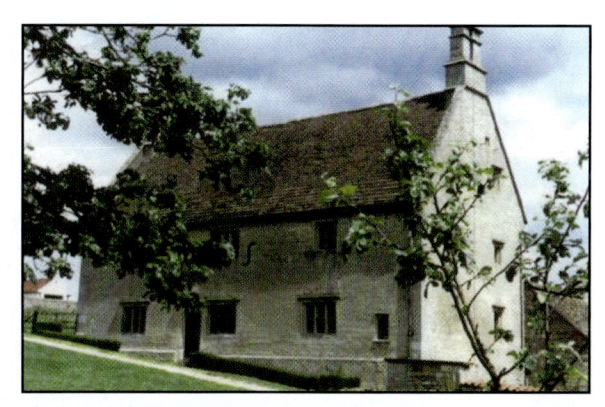

Birthplace of Sir Isaac Newton, near where Dr. Ridley is buried.
LEFT: Artist's rendition of the structure.
RIGHT: Sir Isaac Newton's birthplace as it appears today.

WORDS OF RESPECT

Dr. Charles Letocha of Pennsylvania has been and remains a staunch supporter of Harold and his work. He has been instrumental in collecting material and information about Harold's life. This includes clinical data on several patients who had benefited from the Ridley lens implants for many years. His data further helped verify the quality and safety of the IOL that we all take for granted today.

Letocha's words of respect for Sir Harold, forwarded to Donald Munro, were poignant. They were also appropriate coming from Pennsylvania, where, along with Miami, fine clinical work on the early implants was carried out. Letocha, who was familiar with the early work of Warren Reese, the first American to perform an implant, having received a few lenses from Sir Harold himself in Chicago; Turgut Hamdi, who, no doubt, implanted more original IOLs than any other American; and other doctors took the time to write the following comments. Most important from a medical standpoint is the fact that Letocha's findings verified the truly excellent results that could be obtained with the original Ridley lens. Clearly, it was not the failure it had been made out to be by many during those early, bleak years.

He wrote:

> *"I recently analyzed the published results of the North American experiences with cases done mainly at Wills Eye Hospital in Philadelphia by Drs. Warren Reese, Turgut Hamdi and Cyril Luce, and in Toronto by Drs. J. P. Harshman and Morris Shusterman. In addition, I examined three living patients, following their operations. It is great news that Harold Ridley has now been honored in his own country. American eye surgeons are indebted to this man for the great last step he took in daring to invent and implant this wonderful lens. Tens of millions of Americans would otherwise be living a life of visual impairment caused by the results of cataract treatment without lens implantation. Ridley's invention changed life for the better worldwide—but nowhere more so than here in the US. Deeply felt thanks from your American colleagues and their patients, Sir Harold!"*

A Fitting Place for a Memorial Service

Several weeks after Ridley's funeral at St. Mary's Chapel, a memorial service was held for him at the beautiful chapel in St. Thomas' Hospital, only a few feet from the clinical area. The service was well attended. Harold's oldest son spoke, as well as the minister.

Most of those in attendance were elderly friends of the Ridleys, especially nonmedical coworkers such Doreen Clarke, now Doreen Ogg, his nurse for the first operation in 1949; Christine, his administrator; and many other family members and friends.

Even though the service was in the middle of a workday, I was somewhat surprised that very few physicians or surgeons were present. I wondered if some of the longstanding negative attitudes had persisted, or if (most likely) many of those who disagreed with Harold in earlier years did not come because they felt embarrassed or ashamed. Sadly, it is also quite possible that some did not come because they still harbored negativity toward Harold. However, there was an outpouring of respect, affection, and admiration from those who did come.

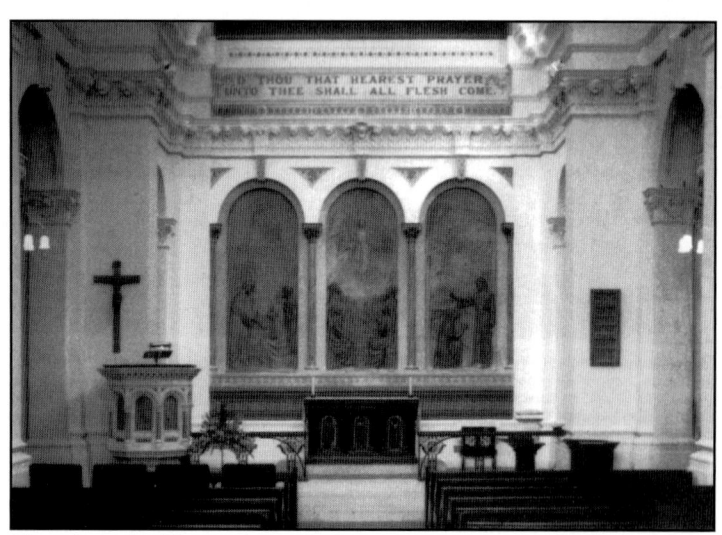

Chapel at St. Thomas' Hospital, where a memorial service was held for Sir Harold Ridley shortly after his death.

Numerous obituaries were written and published around the world, including in the *New York Times*. Mr. John Winstanley, an ophthalmologist and close associate of Harold's, represented the British ophthalmic press, writing a beautiful obituary that was printed in the *British Medical Journal*. I had the privilege of writing five separate obituaries in response to requests from editors of various ophthalmic journals. These obituaries, along with Winstanley's, attempted to bring credit to a man who, for most of his life, received so much scorn despite his remarkable contributions to humanity.

WESTMINSTER ABBEY

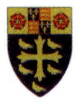

A Service of
Thanksgiving and Rededication
on
Battle of Britain Sunday

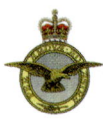

Sunday 18 September 2005
11.00 am

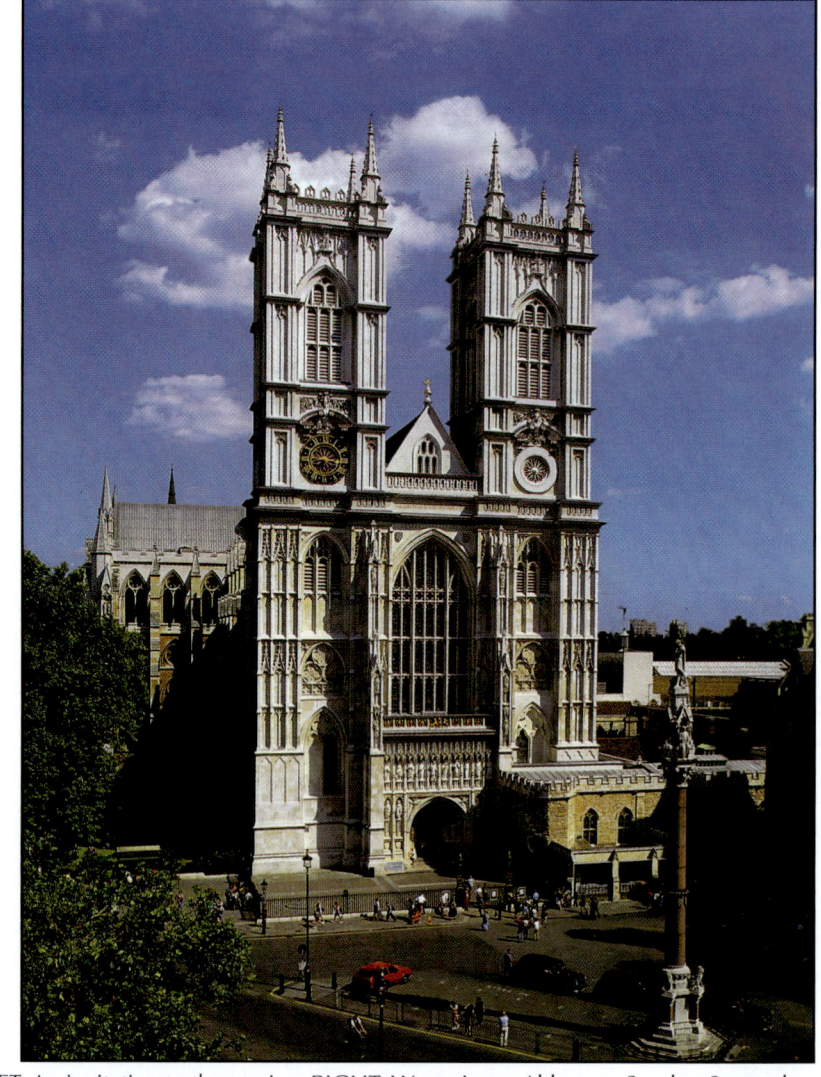

Service of Thanksgiving and Redemption. LEFT: An invitation to the service. RIGHT: Westminster Abbey on Sunday, September 18, 2005.

19

A Service of Thanksgiving and Redemption on Battle of Britain Sunday, September 18, 2005

> *"The specialty of ophthalmology, indeed medicine in general, advanced into a new era when a volley of bullets from a Luftwaffe aircraft smashed into the cockpit canopy of Flight Lieutenant 'Mouse' Cleaver's Hawker Hurricane during the 'Adlertag' phase of the Battle of Britain."*
>
> *David Apple, MD, Salt Lake City, August 2006*

It had been 4 years since Harold Ridley's death. My wife, Ann, and I were busy at work on this book. She is a talented photographer who took some of the photographs for this book.

I received a telephone call from my good friend, Reggie Spooner, former adjutant (administrator) of the 601 Squadron during the period just after the great air battle of Adlertag (see Chapter 5). He did not fly in combat but trained many pilots who did. He told me there was going to be an important ceremony in London the following month, on September 18th. In the United Kingdom, this is officially known as Battle of Britain Day, celebrating the RAF's victory over the enemy in the battle. Extensive fighter plane action, of course, continued in Britain and worldwide throughout the war, but at last, the RAF fighters had some opportunity to recover from the incessant, deadly action. Unfortunately, the bombing (Blitz) phase of the battle began to increase in intensity about that time, lasting for 3 more years. An annual remembrance has been held on this September date ever since the war; 2005 was special in that it marked the 65th anniversary of the battle and the planned dedication of a monument for those who died in the conflict. Reggie had obtained two extra tickets to the event and invited Ann and me to accompany him to the service being held in Westminster Abbey.

CHAPTER 19

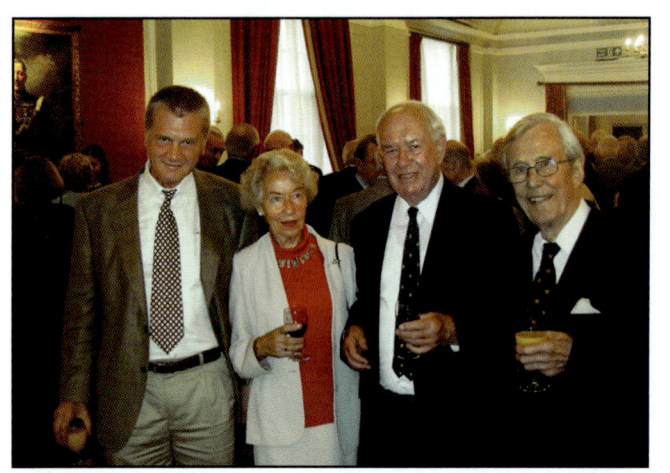

LEFT: The Royal Air Force (RAF) Club on Picadilly Street, London. RIGHT: David and Ann enjoy the day with Reggie Spooner, adjutant administrator for 601 Squadron.

Sharing memories at the RAF club. Left to right: the author, 601 Squadron pilot John and Mrs. Foster, and Reggie Spooner.

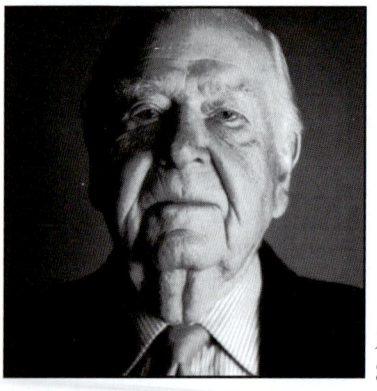

Jack Riddle (see Chapter 6) could not attend the small gathering, but we saw him later after the ceremony.

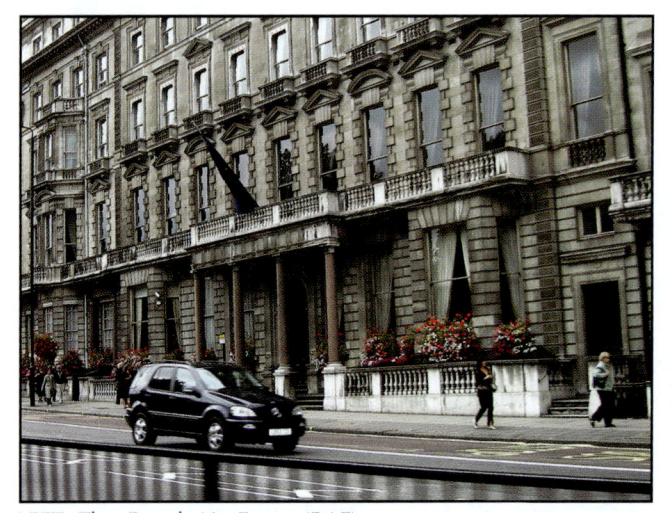

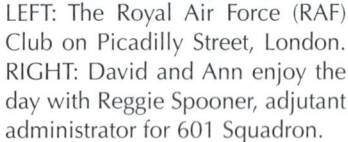

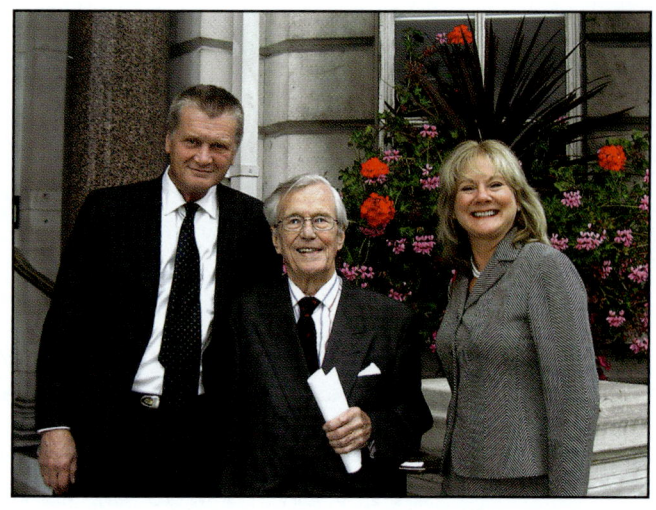

I had already committed to give a lecture in New York. However, I definitely did not want to miss the commemorative event in London. I had a feeling that this would represent a closure to many of the events described in this book. I contacted the physician who was in charge of the scheduled program in New York, Dr. Pricilla Perry, and she graciously, indeed enthusiastically, excused me from that obligation, agreeing that under no circumstances should we miss the London event.

Ann and I flew to London and met Reggie at the RAF Club on Piccadilly Street. This national club has been in existence for pilots of the RAF for many, many decades, although I had never seen or heard of it prior to this. As we walked in through the front door, a petite lady seen in the photograph on this page saw Ann and me and walked over to ask who these "young people" were. I had just turned 64 a few days earlier; Ann is significantly younger. The gracious lady was the wife of a highly decorated former pilot, John Foster. Meeting such a hero filled me with admiration, and this feeling continued to build as the day's events passed by.

Our admiration for these old warriors grew as we walked to the Abbey, for the Service of Remembrance. Many were laden with ribbons and medals. Only a few hundred of the original thousands who fought the battle are now left. Police and security people increased in number, signaling that Prince Charles and his wife, Camilla, were about to arrive. We entered the sanctuary and took our seats directly adjacent to the aisle where the procession passed. The prince and his wife marched within 2 feet of us as they moved to assume their designated positions. We were impressed with their stately appearance and the pleasant feeling they exuded.

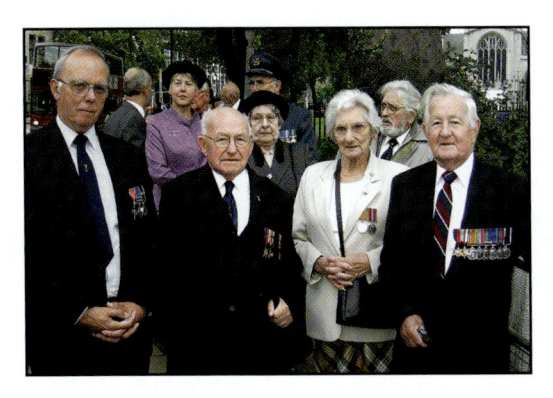

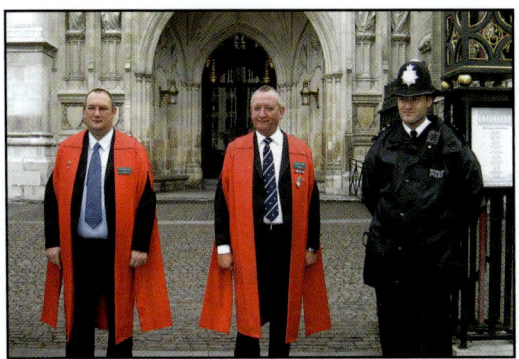

A SERVICE OF THANKSGIVING AND REDEMPTION ON BATTLE OF BRITAIN SUNDAY, SEPTEMBER 18, 2005

It was wonderful to see all these old heroes.
LEFT: Former pilots laden with medals.
RIGHT: As Prince Charles and Camilla arrived the security increased.

After the ceremony, Ann and I walked a few blocks to the Westminster Embankment. It fronts on the Thames River adjacent to the Savoy Hotel, near the famous obelisk that had been brought to England from Egypt. This was also the site where Monet had worked over a century ago, carrying his canvas between this site and the studio-apartment he had set up across the river in St. Thomas' Hospital. The Battle of Britain monument had been erected there.

After viewing the newly dedicated monument, we strolled up to the Westminster Bridge and mused again about many of the pivotal events that occurred during Ridley's time and pondered on how the buildings must have looked before and during the bombing, as compared to today. Now, a significant part of the hospital consists of a large, square block. We could not resist taking a taxi over to the Royal Albert Museum where

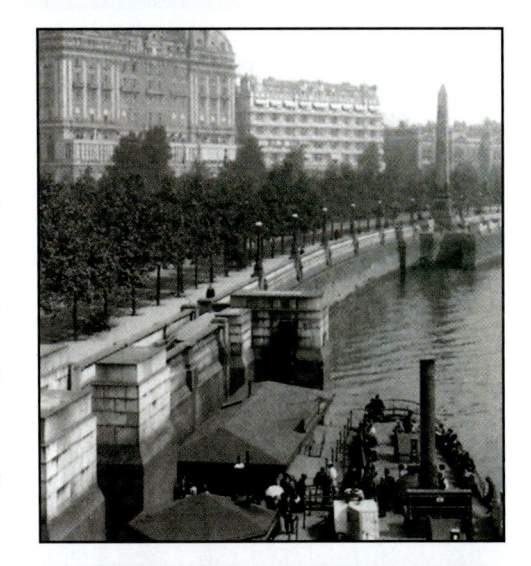

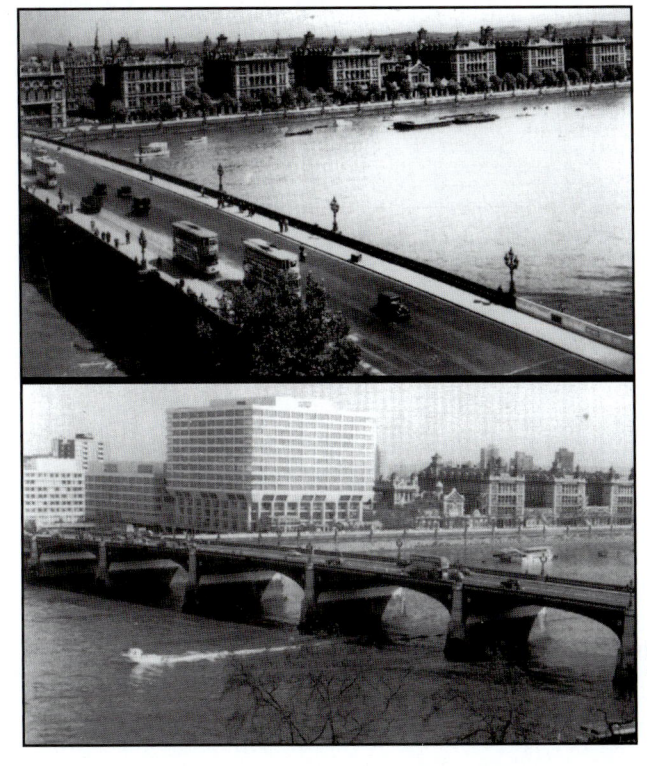

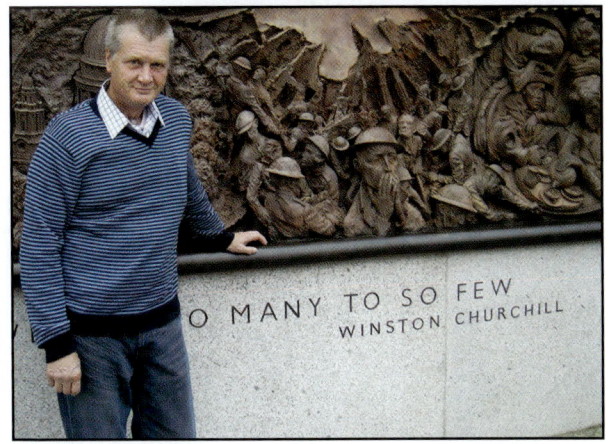

TOP: Thames River adjacent to the Savoy Hotel near the famous obelisk that was brought to England from Egypt.
BOTTOM: David Apple poses before the Battle of Britain Monument.

St. Thomas' Hospital, site of the now-famous Ridley operation.
TOP: St. Thomas' Hospital in the late 1930s.
BOTTOM: St. Thomas' Hospital as it appeared in 2005. Note the new, square block building.

CHAPTER 19

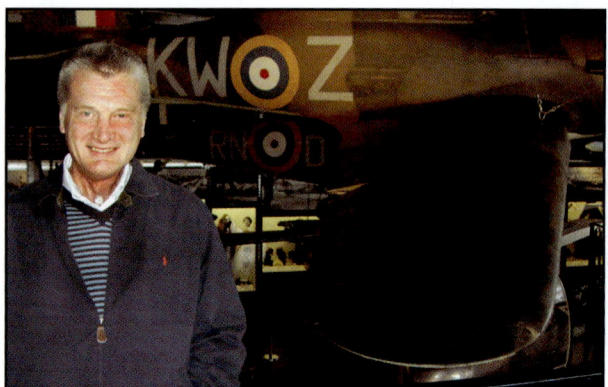

I climbed around like a child on the Hurricanes and Spitfires as I visited the Royal Albert Science Musuem.

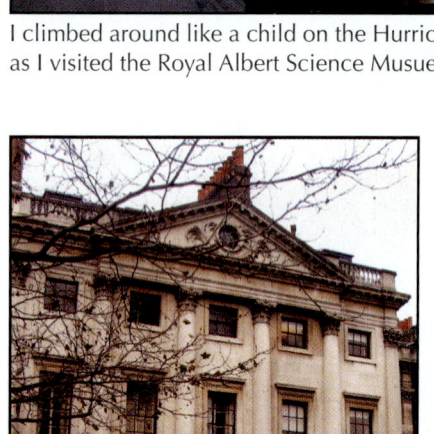

the Science Museum is located. I went to the section where the gala event celebrating the 50th anniversary of Ridley's invention had been held in 1999. I had always been sorry that my illness had prevented me from attending that Rayner & Keeler, Ltd-sponsored event, which I had been asked to chair. Ann had taken my place and done a wonderful job with a moving speech, which has been preserved on videotape. I climbed about on the planes in the museum like a child in a playground. Ann took a photo of me.

Next, we journeyed to Cavendish Square, where the initial discussions on the implant occurred in Harold's automobile with the now-renowned Mr. Pike of Rayner, Ltd. Then, we walked the few blocks to 53 Harley Street, where Ridley had resided for many years. Walking just a few steps further to 63 Harley Street, the home of Sir Stewart Duke-Elder, we noticed a blue circular plaque on the front stonework of the second floor inscribed with his name and dates. This is an honor given to special people in England. They are eligible to receive it no sooner than 100 years after their birth. With Harold's 100-year birthday on July 10, 2006, we committed to do what we could to make sure that a plaque would be applied to his former dwelling in his honor.

Cavendish Square, where the original discussions regarding intraocular lens (IOL) implantation took place with Mr. Pike, of Rayner & Keeler, Ltd., in Sir Harold's prized Bentley.

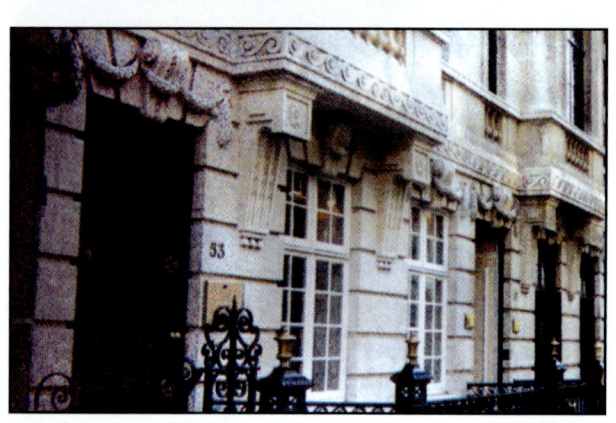

Townhouse at 53 Harley Street today, where Sir Harold resided for many years.

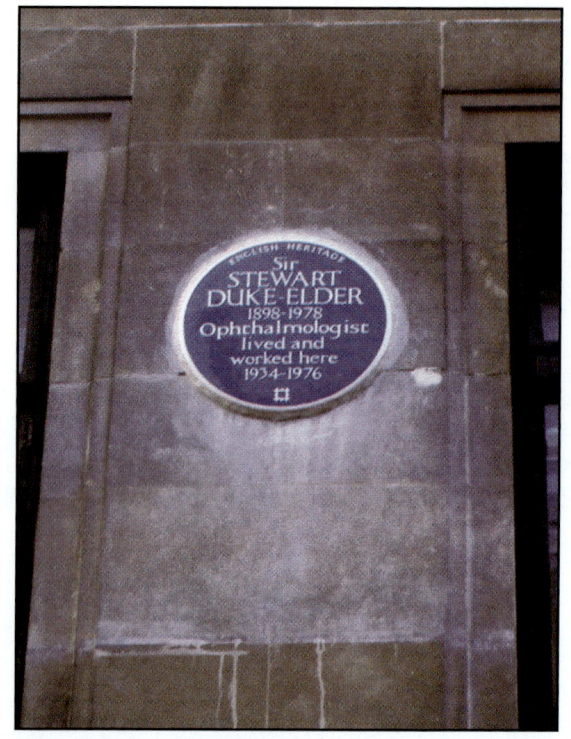

This plaque commemorates the work of Sir Stewart Duke-Elder at 63 Harley Street, a few feet away from Sir Harold Ridley's residence.

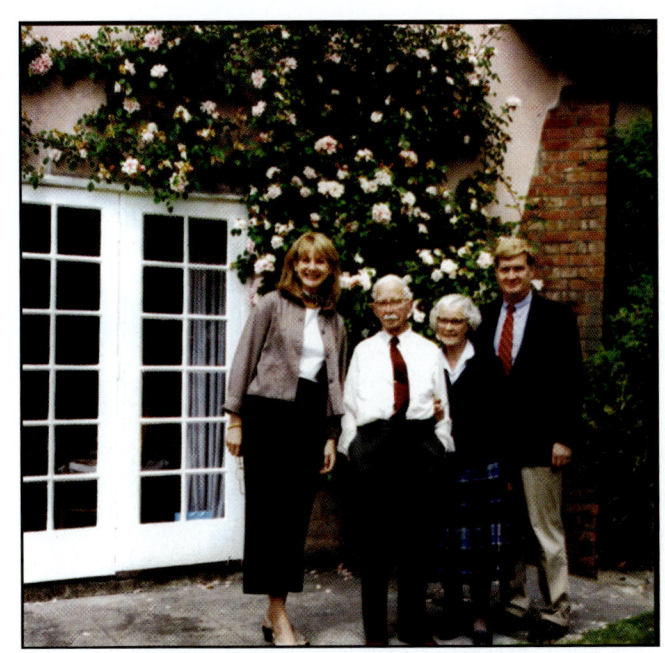

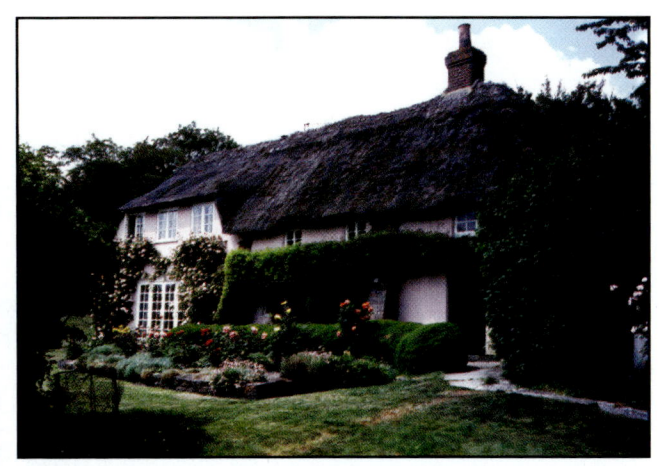

A SERVICE OF THANKSGIVING AND REDEMPTION ON BATTLE OF BRITAIN SUNDAY, SEPTEMBER 18, 2005

LEFT: One of the last photos of Ann and myself with Harold and Elisabeth at Keeper's Cottage in 2000.
RIGHT: Keeper's Cottage, country home of Sir Harold and Mrs. Ridley.

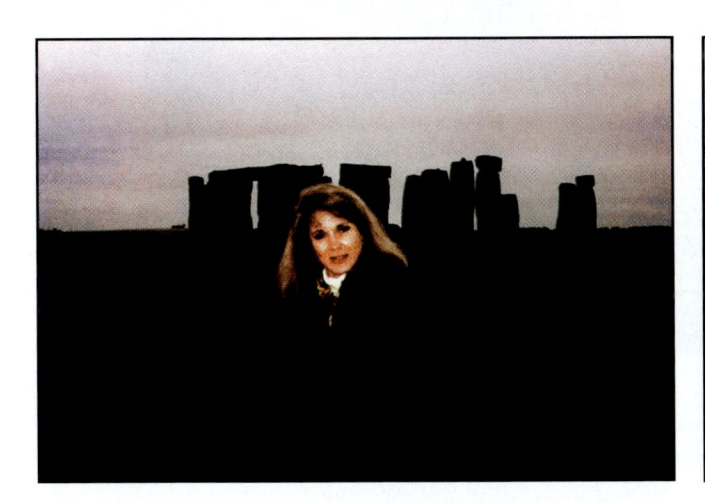

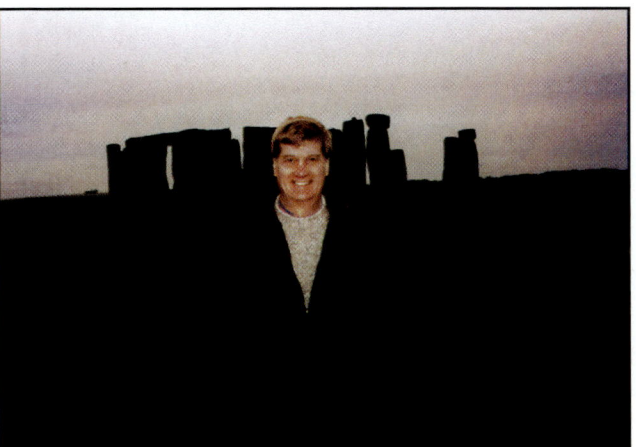

Many memories of Harold are at Stonehenge.
LEFT: Ann Apple.
RIGHT: The author.

As Ann and I finished our walk in downtown London, we went back to the hotel and could do no more than reminisce about the wonderful times we shared with the Ridleys. Our thoughts turned to their country home at Keeper's Cottage and to Stonehenge, just a few miles from the cottage, where Harold often simply walked and meditated. We took a long look at a photo that had been taken of us at the cottage—the last photo of us together.

CHAPTER 19

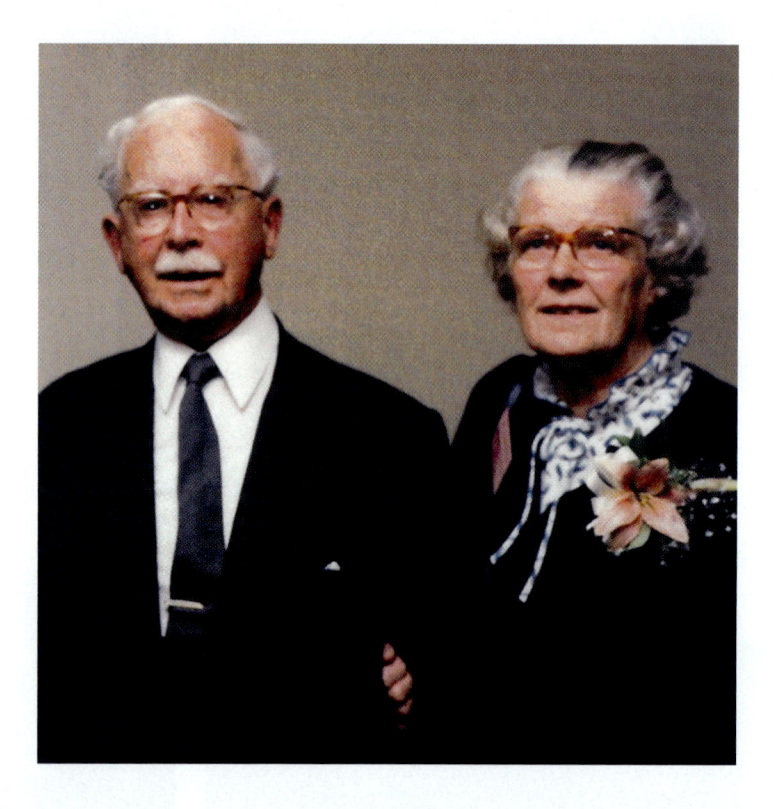

Harold once said, "I would have on my tombstone, 'He cured aphakia.'" He then questioned his own suggestion by musing, "And people will ask, 'Who was Mr. Aphakia?'" Such was the self-effacing humor of a modest genius—a man who in a very real sense gave his life to bring sight to countless millions for untold generations to come.

I am honored to have known him.

Glossary

accommodation: The process by which the eye changes its focusing power by a brain-regulated contraction/relaxation of the ciliary muscle which in turn transmits tension through the zonules into the lens causing it to either thicken or thin for near and far vision.

age-related macular degeneration (ARMD): A degeneration of the central retina occurring most commonly in elderly individuals due to problems with the underlying vasculature. The main symptoms are central vision loss ranging from a blind spot to scotoma. Irregular shape on the Amsler grid caused by macular edema.

It is an important disease causing problems with central vision, but fortunately, it very seldom progresses in the periphery to cause complete blindness.

amblyopia: Reduced vision in any eye not known to be caused by any disease of the eye itself. Amblyopia may occur in young children (1) as a result of misalignment of the two eyes, (2) when the difference between the refractive errors of the two eyes is large, or (3) when an eye has been prevented from seeing because it has been kept covered for an extended period or because of opacities in certain parts of the eye. Some amblyopia may be caused by malnutrition or due to toxic substances (eg, so called tobacco-alcohol amblyopia). Nutritional amblyopia and amblyopia due to mustard gas were seen in the world wars of the last century.

angle: The anterior chamber angle is a junction of the cornea with the iris, where the trabecular meshwork is located. A narrow angle may predispose a person to angle-closure glaucoma.

aphakia: The Gr. a = without; phakia = lens.

aphakic IOL: Aphakic correction may be provided by spectacles, contact lenses, or IOLs that provide the lens power that is lost because of surgical extraction of a cataractous lens. Contact lenses and especially the thick aphakic spectacles are very unsatisfactory since they cause marked visual aberrations; the IOL is by far the best.

anterior chamber IOL: The haptics (footplates) or loops of the lens are situated in the anterior chamber, fixated in the anterior chamber angle. This is a type of lens useful in conjunction with intracapsular cataract extraction (ICCE), but is used much less commonly today.

GLOSSARY

anterior chamber: Space in front portion (anterior segment) of the eye between the cornea and the lens-iris diaphragm, which is filled with aqueous humor.

aqueous humor: Clear, watery fluid that fills the anterior and posterior chambers in the anterior segment of the eye. The aqueous humor is formed in the ciliary processes, passes through the anterior segment providing nutrition, and exits the eye via the canal of Schlemm and trabecular meshwork.

aqueous outflow pathway: The main exit of aqueous humor from the eye is via Schlemm's canal and the trabecular meshwork.

astigmatism: Nonspherical curvature of the cornea (often in the shape of a spoon) resulting in a distorted image because light rays are not focused on a single point on the retina in both major meridians (usually at 90° to each other). These can be corrected by special spectacles or use of a toric lens.

bifocal IOL: An IOL with two built in powers to facilitate both distance and near vision.

binocular vision: Coordinated use of the two eyes to see a single fused three-dimensional image.

blindspot: The dark spot (scotoma) that is a normal finding, caused by the optic nerve-head as it enters the eye. This is a physiologic or normal blind spot and should be differentiated from abnormal scotomas caused by various diseases.

blood aqueous barrier: A physiologic barrier caused by cell modifications of the epithelium of the anterior segment of the eye which in effect separates the aqueous from the circulation of the body. Every time the eye is disturbed, either by surgery or trauma, there is a breakdown of the blood aqueous barrier, which in most cases rapidly disappears, but in some cases may persist and form a disease process.

capsulorrhexis: A technique to open the anterior capsule (a form of anterior capsulotomy) in order to surgically enter the lens during cataract surgery to have access to the cataractous material that must be expressed out of the eye or removed by phacoemulsification. In previous years the capsule was opened by irregular tearing methods such as horizontal slits or the "can opener" or "Christmas tree," but the capsulorrhexis provides a nice smooth edge to the opening (continuous circular curvilinear capsulorrhexis [CCC]) that is efficacious in preventing unwanted tears to the capsule during and after surgery.

cataract: (Ger.= gray stare, Gr. = waterfall, Latin = catarr = flowing substance) These are the various names given to the clouding of the lens, with or without discoloration.

cataract extraction: Removal of the eye's lens by surgery, either couching (pushing the lens into the eye) or, much more modern, removal of the lens from the eye.

central retinal artery: The main artery that enters the eye through the optic nerve and supplies the inner layers of the retina.

central retinal vein: The main venous channel that drains the inner layers of the retina and exits the eye via the optic nerve.

central visual field: The field of space seen centrally, corresponding to an area of 30° within the fixation point (fovea and macular region). This contrasts with the peripheral visual field.

choroid: A component of the uvea. It is the blood vessel-rich central layer of the eye between the sclera and retina, supplying blood to the outer layers of the retina and pigment epithelium. These vessels and their associated choriocapillaris are important in the pathogenesis of age-related macular degeneration (ARMD).

ciliary body: The central portion of the uveal tract of the eye situated between the iris (anteriorly) and the choroid (posteriorly). It has two functions: to secrete aqueous humor into the eye (too much secretion or poor outflow of the aqueous causes glaucoma) and also functions via the ciliary muscle, in the process of accommodation.

color vision deficiency (color blindness): Inability to recognize certain colors, primarily red or green, but also blue.

GLOSSARY

cones: Cone-shaped light-sensitive cells in the retina particularly in the macula area; cone function predominates in daylight with a small pupil allowing one to make out details and shapes, especially colors.

congenital: Present at birth. It is not synonymous with inherited or genetic.

conjunctiva: The transparent-translucent mucous membrane that covers the sclera toward the front of the eye over the limbus. The front portion of the conjunctiva merges with the front portion of the cornea at the limbus.

contact lens: A rigid or soft contact lens that fits over the cornea/sclera and is a refractive appliance, in lieu of other spectacles or an intraocular lens.

cornea: The transparent, watch glass cover-shaped structure at the front of the eye continuous with the sclera (white of the eye) around it for 360 degrees. The cornea is responsible for major focusing of rays as they enter the eye. The ophthalmologist must keep the cornea clear to retain good vision. A corneal opacity (treated by corneal transplant or keratoplasty) must be differentiated from a cataract, an opacity of the lens, which of course is treated by lens extraction. Many healthcare providers still mix up these two conditions.

corneal transplant: An operation in which the central portion of the cornea (corneal button) from a diseased eye is removed and replaced by a donor cornea. Also known as a penetrating keratoplasty.

cataract: A cloudiness of lens substance. The lens substance consists of the central nucleus and surrounding cortex, both can be involved in the cataract formation.

corticosteroid: A class of medications used to treat inflammation. Cortisone is the body's natural form; prednisone, prednisolone, and dexamethasone are examples of commonly used synthetic forms. The natural hormone, cortisone, is produced by the adrenal gland and has anti-inflammatory properties.

cycloplegic: A medication, usually in eye drop form, that temporarily paralyzes the ciliary muscle and dilates the pupil.

decentration: A malposition of a structure, in particular an IOL. Downward malposition is termed a sunset syndrome. Upward decentration is termed a sunrise syndrome. Left or right decentrations are termed east-west syndromes. Today, these are fairly unusual and are usually caused by problems with surgical technique as opposed to the IOL manufacture.

diopter: Metric unit used to denote the refractive power or error of an eye system or lens.

diplopia: Double vision.

direct ophthalmoscope: A variation of the instrument invented by von Helmholtz/Babbage designed to provide the observation of an upright or erect image of the interior of the eye. The original ophthalmoscope was the indirect type.

distance vision: The ability to distinctly perceive objects at a distance, usually tested at 20 feet (6 meters). The condition where one has an inability to see objects at a distance is termed myopia.

endophthalmitis: An infection caused by microorganisms that affects the central tunics of the globe, the uvea, and the retina/vitreous. In advanced cases, a vitreous abscess (a virulent exudate or pus) may occur centrally. When all layers of the eye are affected, it is called a pan ophthalmitis.

endothelium: The cell layer forming the inside lining of certain structures, such as the cornea or the blood vessels. In the cornea, this cell layer helps prevent fluid from getting into the cornea and causing edema, or fluid buildup.

enucleation: Surgical removal of the entire eyeball; fortunately, a rare treatment today in this era of improved treatment.

epithelium: The outermost layer (surface layer) of cells on structures such as the cornea, the surface of the eye.

farsightedness: (hyperopia) A refractive error in which the focal point for light rays is behind the retina; distant objects are seen more clearly than near objects. To correct this requires the addition of a convex (positive) lens in the visual axis, whether it be spectacles, contact lenses or an IOL.

GLOSSARY

floaters: Spots, lines, or "cobwebs" that people may see in their vision. Caused by clumps of cells or other material in the vitreous. They may occur as part of posterior vitreous face detachment, a normal part of aging, but may also occur with retinal tears or detachment, vitritis, or other problems in the vitreous.

fluorescein: A yellow dye used to evaluate the status of various blood vessels and circulation of the eye and to evaluate for abnormal depositions of fluid. A fluorescein angiogram is in essence an x-ray of the eye's vessels.

focus: The point at which light rays meet after passing through the cornea and lens. In normal eyes this point is on the fovea of the retina.

fovea centralis: The site of central vision, normally 20/20 (6/6).

fundus (fundus oculi): The structures on the inside surface of the back wall of the eye, and include the optic disk, the retina, and the retinal blood vessels.

glaucoma: An acute or chronic disease with a common denominator is retinal and optic nerve degeneration and possible eventual blindness; usually based on increases of intraocular pressure caused by various tissue changes.

hereditary (inherited, genetic): Appearing in, or characteristic of successive generations; individual differences in human beings passed from parent to offspring.

hydrodissection: An important technique introduced in the 1980s to be used in cataract surgery. It is done at the step of the operation after the anterior capsule is opened (anterior capsulotomy). Fluid, usually a balanced saline solution, is injected into the lens in several quadrants beneath the capsule. The pressure of this stream of fluid breaks up the lens material and is helpful in two ways. 1) By breaking up the lens material it eases the process of cataract removal and 2) for the long term, it helps in the more complete removal of cells from within the lens and thus is useful in reducing the long term incidence of secondary cataract (posterior capsular opacification, PCO). The term was coined by Kenneth Faust of Virginia, Dr. Fine coined the term cortical cleaving hydrodissection, and we use the term subcapsular injection based on our laboratory studies. It is an underemphasized, under-rated, and very important component of the extracapsular cataract extraction (ECCE) procedure.

hyperopia: A refractive error in which light rays focus behind the retina, commonly known as farsightedness. It can be corrected by applying a minus lens onto spectacles, contact lenses, or (best) an IOL. It can also be corrected by correct use of special IOLs such as multifocal lenses.

hypertension: High systemic blood pressure. Ocular hypertension connotes increased blood pressure from the aqueous in the eye but not yet sufficient to cause overt glaucoma.

hyphema: Bleeding into the anterior chamber of the eye, often forming an inferior layered deposit of blood usually caused by trauma.

incidence: Number of new cases of a particular problem or disease that occurs within a period of time.

indirect ophthalmoscopy: The type of ophthalmoscope invented by Helmholtz/Babbage in which the observed image is inverted as one views the interior of the eye. This type is best for seeing a broad overview of the entire visual field, as opposed to the direct ophthalmoscope which provides a more centralized image.

intraocular lens (IOL, pseudophakos, artificial lenticulus): A substitute lens invented by Sir Harold Ridley designed to be placed in the eye for a long term to take the place of the surgically removed natural lens. Depending on mode of fixation of the haptics (footplates) or loops, IOLs can be anterior chamber, iris fixated, or posterior chamber. (synonym, lens implant: An artificial lens is placed inside the eye during cataract surgery to take the place of the eye's natural lens.)

intraocular pressure: The fluid pressure inside the eye, regulated by the secretion of aqueous humor from the tips of the ciliary processes into the eye and drainage of the humor through the canal of Schlemm and trabecular meshwork. Elevated intraocular pressure is the main cause of glaucoma.

IOL haptic: An extension from the lens optic, usually in pairs designed to enhance fixation of the IOL. Some types of haptics may assume the appearance of a broad footplate of the type designed by Peter Choyce. Haptics should be distinguished from loops, which are basically relatively large, round sutures that have been applied to the IOL as fixation elements.

IOL loop: An optic loop has the same function as a haptic but usually consists simply of a small diameter round structure, usually derived from a suture.

IOL optic: The central component of the intraocular lens that functions as the replacement for the extracted cataractous lens. Like any lens (camera, microscope, telescope) it has dioptic or refractive power to bend light rays to assure proper focus on the retina.

iris: The most anterior part of the uvea, surrounding the pupil. It is a colored circular membrane that is situated directly in front of the lens and controls the size of the pupil, thus regulating the amount of light entering the eye.

iris fixated intraocular lens: An implant style in which the haptics (footplates) or loops are situated in contact with iris tissue to enhance fixation. Sometimes excess iris (uveal) contact is deleterious and may sometimes cause inflammation due to scratching or chafing.

iritis: A form of uveitis in which the iris is inflamed. Characterized by inflammatory cells and protein in the aqueous humor.

keratitis: Inflammation of the cornea.

keratoconus: An eye disease marked by central bulging and thinning of the cornea.

keratopathy: A disease or problem of the cornea.

keratoplasty (penetrating): A corneal transplant.

lacrimal gland: The tear gland. Produces tears to lubricate the eye.

laser: Surgical tool using an intense beam of light energy for many purposes: to close rips, make holes, ablate tissues, to mold tissues for refractive tissues, destroy new vessels (photocoagulation), or to open channels as in the treatment of glaucoma.

LASIK: (Laser in Situ Keratomileusis, also Laser Assisted Intrastromal Keratoplasty). This is a combined laser refractive and surgical (incisional) refractive procedure. It is a type of lamellar refractive surgery in which the cornea is reshaped to change its optical power while a disc of cornea (the button) is raised as a flap. The laser is used (usually an excimer laser) to reshape the intrastromal bed, producing surgical flattening of the cornea, commonly used for correcting various refractive errors, especially myopia.

legal blindness: Visual acuity that does not exceed 20/200 in the better eye with correcting lens; field of vision no greater than 20 degrees in its widest angle (visual acuity of 20/200 means that a person can see at a distance of 20 feet what one with "normal" sight can see at 200 feet).

lens: The normally "lens shaped" structure behind the pupil in the posterior chamber. The cornea is responsible for major focusing and the lens is responsible for fine tuning the focus of light rays on the retina.

lens capsule: The outer cellophane-like membrane of the lens. If you compare the lens to an M & Ms candy, the anterior lens substance is a chocolate material and the outer colored shell of M & Ms candy is analogous to the capsule. The entire lens (capsule and anterior lens substance) are removed during ICCE. The lens capsule is left in the eye during ECCE.

lens nucleus: (see lens).

limbus: The junction between the cornea an sclera, an important surgical marker, eg, needed to place incision that opens the eye.

GLOSSARY

low-vision aids: Optical devices of varying power useful to treat persons with visual impairments that cannot be successfully corrected by the usual therapies.

macula: A rod-free area at the center of the retina that includes the fovea responsible for best central vision (20/20).

macular degeneration: (see age-related macular degeneration.)

macular region: The central portion of the retina.

macular edema: Macular edema can be tested with the Amsler grid.

malignant melanoma: A pigmented tumor affecting the uveal layers of the eye, one of the most common primary tumors in the eye.

metastatic tumor: A tumor that has spread to the eye from elsewhere may be a cause of death. The most common metastatic tumors to the eye are from the lung (males) and breast (females).

Miyake-Apple Technique: A technique first invented by Dr. Kensaku Miyake in Nagoya, Japan who did a study of an IOL implanted into a cadaver eye and was able to view it from behind. The technique was modified by Dr. David Apple and colleagues in Salt Lake City in order to do special studies on human eyes postmortem. It is particularly valuable in assessing the quality of lenses in eyes and also in studying complications of IOLs in eyes obtained postmortem.

multifocal device (spectacles, contact lenses, IOL): Specialized lenses that are receiving much attention now are the new multifocal IOLs that are useful for various techniques such as refractive lens exchange. Multifocal IOLs have rings on the anterior surface, using highly technical optical calculations may allow for distant, middle, and near vision all in the same lens. Successful multifocal IOLs placed into the eye via small incision should be highly efficacious as they are continuously approved.

muscles (extraocular) musculus rectus externus (lateralis): There are four so-called rectus muscles (lateral, internal, inferior, superior), as well as two oblique muscles which help move the eye in all directions of gaze. Sometimes these muscles need to be manipulated during various types of surgery.

myopia (nearsightedness): A very common refractive error in which the incoming light rays focus in front of the retina (in the vitreous). This condition, commonly termed nearsightedness, is treated by addition of a minus (concave) IOL, best applied to an intraocular lens in terms of having minimal visual aberrations. This moves the image from the vitreous onto the retina.

near vision: The perception of objects distinctly at normal reading distance (usually about 14 inches from the eye).

neoplasm (tumor): See tumor and see malignant melanoma, retinoblastoma, and metastatic tumor.

neovascularization: A condition in which abnormal blood vessels may develop, sometimes in response to a lack of oxygen from poor circulation. When it occurs in the retina, as in diabetics, it may cause both background and may lead to a state known as proliferative retinopathy, sometimes in association with neovascularization of the iris (rubeosis iridis). Neovascularization is also a problem in diseases of the posterior pole. New vessels may form in ARMD.

night blindness: Condition in which sight is good by day but deficient at night (scotopic vision) or in faint light.

normal sighted (emmetropia): The state in which entering light rays focus directly on the retina without the assistance of any artificial device such as glasses.

nuclear sclerosis: A form of cataract in which most of the opacity is in the center at the nuclear portion of the lens.

onchocerciasis (river blindness): A disease transmitted by flies that exists in various parts of the world, including Africa. Sir Harold Ridley studied this disease in Ghana. It is one of the most common causes of blindness in the world and is now slowing becoming treatable.

GLOSSARY

ophthalmologist: A physician (MD) who specializes in many aspects of care of the eye, including medical and surgical care.

ophthalmoscope: A special instrument invented by Hermann von Helmholtz in Germany and Charles Babbage in England in order to clearly view the fundus, posterior pole, and retina-optic nerve of the eye.

ophthalmoscopy: The examination of the interior of the eye with the ophthalmoscope.

optic atrophy: Degeneration of the optic nerve fibers are due to many causes including glaucoma, nutritional and toxic casues, and many others.

optic disk (optic nerve head, papilla): The site formed by the meeting of all retinal fibers at the beginning of the optic nerve as it courses back to the brain. This is the site of the physiologic blind spot or scotoma.

optic nerve: Special nerve of sight beginning in the retina as the optic disk, which carries messages from the retina to the brain, resulting in visual images.

optic neuritis: Inflammation of the optic nerve.

optician: A specially trained professional who fills prescriptions for eyeglass lenses.

optometrist: A non-MD specialist who performs refractions and determines contact lens prescriptions, examines eyes to detect disease, and in certain states, where permitted by law, may treat certain eye problems.

phakic lens (spectacles, contact lenses, IOL): Any lens that is provided to a patient who still has his or her own lens in the eye. A phakic IOL, for example, can be implanted next to the patient's own IOL for the sole purpose of changing refractive power.

perimetry: Determination of the visual field using special instruments known as perimeters.

peripheral vision: The ability to perceive the presence or motion of objects outside of the realm of central vision, including the far periphery.

phacoemulsification: A technique invented by Charles Kelman and used for removal of a cataractous lens during cataract surgery. The ultrasonic power of the phaco tip is applied to the lens substance and is then pulverized by the high-frequency sound wave energy. This technique has made possible the modern era of foldable incision IOLs and much better results with cataract IOL surgery.

posterior capsule opacification (PCO, secondary cataract, after cataract): When, during initial surgery, there is incomplete removal of cells and lens material, there is a potential for the retained cells to re-grow and form a secondary mass that covers over the visual axis. This is termed a posterior capsule opacification or secondary cataract. The membrane can be broken with the Nd:YAG laser. This is relatively common in children. One of the best and simplest means to reduce the incidence of this complication, among several, is to do copious hydrodissection.

posterior chamber intraocular lens (PC-IOL): An IOL implant in the posterior chamber with haptic (footplate) or a loop fixation in one of two sites, either in the ciliary sulcus, just behind the iris, or preferably, in the residual lens capsular bag after ECCE.

posterior chamber: The small, almost potential space between the crystalline lens and iris, containing aqueous humor.

posterior pole (fundus, fundus oculi): The region of the retina and optic nerve, best viewed with the ophthalmoscope.

posterior subcapsular cataract: A type of cataract where the most opacification is localized in the central back region of the lens. This is a very common form.

presbyopia: Decreased elasticity of the lens due to advancing age, which moves the near point of vision farther from the eye, making it difficult to focus on near objects up close (difficulty in reading). This is usually corrected by plus (convex) spectacles or can be corrected with special IOLs.

primary position of gaze: Position of the eyes when looking straight forward.

GLOSSARY

prism: A special lens that bends light rays, sometimes used to treat strabismus. A triangular lens that splits a ray of light into its constituent colors and turns or deflects light rays towards its base.

proliferative diabetic retinopathy: Growth of abnormal blood vessels and fibrous tissue on and in front of the retina and optic nerve of diabetics. These vessels may bleed into the vitreous and cause serious scarring and other problems.

pupil: The clinically dark opening in the center, bounded by the iris. It is the opening through which light enters the eye towards the retina.

radial keratotomy: A form of corneal incisional refractive surgery, first performed experimentally by Lans in Holland, in which several radial cuts are placed in the anterior cornea, which tends to flatten it to provide a diminution of myopia or nearsightedness.

refractive surgery: A means of doing refraction on a patient so that the light rays focus precisely on the retina, providing good focus. This can be done simply by spectacles or by refractive surgery, which entails, for example, making cuts in the cornea, or using also the laser.

refraction: Measurement of the focusing characteristics of the eye to determine refractive error and the need for prescription glasses.

refractive error: A problem in which the light rays entering the eye fail to come to a focus on the retina, thereby causing blurred vision. Hyperopia, myopia, astigmatism, and presbyopia are forms of refractive errors.

retina: Structure of the eye, formed by transition of the optic nerve where the fibers span out and cover the entire back portion of the eye (the fundus). The retina consists of several layers, including the photoreceptors.

retinal detachment: A disorder in which the retina balloons forward, separating itself from its deepest layer, the pigment epithelium. Retinal detachments are most commonly caused by fluid that travels through retinal tears and then dissects between the pigment epithelium and the other layers. Retinal detachments may occur when a hole forms, allowing passage of fluid or when scar tissue forms pulling the retina forward towards the vitreous.

retinitis pigmentosa: Progressive retinal degeneration with pigmentation and atrophy. It is accompanied by contraction of the visual field so that the vision contracts down to a central focus, like looking through the barrel of a shotgun. There are star-shaped deposits of pigment in the retina and the retinal vessels may become obliterated.

retinoblastoma: A tumor of the retina most commonly affecting children; a cause of tumor death in childhood.

retinopathy: A disease or disorder of the retina.

rods: Light-sensitive cells in the retina that work best in darkness or dim illuminations.

rubeosis iridis: Neovascularization (abnormal blood vessel growth) on the iris, often seen with diabetes and with retinal vein occlusions. May cause neovascular glaucoma.

scanning laser ophthalmoscope (SLO): An ultramodern means of imaging the posterior structures of the eye (retina and optic nerve) by digital means, as opposed to having to excise tissues surgically and look under the pathology microscope. Sir Harold Ridley developed theorectical basis for this technique, even before the laser was invented.

sclera: The white part of the eye; a tough outer covering that along with the cornea forms the external protective layer of the eye.

scleral buckle: A surgical procedure used to repair retinal detachments in which a band or sponge is sewn onto the sclera to indent it.

scotoma: A blind area in the visual field. The optic nerve forms a physiologic or normal scotoma; other scotomas, for example, caused by glaucoma, are certainly pathologic.

secondary position of gaze: Position of the eyes when looking to the right or left, downwards, or upwards.

GLOSSARY

severe visual impairment: Inability to read ordinary newspaper print, even with the aid of glasses, and impairment indicating no useful vision in either eye; includes those who are legally blind.

spherical lens: Lens that is the segment of a sphere. There are no corrections for astigmatism or other nonspherical problems.

stereoscopic vision: Perception of the relief of objects or of their depth, so that they appear as solid objects and not as flat pictures.

telescopic intraocular optic lens: This is a device used for patients with low vision, used by D. Peter Choyce in the 1950s. He implanted an anterior chamber IOL and positioned a second lens outside of the eye, thus creating a Galilean telescope. The modern telescopic IOL has two lenses, ie, the entire Galilean telescope is situated totally within the eye, within the framework of a posterior chamber lens.

toric lens: Refers to either spectacles, contact lenses, or intraocular lenses in which the correction in the optic is not only spherical, but also corrects the astigmatic error at 90 degrees to each other.

trabecular meshwork: The sponge-like tissue that separates the anterior chamber aqueous from the outflow channels that send the aqueous back into the venous system of the body from the anterior chamber. Any blockage of the trabecular meshwork could lead ocular hypertension or glaucoma.

tumor (neoplasm, cancer): In general there are three types of cancer that affect the eye: uveal (malignant melanoma), retinal (retinoblastoma), and metastatic (usually spreading from the breast or lung).

twenty/twenty vision (20/20): Normal visual acuity expressed in feet or with the metric system (6m/6m vision).

ultrasound: High-frequency sound waves that sometimes can be used in a manner similar to X rays for diagnosis and are also used in phacoemulsification. It is used by the dentist for dental procedures and from there it became phacoemulsification.

ultraviolet: A portion of the spectrum that becomes manifest in solar rays. These type of rays may cause tumors of the skin and also are responsible for cataracts, and perhaps ARMD.

uveal tract: The iris, ciliary body, and choroid. These heavily pigmented structures of the eye are also known collectively as the uvea (uvea = grape).

uveitis: Inflammation of part or all of the uveal tract. Forms of uveitis include iritis, iridocyclitis, cyclitis, choroiditis, and others associated with retinitis, vitritis, and endophthalmitis. A through and through infection of the eye is called a pan ophthalmitis.

vascular coat: (see uveal tract).

virus: An infectious particle consisting of DNA or RNA with a protein coating.

visual acuity: The standard measurement is based on a system devised by the Dutch ophthalmologist, Snellen. Snellen visual acuity implies the ability to correctly perceive an object or letter of a designated size that should be readable at a distance of 20 feet (6 meters). Modern determination of visiual acuity should include contrast sensitivity testing and wavefront aberrometry in order to get an accurate determination.

visual axis: The visual line or ray that light follows as it enters the eye through the cone, passes through the pupil and lens, and reaches the retina. It is the ophthalmologist's job to keep the visual axis (the ocular media) free of opacity, eg, corneal opacities or of course cataract.

visual field: The full extent or field of one's vision, including both central vision and peripheral vision measured by varying types of simple of complex perimetry.

GLOSSARY

visually impaired: Persons who have some difficulty seeing with one or two eyes even when wearing a correction.

vitrectomy: An operation that removes vitreal tissue that may contain pathologic materials that can block vision. Sometimes performed in diabetics to remove blood and scar tissue, but also used for other indications.

vitreous body: The largely transparent colorless mass of soft, gelatinous material filling the globe of the eye between the lens and the retina. It is composed of hyaluronic acid on a delicate fibril framework. It must be clear to obtain vision. It usually partially liquefies with age.

vitreous humor: The gel-like material that fills the cavity of the eye between the retina and the lens. Partially liquefies with age. Usually called "vitreous" for short.

vitritis: Inflammation in the vitreous caused by uveitis.

yellow spot (Macula lutea): An oval depression in the central region of the macula, temporal (towards the ear) to and slightly below the papilla of the optic nerve (optic nerve head). This is the point where the clearest (20/20 vision) is generated.

Zonules of Zinn: Tiny fibrils that attach the ciliary body to the lens capsule. They must be mobile for the appropriate accommodation (thickening and thinning of the lens) to occur.

Map of England

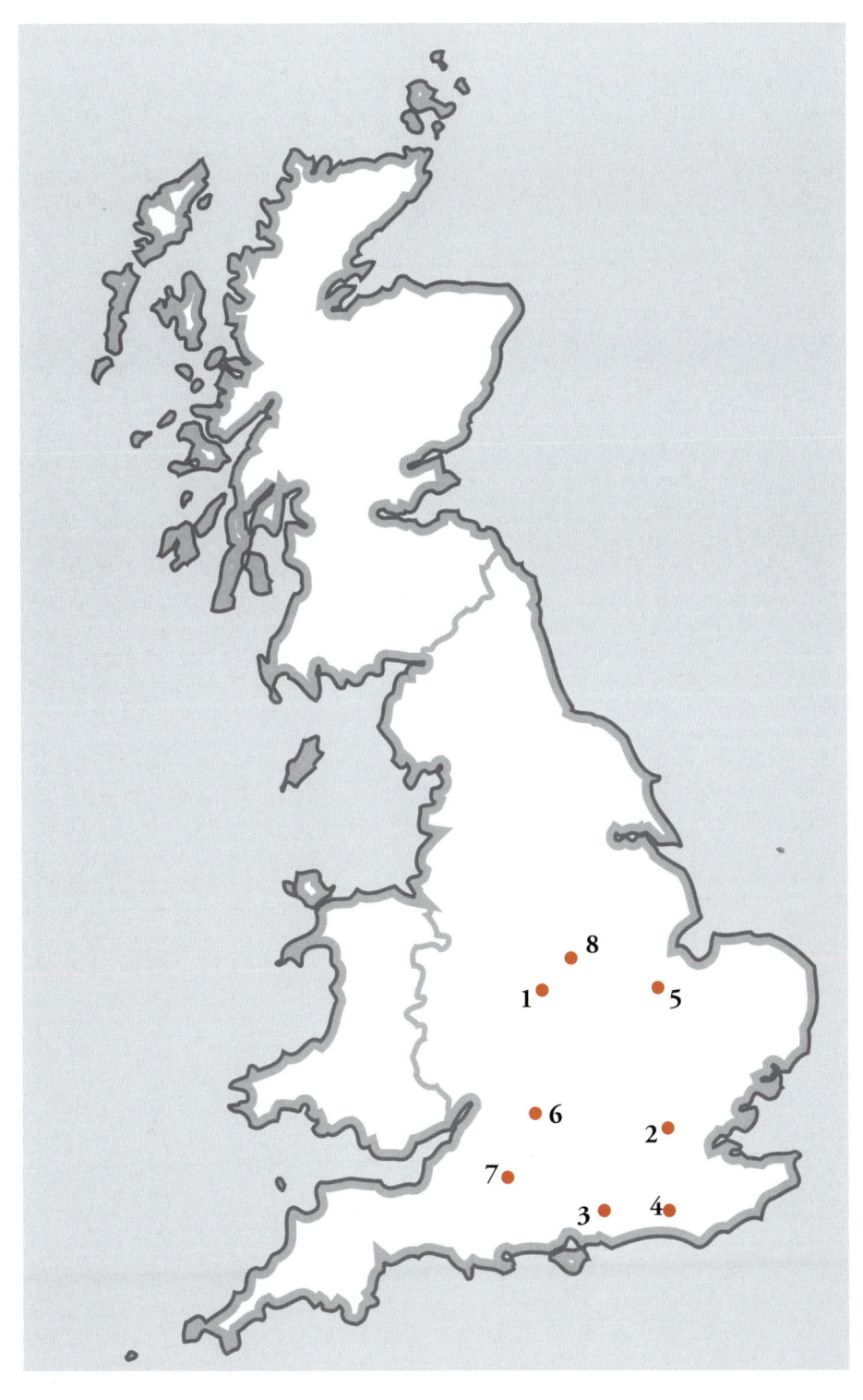

1. Leicestershire. Harold was born here and his childhood home is still standing. His father had a practice at the Leichester Royal Infirmary until his death in 1937.

2. London. The main site of his adult activities, both professional and personal.

3. South England, near the English Channel. This is the site of several satellite hospitals of St. Thomas' Hospital prior to and during World War II and the site of RAF Tangmere.

4. Brighton/Hove. The site of Rayner Intraocular Lenses, Ltd. Harold also attended grammar school here.

5. Cambridgeshire. Harold and his colleagues did some work on electronics at the Marconi Wireless facility at Chelmsford near Cambridge.

6. Oxford. Harold delivered his first public lecture on IOLs at the Oxford Ophthalmological Congress in July of 1951.

7. Stapleford (near Salisbury in Wiltshire). This is the location of Keeper's Cottage, Harold's weekend and retirement cottage.

8. Swinstead. The end. The funeral and burial of harold occurred here near the family home of Lauretta and Nicholas Ridley, and not far from the birthplace of Sir Isaac Newton.

Map of London

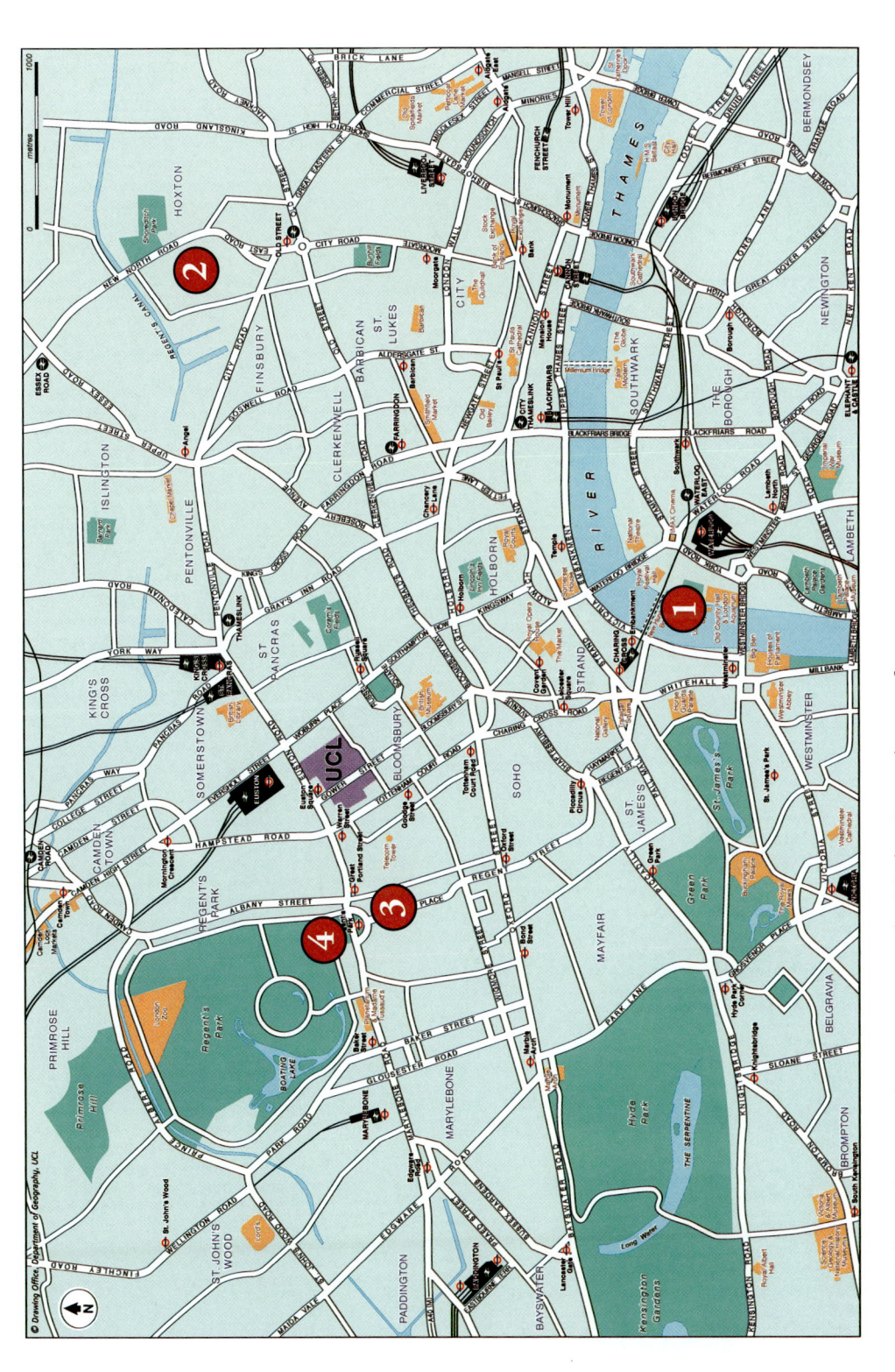

1. St. Thomas' Hospital
2. Moorfields Eye Hospital
3. Cavendish Square
4. Harley Street, home of:
   a. Sir Harold Ridley
   b. Sir Stewart Duke-Elder
   c. Florence Nightingale

Landmark Articles

One of Harold's patients consulted with Frederick Ridley and this "let the cat out of the bag" (see Chapter 9). Harold had to present his results earlier than planned.

He submitted his first paper to the relatively small publication transactions of St. Thomas' Hospital. His first four IOL-related papers, published in rapid succession in 1951-42, were as follows:

1. Ridley NHL. Artificial intraocular lenses after cataract extraction. *St. Thomas' Hospital Reports.* 1951;Vol. 7 (2nd Series):12-14.
2. Intraocular acrylic lenses. Trans. *OSUK.* 1951;Vol. LXXI:617-621. Also, the 1951 Oxford Ophthalmological Congress.
3. Ridley NHL. Intraocular acrylic lenses—A recent development in the surgery of cataract. *British Journal of Ophthalmology.* May 1952;36:113-122. This publication was the "bombshell," the paper that really introduced the world of ophthalmology to a new paradigm, to a new vocabulary, indeed the paper that changed the world.
4. Ridley NHL. Intraocular acrylic lenses after cataract extraction. *Lancet.* January 19, 1952:118-129.

For the first time, many readers would begin to hear about the new terminology associated with IOL implantation. These together created a bombshell that introduced a new vocabulary and a major paradigm shift.

Article 1 (page 286) is from Reference #2.

Article 2 (page 287) is from Reference #4.

INTRA-OCULAR ACRYLIC LENSES AFTER CATARACT EXTRACTION

HAROLD RIDLEY
M.B.Camb., F.R.C.S.

Reprinted from THE LANCET, *January* 10, 1952, p. 118

Article 2.

The Ridley Foundation*

The origins of the Foundation stem from my grandfather, who provided some financial help to the needy workers of Leicester Royal Infirmary during the Great Depression (1929-1932) when their wages were cut and when, before the commencement of the National Health Service (1947), much of the finance for hospitals throughout the UK came from public subscription.

My father formalised the arrangement by creating a charity in 1967. During his lifetime little money was distributed, but instead accumulated. Since my father's death, the Foundation has helped finance some successful clinical research into macular degeneration under Mr. David Wong of Liverpool Royal Victoria Hospital. This course of action would, I am certain, have pleased my father—if for no other reason than it demonstrated to the Charity Commission that the Ridley Foundation was active.

The current trustees of the Foundation are: myself, Mr. Anthony Chignell (formerly senior ophthalmic consultant at St Thomas' Hospital), Mr. Michael Falcon (currently an ophthalmic consultant at St Thomas' Hospital) and Mr. Christopher Morris (formerly a senior partner at the chartered accountant firm of Deloittes).

More recently, the Foundation has provided financial assistance for clinical research into Behcet's Disease, undertaken at the St. John of Jerusalem Eye Hospital and with limited help from St Thomas' Hospital in certain specialist areas. Both Anthony Chignell and I are directors and trustees of the St. John of Jerusalem Eye Hospital, with Anthony having the additional important role of Hospitaller.

The St. John of Jerusalem Eye Hospital is situated in East Jerusalem and caters for the poorest residents of the Holy Land. The Ridley Foundation trustees (all of whom knew my father) firmly believe that the current grant to the Hospital would have fully met with my father's aspirations, he being always keen to undertake research into diseases and to help patients born to third world poverty.

Very ironically, the person that was responsible for the construction of the Hospital was Sir Stewart Duke-Elder. Whilst my father was fully aware of the excellent work undertaken at the Hospital, he was never invited to visit it, even though he was willing to contribute his time gratis.

The Foundation's policy is to continue to assist the very poor people of the Holy Land by undertaking further clinical ophthalmic research in an area where blindness is ten times that of the western world.

Nicholas Ridley
March 7, 2006

---

* Please refer to page 217.

Publications: Sir Harold Ridley, MD, Cantab, FRCS, Eng. FRS*

1. The Diagnosis & Clinical Course of Pituitary Enlargements from the Ophthalmic Standpoint. M.B. Thesis, Cambridge University. 1930.
2. Some practical points in the treatment of simple detachment of the retina. *British Journal of Ophthalmology.* Feb. 1935:101-106.
3. The diagnosis and treatment of detachment of the retina. *The Clinical Journal.* Nov. 1935;Vol LXIV, No. 11:469-470.
4. Cystic Retinal Detachments. *British Journal of Ophthalmology.* Feb. 1936:65-68.
5. Progress in the Treatment of Detachment of the Retina.
6. Aplasia of the Optic Nerves. *British Journal of Ophthalmology.* Nov. 1938:669-671.
7. Broadcast from Accra on Onchocerciasis.
8. The Challenge of Disease. The Empire at War. June 1944;No. 244.
9. Snake Venom Ophthalmia. *British Journal of Ophthalmology.* Nov. 1944:568-572.
10. Penicillin Lamellae. War Office. Jan 1945.
11. Ocular Onchocerciasis. *British Journal of Ophthalmology.* 1945; Monograph Supplement.
12. Ocular lesions in trypanosomiasis. *Annals of Tropical Medicine & Parasitology.* Oct. 1945;Vol. 39, No. 2:66-81.
13. Ocular manifestations of malnutrition in released prisoners of war from thailand. *British Journal of Ophthalmology.* Dec. 1945:613-618.
14. Opening Paper Ophthalmological Society, U.K., Discussions on Amblyopia Trans. *Ophthalmological Society of the United Kingdom.* 1945;LIVI.
15. Toxic Amblyopia. Trans. *OSUK.* Vol. 66:517.
16. Eye—Tropical and nutritional disease. *British Surgical Practice.* London III:6257.

---

* Prepared by Sir Harold Ridley himself, with no modifications.
He did not attempt to arrange his publications, honors, etc in a finished way for publication. Therefore I left them as he had done them.

17. The treatment of glaucoma. *British Encyclopedia of Medical Practice.* London. May 1947; Interim Supplement.
18. Ophthalmic Surgery. B.B.B. Broadcast to the South America. 1948.
19. Toxoplasmosis—A summary of the disease with report of a case. *British Journal of Ophthalmology.* July 1949:397-407.
20. Television in ophthalmology. *St. Thomas' Hospital Reports.* 1949.
21. Metazoan Infections of the Eye—Ocular Complications of the Tropical Diseases for Systemic Ophthalmology. London. 1949. (Also shortened account.)
22. A case of onchocerciasis in london and its treatment with hetrazan. *British Journal of Ophthalmology.* November 1950:688-690.
23. Discussion on Retinal Detachments (opening paper). Annual Meeting Irish Ophthalmological Society. 1950.
24. Television in Ophthalmology. LVI International Congress of Opthalmology. 1950:1397-1404.
25. Undergraduate teaching of Ophthalmology (opening paper). Irish Ophthalmological Society. 1951.
26. Tropical diseases. *Systemic Ophthalmology.* London. 1951:292-298.
27. Metazoan infections. *Systemic Ophthalmology.* London. 1951:275-291.
28. Eye Diseases of Infancy.
29. Intraocular Acrylic Lenses. Trans. *OSUK.* 1951;Vol LXXI:617-621. Also Oxford Ophthalmological Congress 1951.
30. Lenses after cataract extraction. *Lancet.* Jan 19, 1952:118-1929.
31. Artificial intraocular lenses after cataract extraction. *St. Thomas' Hospital Reports.* 1951:Vol. 7(2nd Series):12-14.
32. Intraocular acrylic lenses—A recent development in the surgery of cataract. *British Journal of Ophthalmology.* March 1952:113-122.
33. Intraocular lenses. *Journal International College of Surgeons.* 1952:289-295.
34. Advances in ophthalmology. *The Practitioner.* Oct. 1952:Vol. 169:382-387.

Series 2

35. Recent methods of fundus examination including electronic ophthalmoscopy. Trans. *OSUK.* 1952;Vol. LXXII 497-509.
36. Some surgical technicalities. Intraocular acrylic lenses. *Modern Trends in Ophthalmology: Third Series.* 308-310.
37. Further observations on intraocular acrylic lenses in cataract surgery. J1. *Int. College of Surgeons.* Dec 1952;Vol. XVIII No. 6 825-833.
38. Further observations on intraocular acrylic lenses in cataract surgery. Trans. *American Academy of Ophthalmology.* Jan-Feb. 1953:98-106.
39. Further experiences of intraocular acrylic lens surgery. *British Journal of Ophthalmology.* 1954:38:156-162.
40. Contribution to discussion on the significance of macular changes. Oxford Ophthalmological Congress. Trans. *OSUK.* 1954: LXXIV:61-62 and Film of Operation 345.
41. Keratoplasty in Keratoconus. Section of Ophthalmology. Royal Society of Medicine. November 1955.
42. Five Years Experience of Intraocular Acrylic Lens Surgery. International College of Surgeons, Geneva. 1955.
43. Treatment of Cataract. Annual Meeting Trinity College Dublin Biological Association. 1956.
44. Late Surgical Results of Use of Intraocular Acrylic Lenses. J1. International College of Surgeons. Sept. 1956:Vol. XXVI. No. 3.
45. Artificial lenticulus. Trans. *OSUK.* 1956;LXXVI:549-551.

46. Cataract surgery. *Ophthal Ibero Amer.* Jan 1957:89-106.
47. Further observations on intraocular acrylic lenses. Oxford Ophthalmological Congress. Trans. *OSUK.* LXXVII:527-529.
48. The treatment of cataract. *The Practitioner.* May 1957;Vol. 179.
49. An anterior chamber lenticular implant. *British Journal of Ophthalmology.* June 1957:355-358.
50. Onchocerca—The blinding worm. *Ophthal Ibero Amer.* 1957;19:73-88.

Series 3

51. Retinal photography. Oxford Ophthalmological Congress. 1957. Trans. *OSUK.* LXXVII 417-418.
52. The Graefe Section. Irish Ophthalmological Society, Dublin. May 1958.
53. Cataract surgery with particular reference to intraocular lenticular implants of various types. Trans. *OSUK.* 1958: LXVIII:585-592.
54. The Flying Spot Television Ophthalmoscope. ICIII Concilium Ophthalmologicum. 1958.
55. Intraocular Plastic Lenses. Second International Course, Instituto Barraquer. 1958.
56. Metazoan Diseases of the Eye. Second International Course, Instituto Barraquer. 1958.
57. The improved flying spot electronic ophthalmoscope. Oxford Ophthalmological Congress. Trans. OSUK. 1954;LXXIX:585-589.
58. Discussion on Iris Supported Implants Comment in « Any Questions ? ». Discussion on Melanomata. Oxford Ophthalmological Congress. 1959.
59. Intraocular acrylic lenses—10 years development. *British Journal of Ophthalmology.* Dec. 1960:Vol. 44, No. 12: 705-712.
60. Contribution to the Symposium on Intraocular Acrylic Lenses. Third International Course, Instituto Barraquer. 1961.
61. Intraocular acrylic lenses. *An de Instituto Barraquer III.* 1962:548-554.
62. The Story of Acrylic Lenses. Australian Ophthalmological Society Meeting. November 1962.
63. Experiments with Electronics in Ophthalmology. Australian Ophthalmological Society Meeting. November 1962.
64. Tropical and nutritional diseases. *For Clinical Surgery.* Butterworth & Co; 1963.
65. Contribution to the discussion on Vasculitis Retinae (Scleral buckling for traction detachment). *OSUK.* April 1963.
66. Intraocular Acrylic Lenses—Past, Present & Future.
67. Contribution to the discussion on ocular onchocerciasis. *OSUK.* April 1965.
68. Cataract Surgery in Chronic Uveitis. Oxford Ophthalmological Congress. 1965;85:519-525.
69. The Treatment of Severely Damaged Eyes. Combined Meeting of Irish & New England Ophthalmological Societies, Dublin. April 1967.
70. Intraocular Implants: 1948-68. Ralph I. Lloyd Lecture, Brooklyn Ophthalmological Society. March 1968.
71. Blindness in Leprosy Patients. The Work of the Royal Commonwealth Society for the Blind. Ninth International Leprosy Congress. September 1968.
72. Acrylic lens implants—Current results. *An de Instituto Barraquer 9.* 1969:143-149.
73. Long Term Results of Acrylic Lens Surgery. R.S.M. June 1969. Proceeding of the Royal Society of Medicine. 1970:63:309.
74. Intraocular Acrylic Lenses; Improved Technique & Results XXX International Congress. 771-775.

75. Metazoan Infections. For Systemic Ophthalmology, London. March 1971.
76. The Treatment of Malignant Diseases of the Eye by Radiotherapy & by Logical Excision. European Congress of Ophthalmology, Budapest. 1971.
77. The Origin & Objectives of Intraocular Lenticular Implants. 80th American Academy of Ophthalmology & Otolaryngology, Dallas. September 1975.
78. The Origin of Intraocular Implant Surgery. Congres International et 1er Festival du Film sur l'implantation intraoculaire. Association Francaise des Implants Intra-Oculaires, Cannes. May 1979.
79. (Rosen, Haining and Arnott.) The cure of aphakia, 1949. *Intraocular Lens Implantation.* St. Louis, MO: C.V. Mosby; 1984:37-41.
80. Address to the American Intraocular Implant Society, San Francisco. Nov. 11, 1979.
81. "Would you do anything differently?" International Intraocular Implant Club. April 19, 1980.
82. The True Pioneers of Intraocular Implants. Foreword to book by David Apple et al. Univ. Utah. 1986.
83. Cure of Aphakia. Unpublished. Intended for laymen.
84. Address to open the Moscow Institute of Eye Microsurgery and the First Moscow Symposium of Ophthalmology. 1986. Unpublished in English.
85. Address to Colleagues at St. Thomas' Hospital. Jan. 20, 1987.
86. Address to the European Intraocular Implant Lens Council. Jerusalem 1987.
87. Address to St. Thomas' Hospital Ophthalmic Department "Friends." Nov 14-15 1989.
88. Address to "Trends" St. Thomas' Hospital. Nov. 14-15, 1989.
89. Prenatal Intraocular Acrylic Lenses EIIC. 1989.
90. The Origin of Intraocular Implants.
91. A Novice in Tropical Ophthalmology. 1990.
92. Address in Dublin, presenting the Ridley Medal.
93. The Development of Intraocular Implants. Gullstrand Medal Meeting. Stockholm. Oct. 29, 1992.
94. Gonin Award.
95. Expeditions to Fonsi. 1944.

PUBLICATIONS: SIR HAROLD RIDLEY, MD, CANTAB, FRCS, ENG. FRS

A. Letters from the Patient. *St. Thomas' Hospital Gazette.* April 1958.
B. Report on Some Causes of Blindness in Northern Rhodesia. British Commonwealth Society for the Blind. 1962.
C. Report on Research Visit to Guyana & the West Indies. Royal Commonwealth Society for the Blind. 1967.
D. Indian Ophthalmology as Seen by a British Visitor. 1969.
E. Obituary to the late Mr. P. G. Doyne. *St. Thomas' Hospital Reports.*
F. Obituary to the late Mr. A. C. Hudson. *St. Thomas' Hospital Reports.*
Fa. Obituary to the late A. C. Hudson. *British Journal of Ophthalmology.* 1962.
Fb. Obituary to the late Mr. A. C. Hudson. *The Times.* 1962
G. Obituary to the late Mr. Basil Ward. *St. Thomas' Hospital Gazette.* 1969.
Ga. Obituary to the late Mr. Basil Ward. *The Times.* 1968.
Gb. Obituary to the late Mr. Basil Ward. *Lancet.* December 1968.
H. Obituary to Lieut.-Colonel R. E. Wright, C.I.E.
I. Reminiscences, Royal Buckinghamshire Hospital, Aylesbury.
J. A simple telescope. *Journal of the Flyfishers' Club.* 1951;Vol. XI.
K. A reminder and a warning. *Journal of the Flyfishers' Club.* Spring 1956.
L. A wicked salmon. *Journal of the Flyfishers' Club.* Summer 1973.
M. Getting the salmon home in good condition. *Journal of the Flyfishers' Club.* Winter 1975.

Sir Harold Ridley: Memberships, Presentations, and Honors*

MEMBERSHIPS AND HONORS

1. Founding Member, International Intraocular Lens Implant Club (IIIC), Life President
2. Ophthalmological Society of the United Kingdom
3. Oxford Ophthalmological Congress
4. Royal Society of Medicine
5. American Intraocular Implant Society (now the American Society of Cataract and Refractive Surgery)
6. International College of Surgeons
7. Irish Ophthalmological Society
8. Australian College of Ophthalmologists
9. European Intraocular Lens Implant Club
10. The College of Ophthalmologists, London, 1988
11. Honorary Faculty Miyake-Apple Laboratory in Storm Eye Institute, Charleston, South Carolina
12. Present and Book with signatures of over 4,000 appreciative American ophthalmologists at the annual meeting of the American Academy of Ophthalmology, San Francisco 1978
13. Special Award, European Intraocular Implant Club, Jerusalem, Israel, 1987
14. Inauguration of the Ridley Lecture and Medal, Copenhagen, Denmark, 1988
15. Honorary Degree, Doctor of Human Letters, Medical University of South Carolina, Charleston, South Carolina, USA, 1989
16. Honorary Doctor of Science, University of London, 1990

---

* Prepared by Sir Harold Ridley himself, with no modifications.

17. Gullstrand Medal, Stockholm, Sweden, 1992
18. Gonin Medal, Toronto, Canada, 1994
19. Golden Graefe Knife, Residents of Moorfields Eye Hospital, 1971
20. Plaque, American Implant Society in Dallas, 1975
21. Medallion, Association Francaise des Implantes Intraoculaire, Cannes, 1979
22. Medallion, European Intraocular Implant Society in Jerusalem, 1987
23. Plaque, IIIS 6th Congress in Copenhagen, 1988
24. Plaque, "Quality of Cataract Surgery" in Stockholm, 1999
25. Chicago Medical Society with Insertion of the First Intraocular Implant in North America, 1952
26. American Academy of Ophthalmology and Otolaryngology, Chicago, 1952
27. Life President International Intraocular Implant Club, Budapest, 1966
28. The Lloyd Lecture, Brooklyn, 1968
29. American Academy of Ophthalmology and Otolaryngology, Dallas, 1975
30. Association Française des Implantes Intraoculaire, Cannes, 1979
31. American Academy and American Implant Society, San Francisco, 1979
32. First Moscow Symposium of Ophthalmology & Formal Opening by Harold Ridley, 1986
33. European Implant Lens Council 5th Congress, Jerusalem, 1987
34. European IIIC 6th Congress, Copenhagen, 1988
35. Symposium on "Quality of Cataract Surgery," Stockholm, 1988

David J. Apple, IOL-Related Articles, Early Phase (1984-1986)

Twenty-five IOL-related journal articles, published 1984-1986.

IOL-Related Articles 1984-1986:

1. Apple DJ, Craythorn JM, Olson RJ, Little LE, Lyman JB, Reidy JJ, Loftfield K. Anterior segment complications and neovascular glaucoma following implantation of posterior chamber intraocular lens. *Ophthalmology.* 1984;91:403-419.
2. Apple DJ, Mamalis N, Loftfield K, Googe JM, Novak LC, Kavka-Van Norman D, Brady SE, Olson RJ. Complications of intraocular lenses. A historical and histopathological review. *Surv Ophthalmol.* 1984;29:1-54.
3. Apple DJ, Mamalis N, Brady SE, Loftfield K, Kavka-Van Norman D, Olson RJ. Biocompatability of implant materials: A review and scanning electron microscopic study. *J Am Intraocul Implant Soc.* 1984;10:53-66.
4. Apple DJ, Cameron JD, Lindstrom RL. Loop fixation of posterior chamber intraocular lenses. *Cataract.* 1984;2(1):7-10.
5. Mamalis N, Apple DJ, Brady SE, Notz RG, Olson RJ. Pathological and scanning electron microscopic evaluation of the 91Z intraocular lens. *J Am Intraocul Implant Soc.* 1984;10:191-199.
6. Apple DJ, Mamalis N, Steinmetz RL, Loftfield K, Crandall AS, Olson RJ. Phacoanaphylactic endophthalmitis associated with extracapsular cataract extraction and a posterior chamber intraocular lens. *Arch Ophthalmol.* 1984;102(10):1528-1532.
7. Googe JM, Mamalis N, Apple DJ, Olson RJ. BSS warning (letter to the editor). *J Am Intraocul Implant Soc.* 1984;10:202.
8. Apple DJ. Utah *Center for Intraocular Lens Research. Proceedings of the Research to Prevent Blindness Science Writer's Seminar.* Oct 1984:pp 35-36.
9. Apple DJ, Reidy JJ, Googe JM, Mamalis N, Novak LC, Loftfield K, Olson RJ. A Comparison of ciliary sulcus and capsular bag fixation of posterior chamber intraocular lenses. *J Am Intraocul Implant Soc.* 1985;11:44-63.

10. Kincaid MC, Apple DJ, Mamalis N, Brady SE, Rashid ER. Histopathologic correlative study of kelman-style flexible anterior chamber intraocular lenses. *Am J Ophthalmol.* 1985;99:159-169.

11. Reidy JJ, Apple DJ, Googe JM, Richey MA, Mamalis N, Olson RJ, Mackman G. An analysis of semiflexible, closed-loop anterior chamber intraocular lenses. *J Am Intraocul Implant Soc.* 1985;11:344-352.

12. Gieser SC, Apple DJ, Loftfield K. Richey MA, Rivera RP. Phthisis bulbi after intraocular lens implantation in a child. *Can J Ophthalmol.* 1985;20(5):184-185.

13. Isenberg RA, Weiss RL, Apple DJ, Lowrey DB. Fungal Contamination of Balanced Salt Solution. *J Am Intraocul Implant Soc.* 1985;11:485-486.

14. Apple DJ, Kincaid MC. Histopathology of intraocular lens explantation. *Cataract.* 1985;2(7):7-11.

15. Crandall AS, Richards SC, Apple DJ. Extracapsular cataract extraction: In-the-bag versus ciliary sulcus fixation. In: *Transactions of the Pacific Coast Oto-Ophthalmological Society.* 1985;66:73-79.

16. Apple DJ. Pathology of intraocular lenses: Polypropylene vs PMMA. In: Jeffe MS (ed), *Intraocular Lens Complications; Self-Study Program. Module II: Proceedings of Symposium on IOL Complications.* Stockholm, Sweden. Pharmacia monograph, Aug 17-24, 1985.

17. Isenberg RA, Apple DJ, Reidy JJ, Richards SC, Sumsion MA, Park SB, Allan SA, Deacon J. Histopathologic and scanning electron microscopic study of one type of intraocular lens. *Arch Ophthalmol.* 1986;104:683-686.

18. Richburg FA, Reidy JJ, Apple DJ, Olson RJ. Sterile hypopyon secondary to ultrasonic cleaning solution. *J Cataract Refract Surg.* 1986;12:248-251.

19. Newman DA, McIntyre DJ, Apple DJ, Deacon J, Popham JK, Isenberg RA. Pathologic findings of an explanted silicone intraocular lens. *J Cataract Refract Surg.* 1986;12:292-297.

20. Apple DJ, Park SB, Merkley KH, Brems RN, Richards SC, Langley KE, Piest KL, Isenberg RA. Posterior chamber intraocular lenses in a series of 75 autopsy eyes. Part I: Loop location. *J Cataract Refract Surg.* 1986;12:358-362.

21. Park SB, Brems RN, Parsons MR, Pfeffer BR, Isenberg RA, Langley KE, Apple DJ. Posterior chamber intraocular lenses in a series of 75 autopsy eyes. Part II: Postimplantation loop configuration. *J Cataract Refract Surg.* 1986;12:363-366.

22. Brems RN, Apple DJ, Pfeffer BR, Park SB, Piest KL, Isenberg RA. Posterior chamber intraocular lenses in a series of 75 autopsy eyes. Part III: Correlation of positioning holes and optic edges with the pupillary aperture and visual axis. *J Cataract Refract Surg.* 1986;12:367-371.

23. Apple DJ, Osher RH, Lichtenstein SB, Koch DD. *IOL Materials and Complications. Proceedings of Symposium on IOL Materials and Complications.* Orlando, FL. Jan 31-Feb 2, 1986, Coburn.

24. Apple DJ, Brems RN, Ellis GW, Spencer DA. A review of the histopathology of intraocular lens fixation. *Curr Can Ophthalmic Prac.* 1986;4:54-56 and 78-79.

25. Apple DJ. Intraocular lenses: Notes from an interested observer. *Arch Ophthalmol.* 1986;104:1150-1152.

IOL-Related Books

1. Apple DJ, Geiser SC, Isenberg RA. *Evolution of Intraocular Lenses.* Salt Lake City, UT: University of Utah Printing Services; 1985.

2. Apple DJ, Kincaid MC, Mamalis N. Olson RJ. *Intraocular Lenses. Evolution, Designs, Complications, and Pathology.* Baltimore, MD: Williams & Wilkins; 1989.

3. Apple DJ, Rabb MF. *Ocular Pathology, Clinical Applications, and Self-Assessment.* 4th ed. (Formerly *Clinico-Pathologic Correlation of Ocular Disease: A Text and Stereo Atlas,* 4th ed.) St. Louis, MO: CV Mosby; 1991.

4. Apple DJ, Rabb MF. *Ocular Pathology, Clinical Applications, and Self-Assessment.* 5th ed. St. Louis, MO: Mosby-Year Book, Inc.; 1998.

5. Apple DJ, Ram J, Foster A, et al. Elimination of cataract blindness: A global perspective entering the new century. *Surv Ophthalmol.* 2000; Monograph (Special issue).
6. Apple DJ, Auffarth GU, Peng Q, Vissessok N. *Foldable Intraocular Lenses.* Thorofare, NJ: SLACK Incorporated; 2000.
7. Apple DJ, et al. *Foldable Intraocular Lenses and Specialized Refractive Biodevices: Evolution, Clinicopathologic Correlations, and Complications 25 Years, David J. Apple, M.D. Laboratories For Ophthalmic Devices Research, 1980-2005.* Thorofare, NJ: SLACK Incorporated; In Press.

Articles, Editorials, and Obituaries written by David J. Apple about Sir Harold Ridley

1. Apple DJ, Sims J. Harold Ridley and the invention of the intraocular lens. *Surv Ophthalmol.* 1996;40:279-92.
2. Apple DJ. Harold Ridley MA, MD, FRCS: A gold anniversary celebration and a golden age. *Arch Ophthalmol.* 1999;117:827-28.
3. Apple DJ, Peng Q, Ram J. The 50th anniversary of the intraocular lens and a quiet revolution. *Ophthalmology.* 1999;106:1861-62.
4. Apple DJ. Sir Harold Ridley receives England's highest honor. *Surv Opthalmol.* 2000;44:542.
5. Apple DJ, Peng Q. Harold Ridley knighted. *Ophthalmology.* 2000;107:412-13.
6. Apple DJ, et al. Newly recognized complications of posterior chamber intraocular lenses. *Arch Ophthalmol.* 2001;119:581-82.
7. Apple DJ, Schmidbauer, JM. Sir Nicholas Harold Lloyd Ridley: Pionier der intraokularlinse. *Klin Monatsbl Augenheilkd.* 2001;218:583-585.
8. Auffarth, GU, Schmidbauer, J, Apple DJ. Intraokularlinse. *Der Ophthalmologe.* 2001;98:1001-28.
9. Apple DJ. Pioneering eye care. Guest editorial. *Charleston Post and Courier.* Charleston, SC. June 28, 2000.
10. Apple DJ. Sir Nicholas Harold Ridley: All's well that ends well. *Am J Ophthalmol.* 2002;133:131-33.
11. Traivedi, RH, Apple DJ, Pandey SK, et al. Sir Nicholas Harold Ridley. He changed the world so that we might better see it. *Indian J of Ophthalmol.* 2003;51:211-16.
12. Apple DJ. A pioneer in the quest to eradicate world blindness. *World Health Organization* 2003;81(10):756-761.
13. Apple DJ, Sir Harold Ridley. A pioneer in the quest to eradicate blindness worldwide. *Cataract & Refract Surg Today.* March 2004:1-4.

Total IOL-related books up to 2006, 300 journal articles and 40 book chapters on IOLs were published.

List 1: Visual Acuity Measurements

Equivalent Visual Acuity Measurements

20 Feet	6 Meters	Decimal
20/1200	1/60	0.01
20/400	3/60	0.05
20/200	6/60	0.10
20/160	6/48	0.125
20/125	6/38	0.16
20/100	6/30	0.20
20/80	6/24	0.25
20/60	6/18	0.33
20/50	6/15	0.40
20/40	6/12	0.50
20/30	6/9	0.67
20/20	6/6	1.00
20/16	6/5	1.25
20/10	6/3	2.00

List 2: World Health Organization Classification of Visual Impairment (Simplified)

	Snellen Visual Acuity
Normal	20/20 to 20/200
Visual impairment	2/20 to 200
Severe visual impairment	2/200 to 2/400
Blind	2/400 (no light perception)

In the better eye with correction

PHOTO CREDIT LIST

Books on History of Ophthalmology, Suggested Reading and Photographic/Art Sources.

Albert DM. *Dates in Ophthalmology.* The Parthenon Publishing Group; 2002.
Apple and Associates. *Intraocular Lenses.* Williams & Wilkins; 1989.
Apple and Associates. *Foldable Intraocular Lenses.* SLACK Incorporated; 2000.
Arnott EJ. *A New Beginning in Sight.* Docwife Publications Forest View House, Dockenfield Farnham Surrey; 2005.
Chicago Art Institute.
Choyce P. *Intra-Ocular Lenses and Implants.* H.K. Lewis & Co. Ltd.; 1964.
Duke-Elder S. *System of Ophthalmology.* C. V. Mosby; 1962.
Gallerie dell'Accademia di Venezia. Venice, Ministero per i Beni; 1998.
Gorgin G. *History of Ophthalmology.* Publish or Perish, Inc; 1982.
Grafe-Saemisch Handbuch. *der Augenheikunde.* Leipzig; 1908.
Hirschberg J. *History of Ophthalmology,* translated by F. C. Blodi, J.P. Wayenborgh; 1982-1994.
Leaver PK. *The History of Moorfields Eye Hospital,* Vol III Forty Years On. The Royal Society of Medicine Press, Ltd.; 2004.
Monet's London, Artist's Reflections on the Thames. Snoeck; 2005.
Musee D'Orsay, Paris.
Musee Monmarmottan, Paris.
Museum of Fine Arts, Houston, TX.
Photographs by Gabi Roma.
Tasman W. *The History of Wills Eye Hospital.* Harper & Row; 1980.

Videos on File with the Author

1. Apple DJ. Cataract Surgery: Past, Present and Future.
2. Apple DJ. Harold Ridley—A Pioneer.
3. Implant Performed by Dr. Warren Reese, early 1950s (courtesy William Tassman, MD).

A=Material in possession of Apple-Ridley-Choyce families.
M=Multisource, no copyright found, anonymous, or unknown source.

Chapter 1
A—p2a, p2b; p3a; p5a, p5b, p9a, p12a.
p4a—John Winstanley; p4b Ian Collins.
p6—St. Thomas' Hospital, David Spalton.
p7—Rayner & Keeler, Ltd.
p8a Rayner & Keeler, Ltd., p8b AMO.
p9—late John Pearce.
p10a—AMO; p10b Rayner & Keeler., Ltd; p10c Alcon Laboratories.
p11a—Kevin Buehler, Alcon.
p12a, p12b, p12c—Charles Letocha.

Chapter 2
A—p14, p16a, p16b, p18a, p18b, p20a, p20b, p20c, p20d, p20e, p21a, p21b, p21c, p22a, p22b, p22c, p22d, p22f, p26a, p26b, p28a.
M—p19a, p19b, p21, p23, p25a, p25b, p27, p28a, p28bc.
p14—Museo Nazionale di Capodimonte, Naples.
p16—Bartisch.
p18a, p18b-Holicost Museum, Washington DC.
p23—AAO
p24—Gallerie dell'Accademia di Venezia.
p26—Chicago Art Institute (left and right).
p27—Alcon Laboratories.
p28b, p28e—Musee D'Orsay, Paris.
p28d—Museum of Fine Art, Houston, TX.

Chapter 3
A—p30a, p30b; p32a, p32b; p33a, p33b; p34a, p34b; p38a, p39a, p39b; p40a, p40b, p40c, p40d; p41a, p41b, p41c, p41d, p41e, p41f; p43a, p43b; p44a; p45a; p46a, p46b; p48a, p48b, p48c, p48d, p48e; p49a, p49b, p49c, p49d, p49e; p50a, p50b, p50c, p50d; p51a, p51b, p51c, p51d; p52a, p52b, p52c, p52d; p61a, p61b; p62a, p62b, p62c, p62d, p62e, p62f; p63a, p63b; p64a, p64b, p64c; p66a, p66b, p66c; p67a, p67b, p67c; p68a, p68b; p69a, p69b; p70a, p70b; p71a; p72a, p72b; p73; p73b; p74a, p74b, p74c, p74d; p74e, p74f; p75a, p75b, p75c, p75d, p75e, p75f, p75g.
M—p34a; p36a, p36b; p36c; p36d; p37a, p37b; p38a; p38b; p42a, p42b; p43a.
p40—Mr. and Mrs. David Austin, photograph by Ann Apple.
p44a, p44b, p44c, pp44d—Charterhouse; p44e, p44f—Cambridge University, photograph Ann Apple.
p47—photographs courtesy Dr. Arthur Lim.

Chapter 4
A—p52a, p52b, p52c, p52d; p61a, p61b; p62a, p62b, p62c, p62d, p62e, p62f; p64a, p64b, p64c; p66a, p66b, p66c; p67a, p67b, p67c; p68a, p68b; p69a, p69b; p70; p71a, p71b, p71c, p71d; p72a, p72b; p73; p74a, p74b, p74c, p74d, p74e, p74f; p75a, p75b, p75c, p75d, p75e, p75f, p75g.
M—p70a, p70b; p71a, p71b, p71c.
p55—*Ophthalmology.* 1984:91.
p56—Apple and associates. Anterior segment complications. *Ophthalmology.* 1984:91.
p56—Apple and associates. Complications of intraocular lenses. *Surv Ophthalmol.* 1984:29.
p59—photograph by Dr. John Sims.
p76—Moran Eye Center.

Chapter 5
A—p78a, p78b, p78c, p78d; p79a, p79b; p85a, p85b, p85c; p86a, p86b, p86c; p87a, p87b, p87c, p87d, p87e; p88a, p88b; p90a, p90b, p90c; p91; p92a, p92b, p92c, p92d, p92e, p92f, p92g; p94a, p94b, p94c, p94d; p96a, p96b, p96c, p96d.
M—p80a, p80b; p82a, p82b; p83a, p83b; p84; p85a, p85b, p85c; p86a, p86b; p89a, p89b, p89c, p89d; p91a, p91b; p93a, p93b, p93c, p93d, p93e; p95a, p95b.
p82—Bartisch (left and right).
p83—Bartisch (left, middle, and right), AAO.
p84—AAO (four images).
p90—Harms and MacKensen (left and right), Howatd Gimbel.
p92—Smith (left and right).
p93—D. P. Choyce (left, center, and right).
p95—Charles Letocha (top and bottom).

Chapter 6
A—p98; p100a, p100b; p105a, p105b; p108a, p108b, p108c, p108d; p111a, p111b, p111c, p111d; p112; p114a, p114b; p115; p116a, p116b, p116c; p120a, p120b; p125a, p125b.
M—p100; p102; p107a, p107b, p107c; 109; 110a, 110b; 114a, 114b, 114c, 114d; 115a, 115b, 115c; 116a, 116b, 116c; 118a, 118b; 126; 127.
p99—Jane Adams.
p102—Fechner.
p105—Eric Arnott.
p106—Tangmere Museum.
p107—John Winstanley.
p111—Jane Adams.
p112—Jane Adams.
p114—Rayner & Keeler, Ltd.
p117—Winston Churchill: The Second World War (four).
p118—Winston Churchill: The Second World War; Tangmere Museum.
p119—Tangmere Museum (two); Jane Adams.
p121—Jane Adams; Eric Arnott (two).
p122—Jane Adams.
p125—Joe Thompson (three).
p126—RAF Tangmere.

Chapter 7
A—p131; p133; p135a, p135b; p136a, p136b, p136c.
p128—Mrs. Stephen Perry, Hugh Williams.
p133—Ann Apple.
p134—Rayner & Keeler, Ltd. (three).
p135—Rayner & Keeler, Ltd.
p136—Anil Patel.
p137—Rayner & Keeler, Ltd. (two).
p138—Edward Epstein, Rayner & Keeler, Ltd.

PHOTO CREDIT LIST, CONTINUED

Chapter 8
A—p143a, p143b, p143c, p143d; p144a, p144b, p144c, p144d, p144e; p145a, p145b; p146a, p146b; p147a, p147b, p147c.
M—p140a, p140b.
p140—St. Thomas' Hospital (three).
p142—*London Times*.
p143—*London Times*.
p146—St. Thomas' Hospital, David Spalton (two).

Chapter 9
A—p155a, p155b, p155c; p157a, p157b, p157c; p159; p160; p161.
M—p150a, p150b; p152a, p152b; p153a, p153b; p154a, p154b, p154c; p156; p161; p162a, p162b; p163.
p148—Arthur Lim.
p155—Arthur Lim (two).
p156—*American Journal of Ophthalmology*, Reva Hurtes.
p158—Jane Adams, Eric Arnott.
p159—Arthur Lim (five).
p160—Arthur Lim.
p161—Arthur Lim.

Chapter 10
A—p166; p168; p169a, p169b; p170a, p170b, p170c, p170d, p170e; p171a, p171b, p171c, p171d; p171d; p173a, p173b; p174a, p174b, p174c; p175a, p175b.
M—p173.
p172—Charles Letocha (two).
p175—Robert Drews.
p176—Richard Lindstrom, Richard Kratz.
p177—Stephen Ostbaum, Gabi Roma, 1956.

Chapter 11
A—p180; p181a, p181b; p182; p183; p184a, p184b; p185a, p185b, p185c; p186a, p186b, p186c, p186d; p187a, p187b, p187b, p187c, p187d, p187e, p187f, p187g, p187h; p188a, p188b; p189a, p189b, p189c, p189d, p189e; p190.
p182—AMO (two).

Chapter 12
A—p193; p197; p198a, p198b; p199a, p199b.
M—p194a, p194b; p197, p201a, p201b, p201c.
p197—S. Fyodorov (two).
p200—S. Fyodorov (four).
p201—AMO (two).

Chapter 13
A—p204; p206a, p206b, p206c; p209; p210a, p210b, p210c, p210d, p210e; p212; p213a, p213b; p214a, p214b, p124c; p215a, p215b; p216a, p216b, p216c.

Chapter 14
A—p220a, p220b, p220c, p220d; p224a, p224b.
M—p223a, p223b, p223c, p223d, p223e; p225a, p225b, p225c, p225d, p225e.
p221—*British Journal of Ophthalmology* supplement, December 1945.
p222—*Winston Churchill: The Second World War* (two).
p224—AAO (two).
p225—Bartisch (two).
p226—Bausch & Lomb, Novartis.

Chapter 15
A—p228a, p228b, p228c; p230a, p230b; p232a, p232b, p232c; p233; p234; p235a, p235b; p236.
M—p230, p231a, p231b, p231c.
p228—*British Journal of Ophthalmology* (twice).
p233—GDX (two).
p234—Zeiss, Beth Snodgrass, and James Gilman (two).

Chapter 16
A—p240a, p240b, p240c; p241a, p241b, p241c, p241d, p241e, p241f, p241g.
M—p240a, p240b, p240c.
p242—Ionics Crystalens, Visiogen Synchrony, Telescopic Lens.
p243—Alan Chow.

Chapter 17
A—p244; p246a, p246b; p247; p248a, p248b, p248c, p248d; p249; p250a, p250b, p250c, p250d, p250e, p250f, p250g; p251a, p251b, p251c, p251d, p251e.
p246—Arthur Lim.
p247—Nicholas Ridley, Ann Apple, Arthur Lim.
p249—Eric Arnott.
p250—Nicholas Ridley, St. Thomas' Hospital, ASCRS.

Chapter 18
A—p254a, p254b.
M—p256, p259a, p259b.
p256—Ridley Family, Jan Worst.
p258—Ridley Family, Ann Apple (two).
p259—Ann Apple (two).
p260—St. Thomas' Hospital.

Chapter 19
A—p267a, p267b, p267c, p267d; p268.
M—p264a, p264b; p265a, p265b, p265c;
p262—A Service of Thanksgiving, Westminster Abbey.
p264—Ann Apple (two).
p265—Ann Apple (three).
p266—Ann Apple (four).

Index

Adams, Jane, 105, 111
Adlertag (Eagle Day), 118–121
Africa, Ridley's work in, 205–214
age-related macular degeneration (ARMD), 222–223
Aitken, Max (Lord Beaverbrook), 114
ambylopia, nutritional, 221–224, 226
American Academy of Ophthalmology and Otolaryngology
   A Salute to Dr. Harold Ridley, 244, 246
   57th Session of, 163
American Intraocular Implant Society, tribute to Ridley, 153–154
American Society of Cataract and Refractive Surgery (ASCRS), honoring Ridley, 245, 246
Amsler Grid, 225
anterior chamber lens, 169–170, 198, 201, 216
aphakia, 10–11, 131, 132
   "cure of," 100–101, 129, 133–138
   spectacles for, 100, 193–194
Apple, Ann Addlestone, 71, 74, 79, 250, 258–259, 264–267
Apple, Bob, 62, 63
Apple, David, 10, 72–75, 99, 220, 258–259, 263, 264, 265–267, xxii
   ancestors, childhood, and medical training of, 61–63
   articles on Harold Ridley by, 303
   Harold Ridley and, 51, 58–76, 254
   heroes of, 63–65
   honors received by, 245, 246
   at IOL/Biodevice Research Center, 67–71
   IOL-related articles of, 299–301
   medical career of, 65–67, 196
   at Medical University of South Carolina, Ophthalmology Department of, 248
   at University of Utah, 53–58
Apple, Joseph Bernard, 62, 63
Apple Korps, 67–71, 74, 178, 215–216
Arnott, Eric, 67–68, 96, 105, 110–111, 121, 162–163, 249

Ashton, Norman, 67, 156, 162, 246
Assia, Ehud, 189, 250
Austin, David, 161

Babbage, Charles, 19–20, 81, 232
Barraquer, Joaquin, 169
Barraquer, Jose, 178, 198
Barraquer Dynasty of Barcelona, 95
Bartisch, Georg, 80, 83, 223–224, 225, 235
Battle of Britain, 106, 114, 115, 116–120
   service of thanksgiving and redemption on, 262, 263–268
Bearden, Margaret Josephine, 62, 63
Binkhorst, Cornelius, 171
biocompatibility, 130, 187
biomaterials, 54, 68–69, 171, 191
biomedical engineering, 239–243
Blair, Tony, 254
blindness, 43, xxi
   cataract-induced, 15, 21–24
   cataract-IOL surgery for in developing world, 205–212
Blitzkrieg, 116–120
Blodi, Frederick, 65, 161
Blumenthal, Michael, 96
Bowman, William, 37, 91
Bushell, Roger, 114–115

Cajal, Ramon y, 67
Cambridge University, Pembrook College, 32–34, 44–45
Camm, Sydney, 110
capsular bag, 56
Carriera, Rosalba, 24
Casamata, 102–103
Casanova, Giacomo, stories of, 100–104
Castroviejo, Ramon, 168
cataract-IOL surgery, 95, 165, 194
   in developing world, 205–214, 215–217
   innovations in, 167–178

INDEX

refractive surgery and, 194–196
cataracts, 15, 22, 23–28, xxi
    blindness caused by, 15, 21–24
    clinical diagnosis of, 80–90
    in developing world, 212–214
    formation of, 21–22
    morbidities caused by, 24–25
    search for cure of, 133–138
    secondary, 188–190
    surgical removal of, 91–95
Caudell, John, 99
Caudell, Peter, 122, 136, 137
Cavka, Dr., 102, 103–104
Center for Developing World Ophthalmology, 73
Charleston, SC, 68–71, 248–249
Charterhouse boarding school, 43–44
Chicago meeting, Ridley at, 163
choriocapillaris, 223
Choyce, David Peter, 147, 152, 154, 166, 168–171, 178, 198–200, 216, 224, 242, 251, 266
    International Congress of Ophthalmology Munich meeting, 173–174
    IOL design, 137, 184, 240
Churchill, Winston, 35, 112–113, 116, 117, 125
Clarke (Ogg), Doreen, 5, 88, 138, 142–143, 145–146, 148, 230, 260
Cleaver, Gordon "Mouse," 98, 101, 105–123, 124, 130, 160
    eye injury of, 120–121
    in IOL development, 122–125, 127, 240
Cloud, David S., 194–195
Collins, Ian, 134, 147
complete cataract operation, 79–95, 81, 99–127
contact lenses, 131
continuous circular curvilinear capsulorhexis (CCC), 184, 186
corneal opacities, 21
couching, 16–17, 91, 92, 100, 217

David Apple Center, 73
Daviel, Jacques, 15, 93, 94
DaVinci, Leonardo, anatomic sketches of, 80
Davison, Jim, 250
De Vries, William, 54
Deacon, Jim, 240, 241
decentering problem, 182, 184–186, 189
Derby Royal Infirmary, 46
digital diagnosis, of optic nerve in glaucoma, 234

Dowding, Air Marshall, 117
Doyne, Geoffrey, 45–46
Doyne, Robert, 154–155
Dreadnaught Era, 36–37
Drews, Robert, 178, 199, 253
Duke-Elder, Sir Stewart, 48, 50, 123, 165–166, 174, 246–247
    Choyce and, 168–169
    hostility toward Ridley of, 154–159, 160–161, 233
    Ridley's Ghana assignment by, 207, 208

Edwards, James, 248
electronic devices, 229, 232
endophthalmitis, postimplant, 190–191
Epstein, Edward, 137, 138, 152, 171
Estevez, J.M.J., 122
extracapsular cataract extraction (ECCE) technique, 47, 91, 100
    Daviel's procedure of, 93
    first use of, 3–6, 148
    history of, 15, 94
eye, 82
    anatomy and function of, 7, 17–20, 93
    artificial, 242–243
    bionic, 199, 242–243
    landmarks of, 182
eye-brain connection, 82
eye cancer, 235–236
Eye Operations Using the Microscope, 90
eye pathologists, 66–67, 84–88
eye surgery
    shifting paradigm in, 167–178, xxv
    televising, 230–231
    theory and history of, 15–17
eye tissue measurements, 199

Faust, Kenneth, 189
Findlay, G. M., 210
Fine, Howard, 54, 189, 250, xxi
Fiske, William Meade Lindsley, 115–116
fluorescein angiography, 91
Food and Drug Administration (FDA), IOL implant and, 175–177
Ford, E. B., 136, 137, 247
Forssmann, Werner, 152–153
Foster, John, 104, 159, 264
Frederick Wilhelm III, Kaiser (88-day Kaiser), 38–39
Fuchs, Ernst, 91

fundus examination methods, 232
fundus photography, 228, 230
Fyodorov, Svyatoslav, 152, 171, 197–198, 200

Ghana, Ridley's work in, 48–49, 205–218, 210
Gimbel, Howard, 90
glaucoma, 68, 224, 225, 234
Global Program for the Prevention of Blindness, WHO, 207–208, 212
Goldberg, Morton, 66
Goldsmith, Sir Allen, 156
Green, John, 136, 137
Grosvenor, Edward, 109–110
Gullstrand, Allvar, 84, 86, 136, 137

Hamdi, Turgut N., 8–9, 172, 201
haptics, 180, 184–186, 187
Harms, Heinrich, 88, 89
Hawke Hurricane, 110–111, 119–120
Healon, 186
heart, artificial, 54
histopathological analysis, 232
Hoffer, Ken, 246
Holden, John, 210
Holt, John, 122, 135
Hudson, A. Cyril ("Huddy"), 45–46, 104–105
hydrodissection, 189

Illinois, University of, Eye and Ear Infirmary, 61, 66
IMPACT Program, 208
implant materials, 187, 191
infections, postimplant, 190–191
Ingram, John, 136, 137
International Congress of Ophthalmology meetings, 173–174, 178
Intracapsular cataract extraction (ICCE) technique, 47, 91–93
Intraocular Implant Club/International Intraocular Implant Club, 174–175, 176
intraocular lens (IOL), 7–8, 11, 101, 176, xxi
  acrylic, 158–159
  biocompatibility and safety of, 130, 187, 239–240
  complications of, 54–55, 57, 182–183
  designs and styles of, 7, 8, 88, 137, 138, 182, 184–186
  determining size of, 135
  development of, 102–106, 123–124, 129–138, xxii
    Cleaver's role in, 122–123
    difficulties in, 10–12
  ups and downs in, 181–191
  early quality of, 11–12
  expandable, foldable and injectable, 171, 191, 201, 240–242
  malposition of, 180
  manufacturers of, 58
  multifocal and bifocal, 8–9, 172–173, 201–202
  phakic, 195, 200–201
  single and dual optic accommodative, 242
  telescopic, 224, 242
  50th anniversary of, 249–250
  visual rehabilitation with, 99–127
intraocular lens (IOL) implant operation, 94, 146, 194–202
  declining support for, 161–162
  delayed development of, xxiii–xxiv
  early unveiling of, 151–152
  first, 141–149
  infections after, 190–191
  inserting, 144
  pediatric, 170
  popular press coverage of, 164–165
  problems and questions of, 56, 145–148
  skepticism about in ophthalmologic community, 151–165, 176
  supporters and pioneers of, 168–170, 171–178
intraocular tumors, clinical study of, 235–236
IOL #1/IOL #2, 54–57, xxi
iris claw lens, 201
iris IOL, artificial, 240
iris prolapse, 145–147
irrigation-aspiration apparatus, 147

Jaffe, Norman, 153, 178
Jan Kiewiet de Jonge Medal, 245–246
Jarvik, Dr. Robert, 54
Jimmy Carter Center, 211

Keeler, C. D., 134
Keeper's Cottage, 59, 267
Kelman, Charles, 70, 94–95, 96, 178, 190
keratomileusis, 198
keratoprosthesis, 199
King, Edgar, 121
Kolff, Willem, 54
Kratz, Richard, 176–177
Kronfeld, Peter C., 65

INDEX

Lans, Leendert Jan, 197
laser retinal photocoagulation, 66
laser surgery, 189–190
    corneal, 195
    refractive, 198, 202
LASIK surgery, 202
Law, Frank, 161
Leicester Royal Infirmary, 40
lens, 83, 189
    crystalline, 21
    discoloration of with age, 27
    mushroom, 200
    phacoemulsification and, 96
    photomicrograph of, 87
    stabilization of, 8
lens optic degeneration, 187
Letocha, Charles, 12, 31, 172–173, 259–260
Lim, Arthur, 161
Lindner, Karl, 47, 91
Lindstrom, Richard, 250
Lion's Clubs, International, 210, 211
loops, 184–186, 187
lost generation, 38–39
loupes, 88
Lyman, John, 54

MacDonald, Sir Ramsay, 156
Mackensen, Gunther, 88, 89
macula, images of, 225, 231
macular disease, therapies for, 223–224, 226
malpositioning problems, 184–186
Marconi Wireless Telegraph Co., 230
Masters, Barry, 233
McGill Center for Vision Correction, 69
McIndoe, Sir Archibald, 116, 121
Mectizan, 211
Medical University of South Carolina, honorary degree from, 248–249
Medow, Norman, 181
Meyer-Schwickerath, Gerd, 91
microscope, modern, 87, 88, 90
Mikhailov, Dr., 102–103
Miyake, Kensaku, 69–70, 73, 84, 86, 251
Miyake-Apple technique, 75, 87, 189, 214, 216
Monet, Claude, 4–5, 25–28
Moorfields Eye Hospital (Royal London Ophthalmic Hospital), 49, 121, 160
    Choyce at, 168–169
    current cataract services at, 163

    opposition to IOL implants at, 161–162
    residency training at, 46–47
    Sir Duke-Elder at, 156–158
Moran Eye Center, Salt Lake City, 72, 76
Morgan, Christopher, 254
multivitamin therapy, 223–224
Munich, IOL pioneers in, 173–174
Munro, Donald, 134, 249, 254, 258, 259, 266

Nader, Ralph, 176
Nam, Dr. G., 214
Natchair, Dr. G., 214
Naumann, G.O.H., 67
nerve fiber layer analysis, 233
Newton, Sir Isaac, 19, 81, 83–84, 259
Nightingale, Florence, 42–43
Nitch, Cyril, 45
noninvasive diagnostic technology, 231–236
Northwestern University, 65

Obstbaum, Stephen, 177
ocular pathology, 66–67
Olson, Randall, 53–54, 72, 181
onchocerciasis (river blindness), 204, 205–212
Ophthalmodeulia, 80, 83
ophthalmologic devices, diagnostic, 80–90
ophthalmologic pathology, 66–67
ophthalmology
    in ancient medicine, 80–82
    golden ages in, 37, 60
    subspecialties of, 206
    tropical, 205–218
Ophthalmology Hall of Fame, election to, 251
ophthalmoscopes, 84, 85, 233
    invention of, 81, 222, 232
    laser scanning (LSO, SLO), 229, 231–233, xxiv
optic disc, TV image of, 231
optic nerve, 229
    atrophy of, 222, 224
    noninvasive diagnosis of, 231–236
optical aids, 88
optical coherence tomography (OCT), computerized, 233
organ transplantation, artificial, 239–243
Ostbaum, Steven, 177
Oxford Ophthalmological Congress, 45, 46, 154–155, 156, 158–159, 165

Paris, IOL pioneers in, 174–175

INDEX

Parker family, 34–35
Parsons, John, 84
Pathology of IOLs, 67
Pearce, John, 9–10, 126
Peng, Qun, 251
perimetry, evolution of, 90
Perry, Stephen, 123, 124, 128, 130–131, 132–133
Perspex, 135
phacoemulsification, 95, 96, 100, 178, 190
Philadelphia, IOL pioneers in, 172–173
Phillpot, Jimmy S., 230
photography techniques, retinal and optic nerve, 232
Pike, John, 134–135, 136, 137
PMMA material, 137, 187
polymer materials, injectable, 240–242
posterior capsular opacification, 188–190
posterior chamber IOL, 180
prisoners of war, nutritional amblyopia in, 221–224
Project Focus, 214
prosthetics, 240
Public Citizen, 176
Pye Electronics Co., 230

Queen Mother (Elizabeth II), 126, 249, 252, 266

Rabb, Maurice, 67, 68
radial keratotomy, 197–198
radiation treatment, 235
Ratner, Buddy, 239, 243
Rayner & Keeler, Ltd, 6–7, 133–137, 147, 230, 249, 254, 266, xxiii
Reese, Warren, 8–9, 163, 172, 201, 259–260
refraction, errors of, 83, 84, 145
    medical and surgical correction of, 194–202, 197
refractive surgery, 194
    corneal, 195, 196–198
    incisional versus laser, 198
    IOL, 195, 198–200
Reiner, Jean Baptiste, 134
retina, LSO evaluation of, 231–233
retinal-optic nerve disease, 228
    noninvasive diagnosis of, 229, 231–236
retinal photography techniques, 232
retinitis pigmentosa, 242
Rice, Noel, 161
Riddle, Jack, 105, 111, 112, 115, 116, 120–121, 264
Ridley, Allder, 40, 41–42, 257

Ridley, Bishop Nicholas, 30, 32–34
Ridley, David, 49
Ridley, Elisabeth, 59, 71, 72, 79, 250, xxii
Ridley, Frederick, 150, 151
Ridley, Harold, 3, 70, 72, 79, 98, 268, xxii, xxvi
    aging, 256–257
    in biomedical engineering and artificial organ transplantation, 239–243
    birth and early life of, 35–43
    British airforce pilots and, 105–124
    in cataract surgery evolution, 196
    chronology of, xxix–xxxiii
    on complete cataract operation sequence, 100
    death of, 259–261
    family of, 32–35
    first IOL implants by, 10–11, 141–149
    innovations of in developing world, 205–218
    knighthood of, 252, 253–261
    marriage of, 49
    memberships, presentations, and honors of, 244–251, 297–298
    military service of, 48–49, 221–228
    Oxford Ophthalmological Congress presentation of, 158–159
    professional rejection of, 31, 50, 152–155, xxiii–xxiv
    publications of, 285–287, 291–294
    Rayner & Keeler, Ltd. and, 133–137
    retirement of, 50–51, 162–163
    schooling and medical training of, 43–51
    Sir Stewart Duke-Elder and, 154–161
    supporters of, 168–178
Ridley, Margaret Parker, 40–41, 49, 256, 268
Ridley, Nicholas (brother), 250, 266
Ridley, Nicholas (son), 49
Ridley, Rev. William Charles, 34
Ridley, Sir Nicholas Harold Lloyd (father), 32, 34–35, 39–40
Ridley family coat of arms, 30
Ridley Foundation, 205, 217–218, 289
Ridley fundus, 204, 211
Ridley intraocular lens (IOL), 6–7, 9–10, 12, 136, 138, 182
Ridley Walk (Cambridge University), 32, 34, 45
Ring, Mike, 136
Rofe, Len, 136
Rollo, Ms. Primula, 114
Roper-Hall, Michael, 161

INDEX

Royal Air Force Club, 264
Royal Air Force (RAF), 601 Squadron of, 109–116, 118–121
Royal Albert Science Museum, 249–250, 265–266
Royal Society
    election to, 246–247
    memoirs of, xxii

Sandringham Estates, 35
Schallhorn, Stephen, 193, 195–196
Shearing, Steven, 181, 184–185
Shusterman, David, 173
Sims, John, 148, 230
slip-lamp examination, 86, 210
Smith, Colonel Henry, 92
spectacles, aphakic, 100, 192–194, 214
Spitfire story (airplane story), 104–123, xxii–xxiii
Spooner, Reggie, 105, 111, 264
St. Thomas' Hospital, 2, 140, 260, 265
    first IOL implant operation at, 141–149
    founding of, 4
    medical training at, 45
    Monet at, 25–26
    in wartime, 5, 107–109
Stallard, Henry, 49–50
Storm Eye Institute, 68–71, 73
surgical field illumination, devices for, 88
surgical instruments, 143
Susruta, 16
System of Ophthalmology, 156–157

Tadini, Dr., 102–103
Tangmere, Royal Air Force, 106–109, 126
Taylor, John, 25
technical innovations, post-World War II, 229–235
Theobald, Georgina Dvorak, 164
Thompson, Joe, 125
toric optics, 137
toxic anterior segment syndrome (TASS), 191
Trevor-Roper, Patrick, 161
Trotter, Wilfrid, 132
Troutman, Richard, 88
Tübingen University, Eye Clinic at, 89
TV technology, 229–233
Tylefors, Bjorn, 215–216

United States, IOL pioneers in, 175–177
Utah, University of, IOL/Biodevice Research Center at, 53–58, 67–71

Vail, Derrick, 50, 163, 173, 174, 177
Vallaton, William, 68–69
Venkataswamy, Dr., 214
Verisyse IOL, 201
Viennese School of Ophthalmology, 47
vision anomalies, Newton and, 84
visual acuity measurements, 305
visual loss, pattern of, 23
visual rehabilitation, 95, 99–127
Visudyne, 226
von Bismarck, Otto, 36–37
von Graefe, Albrecht, 37, 91
von Helmholtz, Hermann, 19–20, 84, 85, 232

Weatherhill Ridley, Elisabeth, 49
Wessing, Achin, 91
Wilhelm II, Kaiser, 36–37, 38
Wills Eye Hospital, 172–173
Wilson, John, 207–208, 212, 218
Winstanley, John, 220, 221, 261
Wolfe, Sidney, 176
World Health Organization (WHO)
    Committee on Prevention of Blindness of, 215
    Geneva meeting of, 215–216
    visual impairment classification of, 307
World War I, 35–37, 38–39, 43
World War II, 105–123, 116–120, 125–126
Worst, John, 174
Wright, Pearce, 31

xerophthalmia, 211–212

Yates, Tina, 54
Young, Robert, testimony of, 176–177, 178, 181

Zeiss factory, 89, 137
Zimmerman, Lorenz E., 251
Zirm, Edward, 21